Precision Medicine in Solid Tumors

Precision Medicine in Solid Tumors

Editors

Nandini Dey
Pradip De

MDPI • Basel • Beijing • Wuhan • Barcelona • Belgrade • Manchester • Tokyo • Cluj • Tianjin

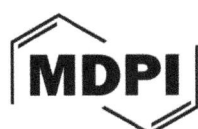

Editors
Nandini Dey
Avera Cancer Institute
USA

Pradip De
Avera Cancer Institute
USA

Editorial Office
MDPI
St. Alban-Anlage 66
4052 Basel, Switzerland

This is a reprint of articles from the Special Issue published online in the open access journal *Cancers* (ISSN 2072-6694) (available at: https://www.mdpi.com/journal/cancers/special_issues/PMST).

For citation purposes, cite each article independently as indicated on the article page online and as indicated below:

LastName, A.A.; LastName, B.B.; LastName, C.C. Article Title. *Journal Name* **Year**, *Volume Number*, Page Range.

ISBN 978-3-0365-4791-6 (Hbk)
ISBN 978-3-0365-4792-3 (PDF)

© 2022 by the authors. Articles in this book are Open Access and distributed under the Creative Commons Attribution (CC BY) license, which allows users to download, copy and build upon published articles, as long as the author and publisher are properly credited, which ensures maximum dissemination and a wider impact of our publications.

The book as a whole is distributed by MDPI under the terms and conditions of the Creative Commons license CC BY-NC-ND.

Contents

About the Editors ix

Nandini Dey and Pradip De
Precision Medicine in Solid Tumors: How Far We Traveled So Far?
Reprinted from: *Cancers* 2022, *14*, 3202, doi:10.3390/cancers14133202 1

Chiaki Inagaki, Daichi Maeda, Kazue Hatake, Yuki Sato, Kae Hashimoto, Daisuke Sakai, Shinichi Yachida, Norio Nonomura and Taroh Satoh
Clinical Utility of Next-Generation Sequencing-Based Panel Testing under the Universal Health-Care System in Japan: A Retrospective Analysis at a Single University Hospital
Reprinted from: *Cancers* 2021, *13*, 1121, doi:10.3390/cancers13051121 7

Valerie Heong, Darwin Tay, Shane Ee Goh, Bernard Wee, Tuan Zea Tan, Ross Soo, Brendan Pang, Diana Lim, Anil Gopinathan, Samuel Ow, Cheng Ean Chee, Boon Cher Goh, Soo Chin Lee, Wei Peng Yong, Andrea Wong, Mohamed Feroz Mohd Omar, Richie Soong and David S.P. Tan
Whole Exome Sequencing of Multi-Regional Biopsies from Metastatic Lesions to Evaluate Actionable Truncal Mutations Using a Single-Pass Percutaneous Technique
Reprinted from: *Cancers* 2020, *12*, 1599, doi:10.3390/cancers12061599 21

Aditi P. Singh, Elaine Shum, Lakshmi Rajdev, Haiying Cheng, Sanjay Goel, Roman Perez-Soler and Balazs Halmos
Impact and Diagnostic Gaps of Comprehensive Genomic Profiling in Real-World Clinical Practice
Reprinted from: *Cancers* 2020, *12*, 1156, doi:10.3390/cancers12051156 39

Hana Noskova, Michal Kyr, Karol Pal, Tomas Merta, Peter Mudry, Kristyna Polaskova, Tina Catela Ivkovic, Sona Adamcova, Tekla Hornakova, Marta Jezova, Leos Kren, Jaroslav Sterba and Ondrej Slaby
Assessment of Tumor Mutational Burden in Pediatric Tumors by Real-Life Whole-Exome Sequencing and In Silico Simulation of Targeted Gene Panels: How the Choice of Method Could Affect the Clinical Decision?
Reprinted from: *Cancers* 2020, *12*, 230, doi:10.3390/cancers12010230 51

Kimberly M. Burcher, Andrew T. Faucheux, Jeffrey W. Lantz, Harper L. Wilson, Arianne Abreu, Kiarash Salafian, Manisha J. Patel, Alexander H. Song, Robin M. Petro, Thomas Lycan Jr., Cristina M. Furdui, Umit Topaloglu, Ralph B. D'Agostino, Wei Zhang and Mercedes Porosnicu
Prevalence of DNA Repair Gene Mutations in Blood and Tumor Tissue and Impact on Prognosis and Treatment in HNSCC
Reprinted from: *Cancers* 2021, *13*, 3118, doi:10.3390/cancers13133118 65

Raed Sulaiman, Pradip De, Jennifer C. Aske, Xiaoqian Lin, Adam Dale, Ethan Vaselaar, Nischal Koirala, Cheryl Ageton, Kris Gaster, Joshua Plorde, Benjamin Solomon, Bradley Thaemert, Paul Meyer, Luis Rojas Espaillat, David Starks and Nandini Dey
A Laboratory-Friendly CTC Identification: Comparable Double-Immunocytochemistry with Triple-Immunofluorescence
Reprinted from: *Cancers* 2022, *14*, 2871, doi:10.3390/cancers14122871 85

Jung-Young Shin, Jeong-Oh Kim, Mi-Ran Lee, Seo Ree Kim, Kyongmin Sarah Beck and Jin Hyoung Kang
A Highly Sensitive Next-Generation Sequencing-Based Genotyping Platform for *EGFR* Mutations in Plasma from Non-Small Cell Lung Cancer Patients
Reprinted from: *Cancers* **2020**, *12*, 3579, doi:10.3390/cancers12123579 . . . . **115**

Jeong-Oh Kim, Jung-Young Shin, Seo Ree Kim, Kab Soo Shin, Joori Kim, Min-Young Kim, Mi-Ran Lee, Yonggoo Kim, Myungshin Kim, Sook Hee Hong and Jin Hyoung Kang
Evaluation of Two *EGFR* Mutation Tests on Tumor and Plasma from Patients with Non-Small Cell Lung Cancer
Reprinted from: *Cancers* **2020**, *12*, 785, doi:10.3390/cancers12040785 . . . . **131**

Pradip De, Jennifer Aske, Raed Sulaiman and Nandini Dey
Bête Noire of Chemotherapy and Targeted Therapy: CAF-Mediated Resistance
Reprinted from: *Cancers* **2022**, *14*, 1519, doi:10.3390/cancers14061519 . . . . **143**

Kimberly M. Burcher, Jeffrey W. Lantz, Elena Gavrila, Arianne Abreu, Jack T. Burcher, Andrew T. Faucheux, Amy Xie, Clayton Jackson, Alexander H. Song, Ryan T. Hughes, Thomas Lycan, Jr., Paul M. Bunch, Cristina M. Furdui, Umit Topaloglu, Ralph B. D'Agostino, Jr., Wei Zhang and Mercedes Porosnicu
Relationship between Tumor Mutational Burden, PD-L1, Patient Characteristics, and Response to Immune Checkpoint Inhibitors in Head and Neck Squamous Cell Carcinoma
Reprinted from: *Cancers* **2021**, *13*, 5733, doi:10.3390/cancers13225733 . . . . **175**

Rumi Higuchi, Taichiro Goto, Yosuke Hirotsu, Yujiro Yokoyama, Takahiro Nakagomi, Sotaro Otake, Kenji Amemiya, Toshio Oyama, Hitoshi Mochizuki and Masao Omata
Primary Driver Mutations in *GTF2I* Specific to the Development of Thymomas
Reprinted from: *Cancers* **2020**, *12*, 2032, doi:10.3390/cancers12082032 . . . . **195**

Tamara Ius, Fabrizio Pignotti, Giuseppe Maria Della Pepa, Giuseppe La Rocca, Teresa Somma, Miriam Isola, Claudio Battistella, Simona Gaudino, Maurizio Polano, Michele Dal Bo, Daniele Bagatto, Enrico Pegolo, Silvia Chiesa, Mauro Arcicasa, Alessandro Olivi, Miran Skrap and Giovanni Sabatino
A Novel Comprehensive Clinical Stratification Model to Refine Prognosis of Glioblastoma Patients Undergoing Surgical Resection
Reprinted from: *Cancers* **2020**, *12*, 386, doi:10.3390/cancers12020386 . . . . **207**

Fokhrul Hossain, Samarpan Majumder, Justin David and Lucio Miele
Precision Medicine and Triple-Negative Breast Cancer: Current Landscape and Future Directions
Reprinted from: *Cancers* **2021**, *13*, 3739, doi:10.3390/cancers13153739 . . . . **227**

Takaharu Jibiki, Hayato Nishimura, Shintaro Sengoku and Kota Kodama
Regulations, Open Data and Healthcare Innovation: A Case of MSK-IMPACT and Its Implications for Better Cancer Care
Reprinted from: *Cancers* **2021**, *13*, 3448, doi:10.3390/cancers13143448 . . . . **249**

Lamorna Brown, Utkarsh Agrawal and Frank Sullivan
Using Electronic Medical Records to Identify Potentially Eligible Study Subjects for Lung Cancer Screening with Biomarkers
Reprinted from: *Cancers* **2021**, *13*, 5449, doi:10.3390/cancers13215449 . . . . **269**

Hiroaki Kuroda, Yusuke Sugita, Katsuhiro Masago, Yusuke Takahashi, Takeo Nakada,
Eiichi Sasaki, Noriaki Sakakura, Rui Yamaguchi, Hirokazu Matsushita and Toyoaki Hida
Clinical Guideline-Guided Outcome Consistency for Surgically Resected Stage III Non-Small Cell Lung Cancer: A Retrospective Study
Reprinted from: *Cancers* **2021**, *13*, 2531, doi:10.3390/cancers13112531 . . . . **281**

About the Editors

Nandini Dey

Nandini Dey MS, Ph.D. is a Senior Scientist and Director of the Translational Oncology Laboratory at Avera Cancer Institute, Sioux Fall, SD, USA. She is an Assistant Professor in the Department of Internal Medicine at the University of South Dakota Sanford School of Medicine. Dey has more than 25 years of experience in translational oncology and has authored or coauthored more than 200 research articles, book chapters, reviews, and abstracts. Currently, Nandini Dey serves as an academic editor of PLOS ONE. Nandini Dey is a Fellow of the Royal Society of Medicine (United Kingdom).

Pradip De

Pradip De MS, Ph.D. is a Senior Scientist of the Translational Oncology Laboratory at Avera Cancer Institute, Sioux Fall, SD, USA. He is an Assistant Professor in the Department of Internal Medicine at the University of South Dakota Sanford School of Medicine. De has more than 25 years of experience in translational oncology and industry research. De has authored or coauthored more than 250 research articles, book chapters, reviews, and abstracts. De currently serves as a consultant in Viecure, Colorado, USA. De is a team member of TRACK (Target Rare Cancer Knowledge, a national patient-centric precision oncology trial for rare cancers).

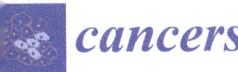

Editorial

Precision Medicine in Solid Tumors: How Far We Traveled So Far?

Nandini Dey [1,2,*] and Pradip De [1,2]

1 Translational Oncology Laboratory, Avera Research Institute, Sioux Falls, SD 57105, USA; pradip.de@avera.org
2 Department of Internal Medicine, University of South Dakota SSOM, USD, Sioux Falls, SD 57105, USA
* Correspondence: nandini.dey@avera.org

The future of disease management in solid tumors will rely heavily on how effectively we understand precision medicine and how successfully we can deliver personalized medicine. In the post-human genome project era, both translational research as well as clinical care in oncology has become functions of knowledge-based deliverance of therapy. The knowledge rides on the technological revolution, next-generation sequencing (NGS), and whole-exome sequencing/whole transcriptome sequencing (WES/WTS), which provide comprehensive genomic data in real-time from the tumor, tumor- microenvironment (TME), and blood. The wealth of information help clinicians interrogate the genomics-driven disease and fuels the decision-making in precision medicine.

During the inception of this Special Issue, entitled "Precision Medicine in Solid Tumors", we promised to present an in-depth review of the topic's current status. We covered (A) the challenges of NGS and WES/WTS in reaching a saturation point for finding a new effective target in oncology; (B) the holistic aspect of tumor biology from the viewpoint of tumor-TME-liquid biopsy; (C) mutation-guided treatment; (D) the enormity and legality of the data, electronic medical record; and (E) the translation of knowledge to patient outcomes and clinical guidelines. The Special Issue presents 11 original research articles, 2 review articles, 1 opinion, and 2 brief reports.

1. NGS & WES/WTS

Precision medicine seeks to use genomic data (alteration, such as mutations, amplifications, copy number variations, chromosomal rearrangements) to help provide the right treatment to the right patient at the right time. In the last 15 years since the invention of this breakthrough technology, NGS technology provided the genetic constitution of different types of cancers. The speed, accuracy, and cost affordability of NGS have helped spur the advent of precision medicine, which involves designing a treatment based on disease-driving molecular alterations [1,2] (Collins F. Precision Oncology: Gene changes predict immunotherapy response (NIH Director's Blog; accessed on 10 November 2017)). In today's world, WES/WTS integrates tumor-normal matched samples. It offers one comprehensive test to rapidly deliver in-depth (>18,000 genes) molecular insight and avoid running multiple sequential panels to unlock the answer to a patient's cancer. WES/WTS-driven comprehensive molecular analysis has identified a relatively high incidence of potentially targetable genomic alterations in solid tumors, predictive of response to targeted and immunotherapies. NGS and tumor mutation profiling have become essential diagnostic/decision-making tools for routine use in oncology clinics, including community-based clinics. In a retrospective study, Inagaki et al. tested the clinical utility of NGS-based panels in the Universal Health-Care System in Japan from a single University hospital in Osaka and reported that the NGS assay should be performed earlier in the clinical course to maximize the clinical benefit. The study revealed that the broader reimbursement for the NGS assay would enhance the delivery of precision oncology to patients. Heong et al. tested the feasibility of a "Multi-Regional" sample biopsy from metastatic lesions

Citation: Dey, N.; De, P. Precision Medicine in Solid Tumors: How Far We Traveled So Far?. *Cancers* **2022**, *14*, 3202. https://doi.org/10.3390/cancers14133202

Received: 23 June 2022
Accepted: 28 June 2022
Published: 30 June 2022

Publisher's Note: MDPI stays neutral with regard to jurisdictional claims in published maps and institutional affiliations.

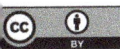

Copyright: © 2022 by the authors. Licensee MDPI, Basel, Switzerland. This article is an open access article distributed under the terms and conditions of the Creative Commons Attribution (CC BY) license (https://creativecommons.org/licenses/by/4.0/).

to evaluate actionable truncal mutations using a Single-Pass Percutaneous Technique by WES. They demonstrated the strength of their evaluation in prioritizing precision-therapy strategies. In debating the implication of NGS in a laboratory setting versus in real-world clinical practice, Singh et al. presented the impact and diagnostic gaps of comprehensive genomic profiling in a study participated by the University of Pennsylvania/Abramson Cancer Center, PA, USA, NYU Langone Perlmutter Cancer Center, New York, USA, and Montefiore Medical Center/Albert Einstein College of Medicine, Bronx NY, USA. Their study concluded that routine use of CGP in the community across all cancer types detects potentially actionable genomic alterations in most patients. In Silico Simulation of targeted gene panels is a powerful tool for the development of technology. Noskova et al. presented a study that evaluated TMB in multiple pediatric tumors by Real-Life Whole-Exome Sequencing and In Silico Simulation of two major targeted gene panels to evaluate the choice of method which affect the clinical decision. Their study confirmed a significant technological variability introduced by different laboratory techniques and various settings of bioinformatics pipelines.

2. Tumor-TME-Blood

Transformed tumor cells reside within their non-transformed host-microenvironment. With the advent of advanced technology to pinpoint both cellular and acellular characteristics of a tumor mass, the relationship between tumor cells and their non-transformed microenvironment has been acknowledged [3,4]. The acknowledgment has come from the translational and clinical research indicating holistic support of TME to tumor cells during the progression of the disease [5,6] by influencing tumor growth, formation of stem cell niches, immunosuppression, metastasis, and drug resistance. The TME encompasses both cellular components, the extracellular space containing both soluble cytokines and insoluble extracellular matrix (ECM) components. The recognition of the undeniable consequence of the 'unholy alliance' of the neoplastic tumor cells and their inherently dynamic non-neoplastic components of the microenvironment [7,8] has led to the incorporation of targeting TME for cancer treatments, including immunotherapy and radiotherapy in recent years [9–11]. As the interaction between the tumor and its TME evolves in a complex bidirectional manner, there was a long-lasting search for finding a "mirror room" that could serve as a surrogate of the actual events at the tumor site. In the last decades, the search has revealed a source-easy sample that can be the "mirror room" for the tumor-TME events in peripheral blood (liquid biopsy). Circulating tumor cells (CTC), ctDNA, cancer-associated fibroblasts (CAF), cell fusions, CAMLS, immune cells, exosomes, soluble proteins (sPD-L1, sPD-L2, sPD-1) from the blood have been beginning to show the reflection of the tumor-TME events about cancer screening, early detection, drug effect, on-treatment monitoring, drug resistance and post-treatment surveillance [12–16]. Burcher et al. demonstrated the prevalence of DNA repair gene mutations in blood and tumor tissue and their impact on prognosis and treatment in HNSCC. A single-institution retrospective study was undertaken to test the profiles of 170 patients with HNSCC and available tumor tissue DNA (tDNA) and circulating tumor DNA (ctDNA). Results were analyzed for mutations in a set of 18 DDR genes as well as in gene subsets defined by technical and clinical significance. This study presents the largest cohort to date to analyze the genomic landscape in both blood and tumor tissue in patients with HNSCC and reports a high prevalence of DDR gene mutations in this tumor type. Patients with DDR gene mutations in ctDNA rather than tDNA had shown significantly worse prognoses, with a more advanced disease burden at the end of the study and with decreased overall survival. Sulaiman et al. provided a method for a user-friendly and cost-effective detection of CTC. The technique's power can be tested as a single-point at the baseline during surgery and in a multi-point longitudinal mode during and after a treatment regimen. To this end, studies showed that meaningful information could be obtained from patients' plasma, offering an avenue for longitudinal surveillance during treatment and post-treatment monitoring period. In a brief report, Shin et al. presented a highly sensitive NGS-based genotyping platform for EGFR mutations in plasma from NSCLC patients. Their study demonstrated that Sel-Cap is a highly sensitive platform for EGFR mutations in plasma, and the timing of the first appearance of T790M mutation in plasma, determined via highly sensitive liquid biopsies, may be useful for the prediction of disease progression of NSCLC around five months in advance. Similarly, Kim et al. evaluated 2 EGFR mutation tests on tumors and plasma from patients with NSCLC. The study reported the interchangeable use of two EGFR mutation tests, cobas v2 and PANAMutyper, in tumor and plasma EGFR testing. Both tests in their study have high diagnostic precision in plasma but are particularly valuable in late-stage disease. Their clinical data in T790M carriers strongly support the clinical benefits of osimertinib treatment guided by both EGFR mutation tests. De et al. interrogated the role of TME in the development of resistance to chemotherapy and targeted therapy. Cancer-Associated Fibroblasts (CAFs) are one of the components of the TME that is used by tumor cells to achieve resistance to therapy. Their review interrogated the irrefutable role of CAFs in the development of resistance that would strategize the ability to design improved therapies inclusive of CAFs in light of currently ongoing and completed CAF-based NIH clinical trials.

3. Mutation-Guided Treatment-ICI Therapy

Since genomic alteration(s) and chromosomal instability are the primary determinants of cells that acquire malignant traits, a cancer-specific genomic map provides the roadmap for the treatment. This treatment philosophy is state-of-art in today's clinics and is called precision oncology, which embraces clinical decisions based on genomic/proteomic data. Today's success in treatment modalities and overall management of cancer, both pathway-targeted and immune-targeted therapy, are empowered by mutation-guided target-specific drugs [17]. Tumors have been known to adopt and bypass the PD-1/PD-L1 axis to achieve immune evasion, and the PD-1/PD-L1 axis has been accepted as an obvious target treated by immune checkpoint inhibitors (ICI). On this basis, PD-L1 protein expression on tumor or immune cells emerged as the first potential predictive biomarker for sensitivity to immune checkpoint blockade. In 2015, PD-L1 was the first FDA-approved predictive biomarker for non-small-cell lung cancer (NSCLC) [18]. Nine FDA approvals have been linked to a specific PD-L1 threshold and companion diagnostics, including bladder cancer (N = 3), non-small cell lung cancer (N = 3), triple-negative breast cancer (N = 1), cervical cancer (N = 1), and gastric/gastroesophageal junction cancer (N = 1) out of which 88.9% have been targeted with ICI monotherapy [19]. Following the IMpower110 (NCT02409342) clinical trial (in May 2020), the inclusion criteria of high PD-L1 expression $\geq$50% of tumor cells or $\geq$10% of tumor-infiltrating immune cells (as defined by an FDA-approved device) were FDA approved for the treatment of adult metastatic NSCLC with no EGFR or ALK genomic aberrations [20]. In the following month, the FDA expanded the approval of pembrolizumab (PD-1 inhibitor), routinely used as immunotherapy in a variety of cancer patients) to include unresectable or metastatic tumors with TMB-H ($\geq$10 mutation/Mb) that have progressed following prior treatment with no satisfactory alternative therapy options, based on the Keynote-158 study (NCT02628067) [21]. Currently, FDA has approved 3 predictive biomarkers, including PD-L1, microsatellite instability (MSI), and tumor mutational burden (TMB), including blood-TMB for patient selection for ICI response in clinical practice. Burcher et al. studied the relationship between TMB, PD-L1, patient characteristics, and response to ICI in HNSCC. Their work demonstrated the utility of TMB as a prognostic variable and predictive marker of response to ICI. The study also pointed to the significant association of high TMB with active tobacco use and primary tumor location in the larynx. In their study, high PD-L1 values were associated with the African American race, high T stage, high overall disease stage, non-/ex-smokers, and non-/ex-drinkers. Higuchi et al. study primary driver mutations in GTF2I specific to the development of thymomas. Their study showed that the majority of thymomas harbor mutations in GTF2I that can be potentially used as a novel therapeutic target in patients with thymomas. Tamara Ius et al. from Italy presented a novel comprehensive clinical stratification model to refine prognosis in GBM. Their prognostic score uses clinical/molecular and images data that can be useful to stratify GBM patients undergoing surgical resection. By using the random forest approach [CART analysis (classification and regression tree)] on Survival time data of 465 cases, they developed a new prediction score resulting in 10 groups based on the extent of resection (EOR), age, volumetric tumor features, intraoperative protocols, and molecular tumor classes. Their score could be helpful in a clinical setting to refine the prognosis of GBM patients after surgery and before postoperative treatment. Hossain et al. discussed tumor heterogeneity and sub-clonal evolution in primary and metastatic TNBC, which still remains a challenge for oncologists to design adaptive precision medicine-based treatment plans.

4. Electronic Medical Record

In today's clinical world, electronic data recording, management, and safety are as important as any branches of disease care. One of the reasons for this is that the Electronic Medical Record (EMR) is viewed as a solution to many of the shortcomings of health care systems, and therefore, its importance is realized to improve patient care [22]. The importance of the electronic health record (EHR) system is highlighted by the promise of substantial benefits, including better patient care and decreased healthcare costs, useability and accessibility of records in one hand, while the poor EHR system design with improper implementation invites EHR-related errors jeopardizing the integrity of the information in the EHR, leading to errors that endanger patients safety or decrease the quality of care and serious unintended consequences in another hand [23]. A limited EMR is often preferred to a faulty EMR from the patients' safety point of view [24–26]. The future will prove the feasibility of a collaborative, noteless EMR design with minimum information chaos, the highest level of patient data protection, and a user-friendly operation for managing team workflows at the clinics [27]. Jibiki et al. investigated a case of Memorial Sloan Kettering-Integrated Mutation Profiling of Actionable Cancer Targets (MSK-IMPACT), a tumor profiling test approved by the U.S. FDA in 2017, to examine what factors would contribute to healthcare innovation. Their study conducted comparative analyses of three tumor profiling tests approved by the U.S. FDA in 2017, hypothesizing that the FDA's regulatory reforms, early application of new technologies to both research and clinical settings, and open data accumulated as a result of large-scale research programs have promoted new drug development in oncology. The study set three parameters to observe cases. First, the FDA regulatory reforms. Second, early application of new technologies, such as NGS, to both research and clinical settings. The third is the accumulation of open data. The study discussed the implications potentially suggested by the outcomes and challenges of the three cases. Brown et al. presented the opinion on the use of EMR to identify potentially eligible study subjects for lung cancer screening with biomarkers which explores the current issues in and approaches to lung cancer screening and whether records can be used to identify eligible subjects for screening and the challenges that researchers face when using EMR data.

5. Clinical Guidelines & Outcome

Any discourse on "Precision Medicine in Solid Tumors" remains incomplete without presenting views on the clinical guidelines and outcomes which embody "response evaluation". Historically, attempts to define the objective response of a tumor to an anticancer agent were made as early as the early 1960s [28]. Following the introduction of specific criteria for the codification of tumor response evaluation in the late 1970s by the International Union Against Cancer and the World Health Organization (the 1979 WHO Handbook), various organizations involved in clinical research reviewed these criteria in 1994 to ready a set of guidelines. Down the road, a model by which response rates could be derived from the unidimensional measurement of tumor lesions instead of the usual bi-dimensional approach was developed, which was validated by the Response Evaluation Criteria in Solid Tumors Group. The philosophic background to clarify the various purposes of "response evaluation" has been presented in an article by Patrick Therasse et al. [29]. The article covers several aspects of response evaluation, including: (1) details of methods of assessing codified tumor lesions within the guidelines; (2) Response Evaluation Criteria In Solid Tumors (RECIST) guidelines; (3) Response Outcomes in Daily Clinical Practice of Oncology; (4) Response Outcomes in Uncontrolled Trials as a Guide to Further Testing of a New Therapy; and (5) Response Outcomes in Clinical Trials as a Surrogate for Palliative Effect. With the advent and success of tumor immunotherapy, attempts have been made to define systematic criteria, designated immune-related response criteria, to include additional response patterns observed with ICI therapy beyond those described by Response Evaluation Criteria in Solid Tumors or WHO criteria, especially in advanced melanoma [30–33]. Among them, Wolchok et al. put forward novel criteria to better capture the response patterns observed with immunotherapies, "Immune-related Response Criteria" (irRC) [33]. The irRC has since then presented a more comprehensive evaluation of immunotherapies in clinical trials, in conjunction with either RECIST or WHO, proving that irRC is a powerful criterion for outcome measurement in clinical investigation. In a retrospective study, Kuroda et al. presented data on the clinical guideline-guided Outcome consistency for surgically resected stage III NSCLC, demonstrating that the guideline-consistent alternatives, which comprise ATSR (adjuvant treatments after surgical resection) or GMT-R (guideline-matched first-line treatment for recurrence), can contribute to survival benefits in pathological stage III NSCLC.

Today's "Precision Medicine in Solid Tumors" is an evolution of medical practice in progress, a perfect example of the power of the interdisciplinary approach. It remains to see how the future liaison of classical medicine and translational research, equipped with technology, bioinformatics, data safety, advocacy, and social media, will shape the deliverance of patient care in medicine.

In this Special Issue, we tried an uphill task to present a scientific interrogation on salient critical features of "Precision Medicine in Solid Tumors." We will consider ourselves immensely humble if our collected reviews on the specific topics are of help to our readers.

Conflicts of Interest: The authors declare no conflict of interest.

References

1. Shin, S.H.; Bode, A.M.; Dong, Z. Addressing the challenges of applying precision oncology. *NPJ Precis. Oncol.* **2017**, *1*, 28. [CrossRef]
2. Schwartzberg, L.; Kim, E.S.; Liu, D.; Schrag, D. Precision Oncology: Who, How, What, When, and When Not? *Am. Soc. Clin. Oncol. Educ. Book* **2017**, *37*, 160–169. [CrossRef]
3. Hernandez-Camarero, P.; Lopez-Ruiz, E.; Marchal, J.A.; Peran, M. Cancer: A mirrored room between tumor bulk and tumor microenvironment. *J. Exp. Clin. Cancer Res.* **2021**, *40*, 217. [CrossRef]
4. Anderson, N.M.; Simon, M.C. The tumor microenvironment. *Curr. Biol.* **2020**, *30*, 921–925. [CrossRef]
5. Quail, D.F.; Joyce, J.A. Microenvironmental regulation of tumor progression and metastasis. *Nat. Med.* **2013**, *19*, 1423–1437. [CrossRef]
6. Hinshaw, D.C.; Shevde, L.A. The Tumor Microenvironment Innately Modulates Cancer Progression. *Cancer Res.* **2019**, *79*, 4557–4566. [CrossRef]
7. De, P.; Aske, J.; Dey, N. Cancer-Associated Fibroblasts in Conversation with Tumor Cells in Endometrial Cancers: A Partner in Crime. *Int. J. Mol. Sci.* **2021**, *22*, 9121. [CrossRef]
8. Hui, L.; Chen, Y. Tumor microenvironment: Sanctuary of the devil. *Cancer Lett.* **2015**, *368*, 7–13. [CrossRef]
9. Wang, J.J.; Lei, K.F.; Han, F. Tumor microenvironment: Recent advances in various cancer treatments. *Eur. Rev. Med. Pharmacol. Sci.* **2018**, *22*, 3855–3864. [CrossRef]
10. Bader, J.E.; Voss, K.; Rathmell, J.C. Targeting Metabolism to Improve the Tumor Microenvironment for Cancer Immunotherapy. *Mol. Cell* **2020**, *78*, 1019–1033. [CrossRef]
11. Jarosz-Biej, M.; Smolarczyk, R.; Cichon, T.; Kulach, N. Tumor Microenvironment as A 'Game Changer' in Cancer Radiotherapy. *Int. J. Mol. Sci.* **2019**, *20*, 3212. [CrossRef]
12. Chen, M.; Zhao, H. Next-generation sequencing in liquid biopsy: Cancer screening and early detection. *Hum. Genom.* **2019**, *13*, 34. [CrossRef]
13. Tay, T.K.Y.; Tan, P.H. Liquid Biopsy in Breast Cancer: A Focused Review. *Arch. Pathol. Lab. Med.* **2021**, *145*, 678–686. [CrossRef]
14. Massihnia, D.; Pizzutilo, E.G.; Amatu, A.; Tosi, F.; Ghezzi, S.; Bencardino, K.; Di Masi, P.; Righetti, E.; Patelli, G.; Scaglione, F.; et al. Liquid biopsy for rectal cancer: A systematic review. *Cancer Treat Rev.* **2019**, *79*, 101893. [CrossRef]

15. Ignatiadis, M.; Sledge, G.W.; Jeffrey, S.S. Liquid biopsy enters the clinic-implementation issues and future challenges. *Nat. Rev. Clin. Oncol.* **2021**, *18*, 297–312. [CrossRef]
16. Alix-Panabieres, C.; Pantel, K. Liquid Biopsy: From Discovery to Clinical Application. *Cancer Discov.* **2021**, *11*, 858–873. [CrossRef]
17. Dey, N.; Williams, C.; Leyland-Jones, B.; De, P. Mutation matters in precision medicine: A future to believe in. *Cancer Treat. Rev.* **2017**, *55*, 136–149. [CrossRef]
18. Wang, Y.; Tong, Z.; Zhang, W.; Zhang, W.; Buzdin, A.; Mu, X.; Yan, Q.; Zhao, X.; Chang, H.H.; Duhon, M.; et al. FDA-Approved and Emerging Next Generation Predictive Biomarkers for Immune Checkpoint Inhibitors in Cancer Patients. *Front. Oncol.* **2021**, *11*, 683419. [CrossRef]
19. Davis, A.A.; Patel, V.G. The role of PD-L1 expression as a predictive biomarker: An analysis of all US Food and Drug Administration (FDA) approvals of immune checkpoint inhibitors. *J. Immunother. Cancer* **2019**, *7*, 278. [CrossRef]
20. Herbst, R.S.; Giaccone, G.; de Marinis, F.; Reinmuth, N.; Vergnenegre, A.; Barrios, C.H.; Morise, M.; Felip, E.; Andric, Z.; Geater, S.; et al. Atezolizumab for First-Line Treatment of PD-L1-Selected Patients with NSCLC. *N. Engl. J. Med.* **2020**, *383*, 1328–1339. [CrossRef]
21. Marabelle, A.; Fakih, M.; Lopez, J.; Shah, M.; Shapira-Frommer, R.; Nakagawa, K.; Chung, H.C.; Kindler, H.L.; Lopez-Martin, J.A.; Miller, W.H., Jr.; et al. Association of tumour mutational burden with outcomes in patients with advanced solid tumours treated with pembrolizumab: Prospective biomarker analysis of the multicohort, open-label, phase 2 KEYNOTE-158 study. *Lancet Oncol.* **2020**, *21*, 1353–1365. [CrossRef]
22. Janett, R.S.; Yeracaris, P.P. Electronic Medical Records in the American Health System: Challenges and lessons learned. *Cien Saude Colet.* **2020**, *25*, 1293–1304. [CrossRef]
23. Bowman, S. Impact of electronic health record systems on information integrity: Quality and safety implications. *Perspect Health Inf. Manag.* **2013**, *10*, 1c.
24. Sittig, D.F.; Ash, J.S.; Singh, H. The SAFER guides: Empowering organizations to improve the safety and effectiveness of electronic health records. *Am. J. Manag. Care* **2014**, *20*, 418–423.
25. Zahabi, M.; Kaber, D.B.; Swangnetr, M. Usability and Safety in Electronic Medical Records Interface Design: A Review of Recent Literature and Guideline Formulation. *Hum. Factors* **2015**, *57*, 805–834. [CrossRef]
26. Stanyon, R. Information technology in health care: Addressing promises and pitfalls. *J. Healthc. Risk Manag.* **2005**, *25*, 25–31. [CrossRef]
27. Steinkamp, J.; Sharma, A.; Bala, W.; Kantrowitz, J.J. A Fully Collaborative, Noteless Electronic Medical Record Designed to Minimize Information Chaos: Software Design and Feasibility Study. *JMIR Form. Res.* **2021**, *5*, e23789. [CrossRef]
28. Gehan, E.A.; Schneiderman, M.A. Historical and methodological developments in clinical trials at the National Cancer Institute. *Stat. Med.* **1990**, *9*, 871–880, discussion 903–876. [CrossRef]
29. Therasse, P.; Arbuck, S.G.; Eisenhauer, E.A.; Wanders, J.; Kaplan, R.S.; Rubinstein, L.; Verweij, J.; Van Glabbeke, M.; van Oosterom, A.T.; Christian, M.C.; et al. New guidelines to evaluate the response to treatment in solid tumors. European Organization for Research and Treatment of Cancer, National Cancer Institute of the United States, National Cancer Institute of Canada. *J. Natl. Cancer Inst.* **2000**, *92*, 205–216. [CrossRef]
30. Wolchok, J.D.; Hoos, A.; O'Day, S.; Weber, J.S.; Hamid, O.; Lebbe, C.; Maio, M.; Binder, M.; Bohnsack, O.; Nichol, G.; et al. Guidelines for the evaluation of immune therapy activity in solid tumors: Immune-related response criteria. *Clin. Cancer Res.* **2009**, *15*, 7412–7420. [CrossRef]
31. Ribas, A.; Chmielowski, B.; Glaspy, J.A. Do we need a different set of response assessment criteria for tumor immunotherapy. *Clin. Cancer Res.* **2009**, *15*, 7116–7118. [CrossRef]
32. Hoos, A.; Wolchok, J.D.; Humphrey, R.W.; Hodi, F.S. CCR 20th Anniversary Commentary: Immune-Related Response Criteria–Capturing Clinical Activity in Immuno-Oncology. *Clin. Cancer Res.* **2015**, *21*, 4989–4991. [CrossRef] [PubMed]
33. Hodi, F.S.; Hwu, W.J.; Kefford, R.; Weber, J.S.; Daud, A.; Hamid, O.; Patnaik, A.; Ribas, A.; Robert, C.; Gangadhar, T.C.; et al. Evaluation of Immune-Related Response Criteria and RECIST v1.1 in Patients with Advanced Melanoma Treated with Pembrolizumab. *J. Clin. Oncol.* **2016**, *34*, 1510–1517. [CrossRef] [PubMed]

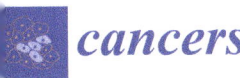

Article

Clinical Utility of Next-Generation Sequencing-Based Panel Testing under the Universal Health-Care System in Japan: A Retrospective Analysis at a Single University Hospital

Chiaki Inagaki [1], Daichi Maeda [2], Kazue Hatake [3], Yuki Sato [4], Kae Hashimoto [4,5], Daisuke Sakai [3], Shinichi Yachida [3,6], Norio Nonomura [3,7] and Taroh Satoh [1,*]

1. Department of Frontier Science for Cancer and Chemotherapy, Graduate School of Medicine, Osaka University, Osaka 565-0871, Japan; cinagaki@cfs.med.osaka-u.ac.jp
2. Department of Clinical Genomics, Graduate School of Medicine, Osaka University, Osaka 565-0871, Japan; daichimaeda@cgp.med.osaka-u.ac.jp
3. Center for Cancer Genomics and Personalized Medicine, Osaka University Hospital, Osaka 565-0871, Japan; k-hatake@mccg.med.osaka-u.ac.jp (K.H.); dsakai@cfs.med.osaka-u.ac.jp (D.S.); syachida@cgi.med.osaka-u.ac.jp (S.Y.); nono@uro.med.osaka-u.ac.jp (N.N.)
4. Department of Genetic Counseling, Osaka University Hospital, Osaka 565-0871, Japan; ysato@hp-gensel.med.osaka-u.ac.jp (Y.S.); kae.h@gyne.med.osaka-u.ac.jp (K.H.)
5. Department of Obstetrics and Gynecology, Graduate School of Medicine, Osaka University, Osaka 565-0871, Japan
6. Department of Cancer Genome Informatics, Graduate School of Medicine, Osaka University, Osaka 565-0871, Japan
7. Department of Urology, Graduate School of Medicine, Osaka University, Osaka 565-0871, Japan
* Correspondence: taroh@cfs.med.osaka-u.ac.jp; Tel.: +81-6-6879-2641

Simple Summary: Next-generation sequencing (NGS)-based assay is widely used in clinical practice due to its reimbursement by Japan's universal health-care system for cancer patients who finished standard treatment in June 2019. To clarify the clinical utility of the NGS assay under the universal health-care system, we retrospectively analyzed patients who underwent NGS assay at our hospital. Since reimbursement of the NGS assay is restricted to patients who complete standard treatment, many patients experience clinical disease progression before receiving results; therefore, they could not use the NGS results for making a therapeutic decision. Broader reimbursement of NGS assays for advanced cancer patients is needed for making optimum use of the NGS assay results. Providing good access to clinical trials and off-label agents is necessary for enabling patients to benefit from NGS assay. Additionally, this study revealed that the disclosure of presumed germline findings is feasible in clinical practice.

Abstract: Next-generation sequencing (NGS) assay is part of routine care in Japan owing to its reimbursement by Japan's universal health-care system; however, reimbursement is limited to patients who finished standard treatment. We retrospectively investigated 221 patients who underwent Foundation One CDX (F1CDx) at our hospital. Every F1CDx result was assessed at the molecular tumor board (MTB) for treatment recommendation. Based on patients' preferences, presumed germline findings were also assessed at the MTB and disclosed at the clinic. In total, 204 patients underwent F1CDx and 195 patients completed the analysis; however, 13.8% of them could not receive the report due to disease progression. Among 168 patients who received the results, 41.6% had at least one actionable alteration, and 3.6% received genomically matched treatment. Presumed germline findings were nominated in 24 patients, and 16.7% of them contacted a geneticist counselor. The NGS assay should be performed earlier in the clinical course to maximize the clinical benefit. Broader reimbursement for the NGS assay would enhance the delivery of precision oncology to patients. Access to clinical trials affects the number of patients who benefit from NGS. Additionally, the disclosure of presumed germline findings is feasible in clinical practice.

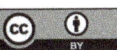

Keywords: next-generation sequencing; solid cancer; universal health-care system; precision medicine; presumed germline findings

1. Introduction

Over the last decade, with the increased knowledge in molecular profiles and mechanisms, there has been significant progress in cancer research and treatment. Next-generation sequencing (NGS) allows the sequencing of a large number of genes in a short time at an affordable cost and therefore contributes to detecting clinically relevant alterations and promoting precision oncology. Several studies have shown that molecular profiling with NGS improves patient response and survival in a selected cohort [1–5].

For example, the Molecular Screening for Cancer Treatment Optimization (MOSCATO 01) study demonstrated that targeted therapy, which was matched to a genomic alteration, improved the survival of 33% (63/193) of the study participants [4]. In addition, in the Targeted Agent and Profiling Utilization Registry (TAPUR) study, genomically matched treatment showed good clinical efficacy in the following five cohorts: pertuzumab and trastuzumab in *ERBB2*-amplified or overexpressed colorectal cancer [6], emurafenib and cobimetinib in *BRAF* V600E/D/K/-mutated colorectal cancer [7], pembrolizumab in metastatic breast cancer with a high mutational burden [8], pembrolizumab in metastatic colorectal cancer with a high mutational burden, and palbociclib in non-small cell lung cancer with *CDKN2A* alteration [9,10].

NGS assay is widely considered a part of the routine care for patients with cancer, and it has been reimbursed in several Western and Asian countries [11]. In June 2019, two types of NGS-based panel testing, Foundation One CDX (F1CDx, developed by Foundation Medicine, Cambridge, MA) and OncoGuide NCC Oncopanel System test (developed by Japan's National Cancer Center; NCC and Sysmex), were reimbursed by Japan's universal health insurance system for patients with advanced cancer who finished standard treatment [12–14]. Although this approval is a big step for advancing precision oncology in Japan, its application is still challenging due to the complexity of the interpretation of genetic profiles and integration of personalized treatment into the health-care system. To investigate the clinical utility of NGS in daily practice, we reviewed patients who underwent F1CDx assay under the universal health-care system at our hospital. Herein, we present precise data of the patient characteristics, genetic alterations, including presumed germline variants nominated by the molecular tumor board (MTB) and subsequent treatment.

2. Results

2.1. Feasibility of Next-Generation Sequencing (NGS) Assay and Patient Characteristics

Samples were received from 213/221 patients, and nine were withdrawn following a pathologist evaluation on tumor volume in the samples (Figure S1). A total of 204 were assayed with F1CDx, and 195 samples (95.6%) were successfully analyzed. Reasons for analysis failure were insufficient tumor volume (n = 4), insufficient DNA quality (n = 4), and contamination (n = 1). A total of 168 (86.6%) patients received their F1CDx results and MTB-approved report at the clinic, while 27 (13.8%) could not due to disease progression (death; n = 10, declining conditions; n = 17). The median turnaround time, which is defined as the duration between the date of sample reception and the date of the MTB, was 43 days (range 35–51 days).

The patient and disease characteristics of 168 patients are listed in Table 1. The median age of the patients was 62 (range 3–92) years, and 163 (97%) patients had an Eastern Cooperative Oncology Group performance status (ECOG PS) of 0–1, while five (3%) patients had an ECOG PS of 2. Most of the patients were heavily pre-treated, and the median number of previous chemotherapy lines was 3 (range 1–11). Nearly half of the patients (n = 75, 44.6%) were referred for NGS from smaller partner community-based hospitals in the region. The most frequent tumor types were colorectal cancer (n = 45, 26.8%), sarcoma (n = 22, 13.1%), and pancreatic cancer (n = 18, 10.7%). The median survival time was 217 days (95% confidence interval; 95%CI 185–262 days).

Table 1. Patient demographics and characteristics.

	Total		168
	Sex	Male (n, %)	87 (51.8)
		Female (n, %)	81 (48.2)
	Age	Median (min/max)	62 (3/92)
	ECOG PS	0 (n, %)	131 (78.0)
		1 (n, %)	32 (19.0)
		2 (n, %)	5 (3.0)
	No. of previous chemotherapy lines	Median (min/max)	3 (1/11)
	Referral to our hospital for NGS assay	Yes, n (%)	75 (44.6)
		No, n (%)	93 (55.4)
	Tissue of Origin	Primary site (n, %)	111 (66.0)
		Metastatic site (n, %)	57 (34.0)
	Turnaround Time	Average (min/max)	43 (35/51)
	Cancer Type	Colorectal	45 (26.8)
		Sarcoma	22 (13.0)
		Pancreatic	18 (10.7)
		Gastric	13 (7.7)
		Ovarian	11 (6.5)
		Bile duct	9 (5.4)
		Esophageal	8 (4.8)
		Breast	7 (4.2)
		Cervical	6 (3.6)
		Small Intestinal	5 (3.0)
		Hepatocellular	3 (1.8)
		Unknown Primary	3 (1.8)
		Endometrial	3 (1.8)
		Non-Small Cell Lung	3 (1.8)
		Brain	3 (1.8)
		Neuroblastoma	3 (1.8)
		Melanoma	3 (1.8)
		Kidney	1 (0.6)
		Prostate	1 (0.6)
		Urinary tract	1 (0.6)

NGS: next-generation sequencing; ECOG PS: Eastern Cooperative Oncology Group performance status.

A summary of the genetic alterations is shown in Figure 1A. The median number of genetic alterations per tumor was 4.72 (range 0–14). The median tumor mutational burden (TMB) was 2.52 (range 0–21.42), and eight patients had TMB–high (TMB-H) (Figure 1B).

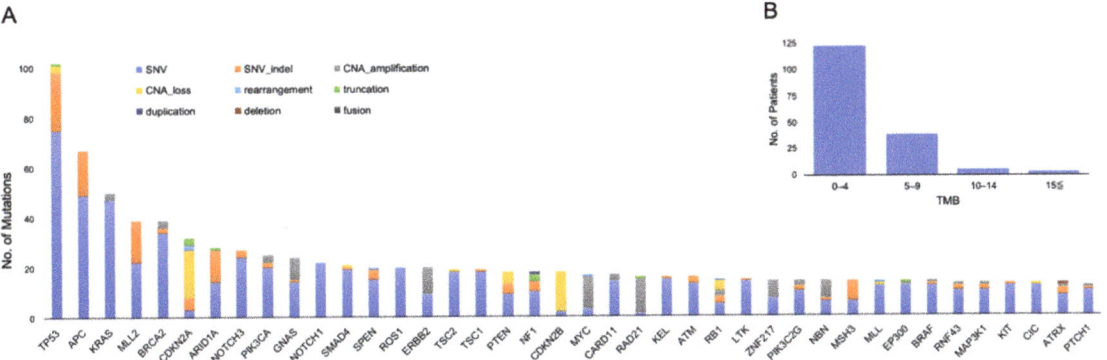

Figure 1. (**A**) Top 40 genomic alterations and (**B**) distribution of tumor mutational burden (TMB) in 168 patients who completed analysis. CAN: copy number alteration; SNV: single nucleotide variant.

2.2. Matched Treatment According to Actionable Mutation

Among the 168 patients who received their results, 107 actionable alterations were found in 70 (41.6%) patients (Figure 2, Table S1). The median number of actionable mutations per person was 1.53 (range 1–5). The frequencies of each OncoKB level of evidence were as follows: level 1A, 8.4% (n = 9); level 2, 5.6% (n = 6); level 3A, 5.6% (n = 6); level 3B, 41.1% (n = 44); and level 4, 15.9% (n = 17). The most frequently annotated genes were *PIK3CA* (n = 18), *TP53* (n = 11), *ERBB2* (n = 9), *MDM2* (n = 6), and *FGFR3* (n = 3) (Figure S2). One patient had a recommendation of off-label treatment only, 13 patients had a recommendation of off-label treatment and clinical trials, and 56 patients had a recommendation of clinical trials. Additionally, 14 patients had a recommendation of mutation-driven clinical trials that were ongoing at our institution. Based on the MTB recommendation, six (3.6%) patients were treated with targeted treatment (Figure 2, Table S2). Four patients were enrolled in five genomically matched clinical trials, four of which were conducted at our institution. Two patients used targeted agents in the off-label treatment, and it was beneficial to one of them (Figure 3). She was a 75-year-old female patient with pre-treated metastatic cholangiocarcinoma harboring an *ERBB2* amplification (Copy number; CN = 114) and treated with dual human epidermal growth factor receptor 2 (HER2) blockage therapy (trastuzumab and pertuzumab), and a good clinical response was observed for 9 months until the appearance of pleural effusion. Following pleural adhesion, the next treatment was initiated with trastuzumab deruxtecan, an HER2-targeting antibody–drug conjugate. She achieved tumor shrinkage after 1.5 months of the treatment, but she requested treatment discontinuation due to grade 3 fatigue, which gradually subsided several weeks following the discontinuation.

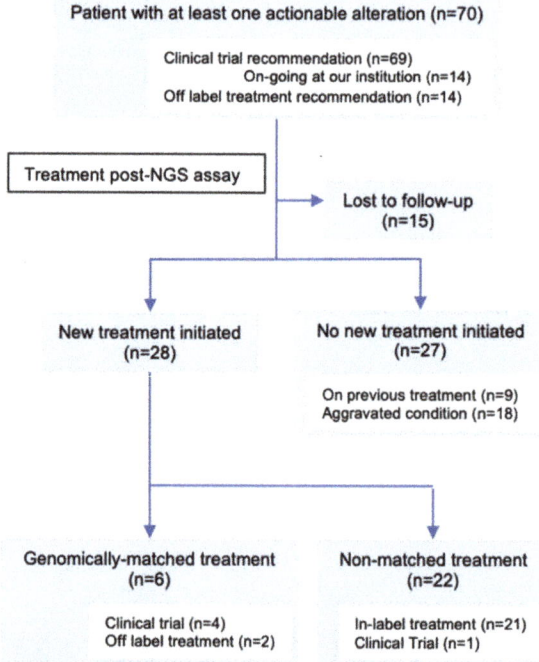

Figure 2. Consort diagram of post-next-generation sequencing (NGS) treatment of patients with at least one actionable alteration on the molecular tumor board (MTB) report. All numbers do not add up because some patients were counted in more than one category (i.e., had an actionable alteration with recommendations of clinical trials and off-label treatment). See Table S2 for detailed information on the patients who received genomically matched treatment.

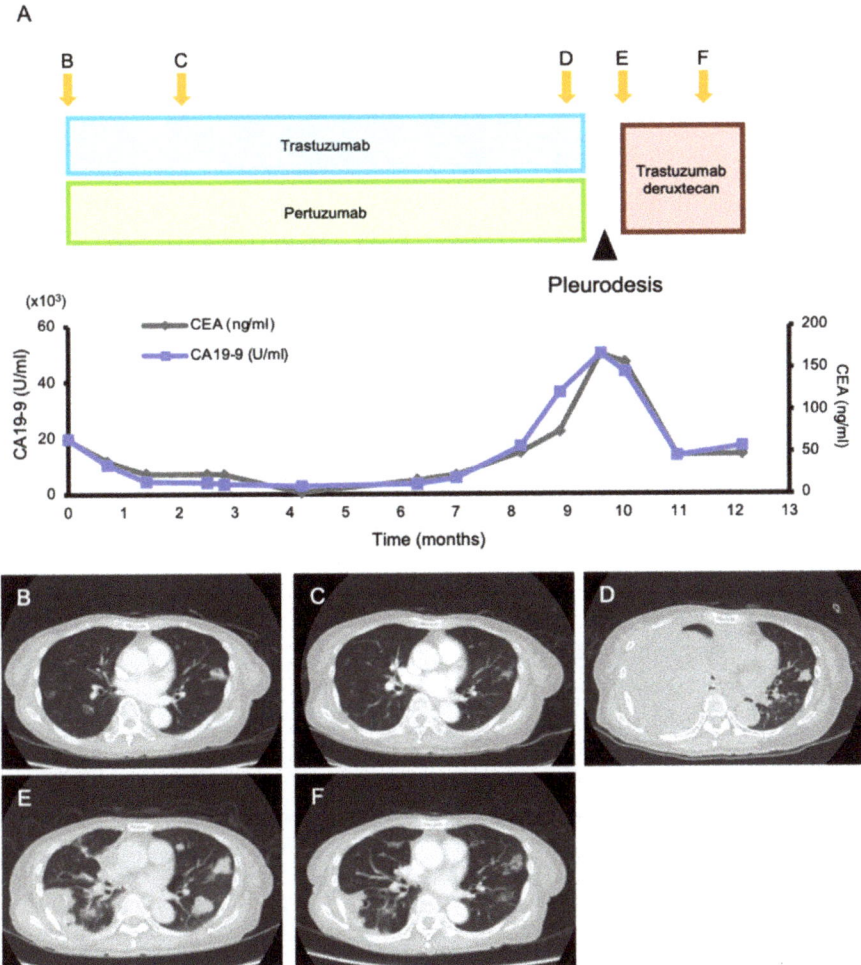

Figure 3. Clinical presentation. (**A**) The course of tumor markers (carcinoembryonic antigen (CEA) and carbohydrate antigen 19-9 (CA 19-9)) and (**B–F**) contrast-enhanced computed tomography (CT) images while receiving treatment with trastuzumab/pertuzumab and trastuzumab deruxtecan. Multiple lung metastases and liver metastases (which is not shown here) were observed when treatment with trastuzumab/pertuzumab was initiated (**B**). Two months after, a good partial response was obtained (**C**). After 9 months of treatment, the tumor became refractory to trastuzumab/pertuzumab, and a massive right pleural effusion was developed (**D**). After improvement of the pleural effusion with pleurodesis (**E**), the next treatment with trastuzumab deruxtecan was initiated, and tumor shrinkage was observed 1.5 months later (**F**).

2.3. Presumed Germline Findings

A total of 166 (98.8%) patients preferred to be informed about the presumed germline findings, and 156 (95.1%) adult patients wanted to share the findings with their family members (Table S3). A total of 26 presumed germline pathogenic variants in 24 patients (14.3%) were nominated by a germline-focused tumor analysis in the following genes: *SMAD4* (n = 6), *BRCA2* (n = 4), *PTEN* (n = 3), *BRCA1* (n = 3), *RB1* (n = 2), *STK11* (n = 2), *ATM* (n = 1), *BRIP1* (n = 1), *MSH6* (n = 1), *RAD51* (n = 1), *TP53* (n = 1), and *TSC2* (n = 1) (Table 2). All the findings were described in the MTB-approved report and returned to the patients. Five of them (20.8%) contacted a genetic counselor, and one patient proceeded for further germline testing.

Table 2. Presumed germline findings nominated on MTB reports.

Gene	Cancer Type	SNV Function	SNV Nucleotide Change	SNV Amino Acid Change	RefSNP Number	CNA Number of Exons	CNA Position
ATM	Small intestinal	frameshift	c.6710dup	p.E2238fs*11	-	-	-
BRCA1	**Ovarian**	**nonsense**	**c.2800C > T**	**p.Q934 ***	rs80357223	-	-
	Small intestinal	missense	c.236T > G	p.F79C	-	-	-
	Ovarian	missense	c.5557T > A	p.Y1853N	-	-	-
BRCA2	Ovarian	nonsense	c.6952C > T	p.R2318*	rs80358920	-	-
	HCC	frameshift	c.5110_5113delAGAA	p.R1704fs*1	-	-	-
	Small intestinal	**missense**	**c.8524C > T**	**p.R2842C**	rs80359104	-	-
	Pancreatic	**nonsense**	**c.7969A > T**	**p.K2657 ***	-	-	-
BRIP1	Ovarian	nonsense	c.1741C > T	p.R581 *	rs780020495	-	-
MSH6	Esophageal	missense	c.1082G > A	p.R361H	rs63750440	-	-
PTEN	Uterine	nonsense	c.733C > T	p.Q245 *	rs786202918	-	-
	Ovarian	missense	c.376G > A	p.A126T	rs1554898129	-	-
	Breast	nonsense	c.295G > T	p.E99 *	-	-	-
RAD51	Gastric	frameshift	c.1dup	p.M1fs	rs55714242	-	-
RB1	Sarcoma	frameshift	c.869delA	p.N290fs*11	rs1131690901	-	-
	Colorectal (CNA_loss)	-	-	-	-	16 of 27	chr13:48881414-49010994
SMAD4	**Colorectal**	**missense**	**c.1487G > A**	**p.R496H**	rs876660045	-	-
	Colorectal	missense	c.1081C > T	p.R361C	rs80338963	-	-
	Colorectal	missense	c.290G > A	p.R97H	rs1555685159	-	-
	Colorectal	frameshift	c.282delC	p.Y95fs*15	-	-	-
	Pancreatic	nonsense	c.346C > T	p.Q116 *	-	-	-
	Bile duct	missense	c.1058A > G	p.Y353C	rs377767346	-	-
STK11	Gastric (CNA_loss) NSCLC	missense	c.580G > A	p.D194N	rs121913315	8 of 9	chr19:1152647-1223171
TP53	Ovarian	splice	c.672 + 1G > A	-	rs863224499	-	-
TSC2	Colorectal	nonsense	c.3412C > T	p.R1138 *	rs45451497	-	-

Bold, patients who contacted a genetic counselor; *ATM*, ataxia telangiectasia mutated; *BRCA1*, breast cancer susceptibility gene 1; *BRCA2*, breast cancer susceptibility gene 2; *BRIP1*, BRCA1 interacting protein C-terminal helicase 1; CNA, copy number alteration; HCC, hepatocellular carcinoma; *MSH6*, mutS homolog 6; MTB, molecular tumor board; NSCLC, non-small cell lung cancer; *PTEN*, phosphatase and tensin homolog; *RB1*, retinoblastoma 1; RefSNP, reference single nucleotide polymorphism; *SMAD4*, mothers against decapentaplegic homolog 4; SNV, single nucleotide variant; *STK11*, serine/threonine kinase 11; *TP53*, tumor protein P53; *TSC2*, tuberous sclerosis complex 2.

3. Discussion

This study presented the real-world data of patients with advanced malignancies who exhausted their standard treatment and underwent NGS at our institution. The NGS assay had a good feasibility in clinical practice with a high success rate and an ordinary turnaround time [15]. MTB recommendations, subsequent genomic-matched treatment, and management of presumed germline findings in daily practice were also presented. Genes that recurrently altered across samples and the percentage of patients who were provided MTB recommendation were similar to that in other series; however, the number of patients who received a targeted agent based on the NGS findings in our cohort is smaller than that in previous reports [16–19]. There are several explanations for the low rate of treatment with the genomically matched drug received in this study.

First of all, the timing for NGS assay appeared to be too late for making optimum use of its results. Under the Japanese universal health-care system, reimbursement of the NGS assay is restricted to patients who have completed their standard treatment and are eligible for palliative treatment. As a result, we found twenty-seven patients (27/204, 13.2%) who experienced disease aggravation or death during the wait for NGS results; the NGS results were not considered for therapeutic decision making. In addition, disease progression is a major limiting factor for the initiation of treatment after NGS assay, as described in previous literature [19]. The optimal timing for NGS assay in patients with cancer has not yet been determined. However, our study suggested that to obtain the maximum therapeutic value of NGS, it should be performed early in the course of the disease. A prospective study on the feasibility and utility of large NGS assays before initial systemic treatment is ongoing, with the aim of reimbursement of NGS assays in the frontline setting for metastatic cancer patients in Japan [20]. Nearly half of the patients who underwent NGS assay were referred from smaller partner community-based hospitals that do not have MTB. To make the best use of NGS, physicians and medical staff need to be encouraged to consider early referral for panel test assessment.

Secondly, limited access to early phase clinical trials is a major barrier for enrolling patients in matched clinical trials, as mentioned in previous articles [17,21]. A recent report from National Cancer Center Hospital (NCCH) demonstrated that 13.3% (25/230) of the patients who underwent NGS after completing their standard chemotherapy were treated with matched targeted agents based on the MTB recommendation; this rate is approximately four times higher than that of our cohort (6/168, 3.6%) [16]. NCCH is a leading facility in early phase drug development in Japan, and it runs the largest number of early phase clinical trials [22,23]. Therefore, they have a greater opportunity for the patients to be enrolled in genomic-driven trials of a drug in development. This leads to a disparity in the number of patients who received matched targeted agents between the hospitals. A new basket/umbrella trial, which is similar to the TAPUR study, was started at our institution in July 2019. It provides 15 targeted agents that were reimbursed in other indications for patients with matched actionable mutations [24]. This trial would partially improve access to targeted therapy. Additionally, consultation via a virtual platform is gradually being adapted in oncology [25,26]. The integration of telemedicine in clinical trials to enhance clinical trial accessibility is anticipated.

Thirdly, it is difficult to access investigational targeted agents outside the clinical trial under the Japanese health-care system. We do not have a system similar to the expanded access program in the United States and Europe. In addition, all the costs related to off-label use generally need to be paid out-of-pocket, and very few patients can afford it. Moreover, each case must be approved by an institutional review committee before prescribing an off-label treatment [27]. Such circumstances make physicians recommend strict off-label use. Consequently, our MTB recommended off-label use in 8.3% (14/168) of the patients in this study, and one of two patients who received off-label treatment had a favorable clinical outcome. Our MTB recommended off-label use for the genetic alterations that responded beneficially to matched treatment in previous clinical trials and case series such as *ERBB2*, *BRCA1*, *BRCA2*, and *BRAF* V600E. The clinical benefit and potential side effects of off-label use are controversial. Previous reports revealed that off-label use without concrete clinical evidence could be harmful to the patients [28,29]. If the indications for off-label use by the MTB are increased, it may increase the number of patients who use off-label agents; however, it is unlikely to be beneficial to several patients. Therefore, we believe that our conservative approach toward off-label use is reasonable in current practice.

The management of presumed germline findings is of increasing importance. A recent recommendation from the European Society of Medical Oncology (ESMO) advocates for the active disclosure of presumed germline findings upon tumor-only sequencing. In addition, the American College of Medical Genetics (ACMG) recommends the reporting of presumed germline findings, even when those found in the genes are unrelated to the primary medical reason for genome sequencing. We found that most of the patients in this study provided consent for reporting presumed germline findings to themselves and their family members. This has been addressed by several Western studies [30,31]. We understand that Japanese and Western patients have similar preferences for presumed germline findings. While 26 presumed germline findings were nominated in 24 individuals, five patients contacted genetic counselors, and one of them underwent further investigation. We learned that our management of presumed germline findings is practically acceptable in the current health-care system. The presence of a genetic specialist is not mandatory when returning presumed germline findings to patients; however, compared to a previous report, this may result in a small number of patients accessing further genetic consultation and testing [32]. We should reconsider and improve our approach for returning presumed germline findings in cooperation with cancer genetic specialists.

This study had several limitations. This was a single-canter, retrospective study. The patient population was heterogeneous, and several patients with extremely advanced disease who waited for approval of the assay were included. Given a short follow-up period of 6 months, the certain number of patients lost to follow-up, and the small number of patients who received targeted treatment, the survival analyses are not statistically reliable and thus are not shown. The presumed germline findings nominated in this study are based on the germline-focused analysis of tumor-only sequencing panel. Therefore, the clear distinction between somatic and germline mutations is difficult, and the interpretation of the findings needs careful consideration.

The strength of the study is that we presented the first real-world data of patients with various cancers who underwent NGS under the universal health-care system.

4. Materials and Methods

4.1. Patients

We retrospectively reviewed the medical records of 221 consecutive patients at Osaka University, who provided their consent to take the F1 CDx *covered* by the Japanese public health *insurance* system from September 2019 to July 2020. The median follow-up period was 179 days (range: 48–439 days). The patients' clinical data were extracted from their medical records.

4.2. The Flow of NGS Assay under National Health Insurance Coverage in Japan

Details of the workflow of the NGS assay under Japan's universal health care are found in previous studies [30–32]. Briefly, patients with a histopathological diagnosis of a solid tumor who finished or have finished their standard chemotherapy were candidates for insurance-covered NGS. Patients aged below 20 years provided their assent, while consent was obtained from their parents/guardians with patients' assent. When consent was obtained, patients (and parents/guardians) were also asked whether they wanted to be informed of the results of the presumed germline variants by the physicians (see Section 4.4). Archival formalin-fixed paraffin-embedded (FFPE) tumor samples (or 20 serial unstained slides) were collected and pre-screened by board-certified pathologists at Osaka University to estimate the duration of storage and tumor content of the specimen, and then, they were sent for NGS assay (F1 CDx), which was carried out following the previously described manufacturer's (Foundation Medicine) instructions [33,34]. Concisely, F1CDx detects 324 genes, including all coding exons of 309 cancer-related genes, one promoter region, one noncoding RNA, and select intronic regions of 34 commonly rearranged genes, the coding exons of 21 of which are also included. F1CDx also simultaneously profiled for TMB as well as microsatellite instability (MSI) status. We sent thin-sectioned FFPE slides to a Clinical Laboratory Improvement Amendments (CLIA)-certified and College of American Pathologists (CAP)-accredited laboratory (Foundation Medicine, Cambridge, MA, USA). After the pathology review of the specimen, DNA was extracted and quantified prior to Library Construction (LC). Libraries passed the quality control were hybridized and then sequenced. Sequence data were analyzed using proprietary software developed by Foundation Medicine, and quality control criteria that included tumor purity, DNA sample size, tissue sample size, library construction size, and hybrid capture yields were employed. Sequence data were mapped to the human genome (hg19) using BWA v0.5.9 [35], PCR duplicate reads were removed, and sequence metrics were collected using Picard 1.47 [36] and SAMtools 0.1.12a [37]. Local alignment optimization was performed using GATK 1.0.4705 [38]. Variant calling was performed only in genomic regions targeted by the test. TMB was measured by counting all coding synonymous and nonsynonymous (SNVs) and indels present at $\geq$5% allele frequency and filtering out potential germline variants according to published databases of known germline polymorphisms, including Single Nucleotide Polymorphism Database (dbSNP) and Exome Aggregation Consortium (ExAC). MSI status was determined by analyzing 95 intronic homopolymer repeat loci (10–20 bp long in the human reference genome) with adequate coverage on the F1CDx assay for length variability and compiled into an overall MSI score via principal components analysis (PCA). The report of the F1CDx as well as variant call file were assessed for the actionability of each alteration by consulting databases, such as ClinVar, Catalogue of Somatic Mutations in Cancer (COSMIC), and availability of genomically matched clinical trials and off-label agents in Japan at our own MTB with primary care clinicians, clinical oncologists, genomic counselor, clinical geneticists, and pathologists, which is a mandatory procedure under the universal health-care system. Subsequently, the MTB-approved report for the assay with the treatment recommendation was provided. The report was returned to the patient and/or their family from his/her primary clinician at the clinic.

4.3. Identification and Classification of Genes with Treatment Recommendation

We defined actionable mutations as mutations for whom genomically matched treatment was recommended by the MTB-approved report. Oncogenic alterations revealed by the previous testing were excluded unless genomically matched therapies beyond the standard of care were available. Genetic alterations that predicted resistance to a targeted agent were also excluded. Additionally, MTB recommendation on the TMB underwent a shift during the study period, reflecting the Food and Drug Administration (FDA)'s approval of pembrolizumab for the treatment of adult and pediatric patients with unresectable or metastatic TMB-H ($\geq$10 mutations/megabase (mut/Mb)) solid tumors. All actionable mutations were classified according to the OncoKB levels of evidence classification as follows [39]: level 1, FDA-approved biomarker predictive of response to an FDA-approved drug in a specific cancer type; level 2A, standard care biomarkers of response to an FDA-approved drug in a specific indication; level 2B, standard care biomarkers predictive of response to an FDA-approved drug in another indication; level 3A, compelling clinical evidence in reported tumor types, which were regarded as biomarkers of therapeutic response for novel targeted agents that are not yet approved in the standard of care; level 3B, compelling clinical evidence reported in other tumor types, which are regarded as the biomarkers of therapeutic response for novel targeted agents that are not yet approved in the standard of care; and level 4; non–FDA-recognized biomarkers that are predictive of response to novel targeted agents based on compelling biologic data.

4.4. Presumed Germline Findings

A germline-focused tumor analysis was carried out after consent was obtained. We assessed the presumed germline findings following the proposal of the Japan Agency for Medical Research and Development (AMED) study group concerning the information transmission process in genomic medicine [40] (Supplementary Figure S3). Briefly, a clinical genetic expert (K.H) extracted the data of 43 genes that were recommended for a presumed germline finding analysis (Supplementary Table S4) from a variant call format file and investigated the variant classification by consulting databases, such as ClinVar and COSMIC. A certified genetic counselor (Y.S) and a clinical geneticist (K.H) assessed the clinical utility of each alteration in terms of allele frequency and correlation to patient and family history as well as clinical findings. For *BRCA1* and *BRCA2*, pathological and likely pathogenic alterations were disclosed as presumed germline findings irrespective of allele frequency of the variants. Pathological and likely pathogenic mutations found in other genes were generally disclosed to be presumed germline variants when the variant allele frequency was $\geq 30\%$ for single nucleotide substitutions and $\geq 20\%$ for small insertions/deletions. Regarding *APC*, *RB1*, *TP53*, and genes of which variant of allele frequency is lower than the threshold described above, the patients' phenotypes were carefully evaluated before disclosure. The assessment was shared and discussed as a way of disclosure at the MTB. Results of the presumed germline findings assessment were described in the MTB-approved report and were returned to the patient and/or their family by his/her primary clinician. Genetic counseling and confirmatory testing are offered to the patient when presumed germline finding is disclosed.

4.5. Statistical Analysis

Statistical analyses were performed using EZR (Saitama Medical Center, Jichi Medical University, Saitama, Japan), which is a graphical user interface for R (The R Foundation for Statistical Computing, Vienna, Austria). Most of our data are descriptive. The Kaplan–Meier method was used to estimate overall survival rates. The study was conducted in accordance with the Declaration of Helsinki and Good Clinical Practice guidelines. The study was approved by the Osaka University Institutional Review Board, and all patients provided written informed consent for the use of their genomic and clinical data for research purposes.

5. Conclusions

In conclusion, this article highlighted the current status and problems of the clinical utility of NGS assay under the universal health coverage system at a single university hospital in Japan. Though it is a top priority in precision oncology to match patients with the appropriate treatment or clinical trials, a small number of patients received genomically matched treatment based on the NGS results. Reimbursement of NGS in the universal health-care system in Japan is restricted to patients who completed their standard treatment, and quite a few patients experience disease progression before they receive their results. This led to a decrease in the number of patients whose results could be used to guide treatment decision-making and administration of matched targeted treatment. NGS assay should be considered earlier in the course of the disease to maximize the therapeutic opportunities after testing. We eagerly hope that NGS reimbursement is done for advanced cancer patients earlier in the course of the disease. The availability of clinical trials in the region is a barrier to patients benefiting from NGS. Our study demonstrated the feasibility of managing presumed germline findings in daily practice. NGS would help bring personalized cancer medicine to routine clinical practice. Adequate integration of NGS in the health-care system is required to promote the efficient clinical application of NGS and advance precision medicine.

Supplementary Materials: The following are available online at https://www.mdpi.com/2072-6694/13/5/1121/s1, Figure S1: CONSORT diagram of patients enrolled in the study, Figure S2: Top 20 frequent genomic alterations with the treatment recommendation, Figure S3: The operation workflow for evaluating and nominating presumed germline findings from tumor-only sequencing panel, Table S1: Actionable alterations according to cancer type, Table S2: List of cases that underwent genomically matched treatment beyond standard of care based on MTB recommendation, Table S3: Patients' preference for receiving presumed germline finding. Table S4: Presumed germline finding gene list used for assessing F1CDx.

Author Contributions: Conceptualization, C.I. and T.S.; data collection, C.I. and K.H (Kazue Hatake).; data analysis, C.I., D.M., K.H. (Kazue Hatake), Y.S, K.H. (Kae Hashimoto), and D.S.; writing—original draft preparation, C.I.; writing—review and editing, T.S., D.M., K.H. (Kazue Hatake), Y.S., D.S., K.H. (Kae Hashimoto), and S.Y.; supervision, N.N.; project administration, T.S.; All authors have read and agreed to the published version of the manuscript.

Funding: This research received no external funding.

Institutional Review Board Statement: The study was conducted according to the guidelines of the Declaration of Helsinki, and approved by Osaka University Hospital Ethics Review Committee for observational studies (20248, date of approval: 5 November 2020).

Informed Consent Statement: Informed consent was obtained from all subjects involved in the study.

Data Availability Statement: Clinical data and all the variant data used in the conduct of the analyses are not publicly available due to the Institutional Review Board restriction in the context of protection of the privacy and confidentiality of patients in this study, but the data are possibly available if a reasonable request is made to the corresponding author.

Acknowledgments: The authors would like to thank T. Ishikawa for helping in data collection. The authors received the generous support and encouragement of H. Kawakami in revising the manuscript.

Conflicts of Interest: Dr. Maeda reports research support from Takara Bio, Inc., outside the submitted work; Dr. Sakai reports grants and personal fees from Chugai Pharma, grants from Yakult Honsha, grants from Ono Pharmaceutical, grants and non-financial support from Daiichi Sankyo, grants from Lilly Japan, outside the submitted work; Dr. Nonomura reports grants and personal fees from Takeda Pharmaceuticals, personal fees from Astellas, personal fees from AstraZeneca, personal fees from Ono Pharmaceuticals, personal fees from Merck Biopharma, grants from Taiho Pharmaceuticals, grants and personal fees from Nihon Shinyaku Pharmaceuticals, outside the submitted work; Dr. Satoh reports grants, personal fees and other from Ono Pharmaceutical, grants, personal fees and other from ChugaiPharmaceutical, grants, personal fees and other from Yakult Honsha, grants and personal fees from Elli Lilly, grants from MSD, grants and other from Bristol Myers, grants from Astellas, grants and personal fees from Daiichi -Sankyo, grants and other from Taiho Pharmaceutical, personal fees from Takara-Bio, grants and other from Sanofi-Aventis, grants from Giliad Sciences, grants from Palexell, outside the submitted work;. All other authors declare no conflict of interest.

References

1. Radovich, M.; Kiel, P.J.; Nance, S.M.; Niland, E.E.; Parsley, M.E.; Ferguson, M.E.; Jiang, G.; Ammakkanavar, N.R.; Einhorn, L.H.; Cheng, L.; et al. Clinical benefit of a precision medicine based approach for guiding treatment of refractory cancers. *Oncotarget* **2016**, *7*, 56491. [CrossRef]
2. Hainsworth, J.D.; Meric-Bernstam, F.; Swanton, C.; Hurwitz, H.; Spigel, D.R.; Sweeney, C.; Burris, H.A.; Bose, R.; Yoo, B.; Stein, A.; et al. Targeted Therapy for Advanced Solid Tumors on the Basis of Molecular Profiles: Results From MyPathway, an Open-Label, Phase IIa Multiple Basket Study. *J. Clin. Oncol.* **2018**, *36*, 536–542. [CrossRef] [PubMed]
3. Mangat, P.K.; Halabi, S.; Bruinooge, S.S.; Garrett-Mayer, E.; Alva, A.; Janeway, K.A.; Stella, P.J.; Voest, E.; Yost, K.J.; Perlmutter, J.; et al. Rationale and Design of the Targeted Agent and Profiling Utilization Registry (TAPUR) Study. *JCO Precis. Oncol.* **2018**, *2018*. [CrossRef]
4. Massard, C.; Michiels, S.; Ferté, C.; Le Deley, M.-C.; Lacroix, L.; Hollebecque, A.; Verlingue, L.; Ileana, E.; Rosellini, S.; Ammari, S.; et al. High-Throughput Genomics and Clinical Outcome in Hard-to-Treat Advanced Cancers: Results of the MOSCATO 01 Trial. *Cancer Discov.* **2017**, *7*, 586. [CrossRef]
5. Sicklick, J.K.; Kato, S.; Okamura, R.; Schwaederle, M.; Hahn, M.E.; Williams, C.B.; De, P.; Krie, A.; Piccioni, D.E.; Miller, V.A.; et al. Molecular profiling of cancer patients enables personalized combination therapy: The I-PREDICT study. *Nat. Med.* **2019**, *25*, 744. [CrossRef]

6. Gupta, R.; Garrett-Mayer, E.; Halabi, S.; Mangat, P.K.; D'Andre, S.D.; Meiri, E.; Shrestha, S.; Warren, S.L.; Ranasinghe, S.; Schilsky, R.L. Pertuzumab plus trastuzumab (P+T) in patients (Pts) with colorectal cancer (CRC) with ERBB2 amplification or overexpression: Results from the TAPUR Study. *J. Clin. Oncol.* **2020**, *38* (Suppl. 4), 132. [CrossRef]
7. Klute, K.; Garrett-Mayer, E.; Halabi, S.; Mangat, P.K.; Nazemzadeh, R.; Yost, K.J.; Butler, N.L.; Perla, V.; Schilsky, R.L. Cobimetinib plus vemurafenib (C+V) in patients (Pts) with colorectal cancer (CRC) with BRAF V600E mutations: Results from the TAPUR Study. *J. Clin. Oncol.* **2020**, *38* (Suppl. 4), 122. [CrossRef]
8. Alva, A.S.; Mangat, P.K.; Garrett-Mayer, E.; Halabi, S.; Alvarez, R.H.; Calfa, C.J.; Khalil, M.F.; Ahn, E.R.; Cannon, T.L.; Crilley, P.A.; et al. Pembrolizumab (P) in patients (pts) with metastatic breast cancer (MBC) with high tumor mutational burden (HTMB): Results from the Targeted Agent and Profiling Utilization Registry (TAPUR) Study. *J. Clin. Oncol.* **2019**, *37* (Suppl. 15), 1014 [CrossRef]
9. Meiri, E.; Garrett-Mayer, E.; Halabi, S.; Mangat, P.K.; Shrestha, S.; Ahn, E.R.; Osayameh, O.; Perla, V.; Schilsky, R.L. Pembrolizumab (P) in patients (Pts) with colorectal cancer (CRC) with high tumor mutational burden (HTMB): Results from the Targeted Agent and Profiling Utilization Registry (TAPUR) Study. *J. Clin. Oncol.* **2020**, *38* (Suppl. 4), 133. [CrossRef]
10. Ahn, E.R.; Mangat, P.K.; Garrett-Mayer, E.; Halabi, S.; Dib, E.G.; Haggstrom, D.E.; Alguire, K.B.; Alvarez, R.H.; Calfa, C.J.; Cannon, T.L.; et al. Palbociclib (P) in patients (pts) with non-small cell lung cancer (NSCLC) with CDKN2A alterations: Results from the Targeted Agent and Profiling Utilization Registry (TAPUR) Study. *J. Clin. Oncol.* **2019**, *37* (Suppl. 15), 9041. [CrossRef]
11. Tan, D.S.; Tan, D.S.; Tan, I.B.H.; Yan, B.; Choo, S.P.; Chng, W.J.; Hwang, W.Y.K. Recommendations to improve the clinical adoption of NGS-based cancer diagnostics in Singapore. *Asia Pac. J. Clin. Oncol.* **2020**, *16*, 222. [CrossRef]
12. Ebi, H.; Bando, H. Precision Oncology and the Universal Health Coverage System in Japan. *JCO Precis. Oncol.* **2019**, *3*, 1–12. [CrossRef] [PubMed]
13. Naito, Y.; Aburatani, H.; Amano, T.; Baba, E.; Furukawa, T.; Hayashida, T.; Hiyama, E.; Ikeda, S.; Kanai, M.; Kato, M.; et al. Clinical practice guidance for next-generation sequencing in cancer diagnosis and treatment (edition 2.1). *Int. J. Clin. Oncol.* **2021**, *26*, 233. [CrossRef]
14. Takeda, M.; Sakai, K.; Takahama, T.; Fukuoka, K.; Nakagawa, K.; Nishio, K. New Era for Next-Generation Sequencing in Japan. *Cancers* **2019**, *11*, 742. [CrossRef]
15. De Falco, V.; Poliero, L.; Vitello, P.P.; Ciardiello, D.; Vitale, P.; Zanaletti, N.; Giunta, E.F.; Terminiello, M.; Caputo, V.; Carlino, F.; et al. Feasibility of next-generation sequencing in clinical practice: Results of a pilot study in the Department of Precision Medicine at the University of Campania 'Luigi Vanvitelli'. *ESMO Open* **2020**, *5*, e000675. [CrossRef]
16. Sunami, K.; Ichikawa, H.; Kubo, T.; Kato, M.; Fujiwara, Y.; Shimomura, A.; Koyama, T.; Kakishima, H.; Kitami, M.; Matsushita, H.; et al. Feasibility and utility of a panel testing for 114 cancer-associated genes in a clinical setting: A hospital-based study. *Cancer Sci.* **2019**, *110*, 1480. [CrossRef]
17. Dalton, W.B.; Forde, P.M.; Kang, H.; Connolly, R.M.; Stearns, V.; Gocke, C.D.; Eshleman, J.R.; Axilbund, J.; Petry, D.; Geoghegan, C.; et al. Personalized Medicine in the Oncology Clinic: Implementation and Outcomes of the Johns Hopkins Molecular Tumor Board. *JCO Precis. Oncol.* **2017**, *1*, 1–19. [CrossRef] [PubMed]
18. Hoefflin, R.; Geißler, A.-L.; Fritsch, R.; Claus, R.; Wehrle, J.; Metzger, P.; Reiser, M.; Mehmed, L.; Fauth, L.; Heiland, D.H.; et al. Personalized Clinical Decision Making Through Implementation of a Molecular Tumor Board: A German Single-Center Experience. *JCO Precis. Oncol.* **2018**, *2*, 1–16. [CrossRef] [PubMed]
19. Sadaps, M.; Funchain, P.; Mahdi, H.; Grivas, P.; Pritchard, A.; Klek, S.; Estfan, B.; Abraham, J.; Budd, G.T.; Stevenson, J.P.; et al. Precision Oncology in Solid Tumors: A Longitudinal Tertiary Care Center Experience. *JCO Precis. Oncol.* **2018**, *2*, 1–11. [CrossRef]
20. Prospective Study for Evaluating Feasibly and Utility of Comprehensive Genomic Profiling Test before Initial Systemic Treatment in Advanced Malignant Solid Tumor Patients. Available online: https://upload.umin.ac.jp/cgi-open-bin/ctr_e/ctr_view.cgi?recptno=R000046492 (accessed on 24 January 2021).
21. Kurnit, K.C.; Dumbrava, E.E.I.; Litzenburger, B.; Khotskaya, Y.B.; Johnson, A.M.; Yap, T.A.; Rodon, J.; Zeng, J.; Shufean, M.A.; Bailey, A.; et al. Precision Oncology Decision Support: Current Approaches and Strategies for the Future. *Clin. Cancer Res.* **2018**, *24*, 2719. [CrossRef] [PubMed]
22. Mizugaki, H.; Yamamoto, N.; Fujiwara, Y.; Nokihara, H.; Yamada, Y.; Tamura, T. Current Status of Single-Agent Phase I Trials in Japan: Toward Globalization. *Int. J. Clin. Oncol.* **2015**, *33*, 2051–2061. [CrossRef]
23. Loong, H.H.; Tan, D.S.W.; Shimizu, T. Challenges and insights of early phase oncology drug development in the Asia-Pacific region. *Chin. Clin. Oncol.* **2019**, *8*, 5. [CrossRef] [PubMed]
24. Ishimaru, S.; Shimoi, T.; Sunami, K.; Shibata, T.; Okamura, N.; Mori, M.; Kawabata, S.; Okita, N.; Nakamura, K.; Yamamoto, N. A novel approach for improving drug access using patient-proposed healthcare service. *ABSTRACTS Pediatr. Blood Cancer* **2019**, *66*, e28049. [CrossRef]
25. Broom, A.; Kenny, K.; Page, A.; Cort, N.; Lipp, E.S.; Tan, A.C.; Ashley, D.M.; Walsh, K.M.; Khasraw, M. The Paradoxical Effects of COVID-19 on Cancer Care: Current Context and Potential Lasting Impacts. *Clin. Cancer Res.* **2020**, *26*, 5809–5813. [CrossRef]
26. Tolaney, S.M.; Lydon, C.A.; Li, T.; Dai, J.; Standring, A.; Legor, K.A.; Caparrotta, C.M.; Schenker, M.P.; Glazer, D.I.; Tayob, N.; et al. The Impact of COVID-19 on Clinical Trial Execution at the Dana-Farber Cancer Institute. *JNCI J. Natl. Cancer Inst.* **2020**, djaa144. [CrossRef]

27. Bun, S.; Yonemori, K.; Sunadoi, H.; Nishigaki, R.; Noguchi, E.; Okusaka, T.; Nishida, T.; Fujiwara, Y. Safety and Evidence of Off-Label Use of Approved Drugs at the National Cancer Center Hospital in Japan. *JCO Oncol. Pract.* **2020**, OP2000131. [CrossRef] [PubMed]
28. Saiyed, M.M.; Ong, P.S.; Chew, L. Off-label drug use in oncology: A systematic review of literature. *J. Clin. Pharm. Ther.* **2017**, *42*, 251–258. [CrossRef]
29. Eguale, T.; Buckeridge, D.L.; Verma, A.; Winslade, N.E.; Benedetti, A.; Hanley, J.A.; Tamblyn, R. Association of Off-label Drug Use and Adverse Drug Events in an Adult Population. *JAMA Intern. Med.* **2016**, *176*, 55. [CrossRef]
30. Wynn, J.; Martinez, J.; Duong, J.; Chiuzan, C.; Phelan, J.C.; Fyer, A.; Klitzman, R.L.; Appelbaum, P.S.; Chung, W.K. Research Participants' Preferences for Hypothetical Secondary Results from Genomic Research. *J. Genet. Couns.* **2017**, *26*, 841. [CrossRef]
31. Murphy Bollinger, J.; Bridges, J.F.P.; Mohamed, A.; Kaufman, D. Public preferences for the return of research results in genetic research: A conjoint analysis. *Genet. Med.* **2014**, *16*, 932. [CrossRef]
32. Sapp, J.C.; Johnston, J.J.; Driscoll, K.; Heidlebaugh, A.R.; Miren Sagardia, A.; Dogbe, D.N.; Umstead, K.L.; Turbitt, E.; Alevizos, I.; Baron, J.; et al. Evaluation of Recipients of Positive and Negative Secondary Findings Evaluations in a Hybrid CLIA-Research Sequencing Pilot. *Am. J. Hum. Genet.* **2018**, *103*, 358–366. [CrossRef] [PubMed]
33. FoundationOne® CDx Full Specification Information. Available online: https://www.acessdata.fda.gov/cdrh_docs/pdf17/P170019C.pdf (accessed on 19 February 2021).
34. FoundationOne® CDx: Summary of Safety and Effectiveness Data (SSED). 2020. Available online: https://www.acessdata.fda.gov/cdrh_docs/pdf17/P170019S016B.pdf (accessed on 19 February 2021).
35. Li, H.; Durbin, R. Fast and accurate long-read alignment with Burrows-Wheeler transform. *Bioinformatics* **2010**, *26*, 589–595. [CrossRef] [PubMed]
36. Picard. A Set of Command Line Tools (in Java) for Manipulating High-Throughput Sequencing (HTS) Data and Formats Such as SAM/BAM/CRAM and VCF. Available online: http://broadinstitute.github.io/picard/ (accessed on 19 February 2021).
37. Li, H.; Li, H.; Handsaker, B.; Wysoker, A.; Fennell, T.; Ruan, J.; Homer, N.; Marth, G.; Abecasis, G.; Durbin, R. 1000 Genome Project Data Processing Subgroup. The Sequence Alignment/Map format and SAMtools. *Bioinformatics* **2009**, *25*, 2078–2079. [CrossRef] [PubMed]
38. DePristo, M.A.; Banks, E.; Poplin, R.; Garimella, K.V.; Maguire, J.R.; Hartl, C.; Philippakis, A.A.; del Angel, G.; Rivas, M.A.; Hanna, M.; et al. A framework for variation discovery and genotyping using next-generation DNA sequencing data. *Nat. Genet.* **2011**, *43*, 491–498. [CrossRef]
39. Chakravarty, D.; Gao, J.; Phillips, S.; Kundra, R.; Zhang, H.; Wang, J.; Rudolph, J.E.; Yaeger, R.; Soumerai, T.; Nissan, M.H.; et al. OncoKB: A Precision Oncology Knowledge Base. *JCO Precis. Oncol.* **2017**, *1*, 1–16. [CrossRef]
40. Proposal Concerning the Information Transmission Process in Genomic Medicine. Available online: https://www.amed.go.jp/en/news/seika/20200706.html (accessed on 19 February 2021).

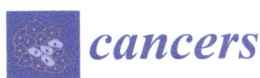

Article

Whole Exome Sequencing of Multi-Regional Biopsies from Metastatic Lesions to Evaluate Actionable Truncal Mutations Using a Single-Pass Percutaneous Technique

Valerie Heong [1,†], Darwin Tay [2,†], Shane Ee Goh [2], Bernard Wee [3], Tuan Zea Tan [2], Ross Soo [1], Brendan Pang [4], Diana Lim [4], Anil Gopinathan [3], Samuel Ow [1], Cheng Ean Chee [1], Boon Cher Goh [1,2], Soo Chin Lee [1,2], Wei Peng Yong [1], Andrea Wong [1], Mohamed Feroz Mohd Omar [2], Richie Soong [2,4] and David S.P. Tan [1,2,*]

1. Department of Haematology-Oncology, National University Cancer Institute, Singapore 119074, Singapore; valerie_ym_heong@ttsh.com.sg (V.H.); ross_soo@nuhs.edu.sg (R.S.); samuel_ow@nuhs.edu.sg (S.O.); cheng_ean_chee@nuhs.edu.sg (C.E.C.); phcgbc@nus.edu.sg (B.C.G.); soo_chin_lee@nuhs.edu.sg (S.C.L.); Wei_Peng_YONG@nuhs.edu.sg (W.P.Y.); Andrea_LA_WONG@nuhs.edu.sg (A.W.)
2. Cancer Science Institute of Singapore, National University of Singapore, Singapore 117599, Singapore; dwintay@gmail.com (D.T.); shanegoh8@gmail.com (S.E.G.); csittz@nus.edu.sg (T.Z.T.); feroz.omar@u.nus.edu (M.F.M.O.); richiesoong@gmail.com (R.S.)
3. Department of Radiology, National University Hospital, Singapore 119074, Singapore; bernard_bk_wee@nuhs.edu.sg (B.W.); anil_gopinathan@nuhs.edu.sg (A.G.)
4. Department of Pathology, National University of Singapore, Singapore 119077, Singapore; brendan.pang@parkwaypantai.com (B.P.); diana_gz_lim@nuhs.edu.sg (D.L.)
* Correspondence: david_sp_tan@nuhs.edu.sg; Tel.: +65-67795555; Fax: +65-67775545
† These authors contributed equally to this paper.

Received: 17 April 2020; Accepted: 7 June 2020; Published: 17 June 2020

Abstract: We investigate the feasibility of obtaining multiple spatially-separated biopsies from a single lesion to explore intratumor heterogeneity and identify actionable truncal mutations using whole exome sequencing (WES). A single-pass radiologically-guided percutaneous technique was used to obtain four spatially-separated biopsies from a single metastatic lesion. WES was performed to identify putative truncal variants (PTVs), defined as a non-synonymous somatic (NSS) variant present in all four spatially separated biopsies. Actionable truncal mutations—filtered using the FoundationOne panel—were defined as clinically relevant PTVs. Mutational landscapes of each biopsy and their association with patient outcomes were assessed. WES on 50 biopsied samples from 13 patients across six cancer types were analyzed. Actionable truncal mutations were identified in 9/13 patients; 31.1 ± 5.12 more unique NSS variants were detected with every additional multi- region tumor biopsy (MRTB) analyzed. The number of PTVs dropped by 16.1 ± 17.9 with every additional MRTB, with the decrease most pronounced (36.8 ± 19.7) when two MRTB were analyzed compared to one. MRTB most reliably predicted PTV compared to in silico analysis of allele frequencies and cancer cell fraction based on one biopsy sample. Three patients treated with actionable truncal mutation-directed therapy derived clinical benefit. Multi-regional sampling for genomics analysis is feasible and informative to help prioritize precision-therapy strategies.

Keywords: intratumor heterogeneity; multiple biopsies; tumor evolution; clonality classification; strategic therapeutic intervention

1. Introduction

Intratumor heterogeneity is a key challenge in precision cancer therapy, contributing to treatment resistance, therapeutic failure and poor prognosis [1,2]. With the growing use and reducing cost of next generation sequencing, the full extent of the complexity and genomic diversity within tumors are becoming more apparent [1,3,4]. Genotype-directed targeted therapies are becoming the standard of care, and as tumor molecular profiling becomes more widely used in routine practice, physicians will require the necessary tools to translate genomic information into clinically actionable results. The consequences of intratumor heterogeneity, such as resistance to drug therapy [3–5] leading to disease recurrence and death, is at least partially the result of limitations in the ability to define the clonal frequency of driver events for prioritization of drug targeting in tumors. Furthermore, it has been demonstrated that high levels of ITH results in poorer survival outcomes across a wide range of cancer types [6,7]. To mitigate this challenge, a more comprehensive view of the mutational diversity of each tumor lesion is required.

The mutational diversity attributed to ITH limits our ability to resolve the full spectrum of cancer pathway aberrations through a single biopsy of the tumor lesion and may under/overestimate driver alterations [4,8,9]. Therefore, multi-region tumor biopsies (MRTBs) are highly beneficial to attenuate the challenge of estimating the prevalence of oncogenic clonal driver mutations. Targeting clonal driver (truncal) mutations would potentially be more effective than targeting subclonal (branch) mutations in a tumor [10,11]. Yap et al. proposed the targeting of genetic alterations located on the trunk of an individual's phylogenetic tree as a more effective clinical strategy [10] as truncal mutations are more likely to represent the core driver mutations within the tumor [10]. In view of the importance of identifying truncal mutations, in silico approaches such as the ABSOLUTE algorithm [12] have been developed to predict truncal variants from a single biopsy sample. However, their ability to identify actionable truncal mutations that would be clinically relevant is hitherto unknown. Similarly, various gene panels have been utilized for diagnostic purposes but the minimum number of MRTB samples needed to address issues associated with ITH remains unknown. This study—conducted across six major cancer types—aims to outline: (a) the safety and significance of MRTB to help navigate the complexities of ITH, (b) the minimum number of MRTB samples required when different gene panels were used for clinical assessment, and (c) the feasibility and clinical efficacy of the approach for identifying clinically actionable truncal mutations (i.e., mutations present in all MRTB obtained from a single tumor lesion) and their outcomes when targeted for strategic therapeutic intervention.

2. Results

A cohort of 15 patients with metastatic colorectal carcinoma (CRC; $n = 1$), non-small cell lung cancer (NSCLC; $n = 6$), ovarian carcinoma (OV; $n = 3$), breast carcinoma (BC, $n = 1$), uterine carcinoma (UC, $n = 2$), hepatocellular carcinoma (HCC; $n = 1$), or cervical cancer (CC, $n = 1$) were recruited to the study. A single-pass radiologically-guided percutaneous biopsy technique was used to obtain MRTBs from a dominantly-progressing metastatic lesion in each patient with core biopsies taken at least 2 mm apart within the same metastatic lesion. Two patients (one with NSCLC and another with cervical cancer) were excluded from analysis as all the MRTB samples collected from them failed quality control (QC). One patient (UC) (P11; Figure 1) had two (out of four) biopsy samples that failed QC which were subsequently excluded from the analysis. Similarly, one patient's (P01) germline sample (i.e., buccal swab) failed QC and was replaced with whole blood sample. All 15 patients tolerated the procedure well with no significant adverse events, except for one patient (P09) who developed a moderately-sized right sided pneumothorax requiring observation overnight and serial imaging to ensure spontaneous resolution of the pneumothorax.

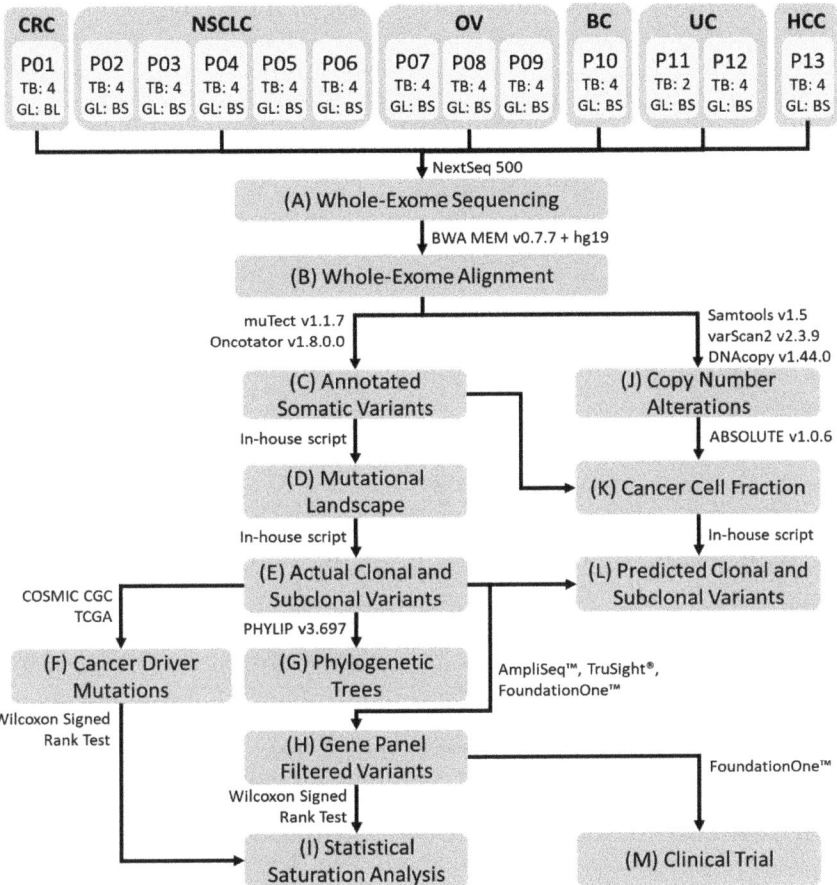

Figure 1. Representative workflow of the processing pipeline. (**A**) Whole-exome sequencing was performed on all germline and MRTB samples obtained from each patient. Bioinformatics analysis was subsequently performed: (**B**) alignment of sequence reads; (**C**) somatic variant calling and variant annotation; (**D**) generation of non-synonymous somatic mutational landscape across all patients; (**E**) identification of truncal and branch variants present in each patient; (**F**) curation of statistically significant somatic cancer driver mutations; (**G**) construction of phylogenetic trees from non-synonymous somatic variants; (**H**) filtering of genetic variants using AmpliSeq™, TruSight®and FoundationOne™ cancer gene panels; (**I**) statistical saturation analysis to determine the minimum number of MRTB samples needed (to alleviate challenges associated with ITH) in relation to the gene panel used; (**J**) copy number alterations analysis; (**K**) estimation of cancer cell fraction (CCF); (**L**) prediction of putative truncal variants using two different threshold metrics, namely variant allele frequency and CCF; (**M**) informed targeted therapies were performed based on patients' mutational profile that reflects genes from the AmpliSeq™ cancer gene panel. MRTB: multi- region tumor biopsy; ITH: intratumor heterogeneity; TB: the number of MRTB samples resected from the patient; GL: the type of germline sample; BL: whole blood sample; BS: buccal swab sample. CRC: Colorectal cancer; NSCLC: Non-small cell lung cancer; OV: Ovarian Cancer; BC: Breast cancer; UC: Uterine Cancer; HCC: Hepatocellular Carcinoma; P: Patient.

The investigation pipeline adopted for analyzing whole-exome sequencing (WES) data that passed QC is illustrated in Figure 1. All processed samples had a DNA concentration greater than 4 ng/μL.

Average sequencing depth, Q30 percentage and uniformity of coverage obtained were 128X ± 29.2, 87.5% ± 4.35, and 91.2% ± 1.94 respectively.

2.1. Tumour Variant Load

The mutational landscape of each patient was examined to evaluate the extent of ITH across different cancer types. The non-synonymous somatic mutational load (nssML)—defined as the total number of non-synonymous somatic (NSS) variants present—was scrutinized for each biopsy sample (Figure 2A). Results indicate that patient P04 has the highest average non-synonymous somatic mutational load (608.0 ± 41.7), while patient P05 with NSCLC has the highest diversity (i.e., difference in non-synonymous somatic mutational load) among the four MRTB samples analyzed (104.3 ± 49.3). The median diversity across all patients was 7.46 (range: 0.957 to 49.3). Friedman test of difference among the different MRTB samples indicated no statistically significant difference between the number of non-synonymous somatic variants present in each MRTB sample ($p = 0.691$).

2.2. Intratumor Heterogeneity

To investigate the extent of the intratumoral heterogeneity, the amount of truncal (i.e., ubiquitous non-synonymous somatic variants that occur in all MRTB samples analyzed) and branch (i.e., non-synonymous somatic variants that do not occur in all MRTB samples) variants were analyzed (Figure 2B). Phylogenetic trees were also constructed to illustrate this phenomenon graphically (Figure 2C, Figure S1). As demonstrated, two patients (P01 and P05) did not have any truncal variants while patients P03 and P13 only had two and one truncal variant(s), respectively. On average, 24.1% ± 20.7, 14.7% ± 13.7 and 61.2% ± 20.6 of non-synonymous somatic variants were truncal, branch and private mutations, respectively. A high level of intratumoral heterogeneity (75.5% ± 34.6) across different tumors was observed, with private mutations dominating the mutational landscape ($p < 0.05$). When copy number alterations (CNAs) were interrogated, a moderate degree of diversity (branch amplification: 54.3% ± 34.7, $p = 0.083$; branch deletion: 59.4% ± 34.8, $p = 0.050$) was observed (Figure 2D, Figure S2).

Statistically significant somatic cancer driver mutations (ssCDMs) were juxtaposed with non-synonymous somatic variants identified in our study cohort. Results indicate that detectable somatic cancer driver mutations were more likely to be truncal variants (68.2%; Figure 2E, Figures S3 and S4); however, the difference was not statistically significant ($p = 0.177$). Truncal somatic cancer driver mutations across this study cohort include *AKT1*, *ATM*, *BCOR*, *CHD4*, *KRAS*, *MAP3K1*, and *PIK3CA*; conversely, branch somatic cancer driver mutations include *ERBB2*, *FOXA1*, and *PPM1D*. In our cohort, *EGFR* mutations were confined to lung cancers, with three out of four (75%) NSCLC patients found to harbor a truncal variant in at least one reportable mutation in *EGFR* [13].

2.3. Statistical Saturation Analysis

The relationship between truncal variants and the number of MRTB samples analyzed was examined. A unique variant in this case refers to a distinct non-synonymous somatic variant that appears in at least one of the MRTB samples analyzed simultaneously. In general, with an increasing number of MRTB samples, a monotonically increasing trend in the number of unique variants and correspondingly decreasing number of truncal variants can be observed (Figure S5).

At the exome level (i.e., WES NSS gene panel), on average 31.1 ± 5.12 more unique non-synonymous somatic variants were detected with every additional MRTB sample analyzed. Conversely, using the number of MRTB samples analyzed simultaneously as the baseline reference to determine putative truncal variants (PTVs), a monotonically decreasing number of PTVs can be observed with an increasing number of MRTB samples. The number of PTVs dropped by 16.1 ± 17.9 on average with every additional MRTB sample, with the decrease most pronounced (36.8 ± 19.7) when two MRTB samples were analyzed compared to just one. Similar trends were observed from filtered variants when the WES data was mapped to genes matching four cancer gene panels—namely COSMIC Cancer

Gene Census (CGC), Ion AmpliSeq™ Cancer Hotspot Panel v2 (Life Technologies, Carlsbad, CA, USA), TruSight®Cancer panel (Illumina Inc, San Diego, CA, USA) and FoundationOne™ cancer gene panel (Foundation Medicine, Cambridge, MA, USA) (Figure S5, Tables S1 and S2). However, the change in the number of unique/truncal mutations with increasing MRTB samples was less pronounced (<2 variants on average).

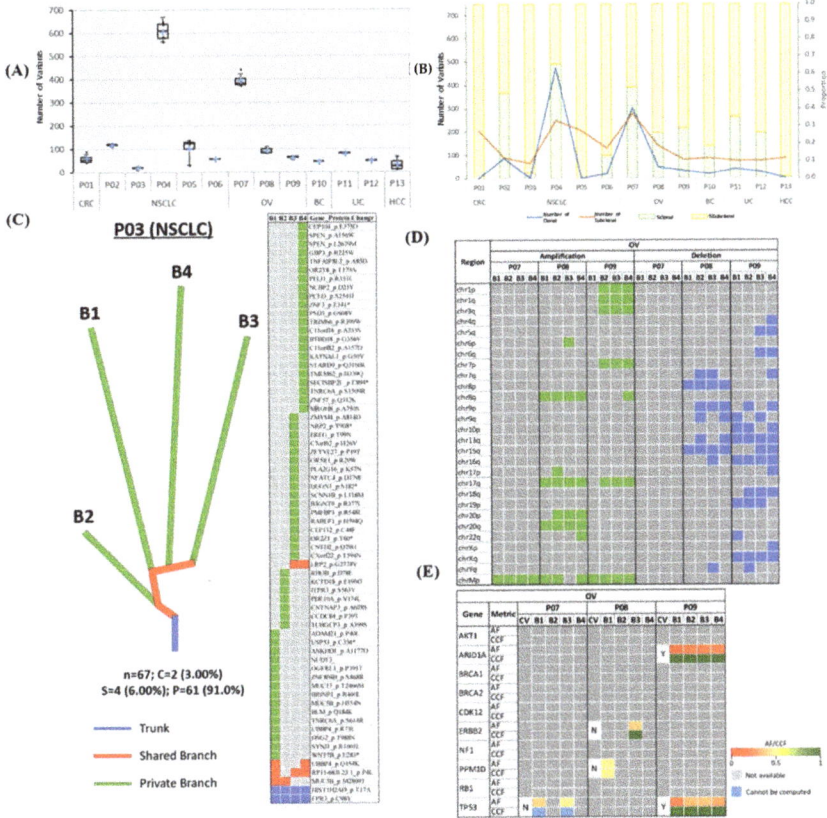

Figure 2. Mutational landscape of patients across six cancer types. (**A**) Boxplot illustrating nssML. A cross (+) represents the mean value of the data. (**B**) Line chart and stacked bar chart representing the number and proportion of truncal/branch variants, respectively. (**C**) Representative phylogenetic tree and mutation heatmap for patient P03. Trunk, branch and private branches of the tree signify mutations that occur in all, in some but not all, and only one MRTB sample(s) resected from the patient, respectively. Heatmap demonstrates the presence (green: private; red: branch; blue: trunk) or absence (gray) of NSS mutations in each MRTB sample. Bx denotes an MRTB sample with identification number x. The total number of NSS, truncal (percentage), branch (percentage), and private (percentage) mutations are denoted by 'n', 'C', 'S', and 'P', respectively. (**D**) Heatmap illustrating the presence and absence (gray) of CNAs for patients with OV. Large-scale amplifications and deletions are represented with areas filled with green and blue, respectively. (**E**) ssCDMs for OC and their associated AF and CCF. CV: clonal (truncal) variant; Y: yes; N: no; AF: allele frequency; CCF: cancer cell fraction.

To quantitatively corroborate the minimum number of MRTB samples required across different gene panels, statistical saturation analysis was conducted. Results (Figure S6) indicate that every additional MRTB sample analyzed increases the ability to detect unique variants when WES non-synonymous somatic, TruSight®and FoundationOne™ gene panels were used; as for CGC and AmpliSeq™ gene panels, at least two or three MRTB samples (depending on the panel used) were required, respectively, before changes in the number of unique variants became statistically not significant. To identify PTVs, results (Figure 3A) suggest that at least two MRTB samples were required for the CGC, AmpliSeq™ and TruSight®gene panels, and three samples were required for the FoundationOne gene panel; the WES NSS gene panel, on other hand, required four or more MRTB samples based on our analysis. In addition, the positive predictive value (PPV) was determined to evaluate the extent to which truncal variants (defined using four MRTB samples as the baseline reference) can be identified among all variants found in a set of less than four MRTB samples. Results (Figure 3B) indicate that four (or more) and two MRTB samples are needed for WES NSS and FoundationOne™ gene panels, respectively, while CGC, AmpliSeq™ and TruSight®cancer gene panels only require a single biopsy sample. The greatest significant increase in PPV based on WES NSS and FoundationOne panels were from one analyzed sample to two samples (Figure 3B).

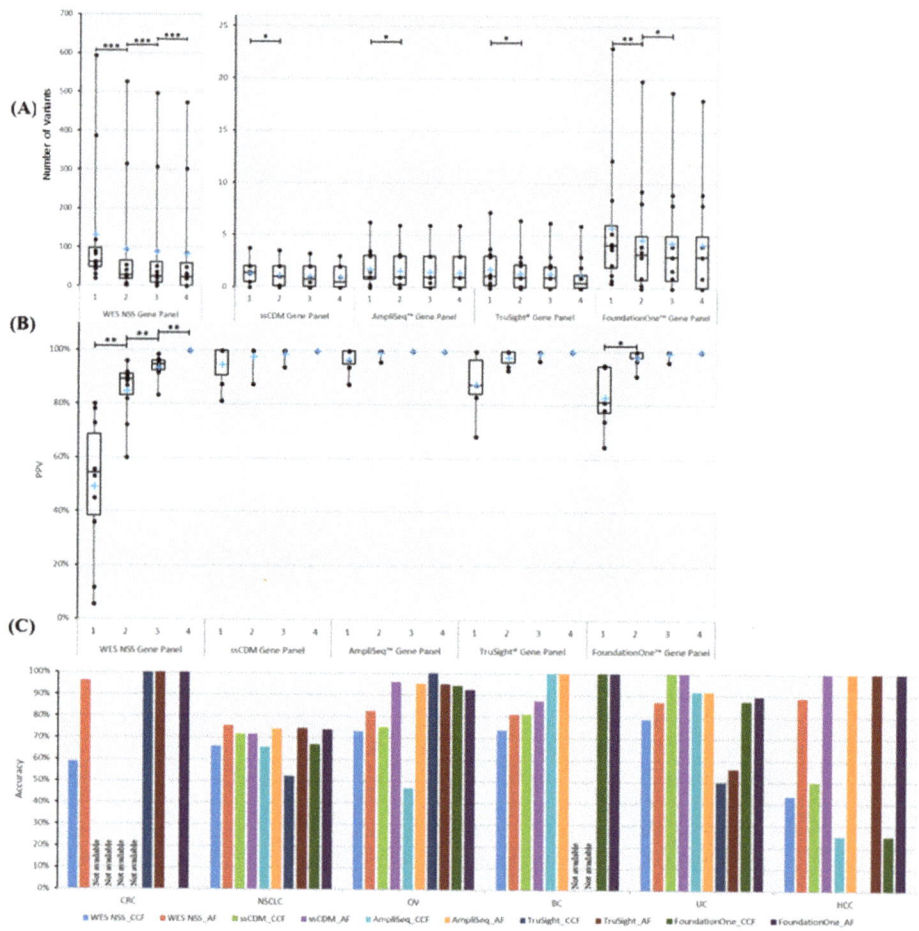

Figure 3. Number, PPV and in silico prediction accuracy of truncal variants across different gene panels. Five gene panels were scrutinized, namely WES NSS, CGC, AmpliSeq™, TruSight®and FoundationOne™ cancer gene panels. (**A**) Boxplot illustrating the number of PTVs across different numbers of MRTB samples analyzed concurrently. (**B**) PPV of PTVs in relation to the number of MRTB samples interrogated simultaneously. (**C**) Best average prediction accuracy of PTVs across different cancer types. Two types of thresholds were used to classify variants into either truncal or branch, namely AF and CCF. Based on the respective threshold, the best average prediction accuracy achievable (within the defined search domain) among all patients with the same cancer type (across different gene panels) is portrayed above. A single asterisk (*) denotes $p < 0.05$, double asterisks (**) signify $p < 0.01$, while triple asterisks (***) indicate $p < 0.001$. A cross (+) represents the mean value of the data. 'Not available' signifies that no variants that are associated with the specific gene panel were found.

2.4. Prediction of Truncal Mutations

To evaluate the ability to identify truncal variants (defined based on four MRTB samples) using a single biopsy sample, two metrics were used as classification thresholds, namely allele frequency (AF) and cancer cell fraction (CCF). Computation of CCF values—the proportion of cancer cells within which the variant is present—for patient P07 (OV) was unable to be performed due to inadequate information related to somatic copy number alteration. Hence, patient P07 was excluded for the purpose of this analysis.

First, the threshold value (for each respective metric) that produces the best average prediction accuracy across all patients was examined. Results, as illustrated in Figure S7, suggest that AF generally outperformed CCF across different patients. Average prediction accuracy improved between 2.7% and 15.3% (across different gene panels) when AF was used as the classification threshold. However, statistical significance of difference was achieved for the WES NSS gene panel only ($p = 0.021$).

Next, the threshold value (for each respective metric) that produces the best average prediction accuracy across patients with the same cancer type was scrutinized. Results, as demonstrated in Figure 3C, show that AF outperformed CCF by 15.6% to 30.4% across the different gene panels, with the FoundationOne™ cancer gene panel having the largest difference. Statistical significance of difference was achieved for the WES NSS gene panel only ($p = 0.031$).

2.5. Clinical Therapeutic Intervention

Three (23.1%) patients (P06, P10, and P11) received an inhibitor targeting an actionable truncal mutation based on molecular profiling while another six (46.2%) patients were treated with non-actionable truncal mutation-directed therapy either because they did not have any actionable truncal mutations or there was no available therapy to target the actionable truncal mutation at our center (Table 1). An illustrative example of the patients' mutational profile can be found in Figures S8 and S9.

Table 1. Clinical details of patients who received therapy targeting their actionable truncal mutation.

Cancer Type	Patient	Age	Sex	No. of MRTB Samples with Abnormality of Interest	No. of MRTB Samples that CCF Metric Classified as Clonal	Targeted Abnormality	Therapeutic Intervention	PFS (Months)			Radiological RECIST (v1.1) Response
								Initial Therapy	Actionable Truncal Mutation-Directed Therapy	PFS Ratio	
NSCLC	P06	74	M	4/4	3/4	EGFR T790M	T790M inhibitor	2.5	25.5	10.2	PR
NSCLC	P05	43	M	3/4	NA	EGFR T790M	T790M inhibitor	2.1	3.6	1.71	SD
BC	P10	41	F	4/4	4/4	PIK3CA H1047R	PI3Kα/β inhibitor	2	1.9	0.95	PD
UC	P11	46	F	2/2	2/2	AKT1 E17K	pan-AKT inhibitor	4	6.1	1.53	SD

M: male; F: female; SD: stable disease; PR: partial response; PD: progressive disease (based on RECIST v1.1); PFS: progression free survival. RECIST: Response evaluation criteria in solid tumors; EGFR: Epidermal growth factor receptor; PIK3CA: phosphoinositide-3-kinase catalytic alpha polypeptide; AKT: RAC-alpha serine/threonine-protein kinase.

Using each patient as his/her own control as a strategy to attenuate confounding factors resulting from the diverse patient population and tumor types, we assessed the clinical efficacy of actionable truncal mutation-directed therapy by comparing progression free survival (PFS) on actionable truncal mutation-directed therapy (PFS-actionable truncal mutation-directed therapy) or non-actionable truncal mutation-directed therapy with the PFS for the most recent prior therapy (PFS-A) in each of these patients [14]. Two NSCLC patients harboring an Epidermal growth factor receptor (EGFR)_T790M mutation were treated with a single agent EGFR_T790M specific tyrosine kinase inhibitor [15] with differing clinical outcomes. Patient P06 had a truncal EGFR_T790M mutation while patient P05 had an EGFR_T790M mutation as a branch mutation. Patient P06 had a partial response and was still on active treatment at last review with a PFS of >25 months (Figure S10a), while patient P05 developed worsening neuro-cognitive defects resulting in cessation of treatment after two months. The PFS ratio for patients P05 and P06 was 0.06 and 10.2, respectively.

Patient P10 with breast cancer and a phosphoinositide-3-kinase catalytic alpha polypeptide (PIK3CA)_H1047R truncal mutation was enrolled into a highly selective PI3Kα/β inhibitor phase 1 (dose escalation) trial [16], but progressed shortly after with a PFS of 1.9 months and PFS ratio of 0.95 despite deriving symptomatic benefit while on the trial. Lastly, patient P11 with uterine carcinoma harbored a truncal RAC-alpha serine/threonine-protein kinase (AKT1) E17K mutation in two out of two of her MRTB cores analyzed (only two of four cores had DNA of sufficient quality for analysis in her case). She had significant sacral bone pain from bone metastasis and received a pan-AKT inhibitor. Strikingly, her pain significantly improved and subsequent scans revealed a 21% reduction in the sum of target lesions with a PFS of 6.1 months (Figure S10b). When compared to the PFS from her most recent physician's choice therapy, a PFS ratio of 1.5 was observed.

It is noteworthy that the CCF metric performed relatively well in predicting the truncal status of the variants targeted. The median PFS-actionable truncal mutation-directed therapy for the small number of patients treated with actionable truncal mutation-directed therapy was 6.1 months, with a median PFS ratio of 1.5. These findings do suggest that the truncal status of tumors influences response and, if validated, could potentially be used in personalized cancer treatment to help prioritize therapeutic strategies.

3. Discussion

ITH represents a significant challenge to precision medicine and contributes to drug resistance. Several studies employing multi-region tumor sampling from post-surgical samples have greatly increased our understanding of tumor evolution and highlighted the importance of tumor sampling from spatially distinct areas in order to avoid erroneous interpretation of genomic data from single sampling bias [8–10]. In clinical practice, however, a systematic regional analysis of resected tumor specimens is unfeasible in the majority of patients with metastatic or recurrent cancer who may only have limited accessible intracorporeal tissue for sampling/biopsy. Hence, high quality patient samples across six major cancer types were analyzed to address certain exigent issues related to ITH and devise a potential novel solution to tackling the complexities of tumor heterogeneity when confronted with the reality of treatment decision-making based on limited access to tumor tissue.

Results in our small cohort demonstrate a high degree of ITH (>65% branch mutations) across the majority of patients, with private mutations dominating the mutational landscape. Clearly, this indicates that ITH is a ubiquitous issue that would confound the ability to identify bona fide truncal variants. Statistical saturation analysis demonstrates that for small targeted cancer gene panels like CGC, AmpliSeq™ and TruSight®, a minimum of two MRTB samples are required to identify PTVs; for a larger cancer gene panel like FoundationOne™, at least three MRTB samples are needed. The determination of the minimum number of MRTB samples required is highly valuable as it enables clinicians to find the equilibrium between cost and accuracy (of identifying bona fide truncal variants), and allows the choice of which cancer gene panel to use with the amount of tumor tissue available.

Examination of the nssML of each patient indicates that individual intratumor biopsy samples comprise a similar amount of NSS variants (Figure 2A) while the aggregated nssML shows that every additional MRTB sample would offer a statistically significant increment in the total number of NSS variants (Figure S6). Correlation analysis indicates a strong correlation between the average number of NSS variants among individual intratumor biopsy samples and aggregated NSS variants across all four MRTB samples (Pearson's rho = 0.975, $p < 0.001$). This suggests minimal intratumoral variation in the ML based on our series and that mutational burden is less likely to be impaired by sampling bias.

Given the coveted utopia of making informed clinical decisions based on a single biopsy sample, in silico methods for predicting truncal variants are of particular interest. AF and CCF are two favored metrics commonly used. Empirical experiments indicate that when AF was used as the threshold to classify truncal variants, it achieved comparable, if not better, accuracy compared to CCF; although both approaches were less compelling for some cancer types. Of note, different cancer types (at the whole-exome level) favor different threshold values for segregating truncal from branch variants, suggesting that each tumor type exhibits distinct biological characteristics that require dedicated data analytics.

Improved clinical outcomes were observed in two out of three patients whose truncal mutations were selectively targeted. Remarkably, all patients in our series treated with actionable truncal mutation-directed therapy derived symptomatic benefit with improvement in their performance status. The small patient numbers across a diverse spectrum of tumors limits our ability to draw significant conclusions within each tumor type, but nonetheless demonstrates its applicability in a variety of tumor types and preliminary evidence of clinical benefit when used for therapeutic prioritization in selected patients. It is noteworthy that patient P05—who had an EGFR_T790M branch mutation that was targeted—did not respond well to the treatment (Table 1). This reaffirms the hypothesis that increased therapeutic efficacy can be achieved by targeting truncal mutations within a tumor, and that targeting branch mutations may result in only partial treatment efficacy and/or accelerated growth in non-targeted subpopulations [17]. Undeniably, the cost per patient of this approach is high; it has been estimated at USD$5000 per patient for the acquisition of biopsy samples and profiling of four biopsy core samples as well as a germline control, but this is likely to be mitigated in the future as next generation sequencing technologies become more widely used and cost of sequencing gradually decreases. Crucially, the data provided by multi-region sequencing of a tumor could have important implications for the prioritization of druggable targets in the clinical setting. To the best of our knowledge, this is the first study assessing the feasibility and utility of obtaining tissue biopsies from multiple spatially separated regions from a single metastatic site percutaneously. A limitation of this study is the small sample size. Nevertheless, it provides adequate resolution into the complexity and management of ITH. In addition, the ITH analysis performed in this study is based on the construction of phylogenetic trees with the implicit assumption that a tumor sample can be meaningfully summarized as the collection of mutations observed in that sample, or that only a single or dominant clone exists per sample that carries all mutations, which could lead to biased inferences.

In our study, we only analyzed single nucleotide variants (SNV) which may potentially underestimate the frequency of clinically actionable mutations and the mutational load of the tumor. We focused solely on SNV mainly because they make up the majority of pathogenic variants relevant in solid tumor malignancies (59.39%) compared to other genomic alterations such as indels, structural variants and copy number loss [18]. Indeed, the majority of annotated variants in oncogenic and actionable target databases such as OncoKB and cancer hotspots consist of predominantly SNV. In addition, the majority of approved targeted inhibitors available for solid cancers currently are also mainly directed at aberrations associated with SNV. As our results relied entirely on WES analysis, and so one of the limitations of our study is the dependence on the size of the panel testing. As the number of variants being considered increases, so does the required number of samples. Our study also used fresh frozen tissue for WES analysis, which resulted in 13 of the 81 samples collected failing quality assurance due to degradation of DNA. As we continue to expand our taxonomy of tumors and seek to enhance the applicability of this approach in clinical practice, it would be ideal to optimize this approach for the clinical grade analysis of formalin-fixed, paraffin-embedded tumor samples, to enable histological and immunohistochemical analyses of samples to be performed in parallel with genomic analysis in the future. It has been suggested that liquid biopsies based on genomic analyses of circulating cell-free tumor DNA (ctDNA) and circulating tumor cells (CTC) may obviate the need for tumor biopsies [19]. Liquid biopsy platforms offer the potential for real-time sampling and resampling of tumor material for monitoring of therapeutic efficacy [20] and early detection of resistance subclones [21]. Furthermore, the MRTB approach we have used in this study will not be feasible in patients with inaccessible lesions. However, the inability to characterize liquid biopsies histologically limits the extent of biomarker analyses, particularly where tumor microenvironmental features (e.g., programme cell death-1/programme cell death ligand-1(PD1/PDL1) protein expression), immune cell infiltrates and stromal content are concerned. Further studies comparing the clinical utility of multi-spatial or multi-lesional biopsy approaches with that of liquid biopsies in monitoring the emergence of resistance and therapeutic efficacy are eagerly awaited

4. Materials and Methods

4.1. Patients and Specimens Collection

All patients were recruited and treated at the National University Cancer Institute (NCIS), Singapore, between December 2014 and May 2016. WES and data analytics were performed at the National University of Singapore (NUS), Singapore. All procedures were conducted in accordance with the approved protocols and written informed consent was provided by the patients (File S1). Eligible patients were at least 21 years of age, had a histological or cytological diagnosis of advanced or metastatic solid malignancy and had recurrent disease for which tissue biopsy was indicated as part of routine clinical practice. This study was approved by the National Health Group Domain Specific Review Board IRB number 2014/00665

Each patient had 5 tumor biopsy samples obtained from one metastatic lesion using a single-pass radiologically-guided percutaneous biopsy technique. This technique involves the insertion of a coaxial needle together with its trocar into a lesion. The trocar is subsequently removed to allow for the introduction of a biopsy device that is composed of a needle with a 1.5 cm throw to facilitate multiple passes along acute angles from a single lesion via a single percutaneous access. Each biopsy sample was obtained at least 2 mm apart. One biopsy core was sent to the histopathology lab as part of routine clinical management while the remaining four tumor biopsy samples were analyzed using WES. Four patients had biopsies obtained from the lung (P3, P4, P5 and P6), four had peritoneal nodes biopsied (P1, P7, P8 and P9), three patients underwent a liver biopsy (P10, P11 and P12) and one patient each had a bone (P13) and supraclavicular lymph node (P2) biopsied. Germline samples were collected from each patient in the form of a buccal swab. If the germline sample failed quantitative QC, whole blood would be used as replacement. Samples with DNA concentration <4 ng/μL would be deemed to have failed QC. Radiological images were obtained as part of clinical care.

4.2. Whole-Exome Sequencing

Extraction of genomic DNA from tumor samples was carried out using the Qiagen Allprep DNA/RNA Micro Kit (Qiagen, Hilden, Germany). The MasterAmp Buccal Swab Kit (Epicenter, Madison, WI, USA) was used to extract DNA from buccal swab samples while the Qiagen EZ1 DNA Blood 350 μL Kit (Qiagen, Hilden, Germany) was used to process whole blood samples. An Illumina NextSeq 500 Sequencing System (Illumina, San Diego, CA, USA) was utilized to perform 150 base pair paired-end WES. All experiments were conducted in accordance to manufacturer guidelines at the Cancer Science Institute of Singapore, NUS. Full patient data can be found in the National Centre for Biotechnology Information (NCBI) Sequence Read Archive (SRA) under accession number SRP137039

4.3. Sequencing Reads Alignment and Somatic Variant Detection

Sequence reads were aligned to the hg19 reference genome using the Burrows–Wheeler Aligner (BWA) v0.7.7 [22] and realignment to the hg19 reference genome was performed by using the Genome Analysis ToolKit (GATK) v3.3.0 [23]. Variant calling was performed with duplication removal and base recalibration prior to variant calling using MuTect somatic variant caller v1.1.7 [24] and annotated using Oncotator v1.8.0.0 [25]. Only NSS variants were filtered out for analysis independent of CCF or AF. All sequencing data have been made available in the NCBI Sequence Read Archive (SRA) under accession number SRP137039.

4.4. Copy Number Alterations

Somatic CNAs were detected using several algorithms. Succinctly, the computation of raw copy number calls and the adjustment of GC content of the raw copy number calls were performed using VarScan2 v2.3.9 [26]. Re-centering and segmentation of the adjusted copy number calls were conducted using DNAcopy v1.44.0 [27]. Sample purity was assessed using the ABSOLUTE algorithm (Appendix A, Table A1).

4.5. Cancer Gene Panels

Five gene panels—WES NSS, COSMIC Cancer Gene Census (CGC), the Ion AmpliSeq™ Cancer Hotspot Panel v2, the TruSight®Cancer panel and the FoundationOne™ cancer gene panel—were examined. The WES NSS gene panel comprises of all protein-coding genes (with NSS property) in the genome, while the CGC gene panel consists of all statistically significant cancer-specific genes curated from the COSMIC Cancer Gene Census (CGC) [28,29] and The Cancer Genome Atlas (TCGA) [30,31]. The complete list of CGC interrogated genes for CRC ($n = 29$), NSCLC ($n = 30$), OV ($n = 10$), BC ($n = 52$), EC ($n = 58$), and HCC ($n = 26$) is available in Figures S3 and S4. Commercial cancer gene panels like AmpliSeq™, TruSight®and FoundationOne™ are comprised of 50, 94, and 315 cancer-related genes, respectively; their interrogated gene lists are available at ThermoFisher [32], Illumina [33], and Foundation Medicine [34], respectively.

All NSS variants identified in the WES NSS gene panel were subsequently juxtaposed with individual targeted cancer gene panels (i.e., CGC, AmpliSeq™, TruSight®and FoundationOne™) and variants from mismatched genes were winnowed out. The resulting list of variants for each cancer gene panel was used for subsequent downstream analysis.

4.6. Construction of Phylogenetic Trees

The construction of phylogenetic trees was carried out based on a binary table that represents the presence or absence of variants across all MRTB samples. Using the PHYLogeny Inference Package v3.695 (PHYLIP) [35] and matched germline information as the outgroup root, discrete character parsimony was used to generate the topology of the phylogenetic trees. Based on the computed mutation counts, the length of the trunk, shared and private branches were drawn accordingly.

4.7. Statistical Saturation Analysis

The computation of the average number of unique variants present when 'k' number of MRTB samples were analyzed concurrently was performed based on the following Formula (1):

$$Average\ unique\ variants_k = \frac{1}{n}\sum_{i=1}^{n} x_i, \quad (1)$$

where 'n' denotes the number of permutation combinations available when 'k' number of MRTB samples were selected from 4 MRTB samples, and 'x_i' refers to the number of variants that are present in at least one of the MRTB samples examined in combination set 'i'. Similarly, the average number of PTVs was calculated based on the formula above but with 'x_i' defined as the number of variants present in all MRTB samples scrutinized in combination set 'i'.

PPV, on other hand, was computed based on the following Formula (2):

$$Average\ PPV_k = \frac{1}{n}\sum_{i=1}^{n}\frac{C}{PCV_{i,k}}, \qquad (2)$$

where 'n' denotes the number of permutation combinations available when 'k' number of MRTB samples were selected from 4 MRTB samples, 'C' represents the number of variants that occur in all 4 MRTB samples, and '$PTV_{i,k}$' (i.e., putative truncal variant) refers to the number of variants present in all 'k' number of MRTB samples examined simultaneously in combination set 'i'.

All statistical hypothesis tests were conducted using the Wilcoxon signed rank test unless otherwise stated. Statistical significance is considered when the p-value is less than 0.05.

4.8. Cancer Cell Fraction and Allele Frequency

The CCF value was estimated using the ABSOLUTE algorithm [13] for each somatic single nucleotide variant (SNV) site based on its AF, CNAs, ploidy and purity of the tumor tissue analyzed. Based on the computed CCF values, a range of thresholds—from 0.90 to 1.00 incremented at a step size of 0.01—were used to classify variants into either truncal or branch.

AF was calculated by dividing the number of alternative sequence read counts with the total number of (alternative and reference) sequence read counts. Likewise, the clonality of variants was determined by comparing the variant's AF with a range of thresholds (from 0.01 to 0.55 incremented at a step size of 0.01). The respective thresholds used for both the cancer cell fraction and allele frequency analysis according to the individual panels are shown in Table 2 below:

Table 2. Thresholds used to determine the clonality of the variants.

Panel	CCF	AF
FoundationOne	0.92	0.13
AmpliSeq	0.92	0.15
TruSight	0.96	0.13
WES	1	0.16

4.9. Prediction of Truncal Mutations

To stratify variants into either truncal or branch based on a single biopsy sample, different (AF and CCF) threshold values were investigated. For each threshold value examined, the following formula was employed to compute the average classification accuracy, by which 4 MRTB samples were used as the baseline reference for defining bona fide truncal variants (3).

$$Average\ Accuracy_k = \frac{1}{4}\sum_{i=1}^{4}\frac{x_{i,k}}{y_i}, \qquad (3)$$

where 'k' denotes the examined threshold value, '$x_{i,k}$' represents the number of correct classification made for biopsy sample 'i' using threshold value 'k', and 'y_i' refers to the total number of variants assessed for biopsy sample 'i'.

4.10. Assessing Targeted Therapy Outcomes

Treatment decisions were made using molecular profiling results from one core biopsy, as reported in the Intergrated Molecular Analysis of Cancer (IMAC) study [14] while the remaining four core biopsies were analyzed for this study. Using each patient as his/her own control as a strategy to attenuate confounding factors resulting from the diverse patient population and tumor types, we assessed the clinical efficacy of actionable truncal mutation-directed therapy by comparing the PFS for each patient who received actionable truncal mutation-directed therapy (PFS-actionable truncal mutation-directed therapy) with the PFS for the therapy immediately before actionable truncal mutation-directed therapy (PFS-A) [36]. If the PFS of PFS-actionable truncal mutation-directed therapy/PFS-A ratio was ≥1.3, then the molecular profiling-selected actionable truncal mutation-directed therapy was defined as having benefit for the patient compared to the physician's choice chemotherapy. The PFS ratio was defined as $\frac{\text{PFS–actionable truncal mutation–directed therapy}}{\text{PFS for the therapy immediately before actionable truncal mutation–directed therapy (PFS–A)}}$ and was used to evaluate the efficiency of the therapeutic intervention [36].

5. Conclusions

In conclusion, this study has demonstrated: (i) the importance of performing multiple biopsies despite extant in silico prediction methods, (ii) the minimum number of MRTB samples required to alleviate challenges related to ITH is dependent on the tested hypothesis and the examined gene panel, but that at least two biopsies should be submitted for analysis to achieve a PPV of >90% identifying AT mutations, and (iii) the feasibility and clinical efficacy of adopting the proposed approach for strategic therapeutic intervention. Further validation of this approach for identifying and targeting AT mutations in larger cohorts will be required to fully assess its potential value as a precision medicine strategy to circumvent the challenges of intratumoral heterogeneity in cancer therapy.

Supplementary Materials: The following are available online at http://www.mdpi.com/2072-6694/12/6/1599/s1, Figure S1: Phylogenetic trees constructed from NSS mutations, Figure S2: Heatmap visualization illustrating the presence/absence of copy number alterations in relation to each region, Figure S3: ssCDMs for CRC, NSCLC, and OV, Figure S4: ssCDMs for BC, UC, and HCC, Figure S5: Mutational characteristics across different number of MRTB samples and gene panels, Figure S6: Boxplot illustrating the average number of unique variants across different gene panels and number of MRTB samples, Figure S7: Best average prediction accuracy of PTVs across different patients, Figure S8: Illustrative example of patients P01-P06 mutational profile, Figure S9: Illustrative example of patients P07-P13 mutational profile, Figure S10: Pre - treatment and 8- week post treatment images from, Table S1: Average number of unique variants detected across different number of MRTB samples and gene panels, Table S2: Average number of PTVs detected across different number of MRTB samples and gene panels, File S1: Study Protocol.

Author Contributions: Conceptualization, D.S.P.T., R.S. and A.G.; methodology, A.G., R.S., M.F.M.O. and D.S.P.T.; software, D.T., V.H., T.Z.T. and S.E.G.; validation, D.T., T.Z.T. and S.E.G.; formal analysis, D.T., V.H., T.Z.T., S.E.G., A.G., R.S. (Richie Soong), M.F.M.O. and D.S.P.T.; investigation, V.H., D.T., T.Z.T., S.E.G., B.W., A.G., R.S. (Richie Soong), M.F.M.O., D.S.P.T., D.L., B.P., A.W., R.S. (Ross Soo), B.C.G., S.C.L., C.E.C., W.P.Y. and S.O. resources, A.G., R.S. (Richie Soong) and D.S.P.T.; data curation, V.H., D.T., T.Z.T., S.E.G., R.S. (Richie Soong), M.F.M.O. and D.S.P.T.; writing— V.H., D.T., S.E.G., R.S. (Richie Soong) and D.S.P.T.; writing—review and editing V.H., D.T., T.Z.T. and D.S.P.T.; visualization D.S.P.T., R.S. (Richie Soong) and A.G. supervision, D.S.P.T., R.S. (Richie Soong) and A.G.; project administration V.H., D.T., T.Z.T., S.E.G., R.S. (Richie Soong), M.F.M.O. and D.S.P.T.; funding acquisition, D.S.P.T., R.S. (Richie Soong) and A.G. All authors have read and agree to the published version of the manuscript.

Funding: This study was supported by the National Medical Research Council Singapore, National Research Foundation Singapore and the Singapore Ministry of Education under its Research Centres of Excellence initiative and a Yong Loo Lin fellowship grant as well as the Singapore Ministry of Health's National Medical Research Council Clinician Scientist Award (NMRC/CSA-INV/0016/2017) to DSPT.

Conflicts of Interest: D. Tan consultancy fees from Astra Zeneca, Roche, MSD, Merck Serono, Tessa Therapeutics, Eisai and Genmab. Reasearch funding from AstraZeneca, Bayer and Karyopharm and V. Heong consult on the advisory board for Astra Zeneca and Pfizer; the sponsor had no involvement in the design and conduct of the study; collection, management, analysis and interpretation of the data; preparation, review, or approval of the manuscript; or the decision to submit the manuscript for publication.

Appendix A

Table A1. Assessment of tumor purity for each sample using ABSOLUTE algorithm. Abbrev: VAF, variant allele frequency; BRCA, breast carcinoma; CRC, colorectal carcinoma; OV, ovarian carcinoma; UCEC, uterine carcinoma; LIHC, hepatocellular carcinoma; NaN, not computable.

Sample	Patient	Patient label	Disease	ABSOLUTE call Status (Called = Clonal)	ABSOLUTE purity	ABSOLUTE ploidy	ABSOLUTE Cancer DNA Faction	ABSOLUTE Coverage for 80% Power	VAF Range-All Variants	VAF Range-Putative Truncal Variants	VAF Range-Private Variants	VAF Range-Branch Variants	Mclust-wCN Cluster#	Mclust-noCN Cluster#	VAF_ROC_AUC_Truncal VsNon Truncal	VAF Youden Threshold Truncal VsNon Truncal	VAF Youden Threshold Truncal Vs Non Truncal_Accuracy	Mclust en. threshold clusterW HighestVAF	Mclust en. threshold Truncal VsNon Truncal_Accuracy	Remark
RE3F1	RE3	P01	CRC	called	0.25	5.86	0.49	64	0.14038	NaN	0.135631915	0.2446	2	2	NaN	NaN	NaN	0.241285714	NaN	No Truncal Mutation detected
RE3F2	RE3	P01	CRC	called	0.21	1.94	0.2	52	0.134576087	NaN	0.099253968	0.152966942	1	2	NaN	NaN	NaN	0.1086	NaN	No Truncal Mutation detected
RE3F3	RE3	P01	CRC	called	0.28	4.02	0.44	49	0.146170833	NaN	0.143824176	0.2004	2	2	NaN	NaN	NaN	0.348666667	NaN	No Truncal Mutation detected
RE3F4	RE3	P01	CRC	high non-clonal	1	2.06	1	8	0.383224409	NaN	0.301089313	0.467715447	2	2	NaN	NaN	NaN	0.447333333	NaN	No Truncal Mutation detected
RE4F1	RE4	P02	LUNG	called	0.39	3.83	0.55	36	0.183591928	0.191490909	0.163944444	0.1565	2	2	0.675130617	0.076	62.27795193	0.419666667	50.49111808	—
RE4F2	RE4	P02	LUNG	called	0.5	3.81	0.65	29	0.205012195	0.226848485	0.145166667	0.177076923	2	2	0.688477366	0.091	68.24913825	0.2135	57.35129068	—
RE4F3	RE4	P02	LUNG	called	0.22	5.43	0.43	68	0.176941909	0.192266667	0.123045455	0.17203125	1	3	0.686582137	0.089	68.12599681	0.20675	56.2830941	—
RE4F4	RE4	P02	LUNG	called	0.42	3.85	0.38	34	0.180034043	0.194039394	0.1438125	0.149815789	2	2	0.714545455	0.096	67.70562771	0.5995	49.89177489	—
RE6F1	RE6	P03	LUNG	called	0.2	4.03	0.33	66	0.106431818	0.156	0.085482759	0.1505	0	2	0.699375	0.364	50	0.173	68.75	Only 2 Truncal Mutations detected
RE6F2	RE6	P03	LUNG	called	0.16	1.96	0.16	66	0.106794118	0.12125	0.102037037	0.130333333	0	3	0.575	0.5	50	0.1345	63.33333333	Only 2 Truncal Mutations detected
RE6F3	RE6	P03	LUNG	called	0.23	2.12	0.24	47	0.105985366	0.236	0.0839	0.124	0	2	0.692567568	0.524	62.5	0.327333333	73.64864865	Only 2 Truncal Mutations detected
RE6F4	RE6	P03	LUNG	called	0.16	1.07	0.09	61	0.106481481	0.21825	0.079666667	0.191375	1	2	0.7325	0.52	50	0.072	60.5	Only 2 Truncal Mutations detected
RE8F1	RE8	P04	LUNG	called	0.32	4.21	0.49	46	0.222009821	0.225307027	0.210836364	0.204115108	2	2	0.589963247	0.052	50.40747256	0.296918919	53.80586048	—
RE8F2	RE8	P04	LUNG	high non-clonal	0.58	4.34	0.75	28	0.29151633	0.316179459	0.201833333	0.234288194	2	3	0.655037957	0.084	55.15448764	0.5657333333	54.26539677	—
RE8F3	RE8	P04	LUNG	high entropy called	0.46	4.39	0.65	35	0.255151779	0.275265946	0.156716418	0.210709599	3	4	0.68003466	0.083	53.60034914	0.3599683051	57.10528998	—
RE8F4	RE8	P04	LUNG	called	0.27	3.33	0.38	47	0.192184165	0.198313514	0.113367419	0.187166667	3	4	0.619140554	0.049	50.58159754	0.332263636	51.06664348	—
RE9F1	RE9	P05	LUNG	called	0.22	3.87	0.36	98	0.152	0.408	0.117938776	0.157363095	1	3	NaN	NaN	NaN	0.117214286	NaN	No Truncal Mutation detected
RE9F2	RE9	P05	LUNG	called	0.31	5.63	0.56	55	0.229921642	0.414333333	0.141388235	0.268655556	2	3	NaN	NaN	NaN	0.416	NaN	No Truncal Mutation detected
RE9F3	RE9	P05	LUNG	called	0.25	3.94	0.4	53	0.12454386	0.407	0.111263306	0.0852	2	2	NaN	NaN	NaN	0.08	NaN	No Truncal Mutation detected
RE9F4	RE9	P05	LUNG	called	0.3	4.85	0.51	51	0.156135739	0.408833333	0.112022222	0.162778378	1	2	NaN	NaN	NaN	0.1255	NaN	No Truncal Mutation detected
RE10F1	RE10	P06	LUNG	called	0.35	6.42	0.63	55	0.233989474	0.420242424	0.186076923	0.2807	2	4	0.9335	0.2235	89.71	0.4315	71.11	—
RE10F2	RE10	P06	LUNG	called	0.24	3.98	0.38	56	0.15439216	0.229876786	0.117741985	0.126333333	2	2	0.8384787	0.167	88.57	0.193142857	72.99	—
RE10F3	RE10	P06	LUNG	called	0.26	5.3	0.48	60	0.2057619195	0.402121212	0.103966516	0.1735	2	2	0.962121212	0.311	88.13131313	0.326714286	82.07070707	—
RE10F4	RE10	P06	LUNG	called	0.35	4.34	0.54	43	0.203847826	0.376272727	0.08216	0.247666667	2	2	0.942218798	0.273	91.88495121	0.332857143	76.91319979	—

Table A1. Cont.

Sample	Patient	Patient label	Disease	ABSOLUTE call Status (Called = Clonal)	ABSOLUTE _purity	ABSOLUTE _ploidy	ABSOLUTE Cancer DNA Faction	ABSOLUTE Coverage for 80% Power	VAF Range-All Variants	VAF Range-Putative Truncal Variants	VAF Range-Private Variants	VAF Range-Branch Variants	McLust.nCN Cluster#	McLust. noCN. Cluster#	VAF_ROC AUC Truncal VsNon Truncal	VAF Youden Threshold VsNon Truncal	VAF Youden Threshold Truncal VsNon Truncal_Accuracy	Mclust.cn. threshold clusterW HighestVAF	Mclust.cn. threshold_Truncal VsNon Truncal_Accuracy	Remark
RE5F1	RE5	P07	OV	non-aneuploid	NaN	NaN	NaN	NaN	0.341515366	0.456792381	0.119782946	0.288920635	4	3	0.953009939	0.278	93.77748109	0.547	55.3600356	–
RE5F2	RE5	P07	OV	non-aneuploid	NaN	NaN	NaN	NaN	0.351859281	0.38549743	0.176089109	0.354071429	3	3	0.767505628	0.188	76.35164835	0.364184211	67.12687213	–
RE5F3	RE5	P07	OV	non-aneuploid	NaN	NaN	NaN	NaN	0.372459689	0.42759619	0.138438895	0.3154951	3	3	0.859644689	0.258	82.34065934	0.378807692	79.35531136	–
RE5F4	RE5	P07	OV	non-aneuploid	NaN	NaN	NaN	NaN	0.391212257	0.431544762	0.17428125	0.3839375	6	3	0.81883254	0.28	78.18085956	0.424096774	68.52380952	–
RE1F1	RE11	P08	OV	called	0.27	3.6	0.4	48	0.182677632	0.214707071	0.109380952	0.174272727	2	3	0.825995807	0.093	80.05526968	0.458	53.09700781	–
RE1F2	RE11	P08	OV	called	0.25	3.02	0.34	48	0.222996988	0.227321211	0.119104167	0.206105263	2	3	0.80830695	0.122	79.69924921	0.383	57.59837178	–
RE1F3	RE11	P08	OV	called	0.25	5.06	0.46	59	0.219164894	0.279626263	0.13537134	0.202272727	4	3	0.806037907	0.123	79.04891613	0.15175	77.1422086	–
RE1F4	RE11	P08	OV	called	0.22	4.74	0.4	65	0.225337079	0.294050505	0.11910167	0.220416667	1	3	0.857424882	0.138	80.39253292	0.2655	67.40825981	–
RE1F1	RE13	P09	OV	called	0.47	5.47	0.71	41	0.196666667	0.242578125	0.126136364	0.215	1	3	0.783166274	0.229	78.19870283	0.370333333	55.76566132	–
RE1F2	RE13	P09	OV	called	0.32	5.19	0.55	50	0.254631944	0.317359375	0.103151515	0.275674468	1	3	0.741113281	0.229	71.875	0.294411765	66.40625	–
RE1F3	RE13	P09	OV	called	0.31	5.3	0.55	52	0.267333333	0.34478125	0.112880952	0.29809617	1	3	0.73851826	0.172	72.05933989	0.222090909	64.9315309	–
RE1F4	RE13	P09	OV	called	0.33	5.21	0.57	49	0.29585799	0.356515625	0.17261905	0.267886364	1	3	0.7055288462	0.145	69.19471154	0.229583333	64.42307692	–
RE7F1	RE7	P10	BRCA	called	0.82	2.3	0.84	11	0.31790099	0.44826087	0.1773125	0.425285714	3	2	0.852806324	0.289	82.74703557	0.325	79.48616601	–
RE7F2	RE7	P10	BRCA	called	0.78	2.32	0.81	12	0.3082	0.422347826	0.133810811	0.485857143	2	2	0.863142292	0.304	86.56126482	0.2225	83.05339668	–
RE7F3	RE7	P10	BRCA	called	0.29	5.98	0.55	59	0.311952584	0.433630435	0.1119375	0.385818182	1	2	0.861223458	0.3	89.76238625	0.269	86.27401416	–
RE7F4	RE7	P10	BRCA	called	0.22	3.61	0.33	59	0.19171134	0.257972261	0.143681818	0.18957142	1	2	0.8056265598	0.132	83.0150424	0.113666667	81.15942029	–
RE12F1	RE12	P11	UCEC	high non-clonal	0.63	2.24	0.66	14	0.221503448	*0.13232666 6666667	0.112514286	0.18957142	2	2	0.903142857	0.164	88.28571429	0.31075	73.85714286	–
RE12F1	RE12	P11	UCEC	called	0.66	4.45	0.81	26	0.267685185	*0.4072	0.1473793	NaN	3	3	0.863984674	0.194	82.99770115	0.9165	52.2972973	–
RE14F1	RE14	P12	UCEC	called	0.2	4.62	0.37	68	0.217402299	0.27652	0.110096774	0.279166667	4	3	0.885135135	0.121	86.83783784	0.518	51.94945595	–
RE14F2	RE14	P12	UCEC	called	0.26	5.79	0.51	62	0.254321839	0.30418	0.1312	0.303083333	2	3	0.817567568	0.178	82.83783784	0.5225	60.65217391	–
RE14F3	RE14	P12	UCEC	called	0.23	4.9	0.43	62	0.295	0.4168	0.101848485	0.3215	2	3	0.882173913	0.174	85.04347826	0.4595	63.7272273	–
RE14F4	RE14	P12	UCEC	called	0.22	5.48	0.44	68	0.295621277	0.423	0.110857143	0.305444444	1	3	0.888636364	0.197	88.9090909	0.495	63.7272273	–
RE15F1	RE15	P13	LIHC	called	0.43	4.05	0.61	35	0.266176	0.35	0.225596774	0.306672131	1	3	0.62601626	0.75	50	0.2527	46.54471545	Only 1 Truncal Mutation detected
RE15F2	RE15	P13	LIHC	called	0.23	1.96	0.23	46	0.179296296	0.2475	0.176842105	0.164333333	0	4	0.72	0.667	50	0.428666667	73	Only 1 Truncal Mutation detected
RE15F3	RE15	P13	LIHC	called	0.23	2.04	0.23	47	0.166075949	0.3635	0.15	0.163171875	0	0	0.948051948	1	50	NaN	NaN	Only 1 Truncal Mutation detected
RE15F4	RE15	P13	LIHC	called	0.2	3.91	0.32	66	0.1189	0.28	0.084888889	0.1479	0	0	0.946428571	0.667	50	NaN	NaN	

* data analysed based on two sample biopsies instead of four.

References

1. Jamal-Hanjani, M.; Wilson, G.A. Tracking the Evolution of Non–Small-Cell Lung Cancer. *N. Engl. J. Med.* **2017**, *376*, 2109–2121. [CrossRef] [PubMed]
2. Greaves, M. Evolutionary determinants of cancer. *Cancer Discov.* **2015**, *5*, 806–820. [CrossRef] [PubMed]
3. Burrell, R.A.; McGranahan, N. The causes and consequences of genetic heterogeneity in cancer evolution. *Nature* **2013**, *501*, 338–345. [CrossRef] [PubMed]
4. Gerlinger, M.; Rowan, A.J. Intratumor Heterogeneity and Branched Evolution Revealed by Multiregion Sequencing. *N. Engl. J. Med.* **2012**, *366*, 883–892. [CrossRef]
5. Dagogo-Jack, I.; Shaw, A.T. Tumour heterogeneity and resistance to cancer therapies. *Nat. Rev. Clin. Oncol.* **2018**, *15*, 81–94. [CrossRef]
6. Turner, N.C.; Reis-Filho, J.S. Genetic heterogeneity and cancer drug resistance. *Lancet Oncol.* **2012**, *13*, 178–185. [CrossRef]
7. Morris, L.G.T.; Riaz, N. Pan-cancer analysis of intratumor heterogeneity as a prognostic determinant of survival. *Oncotarget* **2016**, *7*, 10051–10063. [CrossRef]
8. McGranahan, N.; Swanton, C. Biological and therapeutic impact of intratumor heterogeneity in cancer evolution. *Cancer Cell* **2015**, *27*, 15–26. [CrossRef]
9. Gerlinger, M.; Horswell, S. Genomic architecture and evolution of clear cell renal cell carcinomas defined by multiregion sequencing. *Nat. Genet.* **2014**, *46*, 225–233. [CrossRef]
10. Yap, T.A.; Gerlinger, M. Intratumor heterogeneity: Seeing the wood for the trees. *Sci. Transl. Med.* **2012**, *4*, 127–137. [CrossRef]
11. Schmitt, M.W.; Loeb, L.A. The influence of subclonal resistance mutations on targeted cancer therapy. *Nat. Rev. Clin. Oncol.* **2016**, *13*, 335–347. [CrossRef] [PubMed]
12. Carter, S.L.; Cibulskis, K. Absolute quantification of somatic DNA alterations in human cancer. *Nat. Biotechnol.* **2012**, *30*, 413–421. [CrossRef] [PubMed]
13. Shi, Y.; Au, J.S.-K. A prospective, molecular epidemiology study of EGFR mutations in Asian patients with advanced non-small-cell lung cancer of adenocarcinoma histology (PIONEER). *J. Thorac. Oncol.* **2014**, *9*, 154–162. [CrossRef] [PubMed]
14. Heong, V.; Syn, N.L. Value of a molecular screening program to support clinical trial enrollment in Asian cancer patients: The Integrated Molecular Analysis of Cancer (IMAC) Study. *Int. J. Cancer* **2018**, *142*, 1890–1900. [CrossRef]
15. Wang, S.; Cang, S. Third-generation inhibitors targeting EGFR T790M mutation in advanced non-small cell lung cancer. *J. Hematol. Oncol.* **2016**, *9*, 34. [CrossRef]
16. Janku, F.; Wheler, J.J. PIK3CA mutation H1047R is associated with response to PI3K/AKT/mTOR signaling pathway inhibitors in early-phase clinical trials. *Cancer Res.* **2013**, *73*, 276–284. [CrossRef]
17. Lohr, J.G.; Stojanov, P. Widespread genetic heterogeneity in multiple myeloma: Implications for targeted therapy. *Cancer Cell* **2014**, *25*, 91–101. [CrossRef]
18. Bailey, M.H.; Tokheim, C. Comprehensive Characterization of Cancer Driver Genes and Mutations. *Cell* **2018**, *173*, 371–385.e18. [CrossRef]
19. Jovelet, C.; Ileana, E. Circulating Cell-Free Tumor DNA Analysis of 50 Genes by Next-Generation Sequencing in the Prospective MOSCATO Trial. *Clin. Cancer Res.* **2016**, *22*, 2960–2968. [CrossRef]
20. Marchetti, A.; Palma, J.F. Early Prediction of Response to Tyrosine Kinase Inhibitors by Quantification of EGFR Mutations in Plasma of NSCLC Patients. *J. Thorac. Oncol.* **2015**, *10*, 1437–1443. [CrossRef]
21. Sorensen, B.S.; Wu, L. Monitoring of epidermal growth factor receptor tyrosine kinase inhibitor-sensitizing and resistance mutations in the plasma DNA of patients with advanced non-small cell lung cancer during treatment with erlotinib. *Cancer* **2014**, *120*, 3896–3901.20. [CrossRef] [PubMed]
22. Li, H.; Durbin, R. Fast and accurate short read alignment with Burrows-Wheeler transform. *Bioinformatics* **2009**, *25*, 1754–1760. [CrossRef]
23. McKenna, A.; Hanna, M. The genome analysis toolkit: A MapReduce framework for analyzing next-generation DNA sequencing data. *Genome Res.* **2010**, *20*, 1297–1303. [CrossRef] [PubMed]
24. Cibulskis, K.; Lawrence, M.S. Sensitive detection of somatic point mutations in impure and heterogeneous cancer samples. *Nat. Biotechnol.* **2013**, *31*, 213–219. [CrossRef] [PubMed]

25. Ramos, A.H.; Lichtenstein, L. Oncotator: Cancer variant annotation tool. *Hum. Mutat.* **2015**, *36*, E2423–E2429. [CrossRef]
26. Koboldt, D.C.; Zhang, Q. VarScan 2: Somatic mutation and copy number alteration discovery in cancer by exome sequencing. *Genome Res.* **2012**, *22*, 568–576.
27. Seshan, V.E.; Olshen, A. DNAcopy: DNA copy number data analysis. R package version 1.62.0. Available online: https://bioconductor.org/biocLite.R (accessed on 14 August 2017).
28. Futreal, P.A.; Coin, L. A census of human cancer genes. *Nat. Rev. Cancer* **2004**, *4*, 177–183. [CrossRef]
29. Wellcome Sanger Institute. Cancer Gene Census. 2011. Available online: http://www.sanger.ac.uk/genetics/CGP/Census/ (accessed on 10 June 2018).
30. Lawrence, M.S.; Stojanov, P. Discovery and saturation analysis of cancer genes across 21 tumour types. *Nature* **2014**, *505*, 495–501. [CrossRef]
31. Ally, A.; Balasundaram, M. Comprehensive and Integrative Genomic Characterization of Hepatocellular Carcinoma. *Cell* **2017**, *169*, 1327–1341.e23. [CrossRef]
32. Thermo Fisher. Ion AmpliSeq Cancer Hotspot Panel v2. Available online: https://www.thermofisher.com/order/catalog/product/4475346 (accessed on 28 November 2018).
33. Illumina. TruSight®Cancer Panel. Available online: https://www.illumina.com/products/by-type/clinical-research-products/trusight-cancer.html (accessed on 26 July 2018).
34. Foundation Medicine. FoundationOneTM Cancer Gene Panel. Available online: https://www.foundationmedicine.com/genomic-testing/foundation-one (accessed on 11 August 2018).
35. Felsenstein, J. *PHYLIP (Phylogeny Inference Package) Version 3.6*; Distributed by the Author; Department of Genome Sciences, University of Washington: Seattle, WA, USA, 2005; Available online: http://evolution.genetics.washington.edu/phylip.html (accessed on 15 August 2017).
36. Von Hoff, D.D.; Stephenson, J.J. Pilot study using molecular profiling of patients' tumors to find potential targets and select treatments for their refractory cancers. *J. Clin. Oncol.* **2010**, *28*, 4877–4883. [CrossRef]

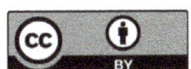

© 2020 by the authors. Licensee MDPI, Basel, Switzerland. This article is an open access article distributed under the terms and conditions of the Creative Commons Attribution (CC BY) license (http://creativecommons.org/licenses/by/4.0/).

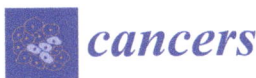

Article

Impact and Diagnostic Gaps of Comprehensive Genomic Profiling in Real-World Clinical Practice

Aditi P. Singh [1], Elaine Shum [2], Lakshmi Rajdev [3], Haiying Cheng [3], Sanjay Goel [3], Roman Perez-Soler [3] and Balazs Halmos [3],*

[1] Division of Hematology and Oncology, University of Pennsylvania/Abramson Cancer Center, Philadelphia, PA 19104, USA; aditi.singh@pennmedicine.upenn.edu
[2] Division of Medical Oncology and Hematology, NYU Langone Perlmutter Cancer Center, New York, NY 10016, USA; elaine.shum@nyumc.org
[3] Department of Oncology, Montefiore Medical Center/Albert Einstein College of Medicine, Bronx, NY 10467, USA; lrajdev@montefiore.org (L.R.); hcheng@montefiore.org (H.C.); sgoel@montefiore.org (S.G.); rperezso@montefiore.org (R.P.-S.)
* Correspondence: bahalmos@montefiore.org; Tel.: +718-405-8404

Received: 22 April 2020; Accepted: 30 April 2020; Published: 4 May 2020

Abstract: Purpose: next-generation sequencing based comprehensive genomic profiling (CGP) is becoming common practice. Although numerous studies have shown its feasibility to identify actionable genomic alterations in most patients, its clinical impact as part of routine management across all cancers in the community remains unknown. Methods: we conducted a retrospective study of all patients that underwent CGP as part of routine cancer management from January 2013 to June 2017 at an academic community-based NCI-designated cancer center. CGP was done in addition to established first tier reflex molecular testing as per national guidelines (e.g., *EGFR/ALK* for non-small cell lung cancer (NSCLC) and extended-*RAS* for colorectal cancer). Results: 349 tests were sent for CGP from 333 patients and 95% had at least one actionable genomic alteration reported. According to the reported results, 23.2% had a Food and Drug Administration (FDA) approved therapy available, 61.3% had an off-label therapy available and 77.9% were potentially eligible for a clinical trial. Treatment recommendations were also reviewed within the OncoKB database and 47% of them were not clinically validated therapies. The CGP results led to treatment change in only 35 patients (10%), most commonly in NSCLC. Nineteen of these patients (54% of those treated and 5% of total) had documented clinical benefit with targeted therapy. Conclusion: we demonstrate that routine use of CGP in the community across all cancer types detects potentially actionable genomic alterations in a majority of patients, however has modest clinical impact enriched in the NSCLC subset.

Keywords: comprehensive genomic profiling; molecular genotyping

1. Introduction

Targeted therapy against driver genomic alterations has improved outcomes for patients with many different cancers, including lung cancer, melanoma, breast cancer, and others [1]. Next-generation sequencing (NGS) based tumor comprehensive genomic profiling (CGP) that detects all classes of genomic aberrations (base pair substitutions, copy number variations, insertions/deletions, and rearrangements) is increasingly being utilized to match patients to relevant targeted therapies against several oncogenic drivers [2,3]. The National Comprehensive Cancer Network (NCCN) guidelines recommend "broad molecular profiling", including *BRAF*, *ERBB2 (HER2)*, *MET*, *RET*, NTRK, and *ROS1*, in addition to *EGFR* and *ALK* for metastatic non-small cell lung cancer (NSCLC) [4–7]. Several in-house as well as commercial testing panels are now available with rapid turnaround times for results [1,8–10]. Several NGS-based platforms are being utilized in the care of cancer patients, since the Food and Drug Administration (FDA) approval of two NGS-based assays in November 2017 for patients with advanced stage cancer and the national coverage determination of the tests by Centers for Medicare and Medicaid Services (CMS) [11,12].

Despite guidelines, the uptake of CGP in the community has not been uniform, even in NSCLC patients and the general impact of CGP as to patient outcomes and cost effectiveness remains unclear [13,14]. A large retrospective study of advanced NSCLC patients treated in the community setting identified gaps in national guideline based genomic testing for *EGFR* and *ALK* [4]. Of 814 patients, 479 (59%) met guideline recommendations for *EGFR* and *ALK* testing and only 63 (8%) underwent testing for all eight NCCN recommended genomic alterations. The barriers cited for under-genotyping included sample handling issues, long turnaround times, confusion about test reimbursement, access to targeted therapies, and insufficient tissue.

Several studies, mostly from large academic centers, have reported successful implementation of CGP and have shown that most patients will have at least one potentially actionable genomic alteration on CGP. In a retrospective study of 125 patients who underwent CGP, clinically relevant genetic alterations were found in 111 (92%) patients [15]. Only 15 (12%) patients received molecularly targeted therapy, with three who derived clinical benefit. The most common reasons for not receiving targeted therapy were ongoing standard of care treatment, poor performance status, stable disease, and lack of access to clinical trials. This trial was smaller than our study, included both adult and pediatric cases, mostly included brain tumors and assessed patients prior to 2016. A prospective trial of 100 patients with rare and/or refractory cancers assessed the clinical actionability of CGP, as determined by recommendations by a molecular tumor board [10]. Ninety-two patients underwent successful genetic sequencing and 96% (n = 88) had at least one genetic alteration. CGP led to change in management in 31% of patients, including targeted therapy, change in diagnosis, and germline testing. However, some of the cases included in this subset were those treated with cytotoxic chemotherapy, due to lack of driver mutations, e.g., a pancreatic tumor with *STK11* mutation treated with pemetrexed. Barriers to change in management were deteriorating patient clinical status and a lack of access to relevant clinical trials. Another prospective study assessed the feasibility of implementing CGP for all cancer patients at the institution and reported the results for the first 3727 patients who were successfully sequenced with their in-house gene panel [1]. Seventy-three percent of cases had at least one clinically actionable genetic alteration and only 19% of these were standard of care therapeutic recommendations at the time. However, this study did not look at actual change in management. A prospective, single arm study enrolled 500 patients with refractory cancers from a phase 1 oncology clinic, of which 339 patients underwent CGP [16]. Of these patients, 317 (93.5%) had at least one potentially actionable molecular alteration. The matching scores were calculated based on the number of drug matches and genomic alterations per patient. 122 of total 500 (24.4%) patients received matched therapy and 66 of 500 (13.2%) received unmatched therapy. High matching scores were associated with a greater frequency of stable disease, partial or complete remission versus low scores (22% vs. 9% respectively, p = 0.024), as well as longer survival (Hazard Ratio = 0.65; p = 0.05). A subsequent analysis of the same patient cohort found that patients on matched therapy had longer time on treatment (1.5 months), longer survival by 2.4 months, and higher drug treatment costs (by $38K) ($p$ < 0.01) [2]. Sixty-six percent of increased drug costs were attributable to longer treatment time, as opposed to higher monthly drug costs. Patients who received matched therapies as an earlier line of treatment (1–3) derived more numerical improvement in the aforementioned areas when compared to those who received them as later line of therapy (4 and above). Although this study provided interesting results, its definition for "matched" therapies was quite liberal—including any drug that had a half maximal inhibitory concentration (IC50) in the low nanomolar range or if the target was the primary one recognized by an antibody. A retrospective review of 439 patients who underwent CGP showed that 393 (90%) patients had at least one potentially actionable molecular alteration [17]. The alteration was targetable by at least an experimental drug in a clinical trial in all cases. The drug was only FDA approved for their tumor (on-label) in 89 patients (20%), requiring off-label use for most recommended drugs. Again, this study did not assess actual change in management.

Recently, another study estimated that 8% of cancer patients in the United States were eligible for genome-targeted therapy and only 4.9% were estimated to actually derive benefit from this therapy (i.e., responders) [18]. The MOSCATO-1 trial prospectively enrolled 1035 patients with advanced cancers, of which 843 (89%) underwent successful molecular profiling [19]. 411 patients (48.7%) had actionable targets and 199 received matched therapy. The outcomes improved (assessed by PFS2/PFS1 score) in 63 patients (7% of total 843 screened) and objective responses were observed in 22 of all 1035 patients (2.1%).

Our study aims to determine the real-world impact of routine incorporation of CGP in the community across all cancer types, regardless of stage or prior lines of therapy, while these studies have shed light on the feasibility as well as actionability in advanced cancers after standard treatments in the setting of clinical trials.

2. Methods

We conducted a retrospective, observational study of all patients that underwent comprehensive genomic profiling from January 1, 2013 to June 30, 2017 at an academic community-based National Cancer Institute (NCI)-designated cancer center. The institution has a multidisciplinary molecular tumor board that was established in September 2015, where some of these cases were referred and reviewed. CGP was performed either on tumor or plasma samples. Our institution, like many others, has a two-tier algorithm for molecular testing. The first-tier included tests that are reflexively sent by the Pathology department based on histology according to established institutional guidelines following national recommendations. For example, this included during the study era extended *RAS* testing for colorectal cancer, *HER2* for breast and esophagogastric cancer, and *EGFR/ALK* for lung adenocarcinoma. CGP constitutes the second tier and these tests are sent at the discretion of the treating oncologist. The assays used for NGS-based genomic profiling included the commercially available Foundation Medicine (Cambridge, MA, USA), Guardant Health (Redwood City, CA, USA), or Genoptix (Carlsbad, CA, USA) multi-gene panels. Testing facilities reported results defining potentially clinically actionable genetic alterations and listed treatment options available in three categories: FDA-approved on-label therapies, FDA-approved off-label therapies, and available clinical trials. Management change included patients in whom targeted therapy was initiated, continued, or withheld based on the results of CGP. Those who had clarification or confirmation of primary tumor or were enrolled on clinical trials based on CGP were also included. Patients already on targeted therapy based on previously known genetic alterations obtained by sequential or first-tier reflex testing were not included. Two independent physicians (A.S. and E.S.) reviewed all patient charts to obtain demographic as well as clinical data.

Next, we utilized the publicly available precision oncology database, OncoKB [20] to assess the supportive evidence behind treatment recommendations for "actionable mutations" labeled by testing platforms. According to the database, each potentially clinically actionable genetic alteration was assigned a level of evidence if applicable. Level 1 denotes FDA-approved targeted therapy available, level 2 denotes the standard of care, but no FDA approved indication, level 3 and 4 are assigned to alterations where therapies are not standard of care, but have compelling clinical or biologic evidence for hypothetical benefit, respectively. Level R1 indicates a standard of care biomarker predictive of resistance to an FDA-approved therapy. In cases where no level of evidence is assigned, alterations are classified as oncogenic, likely oncogenic, oncogenic function unknown, or no information available. All patient information was de-identified. Descriptive statistics and chi-squared analyses were performed using Microsoft Excel. The Institutional Review Board (IRB) of Albert Einstein College of Medicine approved the study (IRB number: 2013-2570).

3. Results

Three hundred and forty-nine tests were sent from 333 adult patients. The median age of patients was 63 years (range 19–98 years). One hundred and ninety-two (56%) of the patients were female. 112 (32%) patients were black and 71 (20.3%) identified as Hispanic. One hundred and twenty-four patients (63.4%) had Medicare or Medicaid and 26% had private insurance. The most common diagnosis for which CGP was sent was NSCLC (n = 107, 31.5%,), followed-by colorectal cancer (n = 58, 16%), ovarian cancer (n = 15, 4.3%), and carcinoma of unknown primary (n = 14, 4%) (a list of all primary oncologic diagnoses is listed in Table 1 in the appendix). 79.9% (n = 279) of tests were sent on tumor tissue samples and 20.1% (n = 70) were sent on plasma samples. The median number of therapies received for metastatic disease at the time of testing was 1 (range 0–5) and the median turnaround time for results was 12 days (range, 6–304 days). In seven cases, the results were not reported due to failed sequencing. At least one clinically actionable genomic alteration was detected in 332 (95%) patients. According to result reports from testing platforms, 23.2% (n = 81) had an FDA approved targeted therapy available for their tumor, 61.3% (n = 214) had an off-label FDA approved targeted therapy available, and 77.9% (n = 272) were potentially eligible for a clinical trial. A total of 408 treatment recommendations were annotated as FDA-approved or off-label therapies and they were reviewed within the OncoKB database. Forty-seven percent of these did not have any level of evidence assigned. Of the 408 actionable alterations, 7.8% were assigned level 1, 9.8% were assigned level 2, 8.6% were assigned level 3, 17.6% as level 4, and 8.6% as level R1. See Table 2 for a list of all actionable alterations and their corresponding OncoKB levels.

Table 1. Primary diagnosis for patients (Appendix, Online only).

Type of Tumor	Number	Type of Tumor	Number
NSCLC	107	Gastric cancer	5
Colon cancer	47	Sarcoma	4
Ovarian cancer	15	Cervical cancer	4
Carcinoma of unknown primary	14	Myelodysplastic syndrome	4
Pancreatic cancer	11	Hepatocellular carcinoma	3
Uterine cancer	11	Thyroid cancer	3
Head and Neck cancer	10	Lymphoma	3
Renal cancer	9	Pancreatobiliary cancer	3
Breast cancer	9	Parotid cancer	3
Brain tumors	8	Multiple myeloma	2
Prostate cancer	7	Small cell lung cancer	2
Gallbladder cancer	7	Thymoma	2
Rectal cancer	11	B-ALL	2
Bladder cancer	6	Melanoma	2
Esophageal cancer	6	Germ cell tumors	2
Cholangiocarcinoma	5	Others	25

The patients had a median follow-up of 1.3 years from the date of the reported CGP results. Despite the high number of listed actionable alterations, management was actually changed based on CGP in only 10% (n = 35) of patients. In another seven patients, treatment change was planned, but the patient either declined treatment or died prior to its initiation. Of these 42 patients, the most common diagnosis was NSCLC (n = 28). CGP-driven management change was observed in 50% (n = 1/2) of thymoma, 40% of head and neck cancer (n = 4/10), 26.2% (n = 28/107) of NSCLC, 27.3% (n = 3/11) of esophagogastric, 25% (n = 1/4) sarcoma, 22.2% (n = 2/9) of breast cancer, 7.1% (n = 1/14) carcinoma of unknown primary, and 3.4% (n = 2/58) of CRC patients. Figure 1 shows patients in whom management changed categorized by diagnoses. We compared the effect of CGP on the two most common patient diagnoses i.e., lung and colorectal cancer using the Chi-squared test. CGP-led management change was significantly higher in lung cancer versus colorectal patients ($p = 0.0002$). Table 3 describes patient information and clinical outcomes of patients where CGP changed management. Nineteen patients (54% of those treated and 5% of total) had documented clinical benefit with targeted therapy based on CGP. Only one patient received immunotherapy based on CGP testing identifying Microsatellite Instability–High (MSI-H) status. It should be mentioned that, given routine Mismatch Repair (MMR) testing at our institution for all colorectal and endometrial cancers, this low frequency is expected.

Table 2. Classification of actionable molecular alterations according to OncoKB levels of evidence (of note, some alterations had more than one level of evidence assigned depending on the alteration and specific therapy involved).

OncoKB Level of Evidence	Number	Percentage
Level 1	32	7.8
Level 2A	9	2.2
Level 2B	31	7.6
Level 3A	4	0.9
Level 3B	31	7.6
Level 4	72	17.6
Level R1	35	8.6
No level assigned, oncogenic	71	17.4
No level assigned, likely oncogenic	57	14.0
No level assigned, oncogenic function unknown	39	9.6
No level assigned, no information available	8	2.0
No level assigned, Tumor mutational burden	8	4.4
No level assigned, Microsatellite Instability	18	0.2

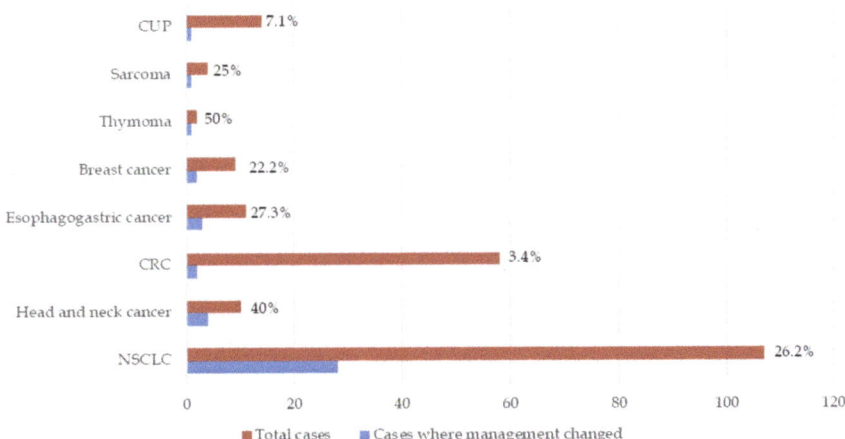

Figure 1. Patients in whom comprehensive genomic profiling changed/potentially changed management (NSCLC, Non-small cell lung cancer, CRC, Colorectal cancer, CUP, Carcinoma of unknown primary).

Of the 81 patients with FDA approved targeted therapies identified by testing platforms, 55 (67.9%) did not result in change in management. Twelve of these had previously known mutations in NSCLC/CRC/gastric/breast cancer as part of established first tier reflex testing. In 37 patients, the recommended targeted therapy was not standard of care, including high tumor mutational burden directed immunotherapy, four patients had early disease where targeted therapy was not indicated, in one patient therapy was reserved for future disease progression, and one patient died. Although 54 patients (15.5%) participated in clinical trials, only five were enrolled in clinical trials based on results from CGP (including two patients on NCI-MATCH).

Table 3. Observed/proposed change in management based on comprehensive genomic profiling (*Documented response or on treatment for at least 3 months).

	Diagnosis	Molecular Alterations	Management Change	Observed Benefit
1.	Lung adenocarcinoma	EML4-ALK fusion (Variant 1)	Crizotinib	Lost to follow-up
2.	Lung adenocarcinoma	EGFR amplification, G719A	Erlotinib continued	Yes
3.	Lung adenocarcinoma	EGFR G719A, Q701L, amplification	Erlotinib continued	Yes
4.	Lung adenocarcinoma	EGFR E746_A750del MET amplification	Crizotinib-Erlotinib	Lost to follow-up
5.	Poorly differentiated NSCLC, sarcomatoid morphology	NTRK1 TPM3-NTRK1 fusion	Died prior to giving Crizotinib	N/A
6.	Lung adenocarcinoma	EGFR amplification, exon 19 deletion	Afatinib	Yes
7.	Lung adenocarcinoma	EGFR exon 19 deletion, T790M	Osimertinib	Yes
8.	Lung adenocarcinoma	ALK EML4-ALK fusion (Variant 1)	Alectinib	Yes
9.	Lung adenocarcinoma	BRCA2 S1099* MET amplification	Declined participation in MATCH study	N/A
10.	Lung adenocarcinoma	EGFR L858R	Died prior to starting EGFR-TKI	N/A
11.	Lung adenocarcinoma	EGFR exon 19 deletion, T790M, L792F, C797S	Osimertinib continued beyond progression	N/A
12.	Medullary thyroid cancer	RET V804M	Cabozantinib Lenvatinib Phase 1 study of MGCD516	Yes
13.	Poorly differentiated NSCLC	MET amplification	Died prior to planned phase 1 trial of MGCD516	N/A
14.	Poorly differentiated NSCLC	MET amplification	Died prior to planned phase 1 trial of MGCD516	N/A
15.	Lung adenocarcinoma	EGFR exon 19 deletion (L747_S752del) T790M	Osimertinib	Yes
16.	Lung adenocarcinoma Urothelial bladder cancer	Numerous	Clarified primary tumor to be urothelial in origin	Yes
17.	Gastric adenocarcinoma	MSI-High	Pembrolizumab	Yes
18.	Lung adenocarcinoma	EGFR exon 19 deletion (E746_A750del), T790M	Osimertinib	Yes
19.	Lung adenocarcinoma	EGFR amplification, L858R, R776C, T790M MET amplification	Osimertinib + crizotinib	Yes
20.	Lacrimal duct carcinoma	ERBB2 amplification	Trastuzumab	No
21.	Nasopharyngeal adenoid cystic carcinoma	PIK3CA H1047R	Taselisib on MATCH study	Yes
22.	Lung adenocarcinoma	EGFR exon 19 deletion	Erlotinib after clearance of T790M	No
23.	Thymoma	CDKN2A/B loss KDM6A W1194*	Phase I/IIa trial of ALRN-6924 in patients with wild typeTP53	Yes
24.	Invasive ductal breast cancer	CCND1 amplification	Abemaciclib	No
25.	Lung adenocarcinoma	RET KIF5B-RET fusion, RET-KIF5B fusion	Phase 1/1b MGCD516	Not documented, patient withdrew from study
26.	Lung adenocarcinoma	BRAF V600E	Vemurafenib Dabrafenib +Trametinib	Yes
27.	Lung adenocarcinoma	EGFR exon 19 deletion	Erlotinib after clearance of T790M	No
28.	Lung adenocarcinoma	EGFR amplification, exon 19 deletion (E746_A750del), T790M	Osimertinib	Yes
29.	Rectal adenocarcinoma	ERBB2 amplification, V777L	Ado-trastuzumab emtansine on MATCH study	Yes
30.	Esophageal adenocarcinoma	ERBB2 amplification	Trastuzumab	Patient lost to follow-up/did not complete treatment
31.	Carcinoma of unknown primary, likely upper GI/pancreaticobiliary origin	MET amplification	Planned for crizotinib but not approved by insurance	N/A
32.	Lung adenocarcinoma	EGFR amplification, L858R, T790M	Osimertinib	Yes
33.	Invasive ductal breast cancer	CCND1 amplification	Palbociclib	No
34.	Lung adenocarcinoma	EGFR exon 19 deletion	Afatinib	Yes
35.	Salivary ductal carcinoma	VEGFA amplification	Sorafenib	No
36.	Colon adenocarcinoma	Numerous	Pembrolizumab based on numerous mutations detected and concern for MSI status	No
37.	Esophageal squamous cell carcinoma	EGFR amplification	Panitumumab	No
38.	Lung adenocarcinoma	ALK EML4-ALK fusion (Variant 3a/b)	Alectinib	Yes
39.	Lung adenocarcinoma	EGFR L964L	Erlotinib	Yes
40.	Follicular dendritic cell sarcoma	AKT2 amplification	Everolimus	Yes
41.	Lung adenocarcinoma	MET H1094R	Died prior to starting crizotinib	N/A
42.	Lung adenocarcinoma	MET exon 14 splice site (D1010N)	Crizotinib	No

(EGFR, Epidermal growth factor receptor; MATCH, Molecular Analysis for Therapy Choice; TKI, Tyrosine Kinase Inhibitor; MSI, Microsatellite Instability).

4. Discussion

In our study, CGP identified at least one potentially clinically actionable genomic alteration in 95% of patients, which is similar to several other reports [1,10,21]. However, management changed based on these results in only 10% of patients. An additional 2% who could have benefited were unable to, as they either died prior to its initiation or declined therapy. Although our numbers were too small to draw any robust conclusion on response rates, 19 patients (54% of those treated and 5% of total) had documented clinical benefit with targeted therapy that was based on CGP, which is similar to that recently predicted by Marquart et al. [18]. Most of the patients who benefited were those who had NSCLC, which was also the most common patient diagnosis. When comparing lung cancer to the next most common diagnosis, colorectal cancer; GCP-led management change was significantly higher in the former ($p = 0.0002$). 28 of 107 (26.2%) NSCLC patients had change/potential change in management based on CGP. As a result of first tier Epidermal Growth Factor Receptor (EGFR)/Anaplastic Lymphoma Kinase (ALK) testing, the majority of EGFR/ALK mutated patients were identified outside of CGP testing. If such first-tier testing results were to be included, the impact of molecular testing would be much higher. In addition, recent studies, for example, with K-Ras G12C inhibitors offer the hope of further expansion of actionable targets [22]. A recent study utilized a decision analytic tool to compare upfront CGP vs. sequential testing for genomic alterations in metastatic NSCLC patients [23]. The study found that upfront CGP led to the same (as panel) or shorter (vs. sequential testing) turnaround time and lowest payer cost in these patients and it is likely to become the preferred approach in most institutions.

In other cancer types in our study, the impact was much less, soberingly with only 14 of 242 patients (5.8%) with change/potential change in management based on CGP results. Again, the impact would be higher if first-tier testing such as *HER2* in breast/upper GI and extended-*RAS* in colorectal cancer are included. The impact of CGP will likely also increase with the tissue/site agnostic approval of pembrolizumab in solid tumors with microsatellite instability and Tropomyosin Receptor Kinase (TRK) inhibitors for Neurotrophic Tropomyosin-Related Kinase (NTRK)-translocation positive malignancies; however, the frequency of these alterations admittedly is low [7,24]. Tumor mutational burden (TMB) as a predictive biomarker for immune checkpoint inhibitors is another emerging use of CGP and it might add to its impact in routine use in clinical practice, although initial results in the context of advanced NSCLC have been disappointing [25,26].

Despite the aforementioned emerging uses of CGP, at present, data to support therapeutic recommendations for many targeted drugs is not robust enough to warrant therapy off a clinical trial, e.g., trastuzumab in (v-erb-b2 avian erythroblastic leukemia viral oncogene homolog 2) ERBB2 amplified lung cancer. Our review of treatment recommendations in the OncoKB database showed that 47% of them did not have strong clinical evidence to support their use. Only 17.6% of recommendations were based on level 1 or 2 evidence. Therefore, the actual actionability of these genomic alterations is currently significantly less than presented. Additionally, an increasing number of commercial as well as institutional multi-gene panels are now being utilized for CGP; however, there is no standardization of therapeutic recommendations based on results [27]. Multidisciplinary molecular tumor boards can certainly help interpret results of CGP, especially in cases where a clinician needs to decide on whether or not to start a patient on an off-label therapy [28,29]. While currently tissue-based CGP utilizing panels, such as ones used in our study, are the most widely utilized, admittedly, further technological advances in circulating tumor DNA (ctDNA), circulating tumor cells (CTC) technology, and the incorporation of whole exome sequencing (WES) and whole genome sequencing (WGS) will provide expansion of information as to tumor heterogeneity, clonal evolution, dynamic assessment of treatment response, and minimal residual disease status that will better inform clinical decision making [30–36].

Our study has certain limitations, particularly because of its retrospective nature. The timing and choice of CGP panel was not standardized and it was at the discretion of the treating oncologist; however, this indeed best captures a "real-world" scenario in the community as compared to other publishes studies. Another drawback is the short follow-up and the proportion of patients with change in management based on CGP would likely increase with time, due to disease progression or more targeted agents becoming standard of care. We did not include patients who benefited from targeted therapy based on first-tier testing. However, this study specifically assessed the impact of CGP in settings such as ours, where there might be a two-step process for genomic profiling, likely representing the majority of practice patterns both in and especially outside of the United States. Another issue is optimal timing for CGP. Whereas some patients with actionable genetic alterations had early stage disease and, hence, not initiated on targeted therapy, some deteriorated clinically prior to the initiation of treatment. This makes a case for obtaining CGP as soon as possible with metastatic disease or locally advanced disease with a high risk of recurrence. Serial liquid biopsies are now being utilized for the real-time assessment of tumor mutations and more studies are needed to inform the decision of ideal timing for CGP. The lack of available molecularly driven protocols was not a factor, with more than 200 open clinical trials, including the NCI-MATCH trial actively recruiting patients at our institution. Moreover, our enrolment rate of 15% was higher than the national average indicating the robustness of our clinical trials program [37]. Our study focused on patients with whom a change in management was possible as a result of CGP. However, we are unable to comment whether such a treatment approach indeed has merit. We realize that the ultimate litmus test of CGP based treatment is to prove that treating a patient based on a specific mutation is actually superior than offering a non-molecularly targeted agent, either on or off a clinical trial. One randomized trial attempting to answer this question is the Therapy Based on Tumor Molecular Profiling Versus Conventional Therapy in Patients With Refractory Cancer (SHIVA) study, which did not show benefit of the molecularly directed therapeutic approach [38]. Recent studies add to this database and offer more promise as to the benefit of CGP in this context [39].

5. Conclusions

Overall, our study provides a real-world experience of the impact of CGP in a community-based academic NCI-designated cancer center serving a highly diverse patient population, where molecular testing is based on a two-tier testing algorithm. While recognizing that a 10% overall rate of management change that is based on CGP is very modest, its use in certain subsets, such as advanced NSCLC, where the impact currently is most significant appears to be justifiable and it has been found to be cost effective [40–42]. In addition, we have identified multiple reasons for the relatively smaller clinical impact of CGP in other tumor types, despite a much larger proportion of patients with actionable genomic alterations reported. The impact however is anticipated to be increasing in light of new advances, e.g., recent studies do suggest expanding impact in breast (PI3kinase inhibitors) and pancreatic malignancies (poly ADP ribose polymerase (PARP) inhibition) [43–46]. Although issues, such as optimal timing, access to clinical trials, and consolidating genomic testing need to be addressed at an institutional level, reports from testing platforms need to be carefully interpreted and ideally discussed in molecular tumor boards to provide the best treatment option possible. More prospective trials are needed that would better inform our choices for personalized treatment by providing assessments of overall survival and quality of life with choosing targeted therapies that are based on CGP when compared to conventional therapies [11].

Author Contributions: Conceptualization, A.P.S. and B.H.; Data curation, A.P.S., E.S and B.H.; Formal analysis, A.P.S. and B.H.; Methodology, B.H.; Supervision, H.C. and B.H.; Validation, S.G.; Writing–original draft, A.P.S.; Writing–review & editing, E.S., L.R., H.C., S.G., R.P.-S. and B.H. All authors have read and agreed to the published version of the manuscript.

Funding: This research received no external funding.

Conflicts of Interest: The authors declare no conflict of interest.

References

1. Sholl, L.M.; Do, K.; Shivdasani, P.; Cerami, E.; Dubuc, A.M.; Kuo, F.C.; Garcia, E.P.; Jia, Y.; Davineni, P.; Abo, R.P.; et al. Institutional implementation of clinical tumor profiling on an unselected cancer population. *JCI Insight* **2016**, *1*, e87062. [CrossRef]
2. Signorovitch, J.; Janku, F.; Wheler, J.J.; Miller, V.A.; Ryan, J.; Zhou, Z.; Chawla, A. Estimated cost of anticancer therapy directed by comprehensive genomic profiling (CGP) in a single-center study. *J. Clin. Oncol.* **2017**, *35*, 6605. [CrossRef]

3. Remon, J.; Steuer, C.; Ramalingam, S.; Felip, E. Osimertinib and other third-generation EGFR TKI in EGFR-mutant NSCLC patients. *Ann. Oncol.* **2018**, *29*, i20–i27. [CrossRef] [PubMed]
4. Gutierrez, M.E.; Choi, K.; Lanman, R.B.; Licitra, E.J.; Skrzypczak, S.M.; Benito, R.P.; Wu, T.; Arunajadai, S.; Kaur, S.; Harper, H.; et al. Genomic Profiling of Advanced Non–Small Cell Lung Cancer in Community Settings: Gaps and Opportunities. *Clin. Lung Cancer* **2017**, *18*, 651–659. [CrossRef]
5. Pennell, N.A.; Arcila, M.E.; Gandara, D.R.; West, H. Biomarker Testing for Patients with Advanced Non–Small Cell Lung Cancer: Real-World Issues and Tough Choices. *Am. Soc. Clin. Oncol. Educ. Book* **2019**, *39*, 531–542. [CrossRef]
6. NCCN Clinical Practice Guidelines in Oncology (NCCN Guidelines®). Non Small Cell Lung Cancer Version 3.2020 [11 February 2020]. Available online: https://www.nccn.org/professionals/physician_gls/pdf/nscl.pdf (accessed on 16 April 2020).
7. Drilon, A.; Laetsch, T.W.; Kummar, S.; Dubois, S.G.; Lassen, U.N.; Demetri, G.D.; Nathenson, M.; Doebele, R.C.; Farago, A.F.; Pappo, A.; et al. Efficacy of Larotrectinib in TRK Fusion-Positive Cancers in Adults and Children. *N. Engl. J. Med.* **2018**, *378*, 731–739. [CrossRef] [PubMed]
8. Sireci, A.N.; Aggarwal, V.S.; Turk, A.; Gindin, T.; Mansukhani, M.M.; Hsiao, S.J. Clinical Genomic Profiling of a Diverse Array of Oncology Specimens at a Large Academic Cancer Center. *J. Mol. Diagn.* **2017**, *19*, 277–287. [CrossRef] [PubMed]
9. Zehir, A.; Benayed, R.; Shah, R.; Syed, A.; Middha, S.; Kim, H.; Srinivasan, P.; Gao, J.; Chakravarty, D.; Devlin, S.M.; et al. Mutational landscape of metastatic cancer revealed from prospective clinical sequencing of 10,000 patients. *Nat. Med.* **2017**, *23*, 703–713. [CrossRef]
10. Hirshfield, K.M.; Tolkunov, D.; Zhong, H.; Ali, S.M.; Stein, M.N.; Murphy, S.; Vig, H.; Vázquez, A.; Glod, J.; Moss, R.A.; et al. Clinical Actionability of Comprehensive Genomic Profiling for Management of Rare or Refractory Cancers. *Oncologist* **2016**, *21*, 1315–1325. [CrossRef]
11. Prasad, V. Why the US Centers for Medicare and Medicaid Services (CMS) should have required a randomized trial of Foundation Medicine (F1CDx) before paying for it. *Ann. Oncol.* **2018**, *29*, 299–301. [CrossRef] [PubMed]
12. Institute NC. Genomic Profiling Tests Cleared by FDA Can Help Guide Cancer Treatment, Clinical Trial Enrollment 2017 [29 May 2019]. Available online: https://www.cancer.gov/news-events/cancer-currents-blog/2017/genomic-profiling-tests-cancer (accessed on 16 April 2020).
13. Inal, C.; Yilmaz, E.; Cheng, H.; Zhu, C.; Pullman, J.; Gucalp, R.; Keller, S.M.; Perez-Soler, R.; Piperdi, B. Effect of reflex testing by pathologists on molecular testing rates in lung cancer patients: Experience from a community-based academic center. *J. Clin. Oncol.* **2014**, *32*, 8098. [CrossRef]
14. Nesline, M.K.; DePietro, P.; Dy, G.K.; Early, A.; Papanicolau-Sengos, A.; Conroy, J.M.; Lenzo, F.L.; Glenn, S.T.; Chen, H.; Grand'Maison, A.; et al. Oncologist uptake of comprehensive genomic profile guided targeted therapy. *Oncotarget* **2019**, *10*, 4616–4629. [CrossRef] [PubMed]
15. Hilal, T.; Nakazawa, M.; Hodskins, J.; Villano, J.L.; Mathew, A.; Goel, G.; Wagner, L.; Arnold, S.M.; DeSimone, P.; Anthony, L.; et al. Comprehensive genomic profiling in routine clinical practice leads to a low rate of benefit from genotype-directed therapy. *BMC Cancer* **2017**, *17*, 602. [CrossRef] [PubMed]
16. Wheler, J.J.; Janku, F.; Naing, A.; Li, Y.; Stephen, B.; Zinner, R.G.; Subbiah, V.; Fu, S.; Karp, D.D.; Falchook, G.S.; et al. Cancer Therapy Directed by Comprehensive Genomic Profiling: A Single Center Study. *Cancer Res.* **2016**, *76*, 3690–3701. [CrossRef]
17. Schwaederle, M.; Daniels, G.A.; Piccioni, D.E.; Fanta, P.T.; Schwab, R.B.; Shimabukuro, K.A.; Parker, B.A.; Kurzrock, R. On the Road to Precision Cancer Medicine: Analysis of Genomic Biomarker Actionability in 439 Patients. *Mol. Cancer Ther.* **2015**, *14*, 1488–1494. [CrossRef]
18. Marquart, J.; Chen, E.Y.; Prasad, V. Estimation of the Percentage of US Patients With Cancer Who Benefit From Genome-Driven Oncology. *JAMA Oncol.* **2018**, *4*, 1093. [CrossRef]
19. Massard, C.; Michiels, S.; Ferté, C.; Le Deley, M.-C.; Lacroix, L.; Hollebecque, A.; Verlingue, L.; Ileana, E.; Rosellini, S.; Ammari, S.; et al. High-Throughput Genomics and Clinical Outcome in Hard-to-Treat Advanced Cancers: Results of the MOSCATO 01 Trial. *Cancer Discov.* **2017**, *7*, 586–595. [CrossRef]
20. Chakravarty, D.; Gao, J.; Phillips, S.; Kundra, R.; Zhang, H.; Wang, J.; Rudolph, J.E.; Yaeger, R.; Soumerai, T.; Nissan, M.H.; et al. OncoKB: A Precision Oncology Knowledge Base. *JCO Precis. Oncol.* **2017**, *1*, 1–16. [CrossRef]

21. Hilal, T.; Nakazawa, M.; Hodskins, J.; Arnold, S.M.; DeSimone, P.A.; Wagner, L.M.; Anthony, L.B.; Chambers, M.D.; Villano, J.L.; Mathew, A.; et al. Utility of comprehensive genomic profiling (CGP) at an NCI-designated cancer center for identifying clinically relevant genomic alterations (CRGA) and implementing genomically directed therapy (GDT). *J. Clin. Oncol.* **2016**, *34*, e18018. [CrossRef]
22. Fakih, M.; O'Neil, B.; Price, T.J.; Falchook, G.S.; Desai, J.; Kuo, J.; Govindan, R.; Rasmussen, E.; Morrow, P.K.H.; Ngang, J.; et al. Phase 1 study evaluating the safety, tolerability, pharmacokinetics (PK), and efficacy of AMG 510, a novel small molecule KRASG12C inhibitor, in advanced solid tumors. *J. Clin. Oncol.* **2019**, *37*, 3003. [CrossRef]
23. Pennell, N.A.; Mutebi, A.; Zhou, Z.-Y.; Ricculli, M.L.; Tang, W.; Wang, H.; Guerin, A.; Arnhart, T.; Culver, K.W.; Otterson, G.A. Economic impact of next generation sequencing vs sequential single-gene testing modalities to detect genomic alterations in metastatic non-small cell lung cancer using a decision analytic model. *J. Clin. Oncol.* **2018**, *36*, 9031. [CrossRef]
24. Administration USFaD. FDA grants accelerated approval to pembrolizumab for first tissue/site agnostic indication. Available online: https://www.fda.gov/Drugs/InformationOnDrugs/ApprovedDrugs/ucm560040.htm (accessed on 16 April 2020).
25. Langer, C.; Gadgeel, S.; Borghaei, H.; Patnaik, A.; Powell, S.; Gentzler, R.; Yang, J.; Gubens, M.; Sequist, L.; Awad, M.; et al. OA04.05 KEYNOTE-021: TMB and Outcomes for Carboplatin and Pemetrexed With or Without Pembrolizumab for Nonsquamous NSCLC. *J. Thorac. Oncol.* **2019**, *14*, S216. [CrossRef]
26. Garassino, M.; Rodriguez-Abreu, D.; Gadgeel, S.; Esteban, E.; Felip, E.; Speranza, G.; Reck, M.; Hui, R.; Boyer, M.; Cristescu, R.; et al. OA04.06 Evaluation of TMB in KEYNOTE-189: Pembrolizumab Plus Chemotherapy vs Placebo Plus Chemotherapy for Nonsquamous NSCLC. *J. Thorac. Oncol.* **2019**, *14*, S216–S217. [CrossRef]
27. Patel, J.M.; Knopf, J.; Reiner, E.; Bossuyt, V.; Epstein, L.; DiGiovanna, M.; Chung, G.; Silber, A.; Sanft, T.; Hofstatter, E.; et al. Mutation based treatment recommendations from next generation sequencing data: A comparison of web tools. *Oncotarget* **2016**, *7*, 22064–22076. [CrossRef]
28. Tafe, L.J.; Gorlov, I.P.; De Abreu, F.B.; Lefferts, J.A.; Liu, X.; Pettus, J.R.; Marotti, J.D.; Bloch, K.J.; Memoli, V.A.; Suriawinata, A.A.; et al. Implementation of a Molecular Tumor Board: The Impact on Treatment Decisions for 35 Patients Evaluated at Dartmouth-Hitchcock Medical Center. *Oncologist* **2015**, *20*, 1011–1018. [CrossRef]
29. Dalton, W.B.; Forde, P.M.; Kang, H.; Connolly, R.M.; Stearns, V.; Gocke, C.D.; Eshleman, J.R.; Axilbund, J.; Petry, D.; Geoghegan, C.; et al. Personalized Medicine in the Oncology Clinic: Implementation and Outcomes of the Johns Hopkins Molecular Tumor Board. *JCO Precis. Oncol.* **2017**, *2017*, 1–19. [CrossRef]
30. Gupta, R.; Othman, T.; Chen, C.; Sandhu, J.; Ouyang, C.; Fakih, M. Guardant360 Circulating Tumor DNA Assay Is Concordant with FoundationOne Next-Generation Sequencing in Detecting Actionable Driver Mutations in Anti-EGFR Naive Metastatic Colorectal Cancer. *Oncologist* **2019**, *25*, 235–243. [CrossRef]
31. Russo, A.; Perez, D.D.M.; Gunasekaran, M.; Scilla, K.; Lapidus, R.; Cooper, B.; Mehra, R.; Adamo, V.; Malapelle, U.; Rolfo, C.D. Liquid biopsy tracking of lung tumor evolutions over time. *Expert Rev. Mol. Diagn.* **2019**, *19*, 1099–1108. [CrossRef]
32. Imperial, R.; Nazer, M.; Ahmed, Z.; Kam, A.E.; Pluard, T.J.; Bahaj, W.; Levy, M.; Kuzel, T.M.; Hayden, D.M.; Pappas, S.G.; et al. Matched Whole-Genome Sequencing (WGS) and Whole-Exome Sequencing (WES) of Tumor Tissue with Circulating Tumor DNA (ctDNA) Analysis: Complementary Modalities in Clinical Practice. *Cancers* **2019**, *11*, 1399. [CrossRef]
33. Kelley, S.; Pantel, K. A New Era in Liquid Biopsy: From Genotype to Phenotype. *Clin. Chem.* **2019**, *66*, 89–96. [CrossRef] [PubMed]
34. Bin Lim, S.; Di Lee, W.; Vasudevan, J.; Lim, W.-T.; Lim, C.T. Liquid biopsy: One cell at a time. *npj Precis. Oncol.* **2019**, *3*, 23–29. [CrossRef]
35. Keller, L.; Pantel, K. Unravelling tumour heterogeneity by single-cell profiling of circulating tumour cells. *Nat. Rev. Cancer* **2019**, *19*, 553–567. [CrossRef] [PubMed]
36. Batth, I.S.; Mitra, A.; Rood, S.; Kopetz, S.; Menter, D.; Li, S. CTC analysis: An update on technological progress. *Transl. Res.* **2019**, *212*, 14–25. [CrossRef] [PubMed]
37. Unger, J.M.; Cook, E.; Tai, E.; Bleyer, A. The Role of Clinical Trial Participation in Cancer Research: Barriers, Evidence, and Strategies. *Am. Soc. Clin. Oncol. Educ. Book* **2016**, *35*, 185–198. [CrossRef] [PubMed]

38. Le Tourneau, C.; Delord, J.-P.; Gonçalves, A.; Gavoille, C.; Dubot, C.; Isambert, N.; Campone, M.; Trédan, O.; Massiani, M.-A.; Mauborgne, C.; et al. Molecularly targeted therapy based on tumour molecular profiling versus conventional therapy for advanced cancer (SHIVA): A multicentre, open-label, proof-of-concept, randomised, controlled phase 2 trial. *Lancet Oncol.* **2015**, *16*, 1324–1334. [CrossRef]
39. Stockley, T.L.; Oza, A.M.; Berman, H.K.; Leighl, N.B.; Knox, J.J.; Shepherd, F.A.; Chen, E.X.; Krzyzanowska, M.K.; Dhani, N.; Joshua, A.M.; et al. Molecular profiling of advanced solid tumors and patient outcomes with genotype-matched clinical trials: The Princess Margaret IMPACT/COMPACT trial. *Genome Med.* **2016**, *8*, 109. [CrossRef]
40. Singal, G.; Miller, P.G.; Agarwala, V.; Li, G.; Kaushik, G.; Backenroth, D.; Gossai, A.; Frampton, G.M.; Torres, A.Z.; Lehnert, E.M.; et al. Association of Patient Characteristics and Tumor Genomics with Clinical Outcomes Among Patients With Non-Small Cell Lung Cancer Using a Clinicogenomic Database. *JAMA* **2019**, *321*, 1391–1399. [CrossRef]
41. Spizzo, G.; Siebert, U.; Gastl, G.; Voss, A.; Schuster, K.; Leonard, R.; Seeber, A. Cost-comparison analysis of a multiplatform tumour profiling service to guide advanced cancer treatment. *Cost Eff. Resour. Alloc.* **2019**, *17*, 23–25. [CrossRef]
42. Signorovitch, J.; Zhou, Z.; Ryan, J.; Anhorn, R.; Chawla, A. Budget impact analysis of comprehensive genomic profiling in patients with advanced non-small cell lung cancer. *J. Med. Econ.* **2018**, *22*, 140–150. [CrossRef]
43. Pezo, R.C.; Chen, T.W.-W.; Berman, H.K.; Mulligan, A.M.; Razak, A.A.; Siu, L.L.; Cescon, D.W.; Amir, E.; Elser, C.; Warr, D.G.; et al. Impact of multi-gene mutational profiling on clinical trial outcomes in metastatic breast cancer. *Breast Cancer Res. Treat.* **2017**, *168*, 159–168. [CrossRef] [PubMed]
44. André, F.; Ciruelos, E.; Rubovszky, G.; Campone, M.; Loibl, S.; Rugo, H.S.; Iwata, H.; Conte, P.; Mayer, I.A.; Kaufman, B.; et al. Alpelisib for PIK3CA-Mutated, Hormone Receptor-Positive Advanced Breast Cancer. *N. Engl. J. Med.* **2019**, *380*, 1929–1940. [CrossRef] [PubMed]
45. Lin, P.; Chen, M.; Tsai, L.; Lo, C.; Yen, T.; Huang, T.Y.; Chen, C.; Fan, S.; Kuo, S.; Huang, C. Using next-generation sequencing to redefine BRCAness in triple-negative breast cancer. *Cancer Sci.* **2020**, *111*, 1375–1384. [CrossRef] [PubMed]
46. Golan, T.; Hammel, P.; Reni, M.; Van Cutsem, E.; Macarulla, T.; Hall, M.J.; Park, J.-O.; Hochhauser, D.; Arnold, D.; Oh, Y.; et al. Maintenance Olaparib for Germline BRCA-Mutated Metastatic Pancreatic Cancer. *N. Engl. J. Med.* **2019**, *381*, 317–327. [CrossRef]

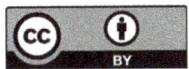

© 2020 by the authors. Licensee MDPI, Basel, Switzerland. This article is an open access article distributed under the terms and conditions of the Creative Commons Attribution (CC BY) license (http://creativecommons.org/licenses/by/4.0/).

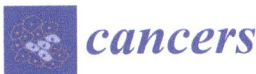

Article

Assessment of Tumor Mutational Burden in Pediatric Tumors by Real-Life Whole-Exome Sequencing and In Silico Simulation of Targeted Gene Panels: How the Choice of Method Could Affect the Clinical Decision?

Hana Noskova [1,2], Michal Kyr [2,3,4], Karol Pal [1,5], Tomas Merta [2,3,4], Peter Mudry [2,3,4], Kristyna Polaskova [2,3,4], Tina Catela Ivkovic [1], Sona Adamcova [1], Tekla Hornakova [1], Marta Jezova [6], Leos Kren [6], Jaroslav Sterba [2,3,4,7,*] and Ondrej Slaby [1,3,6,*]

1. Central European Institute of Technology, Masaryk University, 62500 Brno, Czech Republic; hana.noskova@ceitec.muni.cz (H.N.); pal@mail.muni.cz (K.P.); tina.ivkovic@ceitec.muni.cz (T.C.I.); sona.adamcova@ceitec.muni.cz (S.A.); tekla.hornakova@hotmail.com (T.H.)
2. Department of Pediatric Oncology, University Hospital Brno, 613 00 Brno, Czech Republic; kyr.michal2@fnbrno.cz (M.K.); merta.tomas@fnbrno.cz (T.M.); Mudry.Peter@fnbrno.cz (P.M.); polaskova.kristyna@fnbrno.cz (K.P.)
3. Faculty of Medicine, Masaryk University, 62500 Brno, Czech Republic
4. International Clinical Research Center, St. Anne's University Hospital, 65691 Brno, Czech Republic
5. Department of Hematology, University Hospital Schleswig-Holstein, 24105 Kiel, Germany
6. Department of Pathology, University Hospital Brno, 62500 Brno, Czech Republic; jezova.marta@fnbrno.cz (M.J.); Kren.Leos@fnbrno.cz (L.K.)
7. Regional Centre for Applied Molecular Oncology, Masaryk Memorial Cancer Institute, 60200 Brno, Czech Republic
* Correspondence: Sterba.Jaroslav@fnbrno.cz (J.S.); ondrej.slaby@ceitec.muni.cz (O.S.)

Received: 25 December 2019; Accepted: 11 January 2020; Published: 17 January 2020

Abstract: Background: Tumor mutational burden (TMB) is an emerging genomic biomarker in cancer that has been associated with improved response to immune checkpoint inhibitors (ICIs) in adult cancers. It was described that variability in TMB assessment is introduced by different laboratory techniques and various settings of bioinformatic pipelines. In pediatric oncology, no study has been published describing this variability so far. Methods: In our study, we performed whole exome sequencing (WES, both germline and somatic) and calculated TMB in 106 patients with high-risk/recurrent pediatric solid tumors of 28 distinct cancer types. Subsequently, we used WES data for TMB calculation using an in silico approach simulating two The Food and Drug Administration (FDA)-approved/authorized comprehensive genomic panels for cancer. Results: We describe a strong correlation between WES-based and panel-based TMBs; however, we show that this high correlation is significantly affected by inclusion of only a few hypermutated cases. In the series of nine cases, we determined TMB in two sequentially collected tumor tissue specimens and observed an increase in TMB along with tumor progression. Furthermore, we evaluated the extent to which potential ICI indication could be affected by variability in techniques and bioinformatic pipelines used for TMB assessment. We confirmed that this technological variability could significantly affect ICI indication in pediatric cancer patients; however, this significance decreases with the increasing cut-off values. Conclusions: For the first time in pediatric oncology, we assessed the reliability of TMB estimation across multiple pediatric cancer types using real-life WES and in silico analysis of two major targeted gene panels and confirmed a significant technological variability to be introduced by different laboratory techniques and various settings of bioinformatic pipelines.

Keywords: pediatric tumors; tumor mutational burden; TMB; whole-exome sequencing; gene panel sequencing; immune checkpoint inhibitors

1. Introduction

The cancer cell genome acquires genetic alterations differing from the germline of the host [1]. Somatic mutation rates can be affected by exposure to exogenous factors, such as ultraviolet light or tobacco smoke [2], or by compounding genetic defects, such as DNA mismatch repair deficiency, microsatellite instability, or replicative DNA polymerase mutations [1–3]. These somatic genetic alterations induce and drive carcinogenesis. The type and the number of acquired mutations varies among the cancer types but also among the affected individuals [4]. Some of these mutations lead to the formation of tumor-specific neoantigens, which could be recognized by a patient's immune system as non-self and which are highly clinically relevant since these neoantigens can make the cancer cells sensitive to treatment with immune checkpoint inhibitors (ICIs) against cytotoxic T-lymphocyte-associated protein 4 (CTLA-4), programmed cell death protein 1 (PD-1) and programmed death-ligand 1 (PD-L1) in various cancers including melanoma [5], non–small-cell lung cancer (NSCLC) [6], kidney cancer [7], bladder cancer [8] and others [9]. The genomic landscape of smoking-induced NSCLC and UV light-induced melanoma is often characterized by a high number of acquired alterations, while leukemias and pediatric tumors show the lowest mutations counts.

Rapidly developing genomic methods based on next-generation sequencing (NGS) simplified the detection and quantification of these acquired changes on the level of individual cancer genomes. Tumor mutational burden (TMB) is a quantitative measure of acquired somatic mutations in the cancer cell genome. Initial exploratory analyses of TMB in cancer patients [10,11] were carried out using whole exome sequencing (WES). WES is a comprehensive research tool for assessment of genomic alterations across the entire coding region of the ~22,000 genes in the human genome, comprising of 1–2% of the genome [3,12]. Currently, WES-derived TMB values are considered to be the gold standard, but the high cost and long turnaround time limit routine diagnostic applicability of WES. Therefore, targeted NGS cancer gene panels have been promoted for TMB estimation as a feasible and cheaper alternative to WES [13]. Whereas TMB assessed by WES is typically reported as the total number of mutations per cancer cell exome, TMB assessed by gene panel assays is usually referred to as mutations per megabase (mut/Mb) because it differs in the number of genes and target region size [2,3,14]. The precise calculation of TMB may, however, vary depending on the region of tumor genome sequenced, types of mutations included, methods of subtracting germline variants and other aspects of bioinformatic analysis pipeline of the sequencing data [3,15]. Both the FDA-approved FoundationOne CDx (F1CDx) panel and the FDA-authorized Memorial Sloan Kettering-Integrated Mutation Profiling of Actionable Cancer Targets (MSK-IMPACT) panel used correlation between panel- and WES-based TMB to validate the reliability of panel based TMB estimation, and they claimed that these panels can assess TMB accurately ($R = 0.74$ for F1CDx and $R = 0.76$ for MSK-IMPACT) [2,13,16]. However, as Wu et al. [13] proposed in their recent work, the overall correlation between the panel- and WES-based TMB could be substantially distorted by outliers (i.e., cases with relatively ultra-high TMB within each cancer type) [13], which might lead to overestimation of the reliability of panel-based TMB estimation. Therefore, additional studies are needed to evaluate the significance of correlation between the WES-based and targeted panel-based TMB values.

As already mentioned, TMB is considered to be a proxy for cancer cell neo-antigenicity and therefore could potentially serve as a predictive biomarker of therapeutic response to ICI. Several studies, especially in NSCLC, retrospectively employed WES or larger NGS panels to determine TMB as a potential response predictor [17–19]. Unfortunately, the definition of cut-off values to separate "high TMB" from "low TMB" tumors is not consistent in recent NSCLC trials. For example, in the CheckMate (CM) trials CM012 (nivolumab and ipilimumab) [20], CM227 (nivolumab and ipilimumab) [17] and CM026 (nivolumab only) [21] cut-points of 158 mutations, 199 mutations and 243 somatic missense mutations (number of mutations estimated from a commercial gene panel based cut point of 10 mutations per Mbp) were used, respectively [22].

This is the first study in pediatric oncology that aims to assess the reliability of TMB estimation using real-life WES across multiple cancer types and in silico analysis of two major gene panels, which are widely used for routine diagnostics in clinical practice, where various settings of bioinformatic pipeline were employed. The performance and correlation of WES and panel-based TMB assessment methods were evaluated together with potential consequences for clinical decision making where various cut-offs for ICI indication were used.

2. Results

2.1. Comparison of TMB between Real-Life WES and In Silico Targeted Gene Panels

We successfully performed germline and somatic WES and calculated TMB in 106 pediatric patients of 28 distinct cancer types. We stratified patients based on their diagnosis and expressed TMB for each group of patients as a median (min–max) or as a concrete value in cases where there was only one patient within a group (summarized in Table 1). WES-based TMB for each tumor is depicted in Figure 1. The median TMB ranged widely among diagnoses, from 0.3 mutations/Mb in myeloid sarcoma to 14.2 mutations/Mb in Burkitt lymphoma.

Table 1. Comparison of TMB determined by real-life WES and in silico targeted gene panels.

Diagnosis	TMB WES—M1 * Real-Life (Median/Value)	(Min–Max)	TMB MSK—M1 * In Silico (Median/Value)	(Min–Max)	TMB F1CDx—M2 ** In Silico (Median/Value)	(Min–Max)
HGG glioma H3K27M+	2.9	(1.6–15.7)	4.7	(2.6–17.9)	4.5	(2.6–31)
Rhabdomyosarcoma	3.6	(1.7–6.4)	2.6	(1.7–4.3)	2.6	(0–5.2)
Ewing sarcoma	3.1	(0.2–5.1)	2.6	(0–5.1)	2.6	(0–7.8)
Ependymoma	3.1	(1.3–10.4)	1.7	(0–5.1)	3.2	(1.3–9)
Neuroblastoma	3.8	(1.6–17.2)	3.0	(0.9–7.7)	4.5	(1.3–15.5)
Soft tissue sarcoma	3.6	(1.7–6.7)	3.4	(0–6.8)	3.2	(0–9)
Low-grade glioma	3.5	(1.6–6.8)	2.1	(0.9–4.3)	3.9	(1.3–5.2)
High-grade glioma H3K27M wt	4.5	(1.4–269.8)	3.4	(0.9–294.7)	5.2	(1.3–410.9)
Osteosarcoma	2.2	(1.9–7.5)	3.4	(0–5.1)	5.2	(1.3–6.5)
Burkitt lymphoma	14.2	(6.1–100.7)	19.6	(6.8–46.1)	27.1	(6.5–89.2)
Medulloblastoma	3.8	(3.5–63.6)	3.4	(0.9–61.5)	3.9	(1.3–89.2)
Fibromatosis	6.2	(1.1–56.2)	5.1	(1.7–29)	10.3	(1.3–82.7)
Wilms tumor	3.1	(2.3–3.9)	3.4	(2.6–4.3)	2.6	(1.3–3.9)
Renal cell carcinoma	1.8	(1.5–2.1)	4.3	(2.6–6.0)	4.5	(1.3–7.8)
Adrenocortical carcinoma	0.9	-	0.9	-	1.3	-
Plexus choroideus carcinoma	5.2	-	2.6	-	5.2	-
Hepatocellular carcinoma	3.6	-	0.9	-	3.9	-
Disseminated adenocarcinoma	2.3	-	4.3	-	6.5	-
Familiar infantile myofibromatosis	2.1	-	1.7	-	0.0	-
Myeloid sarcoma	0.3	-	0.0	-	0.0	-
Undifferentiated embryonal tumor of spinal canal	3.1	-	2.6	-	2.6	-
Nongerminomatous Germ Cell tumor CNS	2.3	-	1.7	-	1.3	-
Epithelial hepatoblastoma	0.5	-	0.0	-	0.0	-
Spindle cell hemangioma	2.1	-	0.9	-	2.6	-

Table 1. Cont.

Fibrodysplasia ossificans progressiva	3.1	-	2.6	-	2.6	-
Hepatosplenic T-lymphoma	0.4	-	0.9	-	0.0	-
Multisystemic Langerhans cell histiocytosis	3.1	-	2.6	-	3.9	-
Gastrointestinal stromal tumor	2.7	-	3.4	-	6.5	-

* M1—Method 1 for calculation of TMB excluding synonymous variants and indels; ** M2—Method 2 for calculation of TMB including synonymous variants and indels.

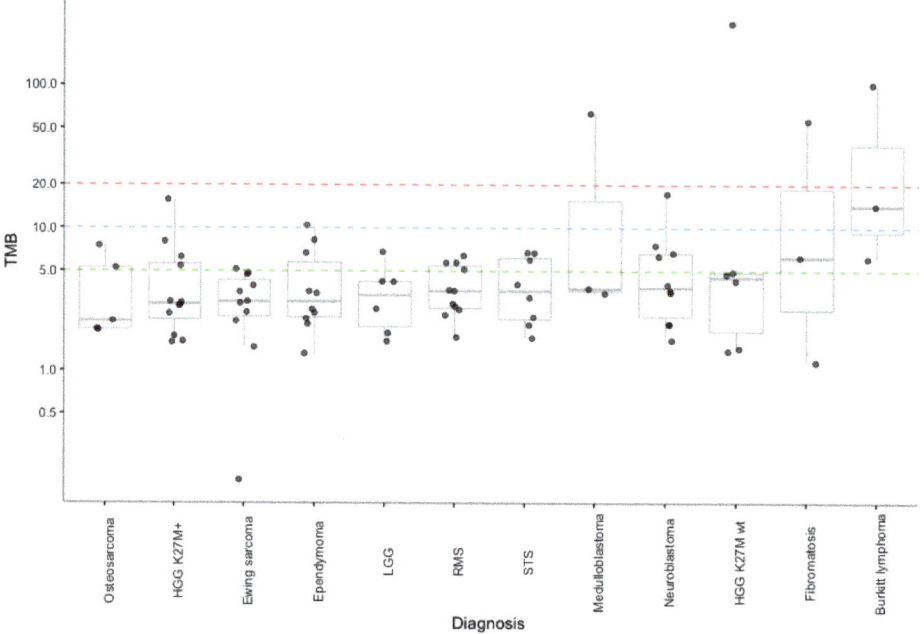

Figure 1. Tumor mutational burden (TMB) values determined in our pediatric cancer patient cohort (WES—Method1) stratified by cancer type. Hypothetical TMB cut-off values are shown as dashed lines (green, TMB ≥ 5; blue, TMB ≥ 10, red, TMB ≥ 20).

Furthermore, we determined, by an in silico approach, whether TMB, as measured by WES, correlates with TMB calculated by the gene sets and bioinformatic approaches used by two commercially available targeted gene panels. Panel-based TMB (MSK-IMPACT and F1CDx) for each group of patients expressed as a median (min–max) or as a concrete value in cases where there was only one patient in a group are summarized in Table 2. We confirmed a strong Pearson correlation of the panel TMB with the WES-based TMB characterized by $R = 0.993$ (F1CDx), and $R = 0.974$ (MSK-IMPACT), respectively (Figure 2A,C). Correlation between MSK-IMPACT and F1CDx panels was $R = 0.993$ (Figure 2B). The TMB assessment method was adapted for each panel accordingly (MSK-IMPACT—Method 1; F1CDx—Method 2). However, when the few hypermutated cases were excluded and only samples with TMB <10 mut/Mb were considered for analysis, the correlation decreased significantly: $R = 0.514$ (F1CDx), and $R = 0.560$ (MSK-IMPACT). Correlation between TMBs determined by the two panels remained remarkably higher ($R = 0.726$).

Table 2. Comparison of TMB determined by real-life WES and the FMI laboratory testing service FoundationOne Heme (F1Heme).

Gender	Age at Diagnosis	Diagnosis	TMB F1Heme Real-Life (Mut/Mb)	TMB WES—M1 * Real-Life (Mut/Mb)	Same Sample (Yes/No)
F	9	Renal cell carcinoma	1.63	1.45	yes
F	7	Diffuse intrinsic pontine glioma H3K27M+	2.44	1.60	yes
M	13	Desmoid fibromatosis	0.81	1.14	yes
M	6	Spindle cell hemangioma	0.81	2.05	yes
F	14	Gastrointestinal stromal tumor	4.07	2.71	yes
F	14	Osteosarcoma	2.44	1.91	yes
M	2	Langerhans cell histiocytosis	2.44	3.11	yes
M	11	Wilms tumor	1.63	2.34	yes
M	11	Ewing sarcoma	1.63	2.57	yes
F	7	Ependymoma	2.44	3.48	yes
M	18	Embryonal rhabdomyosarcoma	4.89	2.82	yes
F	14	Ewing sarcoma	1.63	3.57	yes
F	6	Wilms tumor	0.81	3.91	yes
F	18	Ewing sarcoma	0.81	2.97	yes
M	9	Alveolar rhabdomyosarcoma	3.26	3.62	yes
F	5	Diffuse intrinsic pontine glioma	2.44	2.85	yes
M	10	Ewing sarcoma	1.63	0.17	yes
F	1	Neuroblastoma	1.63	7.53	yes
F	10	Ewing sarcoma	7.33	4.82	yes
M	20	Glioblastoma H3G34R+	7.33	8.02	yes
F	2	Neuroblastoma	5.70	6.33	yes
F	1	Embryonal rhabdomyosarcoma	1.63	6.39	yes
M	3	Burkitt lymphoma	10.59	6.08	yes
M	7	Burkitt lymphoma	19.55	14.18	yes
M	18	Glioblastoma	265.56	269.75	yes
F	10	Low-grade astroblastoma	1.63	1.83	no
M	4	Adrenocortical carcinoma	0.00	0.88	no
M	15	Hepatocellular carcinoma	2.44	3.59	no
M	3	Epithelial hepatoblastoma	2.44	0.46	no
M	5	Embryonal rhabdomyosarcoma	6.52	3.68	no
M	3	Embryonal rhabdomyosarcoma	4.07	5.71	no
F	7	Glioblastoma	0.81	4.48	no
M	1	Anaplastic ependymoma	1.63	6.65	no
F	4	Diffuse intrinsic pontine glioma H3K27M+	9.78	5.39	no

* M1—Method 1 for calculation of TMB excluding synonymous variants and indels.

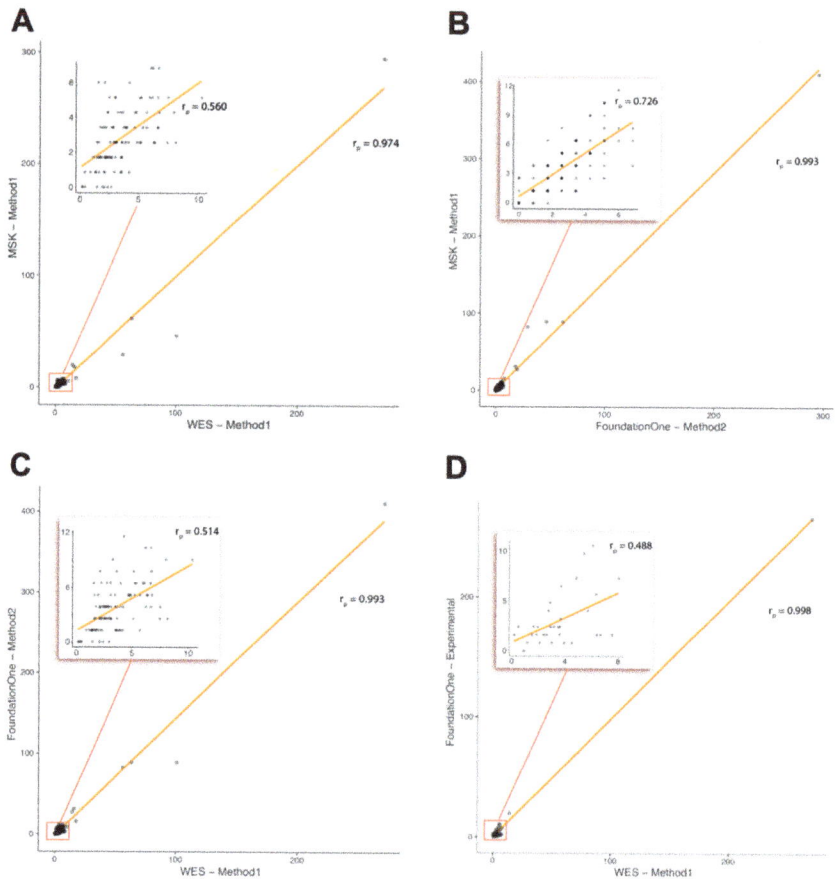

Figure 2. Correlation of tumor mutational burden (TMB) determined by real-life WES and targeted gene panels: real-life WES vs. in silico MSK-IMPACT (**A**), in silico F1CDx vs. MSK-IMPACT (**B**), real-life WES vs. in silico F1CDx (**C**), real-life WES vs. real-life laboratory service F1Heme (**D**).

2.2. Comparison of TMB between Real-Life WES and the Foundation Medicine Inc. (FMI) Testing Service (Subcohort of Patients)

In the subgroup of 34 patients (randomly selected from the patients where a Formalin-Fixed Paraffin-Embedded (FFPE) block with tumor tissue was available), comparative study of real-life WES-based TMB assessment and the FMI testing service was performed. For the WES samples, tumor and normal tissue were each sequenced in order to distinguish germline polymorphisms from somatic mutations. For the targeted FMI testing, no matched normal material was sequenced; rather, genomic variants were stringently filtered to eliminate germline polymorphisms, as declared by the vendor. For TMB determination from WES data, we used Method 1 (excluding indels and synonymous mutations). The FMI testing services are done using Method 2 (including indels and synonymous mutations). In nine cases, different samples from one resection or biopsy collection were used. This is summarized in Table 2. However, the Pearson correlation between TMBs determined by these two real-life approaches was comparable to the correlation of real-life WES and in silico F1CDx panel (R = 0.998 vs. R = 0.993) indicating the relevance of the in silico approach for TMB assessment comparative studies. When hypermutated cases were excluded, correlation decreased to R = 0.488 (Figure 2D), which is similar to the decrease observed in the in silico approach (R = 0.514).

2.3. WES-Based TMB Values during Tumor Progression

In nine cases, we determined the TMB by WES in sequential tumor biopsies or tumor tissues from surgical resection. In five cases, we used tumor tissue from a primary tumor and its relapse. In the remaining four cases, tumor tissue was collected from two consequent local or metastatic relapses. TMB values are summarized in Table 3. In seven out of nine cases, an increase in TMB in the second tumor tissue was observed, with the average increase being 1.6 ± 1.3 mut/Mb.

Table 3. WES-based TMB values during tumor progression in nine patient case cohorts.

Gender	Age at Diagnosis	Diagnosis	Diagnosis/Relapse	Year of Biopsy	TMB (WES M1 *) Real-Life
F	9	Supratentorial ependymoma	local relapse	2016	2.31
			local relapse	2018	3.88
F	1	Neuroblastoma	metastatic relapse	2017	7.53
			metastatic relapse	2018	3.17
M	11	Ewing sarcoma	primary tumor	2017	2.57
			local relapse	2018	4.19
M	5	DIPG	primary tumor	2015	2.51
			local relapse	2018	6.68
F	10	LG astroblastoma	primary tumor	2017	1.83
			local relapse	2018	3.05
M	3	Epithelial hepatoblastoma	primary tumor	2016	0.46
			local relapse	2018	2.48
F	2	Ependymoma	primary tumor	2014	10.38
			metastatic relapse	2018	10.53
M	18	Osteosarcoma	metastatic relapse	2018	7.47
			metastatic relapse	2018	8.10
M	1	Infantile myofibromatosis	metastatic relapse	2015	2.08
			metastatic relapse	2018	1.88

* M1—Method 1 for calculation of TMB excluding synonymous variants and indels.

2.4. Consequence of TMB Assessment Method for ICI Indication

TMB as a predictive biomarker is currently the focus of several clinical trials with ICI. We have evaluated how the sequencing region (WES vs. the gene set used in MSK-IMPACT vs. the gene set used in F1CDx) and method for TMB calculation affect the final TMB and potential ICI indication when various hypothetical cut-off values are applied. Results of this analysis are summarized in Table 4. As expected, the number of patients above a cut-off is always higher with WES-based TMB assessment (compared to panel-based) and when TMB is assessed by Method 2 (including indels and synonymous mutations). Number of patients above a cut-off differs significantly when low TMB cut-off value is applied (cut-off ≥ 5). With the increasing cut-off values, the significance of technological variability introduced by sequencing various genome regions and different TMB calculating methods decreases. However, even with a relatively high cut-off value (cut-off ≥ 20), the number of pediatric patients hypothetically indicated for ICI therapy differs between TMB groups calculated with Method 1 and Method 2 (e.g., four vs. seven pediatric patients with WES).

Table 4. WES-based TMB values during tumor progression in nine patient case cohorts.

	TMB—M1 * In Silico (Number of Cases Above Cut-Off)			TMB—M2 ** In Silico (Number of Cases Above Cut-Off)		
Cut-off for ICIs Indication (mut/Mb)	≥5	≥10	≥20	≥5	≥10	≥20
WES	30	8	4	75	25	7
MSK-IMPACT	23	6	4	61	12	6
F1CDx	24	7	5	42	11	6

* M1—Method 1 for calculation of TMB excluding synonymous variants and indels; ** M2—Method 2 for calculation of TMB including synonymous variants and indels; ICIs—immune checkpoint inhibitors.

3. Discussion

The predictive power of TMB as a biomarker for response to ICI is currently being investigated in many clinical trials across various cancer types. Patients with a higher TMB are more likely to respond to ICI in various settings, including PD-(L)1 blockade in NSCLC [10], CTLA-4 blockade in malignant melanoma [11], and combined PD(L)-1 and CTLA-4 blockade in NSCLC [17]. Studies have shown that TMB is to a large extent independent of the PD-L1 status and might thereby identify additional subgroups of patients who benefit from ICI [17,20,22].

Based on these clinical observations, TMB became an emerging predictive biomarker for ICI in various cancer types, and an urgent need occurred to answer the questions concerning the technological aspects affecting TMB detection by WES and targeted panel sequencing to ensure implementation of lab developed tests that guarantee optimal reference standard quality for patient stratification [19].

In initial studies, WES was widely used to determine TMB and is still considered to be the gold standard; however, targeted sequencing panels are more readily interpretable and are a more pragmatic and potentially cost-effective approach to TMB testing in clinical diagnostics [3]. While in the context of clinical trial, TMB testing is mainly carried out by commercial vendors, many clinical laboratories depending on the regulatory approval context may eventually use in-house designed panels to determine TMB scores [22]. Endris and others have already investigated the minimum required size of a gene panel by comprehensive in silico analyses of available WES data sets and have shown that at least 1 Mbp of exonic and/or intronic region should be sequenced to achieve a similar power in discriminating ICI responders from non-responders comparable to WES [19]. Furthermore, Buchhalter at al. showed that "size does matter", with an optimal panel size being between 1.5 and 3 Mbp, considering the benefit–cost ratio, and that the inclusion of all point mutations (instead of only missense mutations) in the TMB calculation is possible and recommendable to enhance precision [9].

In our study, we focused on the potential technological variability introduced to TMB scoring by the usage of various platforms and bioinformatic pipelines for their assessment in pediatric tumors. As a reference method, we performed WES and subsequently in silico simulated two most frequently used sequencing panels, MSK-IMPACT and F1CDx. We confirmed a strong Pearson correlation of the panel-based TMB with the WES-based TMB; however, when the few hypermutated cases were excluded and only samples with TMB < 10 mut/Mb were considered for analysis, the correlation decreased significantly (Figure 2). This indicates a significant bias introduced to correlation analysis by only a few hypermutated cases included in the study. Correlation between samples with TMB < 10 mut/Mb was not satisfactory and probably lead to significant clinical misclassifications in the routine diagnostic scenario based on the usage of a cut-off value in the range of 5 to 15 mut/Mb. Similar observations were also provided by other authors describing adult tumors [9,19].

In a subgroup of patients, we performed a comparative study of real-life WES-based TMB assessment and the FMI testing service where we observed a similar effect of the hypermutated cases on the correlation significance. In agreement with others [9,19], we observed that the identification of high TMB tumors can be reliably achieved by any of the tested methods (cases with ultra-hypermutated tumors). However, the vast majority of tumors have intermediate TMB values; in these cases, a technological variability interferes with the reliable differentiation between TMB-high and low tumors [9,19].

In nine cases, we determined the TMB by WES in sequential tumor biopsies or tumor tissues from surgical resection. As expected, in seven out of nine cases, there was an increase in TMB in the second tumor with the average increase being approx. 2 mut/Mb. Surprisingly, in two cases, we observed a decrease in TMB, which could be explained mainly by the quality of the tumor tissue specimen and a low content of tumor cells in the second tumor which could decrease detectable mutations used for TMB assessment. It is important to mention that tumor content in the tissue specimens is an important factor affecting TMB scoring and is often not considered in TMB studies.

Finally, we evaluated how the sequencing region (WES vs. the gene set used in MSK-IMPACT vs. the gene set used in F1CDx) and the bioinformatic pipeline used for TMB calculation affect the final TMB and potential ICI indication when various hypothetical cut-off values are applied. In general, as expected, the number of patients above a cut-off is always higher in WES-based TMB assessment (compared to panel-based) and when the TMB is assessed by Method 2 (including indels and synonymous mutations). We also found that with the increasing cut-off values, the significance of technological variability and consequent clinical misclassification decreases. However, certain combinations of settings of TMB assessment methods (e.g., WES-M2 vs. F1CDx-M1), compounded by the use of a cut-off value of 10 mut/Mb, yield extremely different results. While the first approach predicts 25 patients to be good responders to ICI, the second approach predicts only seven patients. This indicates a potentially very strong misclassification issue for routine diagnostics. Based on the currently available results from clinical trials, it is very difficult to judge whether TMB assessed by Method 1 or Method 2 is a more accurate predictive biomarker of response to ICI therapy. Unfortunately, this in silico modeling has not been performed in the context of clinical outcomes from ICI trials.

4. Materials and Methods

4.1. Patients and Biological Specimens

We reviewed tumor mutational burden (TMB) results from 106 patients with pediatric high-risk/recurrent solid tumors (both newly diagnosed and relapsed) who had undergone laboratory WES at Central European Institute of Technology (CEITEC, Masaryk University, Brno, Czech Republic). Informed consent was obtained from all patients and all experiments using clinical samples were performed in accordance with the approved international guidelines. After surgical resection of the tumor or collection of the tumor biopsies, tissue samples were evaluated by an experienced surgical pathologist for the tumor cell content, and only specimens with more than 20% of the tumor cells were included. In addition, peripheral blood was collected to obtain DNA for germline WES. Number of patients stratified according to their diagnoses and related clinical data are summarized in Table 5. In nine cases, we collected two consequent tissue specimens (diagnosis/relapse or two relapses) and both were used for WES and TMB assessment.

4.2. DNA Isolation

Tumor DNA was extracted from the FFPE samples or fresh frozen tissues using QIAmp DNA FFPE Tissue Kit (Qiagen, Venlo, The Netherland) or QIAamp DNA Micro Kit (Qiagen). Germline DNA was extracted from peripheral blood leukocytes using QIAamp DNA Micro Kit (Qiagen). The purified DNA was quantified using Qubit 2.0 Fluorometer and NanoDrop 2000c spectrophotometer (both Thermo Fisher Scientific, MA, USA).

Table 5. Number of patients stratified according to their diagnoses and baseline clinical data.

Diagnosis	Number of Patients	Gender Ratio (F/M)	Age Median	Age (Min–Max)	Type of Sample Ratio (Primary Tumor/Local or Metastatic Relapse)
High-grade glioma H3K27M+	12	8/2	9	4–20	12/0
Rhabdomyosarcoma	11	7/4	5	0–18	6/5
Ewing sarcoma	11	6/5	11	8–18	2/9
Neuroblastoma	10	6/4	2	1–8	1/9
Ependymoma	10	6/4	5.5	1–16	4/6
Non-rhabdomyosarcoma soft-tissue sarcomas	8	2/6	12	8–19	0/8
High-grade glioma H3K27M wt	6	0/6	16	8–23	5/1
Low-grade glioma	6	1/5	9.5	3–19	1/5
Osteosarcoma	5	4/1	18	14–28	0/5
Burkitt lymphoma	3	0/3	7	3–12	0/3
Medulloblastoma	3	0/3	4	2–5	1/2
Fibromatosis	3	1/2	17	13–20	1/2
Wilms tumor	2	1/1	8.5	6–11	1/1
Renal cell carcinoma	2	1/1	13.5	9–18	1/0
Adrenocortical carcinoma	1	F	4	-	primary tumor
Choroid plexus carcinoma	1	M	1	-	primary tumor
Hepatocellular carcinoma	1	M	15	-	primary tumor
Lung adenocarcinoma	1	F	15	-	metastatic relapse
Familiar infantile myofibromatosis	1	M	1	-	primary tumor
Myeloid sarcoma	1	F	5	-	primary tumor
Undifferentiated embryonal tumor of spinal canal	1	M	2	-	local relapse
CNS germ cell tumor	1	M	11	-	primary tumor
Epithelial hepatoblastoma	1	M	3	-	primary tumor
Spindle cell hemangioendothelioma	1	M	6	-	primary vascular malformation
Fibrodysplasia ossificans progressiva	1	F	1	-	primary tumor
Hepatosplenic T-lymphoma	1	M	17	-	diagnostic aspiration/bone marrow
Multiple system Langerhans cell histiocytosis	1	M	2	-	metastasis
Gastrointestinal stromal tumor	1	F	14	-	metastatic relapse

4.3. Whole Exome Sequencing

Libraries for whole exome capture and sequencing were prepared using TruSeq Exome Kit (Illumina, CA, USA) according to manufacturer's recommendations. Quantity and quality of the exome libraries were checked using Qubit 2.0 Fluorometer and NanoDrop 2000c spectrophotometer (Thermo Fisher Scientific). Prepared libraries were loaded onto NextSeq 500/550 Mid Output Kit (150 cycles) and sequenced on the NextSeq 500 instrument (both Illumina). Sequencing coverage for both exomes was >20 × at >90% of captured regions.

4.4. Bioinformatic Analysis

Sequencing reads in FASTQ format were mapped to the human reference genome hg19 with the BWA-MEM algorithm [23] for both the tumor and the healthy control sample. The resulting alignments in BAM format were postprocessed with the SAMBLASTER program [24] for marking PCR duplicates. The final alignment file of the control sample was used to assess single nucleotide variants (SNVs) and short insertions/deletions (indels). Two variant callers were used for germline variant calling; the GATK HaplotypeCaller [25] and VarDict [26]. Reported variants were annotated with Annovar [27] and Oncotator [28] annotation programs. Tumor specific variants were assessed by somatic (paired; tumor vs. control) variant calling. For this purpose, we used GATK MuTect2 (SNVs), Scalpel [29] (Indels), and VarDict (SNVs and Indels) variant callers. The annotation of somatic variants was performed with the addition of the COSMIC database [30]. Overview of the bioinformatic pipeline is depicted in Figure 3.

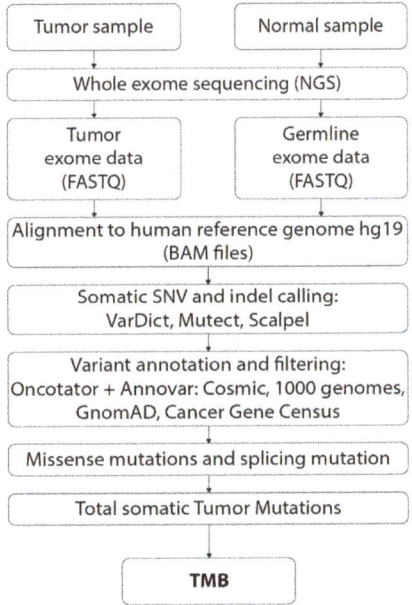

Figure 3. Workflow for tumor mutational burden (TMB) assessment by WES in this study.

4.5. Tumor Mutational Burden Estimation

An annotated list of somatic variants from the previous step was used to assess the TMB. We chose to compare two methods of TMB estimation, both based on publicly available approaches.

Method 1 (M1)—In our laboratory, we only consider somatic single nucleotide variants (SNVs) for TMB calculation from WES data, since indels (short insertions and deletions) tend to be called with high false positive rates and could potentially skew the outcome. Additionally, two bases before and after each exon are considered as splicing mutations. Synonymous variants are filtered out, as they do not fit the definition of TMB. Finally, variants with variant allele frequency (VAF) of less than 5% are also filtered out. This approach is also used by MSK-IMPACT NGS panel.

Method 2 (M2)—This approach, used by the Foundation Medicine Inc. (FMI) targeted panels (e.g., F1CDx [2] as well as F1Heme), defines TMB as the number of SNVs (including synonymous variants) and indels in the coding regions of targeted genes. However, splicing variants are not included. A 5% cut-off for the VAF was also applied.

For the final TMB calculation, in both methods, the sum of variants remaining after application of the all filters, is then divided by the size (in megabases) of the target region from which the variants have been assessed. The target regions together with their sizes are listed below.

Both methods were applied to the three target regions (as shown in Table 5):

1. All coding sequences (whole exome; 35 Mb; using M1 for TMB calculation);
2. The coding sequences of genes analyzed by the FMI (F1CDx panel; 324 cancer-related genes; 0,8 Mbl using M2 for TMB calculation);
3. The coding sequences of genes analyzed by the Memorial Sloan Kettering Cancer Center (MSK-IMPACT; 468 cancer-related genes; 1.22 Mb; using M1 for TMB calculation)

The coding region locations on the hg19 genome were downloaded from the UCSC web site.

4.6. Comparative Study with the Foundation Medicine Inc. (FMI) Sequencing Service

FFPE tumor tissue samples of 34 patients who were previously examined by WES in our laboratory and were sent to the FMI for the FoundationOne Heme (F1Heme) test, which is recommended by vendor for pediatric tumors. In the nine cases, WES was performed using fresh frozen tissue, while different FFPE samples were sent for the F1Heme test. These specimens are indicated in the summarizing tables (Table 3) with the TMB results.

5. Conclusions

We present a study, where, for the first time in the context of pediatric tumors, the reliability of TMB estimation across multiple pediatric cancer types using real-life WES and in silico analysis of two major targeted gene panels was assessed. We confirmed a significant technological variability introduced by different laboratory technologies and various settings of bioinformatic pipelines. These results may provide valuable information for improving the accuracy of TMB estimation based on targeted gene panel sequencing in a diagnostic setting. Our study confirmed previous observations from adult tumors and thus supports the incentive to establish concordance between assay platforms used across different clinical trials in order to achieve a successful real-world implementation of TMB testing. To this end, worldwide efforts to ensure the harmonization of TMB assessment are ongoing [31–33].

Author Contributions: Conceptualization, H.N., K.P., T.H., J.S. and O.S.; data curation, M.K., K.P., T.M., P.M., K.P., T.C.I., S.A., M.J. and L.K.; formal analysis, M.K., K.P. and O.S.; funding acquisition, J.S. and O.S.; Investigation, H.N., M.K., T.M., P.M., K.P., T.C.I., S.A., M.J., L.K. and J.S.; methodology, S.A. and T.H.; project administration, H.N. and O.S.; resources, L.K. and J.S.; supervision, J.S. and O.S.; validation, T.M., P.M., K.P., T.C.I., S.A. and L.K.; visualization, M.J.; writing—original draft, H.N. and O.S.; writing—review and editing, H.N., K.P., T.H., J.S. and O.S. All authors have read and agreed to the published version of the manuscript.

Funding: This work has been supported by Roche supplying FoundationOne Heme tests and by the Czech Ministry of Health, grant no 16-33209A. Roche did not have any role in the study design, data collection and analysis, decision to publish, or preparation of the manuscript.

Conflicts of Interest: The authors declare no conflict of interest.

References

1. Stratton, M.R.; Campbell, P.J.; Futreal, P.A. The cancer genome. *Nature* **2009**, *458*, 719–724. [CrossRef] [PubMed]

2. Chalmers, Z.R.; Connelly, C.F.; Fabrizio, D.; Gay, L.; Ali, S.M.; Ennis, R.; Schrock, A.; Campbell, B.; Shlien, A.; Chmielecki, J.; et al. Analysis of 100,000 human cancer genomes reveals the landscape of tumor mutational burden. *Genome Med.* **2017**, *9*, 34. [CrossRef] [PubMed]
3. Chang, H.; Sasson, A.; Srinivasan, S.; Golhar, R.; Greenawalt, D.M.; Geese, W.J.; Green, G.; Zerba, K.; Kirov, S.; Szustakowski, J. Bioinformatic Methods and Bridging of Assay Results for Reliable Tumor Mutational Burden Assessment in Non-Small-Cell Lung Cancer. *Mol. Diagn. Ther.* **2019**, *23*, 507–520. [CrossRef] [PubMed]
4. Lawrence, M.S.; Stojanov, P.; Polak, P.; Kryukov, G.V.; Cibulskis, K.; Sivachenko, A.; Carter, S.L.; Stewart, C.; Mermel, C.H.; Roberts, S.A.; et al. Mutational heterogeneity in cancer and the search for new cancer-associated genes. *Nature* **2013**, *499*, 214–218. [CrossRef] [PubMed]
5. Hodi, F.S.; O'Day, S.J.; McDermott, D.F.; Weber, R.W.; Sosman, J.A.; Haanen, J.B.; Gonzalez, R.; Robert, C.; Schadendorf, D.; Hassel, J.C.; et al. Improved survival with ipilimumab in patients with metastatic melanoma. *N. Engl. J. Med.* **2010**, *363*, 711–723. [CrossRef] [PubMed]
6. Borghaei, H.; Paz-Ares, L.; Horn, L.; Spigel, D.R.; Steins, M.; Ready, N.E.; Chow, L.Q.; Vokes, E.E.; Felip, E.; Holgado, E.; et al. Nivolumab versus Docetaxel in Advanced Nonsquamous Non-Small-Cell Lung Cancer. *N. Engl. J. Med.* **2015**, *373*, 1627–1639. [CrossRef]
7. Motzer, R.J.; Escudier, B.; McDermott, D.F.; George, S.; Hammers, H.J.; Srinivas, S.; Tykodi, S.S.; Sosman, J.A.; Procopio, G.; Plimack, E.R.; et al. Nivolumab versus Everolimus in Advanced Renal-Cell Carcinoma. *N. Engl. J. Med.* **2015**, *373*, 1803–1813. [CrossRef]
8. Powles, T.; Eder, J.P.; Fine, G.D.; Braiteh, F.S.; Loriot, Y.; Cruz, C.; Bellmunt, J.; Burris, H.A.; Petrylak, D.P.; Teng, S.L.; et al. MPDL3280A (anti-PD-L1) treatment leads to clinical activity in metastatic bladder cancer. *Nature* **2014**, *515*, 558–562. [CrossRef]
9. Buchhalter, I.; Rempel, E.; Endris, V.; Allgauer, M.; Neumann, O.; Volckmar, A.L.; Kirchner, M.; Leichsenring, J.; Lier, A.; von Winterfeld, M.; et al. Size matters: Dissecting key parameters for panel-based tumor mutational burden analysis. *Int. J. Cancer* **2019**, *144*, 848–858. [CrossRef]
10. Rizvi, N.A.; Hellmann, M.D.; Snyder, A.; Kvistborg, P.; Makarov, V.; Havel, J.J.; Lee, W.; Yuan, J.; Wong, P.; Ho, T.S.; et al. Cancer immunology. Mutational landscape determines sensitivity to PD-1 blockade in non-small cell lung cancer. *Science* **2015**, *348*, 124–128. [CrossRef]
11. Snyder, A.; Makarov, V.; Merghoub, T.; Yuan, J.; Zaretsky, J.M.; Desrichard, A.; Walsh, L.A.; Postow, M.A.; Wong, P.; Ho, T.S.; et al. Genetic basis for clinical response to CTLA-4 blockade in melanoma. *N. Engl. J. Med.* **2014**, *371*, 2189–2199. [CrossRef] [PubMed]
12. Warr, A.; Robert, C.; Hume, D.; Archibald, A.; Deeb, N.; Watson, M. Exome Sequencing: Current and Future Perspectives. *G3 Genes Genomes Genet.* **2015**, *5*, 1543–1550. [CrossRef] [PubMed]
13. Wu, H.X.; Wang, Z.X.; Zhao, Q.; Wang, F.; Xu, R.H. Designing gene panels for tumor mutational burden estimation: The need to shift from 'correlation' to 'accuracy'. *J. Immunother. Cancer* **2019**, *7*, 206. [CrossRef] [PubMed]
14. Gong, J.; Pan, K.; Fakih, M.; Pal, S.; Salgia, R. Value-based genomics. *Oncotarget* **2018**, *9*, 15792–15815. [CrossRef] [PubMed]
15. Schumacher, T.N.; Schreiber, R.D. Neoantigens in cancer immunotherapy. *Science* **2015**, *348*, 69–74. [CrossRef] [PubMed]
16. Zehir, A.; Benayed, R.; Shah, R.H.; Syed, A.; Middha, S.; Kim, H.R.; Srinivasan, P.; Gao, J.; Chakravarty, D.; Devlin, S.M.; et al. Mutational landscape of metastatic cancer revealed from prospective clinical sequencing of 10,000 patients. *Nat. Med.* **2017**, *23*, 703–713. [CrossRef]
17. Hellmann, M.D.; Ciuleanu, T.E.; Pluzanski, A.; Lee, J.S.; Otterson, G.A.; Audigier Valette, C.; Minenza, E.; Linardou, H.; Burgers, S.; Salman, P.; et al. Nivolumab plus Ipilimumab in Lung Cancer with a High Tumor Mutational Burden. *N. Engl. J. Med.* **2018**, *378*, 2093–2104. [CrossRef]
18. Yarchoan, M.; Hopkins, A.; Jaffee, E.M. Tumor Mutational Burden and Response Rate to PD-1 Inhibition. *N. Engl. J. Med.* **2017**, *377*, 2500–2501. [CrossRef]
19. Endris, V.; Buchhalter, I.; Allgauer, M.; Rempel, E.; Lier, A.; Volckmar, A.L.; Kirchner, M.; von Winterfeld, M.; Leichsenring, J.; Neumann, O.; et al. Measurement of tumor mutational. burden (TMB) in routine molecular diagnostics: In silico and real-life analysis of three larger gene panels. *Int. J. Cancer* **2019**, *144*, 2303–2312. [CrossRef]

20. Hellmann, M.D.; Nathanson, T.; Rizvi, H.; Creelan, B.C.; Sanchez-Vega, F.; Ahuja, A.; Ni, A.; Novik, J.B.; Mangarin, L.M.B.; Abu-Akeel, M.; et al. Genomic Features of Response to Combination Immunotherapy in Patients with Advanced Non-Small-Cell Lung Cancer. *Cancer Cell* **2018**, *33*, 843–852. [CrossRef]
21. Carbone, D.P.; Reck, M.; Paz-Ares, L.; Creelan, B.; Horn, L.; Steins, M.; Felip, E.; van den Heuvel, M.M.; Ciuleanu, T.E.; Badin, F.; et al. First-Line Nivolumab in Stage IV or Recurrent Non-Small-Cell Lung Cancer. *N. Engl. J. Med.* **2017**, *376*, 2415–2426. [CrossRef] [PubMed]
22. Budczies, J.; Allgauer, M.; Litchfield, K.; Rempel, E.; Christopoulos, P.; Kazdal, D.; Endris, V.; Thomas, M.; Frohling, S.; Peters, S.; et al. Optimizing panel-based tumor mutational burden (TMB) measurement. *Ann. Oncol.* **2019**, *30*, 1496–1506. [CrossRef] [PubMed]
23. Li, H. Aligning sequence reads, clone sequences and assembly contigs with BWA-MEM. *arXiv* **2013**, arXiv:1303.3997.
24. Faust, G.G.; Hall, I.M. SAMBLASTER: Fast duplicate marking and structural variant read extraction. *Bioinformatics* **2014**, *30*, 2503–2505. [CrossRef]
25. Poplin, R.; Ruano-Rubio, V.; DePristo, M.A.; Fennell, T.J.; Carneiro, M.O.; Van der Auwera, G.A.; Kling, D.E.; Gauthier, L.D.; Levy-Moonshine, A.; Roazen, D.; et al. Scaling accurate genetic variant discovery to tens of thousands of samples. *bioRxiv* **2017**, 201178.
26. Lai, Z.; Markovets, A.; Ahdesmaki, M.; Chapman, B.; Hofmann, O.; McEwen, R.; Johnson, J.; Dougherty, B.; Barrett, J.C.; Dry, J.R. VarDict: A novel and versatile variant caller for next-generation sequencing in cancer research. *Nucleic Acids Res.* **2016**, *44*, e108. [CrossRef]
27. Wang, K.; Li, M.; Hakonarson, H. ANNOVAR: Functional annotation of genetic variants from high-throughput sequencing data. *Nucleic Acids Res.* **2010**, *38*, e164. [CrossRef]
28. Ramos, A.H.; Lichtenstein, L.; Gupta, M.; Lawrence, M.S.; Pugh, T.J.; Saksena, G.; Meyerson, M.; Getz, G. Oncotator: Cancer variant annotation tool. *Hum. Mutat.* **2015**, *36*, E2423–E2429. [CrossRef]
29. Fang, H.; Bergmann, E.A.; Arora, K.; Vacic, V.; Zody, M.C.; Iossifov, I.; O'Rawe, J.A.; Wu, Y.; Jimenez Barron, L.T.; Rosenbaum, J.; et al. Indel variant analysis of short-read sequencing data with Scalpel. *Nat. Protoc.* **2016**, *11*, 2529–2548. [CrossRef]
30. Tate, J.G.; Bamford, S.; Jubb, H.C.; Sondka, Z.; Beare, D.M.; Bindal, N.; Boutselakis, H.; Cole, C.G.; Creatore, C.; Dawson, E.; et al. COSMIC: The Catalogue of Somatic Mutations In Cancer. *Nucleic Acids Res.* **2019**, *47*, D941–D947. [CrossRef]
31. Buttner, R.; Longshore, J.W.; Lopez-Rios, F.; Merkelbach-Bruse, S.; Normanno, N.; Rouleau, E.; Penault-Llorca, F. Implementing TMB measurement in clinical practice: Considerations on assay requirements. *ESMO Open* **2019**, *4*, e000442. [CrossRef] [PubMed]
32. Deans, Z.C.; Costa, J.L.; Cree, I.; Dequeker, E.; Edsjo, A.; Henderson, S.; Hummel, M.; Ligtenberg, M.J.; Loddo, M.; Machado, J.C.; et al. Integration of next-generation sequencing in clinical diagnostic molecular pathology laboratories for analysis of solid tumours; an expert opinion on behalf of IQN Path ASBL. *Virchows Arch.* **2017**, *470*, 5–20. [CrossRef] [PubMed]
33. Van Krieken, H.; Deans, S.; Hall, J.A.; Normanno, N.; Ciardiello, F.; Douillard, J.Y. Quality to rely on: Meeting report of the 5th Meeting of External Quality Assessment,c Naples 2016. *ESMO Open* **2016**, *1*, e000114. [CrossRef] [PubMed]

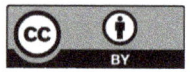

© 2020 by the authors. Licensee MDPI, Basel, Switzerland. This article is an open access article distributed under the terms and conditions of the Creative Commons Attribution (CC BY) license (http://creativecommons.org/licenses/by/4.0/).

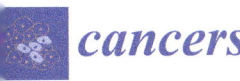

Article

Prevalence of DNA Repair Gene Mutations in Blood and Tumor Tissue and Impact on Prognosis and Treatment in HNSCC

Kimberly M. Burcher [1], Andrew T. Faucheux [1], Jeffrey W. Lantz [1], Harper L. Wilson [2], Arianne Abreu [3], Kiarash Salafian [1], Manisha J. Patel [1], Alexander H. Song [1], Robin M. Petro [1], Thomas Lycan, Jr. [1], Cristina M. Furdui [1], Umit Topaloglu [1], Ralph B. D'Agostino, Jr. [1], Wei Zhang [1] and Mercedes Porosnicu [1,*]

[1] Wake Forest Baptist Medical Center, Winston-Salem, NC 27157, USA; kburcher@wakehealth.edu (K.M.B.); afaucheu@wakehealth.edu (A.T.F.); jwlantz@wakehealth.edu (J.W.L.); ksalafia@wakehealth.edu (K.S.); manisha.patel10@gmail.com (M.J.P.); asong@wakehealth.edu (A.H.S.); rpetro@wakehealth.edu (R.M.P.); tlycan@wakehealth.edu (T.L.J.); cfurdui@wakehealth.edu (C.M.F.); Umit.Topaloglu@wakehealth.edu (U.T.); rdagosti@wakehealth.edu (R.B.D.J.); wezhang@wakehealth.edu (W.Z.)
[2] University of Kentucky Medical Center, Lexington, KY 40536, USA; harper.wilson@uky.edu
[3] Campbell University School of Osteopathic Medicine (CUSOM), Lillington, NC 27546, USA; a_abreu0419@email.campbell.edu
* Correspondence: mporosni@wakehealth.edu

Citation: Burcher, K.M.; Faucheux, A.T.; Lantz, J.W.; Wilson, H.L.; Abreu, A.; Salafian, K.; Patel, M.J.; Song, A.H.; Petro, R.M.; Lycan, T.J.; et al. Prevalence of DNA Repair Gene Mutations in Blood and Tumor Tissue and Impact on Prognosis and Treatment in HNSCC. *Cancers* **2021**, *13*, 3118. https://doi.org/10.3390/cancers13133118

Academic Editors: Nandini Dey and Pradip De

Received: 25 May 2021
Accepted: 16 June 2021
Published: 22 June 2021

Publisher's Note: MDPI stays neutral with regard to jurisdictional claims in published maps and institutional affiliations.

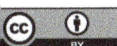

Copyright: © 2021 by the authors. Licensee MDPI, Basel, Switzerland. This article is an open access article distributed under the terms and conditions of the Creative Commons Attribution (CC BY) license (https://creativecommons.org/licenses/by/4.0/).

Simple Summary: The DNA damage repair (DDR) gene profile is largely unexplored in head and neck squamous cell cancer (HNSCC), leaving little known about the treatment of HNSCC with PARP inhibitors. In this retrospective study, the prevalence of mutated DDR genes was studied in the tissue and/or blood samples (tDNA and ctDNA samples, respectively) of 170 patients with HNSCC. These findings were correlated with demographic and outcome data. DDR gene mutations were significantly increased in older patients, patients with primary tumors located in the larynx, patients with more advanced cancers at diagnosis and patients previously treated with chemotherapy and/or radiotherapy. Patients with primary tumors in the oropharynx were less likely to have DDR gene mutations. Patients with DDR gene mutations identified in blood samples were found to have worse survival. The combined mutational analysis in blood and tumor demonstrated a high prevalence and an important prognostic role of DDR gene mutations in HNSCC, supporting further clinical research of PARP inhibitors in the genomic guided treatment of HNSCC.

Abstract: PARP inhibitors are currently approved for a limited number of cancers and targetable mutations in DNA damage repair (DDR) genes. In this single-institution retrospective study, the profiles of 170 patients with head and neck squamous cell cancer (HNSCC) and available tumor tissue DNA (tDNA) and circulating tumor DNA (ctDNA) results were analyzed for mutations in a set of 18 DDR genes as well as in gene subsets defined by technical and clinical significance. Mutations were correlated with demographic and outcome data. The addition of ctDNA to the standard tDNA analysis contributed to identification of a significantly increased incidence of patients with mutations in one or more genes in each of the study subsets of DDR genes in groups of patients older than 60 years, patients with laryngeal primaries, patients with advanced stage at diagnosis and patients previously treated with chemotherapy and/or radiotherapy. Patients with DDR gene mutations were found to be significantly less likely to have primary tumors within the in oropharynx or HPV-positive disease. Patients with ctDNA mutations in all subsets of DDR genes analyzed had significantly worse overall survival in univariate and adjusted multivariate analysis. This study underscores the utility of ctDNA analysis, alone, and in combination with tDNA, for defining the prevalence and the role of DDR gene mutations in HNSCC. Furthermore, this study fosters research promoting the utilization of PARP inhibitors in HNSCC precision oncology treatments.

Keywords: HNSCC; ctDNA; tDNA; DDR genes; PARP inhibitors

1. Introduction

Over the past decade, next generation sequencing (NGS) of genetic material contained in blood and tissue samples (tDNA and ctDNA, respectively) has revolutionized the field of oncology [1–3]. Such discoveries have allowed for the treatment of non-small cell lung cancer with *EGFR*, *ALK* and *MET* inhibitors and basal cell cancer with hedgehog pathway inhibitors with improved outcomes. These studies have also contributed to outcome data, which have improved the management of malignant melanoma found to have mutations in *BRAF*. Many have considered the targeted treatment plans derived from the NGS of tDNA and ctDNA to be oncology's first venture into the world of personalized medicine.

Despite the benefits of NGS in the management of many malignancies, the mutational landscape of squamous cell cancers of the head and neck (HNSCC) remains largely undescribed. This has left the field without targeted management strategies and reliable prognostication based on an individual cancer's genetic profile [4]. Though relatively little is known, early studies regarding mutations in HNSCC have begun to lay the necessary groundwork on which clinical trials may be based. For example, data suggest that loss of function mutations in p53 [5–7], retinoblastoma tumor suppressor [8,9] p16 [5] and activation of p63 (all constituents of the p53 pathway) [10–12] are known to be frequent mutations in HNSCC, with up to 80% of patients with HNSCC experiencing loss of function mutation in p53 [6,7]. Therapies targeted to this pathway (such as adenoviral p53 gene therapy and use of small molecules to restore TP53 function/disrupt inactivation of wild-type p53) have been proposed but are yet to meet fruition [13]. Mutations in the NOTCH pathway are detected less frequently but are estimated to occur in 17% of HPV-positive and 26% of HPV-negative HNSCCs [6]. Clinical trials for patients with *NOTCH1* mutations also remain in early phases [14]. Other mutations, including those in *EGFR*, *MET*, RAS/RAF/MAPK and JAK/STAT pathways, have also been described in HNSCC with respective treatments in various phases of investigation [4].

A recent retrospective analysis studied 75 patients with HNSCC and revealed that 38.8% of patients had alterations in one or more DNA repair genes (limited in that study to *APC*, *ATM*, *BRCA1* and *BRCA2*). Not only was this percentage higher than previous studies would suggest, but the study was also able to demonstrate that patients with such mutations in ctDNA were associated with decreased overall survival in univariate and multivariate analysis [15]. Theoretically, cells without functional copies of these genes (and others) with a direct or an indirect role in homologous recombination repair (HRR) or the Fanconi anemia (FA) pathway are sensitive to poly (ADP-ribose) polymerase (PARP) inhibition. Genes involved in HRR resolve breaks in DNA through a PARP-independent pathway. Defects in HRR result in hypersensitivity to a number of therapeutics, including PARP inhibitors, topoisomerase inhibitors and many other DNA break inducers. The genes that encompass the FA pathway encode similarly PARP-independent DNA repair machinery utilized to resolve interstrand crosslinks. Though classically associated with hypersensitivity to platinum-based chemotherapies, defects in these genes in HNSCC have been shown to create cell lineages that rely on PARP mechanisms for DNA repair [16–20]. When mutations in genes involved in HRR or the FA pathway confer loss of function, PARP inhibitors can be utilized to prevent repair of breaks in DNA, ultimately leading to cell death. All clinical PARP inhibitors inhibit both PARP1 and PARP2. PARP1 repairs double-strand DNA (dsDNA) breaks and single-strand DNA (ssDNA) breaks. PARP2 repairs only ssDNA breaks. The clinical utility of PARP inhibition lies in the concept of "synthetic lethality", in which neither a mutation in HHR genes nor PARP inhibition, alone, would be lethal to a cell, but the combination of the two factors in tumor cells ensures cell death [16].

PARP inhibitors are currently approved for breast, ovarian and pancreatic cancers carrying *BRCA1* or *BRCA2* mutations. The FDA has also approved use of PARP inhibitors for prostate cancers in which *BRCA1* or *BRCA2* or *ATM* mutations have been detected. Investigations regarding the use of PARP inhibitors in HNSCC are currently underway but are hindered by the low reported prevalence of mutations in applicable genes. Perhaps for this reason, these studies focus on their use in combination with traditional chemo- or radiotherapies rather than in cases in which NGS has directed decision making [21–23].

In this retrospective review, the investigators aim to validate previous findings regarding the prevalence and prognostic value of mutated DNA damage repair (DDR) genes in HNSCC utilizing combined genomic analysis performed both in blood and in tumor tissue (ctDNA and tDNA, respectively) in a larger patient population. In addition to the inclusion of a larger sample size, this study also expanded the DDR gene panel investigated based on recent studies involving PARP inhibitors [18]. The investigators aim to demonstrate a significant prevalence of DDR gene mutations in the genomic landscape of HNSCC which may assist in laying groundwork for NGS-guided investigations of PARP inhibitors in HNSCC. Correlation of patient characteristics and outcomes of tDNA and ctDNA sequencing results was also performed to assist in identification of patients with HNSCC likely to benefit from NGS.

2. Materials and Methods

This study is a single-institution retrospective review of adult patients with HNSCC who underwent NGS (tDNA, ctDNA or both) at Wake Forest Baptist Health between August 2014 and October 2020. The Wake Forest School of Medicine Institutional Review Board approved the study (IRB00057787). HNSCC patients were required to have had a valid tDNA and/or ctDNA test to be included in the study. Patients with cutaneous SCC or salivary gland cancers, as well as patients with other active primary cancers, were excluded.

Eighteen DDR genes (*BRCA1, BRCA2, ATM, BRIP1, BARD1, CDK12, CHEK1, CHEK2, FANCL, PALB2, PPP2R2A, RAD51B, RAD51C, RAD51D, RAD51L, APC, ARID1A* and *MLL3*) were selected for this study based on their involvement with HRR or the FA pathway [16–20]. All 18 genes were tested for tDNA mutations (substitutions, insertion and deletion alterations) by the FoundationOne platform (Foundation Medicine, Cambridge, MA, USA) (FM). Mutations in ctDNA (single nucleotide variants, including indels and fusion alterations) were tested for by the Guardant360 platform (G360) (Guardant Health, Redwood City, CA, USA). Variants of unknown significance were included in this analysis. Six of the eighteen genes selected for this study (*APC, ARID1A, APC, BRCA1, BRCA2* and *CDK12*) are included in the G360 platform and were analyzed for ctDNA mutations.

Concordance analysis was performed for the six genes sequenced by both FoundationOne and Guardant360 platforms. Concordance was calculated per patient at the gene level. Full concordance is defined as detection of matching, identical mutations in tDNA and ctDNA per gene, per patient. Partial concordance is defined as detection of identical mutations in tDNA and ctDNA and additional mutations in tDNA and/or ctDNA within a gene. Discordance is defined as detection of different mutations by tDNA and ctDNA in a gene.

Demographic and disease characteristics were collected from the electronic medical record with regard to age (grouped as older and younger than the median age), gender, stage of disease at diagnosis (per cancer staging AJCC 8th edition), HPV status defined by HPV by PCR and/or p16 status, smoking status (grouped as never-smokers vs. ever-smokers where ever smokers were defined as former or current smokers), alcohol use, tumor subsite (oral cavity, oropharynx, larynx, hypopharynx, nasopharynx, paranasal sinuses or unknown primary) and treatment received before tDNA and before ctDNA collection (chemotherapy, radiotherapy or both). Outcome measures included overall survival measured from the time of diagnosis, from the time of tDNA collection or from the time of ctDNA collection. Survival at 1 and 2 years measured from the date of tDNA or ctDNA collection, survival at the end of the study and extent/burden of disease at last visit were also included in outcome data. It should be noted that, for all calculations in which extent of disease was measured, three categories were considered. These were defined as "no evidence of disease", "localized disease" and "metastatic disease." Patients with follow-up shorter than 6 months from the date of last NGS testing were excluded from the outcome analysis.

Subset analysis was performed for the six genes (*ATM, APC, ARID1A, BRCA1, BRCA2* and *CDK12*) for which alterations could be detected in both tDNA and ctDNA via the above methods (6-gene subset). Additional subset analyses were conducted for *BRCA1* and *BRCA2* genes (2-gene subset), for which PARP inhibitors are FDA-approved in patients with mutations present in breast, ovarian and pancreatic cancer, and for *BRCA1, BRCA2* and *ATM* (3-gene subset), for which PARP inhibitors have been recently approved when such mutated genes are identified in prostate cancer. The gene subsets can be reviewed in (Table 1). Patients were considered positive for a DDR gene mutation if they had a mutation in one or more DDR gene mutations in tDNA, ctDNA or tDNA and/or ctDNA.

Table 1. 18-Gene panel and gene subsets.

DNA Damage Repair Genes			
18-Gene Panel (Selected based on literature review)	6-Gene Subset (Genes common to both tDNA and ctDNA assays)	3-Gene Subset (Mutated genes with approved PARP inhibitors in prostate cancer)	2-Gene Subset (Mutated genes with approved PARP inhibitors in ovarian, breast and pancreatic cancer)
BRCA1, BRCA2, ATM, BRIP1, BARD1, CDK12, CHEK1, CHEK2, FANCL, PALB2, PPP2R2A, RAD51B, RAD51C, RAD51D, RAD51L, APC, ARID1A, MLL3	ATM, APC, ARID1A, BRCA1, BRCA2, CDK12	BRCA1, BRCA2, ATM	BRCA1, BRCA2

ctDNA, circulating tumor DNA; tDNA, tumor tissue DNA.

Statistical Analysis

Descriptive statistics of means and standard deviations were calculated for continuous variables. Counts and percentages for categorical variables were also presented. There was notation of the prevalence of mutations in each of the eighteen selected genes. Several sets of these results were created based upon the genetic material in which the mutation was detected (tDNA only, ctDNA only and tDNA ± ctDNA). Composite measures were then created to determine whether mutations were present in any of the gene subsets (2-gene, 3-gene or 6-gene). For each of these dichotomous variables, groups of patients with or without mutated DDR were compared with categorical variables using Fisher's exact tests when both variables were binary. Chi-square tests were used when comparing groups with more than two categories. For analyses comparing mean values of continuous measures, we used two-sample t tests. When comparing survival curves, Kaplan–Meier curves were generated and compared groups of patients with DDR mutations to those without using log-rank tests. For some survival models, groups were compared after accounting for a stratification variable, such as staging at diagnosis or HPV status. Cox proportional hazards regression models were used to examine the relationship of survival (from time of sample collection) to a number of potential risk factors and predictors in the same model. Age, tobacco use, tumor site, nodal stage at diagnosis and previous treatment with combined chemoradiation therapy were included in these adjusted models based on statistical significance and/or clinical importance (i.e., age was included despite not having been found to be statistically significant based on clinical relevance). Hazard ratios and corresponding 95% confidence intervals were estimated from these proportional hazards regression models. In all analyses, two-sided tests with an alpha level of 0.05 were used to determine significance. SAS version 9.4 (SAS Institute, Cary, NC, USA) was used to perform all analyses.

3. Results

3.1. Patient Characteristics

One hundred and seventy total patients met criteria for enrollment. Of these, 139 underwent NGS via tDNA, 146 via ctDNA and 115 via both methods. Demographics and disease characteristics are available for review in Table 2. Age, race, gender and stage in this study are congruent with a standard HNSCC population.

Table 2. Patient Characteristics.

Characteristics	No.	%	Characteristics	No.	%
Age at Diagnosis (Years)			Primary Tumor Location		
Median	60	-	Nasopharynx	14	8.2%
≥60	85	50.0%	Oropharynx	68	40.0%
<60	85	50.0%	Oral Cavity	40	23.5%
			Hypopharynx	10	5.9%
Gender			Larynx	27	15.9%
Male	123	72.4%	Sino–Nasal	6	3.5%
Female	47	27.6%	Unknown	5	3.0%
Race			Disease Stage at Time of Diagnosis		
Caucasian	142	83.5%			
African American	19	11.2%			
Other	9	5.3%	Cancer Stage		
			I	21	12.4%
ETOH Status			II	30	17.6%
Never	92	54.1%	III	37	21.8%
Former	36	21.2%	IV	82	48.2%
Active	72	24.7%			
			Cancer Stage IV		
Smoking Status			IVA	50	29.4%
Never	48	28.2%	IVB	22	12.9%
Former	50	29.4%	IVC	9	5.3%
Active	72	42.4%			
			N Stage		
HPV and/or p16			N0	47	27.6%
Negative	61	35.9%	N1	35	20.6%
Positive	61	35.9%	N2	69	40.6%
Not Tested	48	28.2%	N3	19	11.2%
tDNA Tissue Source			Disease Status At Last Visit		
Primary Tumor	92	54.1%	No Evidence of Disease	61	35.9%
Regional Lymph Node	11	6.5%	Locoregional	44	25.9%
Metastatic Lesion	11	6.5%	Metastatic (only)	17	10.0%
Recurrence	25	14.7%	Locoregional and Metastatic	48	28.2%

ctDNA, circulating tumor DNA; tDNA, tumor tissue DNA.

3.2. Sequencing Results. Prevalence of Mutations in DDR Genes in Study Population

Presence (or absence) of mutated DDR genes was reported per patient, stipulating the specific DDR gene mutated and sample source (ctDNA and/or tDNA). Detailed information about the prevalence of specific mutated DDR genes can be located in Table 3 and in Figure 1, and the allocation of the DDR gene mutations among patients can be viewed in Figure 2.

Table 3. Overall Prevalence of Individual DNA Damage Repair (DDR) Gene Mutations (Any Type of Mutation and Pathogenic or Presumed Pathogenic Mutations).

	Patients with DDR Gene Mutations in tDNA Number (%)		Patients with DDR Gene Mutations in ctDNA Number (%)		Patients with DDR Gene Mutations in tDNA and ctDNA Number (%)		Patients with DDR Gene Mutations in tDNA and/or ctDNA Number (%)	
	Pathogenic Mutation(s)	Any Mutation(s)	Pathogenic Mutation(s)	Any Mutation(s)	Pathogenic Mutation(s)	Any Mutation(s)	Pathogenic Mutation(s)	Any Mutation(s)
All DDR Genes	16 (11.5%)	66 (47.5%)	18 (12.3%)	54 (36.9%)	4 (3.4%)	11 (9.6%)	30 (17.6%)	97 (57.1%)
BRCA1	3 (2.2%)	6 (4.3%)	5 (3.4%)	13 (8.9%)	2 (1.7%)	2 (1.7%)	6 (%)	17 (10.0%)
BRCA2	3 (2.2%)	21 (15.1%)	1 (0.7%)	14 (9.6%)	0	5 (4.3%)	4 (%)	30 (17.6%)
ATM	2 (1.4%)	9 (6.4%)	9 (6.2%)	15 (10.3%)	0	1 (0.9%)	11 (%)	23 (13.5%)
CDK12	1 (0.7%)	11 (7.9%)	1 (0.7%)	2 (1.4%)	0	0	2 (%)	13 (7.6%)
APC	3 (2.2%)	10 (7.2%)	1 (0.7%)	9 (6.2%)	1 (0.9%)	4 (3.4%)	3 (%)	15 (8.8%)
ARID1A	3 (2.2%)	12 (8.6%)	3 (2.1%)	19 (13.0%)	1 (0.9%)	1 (0.9%)	5 (%)	30 (17.6%)
MLL3	1 (0.7%)	10 (7.2%)	-	-	-	-	-	-
BRIP1	0	2 (1.4%)	-	-	-	-	-	-
BARD1	0	3 (2.2%)	-	-	-	-	-	-
CHEK1	0	3 (2.2%)	-	-	-	-	-	-
CHEK2	0	1 (0.7%)	-	-	-	-	-	-
FANCL	0	3 (2.2%)	-	-	-	-	-	-
PALB2	1 (0.7%)	3 (2.2%)	-	-	-	-	-	-
PPP2R2A	0	0	-	-	-	-	-	-
RAD51B	0	1 (0.7%)	-	-	-	-	-	-
RAD51C	0	0	-	-	-	-	-	-
RAD51D	0	2 (1.4%)	-	-	-	-	-	-
RAD51L	0	1 (0.7%)	-	-	-	-	-	-
MLL3	1 (0.7%)	10 (7.2%)	-	-	-	-	-	-
Total Number of Patients Tested	139 patients		146 patients		115 patients		170 patients	

Occurrences are listed as patients with one or more mutations in the specified gene, rather than total number of mutations encountered for each gene. tDNA was analyzed by the FM platform, which assesses for mutations in all 18 genes. ctDNA was analyzed by the G360 platform, which is limited to analysis of ATM, APC, ARID1A, BRCA1, BRCA2 and CDK12. Pathogenic/presumed pathogenic mutations are as defined by FoundationOne and Guardant 360 reports. The number of patients with mutations in any of the DDR genes does not represent the sum of patients with each individual DDR gene mutations, because a patient could have more than one DDR gene mutated. ctDNA, circulating tumor DNA; DDR, DNA damage repair; tDNA, tumor tissue DNA.

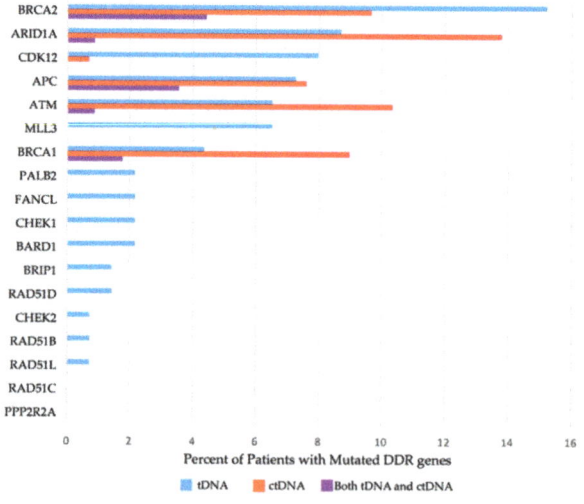

Figure 1. Histogram of Gene Prevalence. ctDNA, circulating tumor DNA; DDR, DNA damage repair; tDNA, tumor tissue DNA.

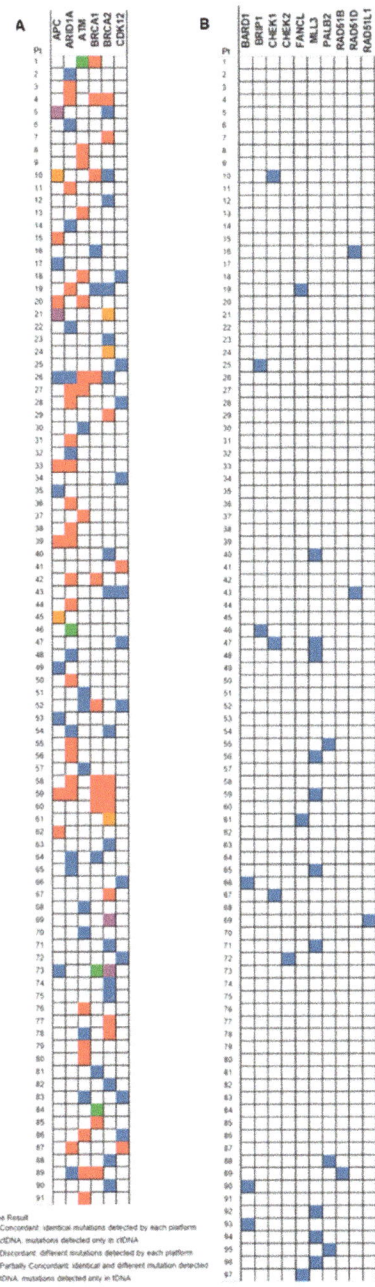

Figure 2. (**A**) Mutated genes tested in both tDNA and ctDNA. (**B**) Mutated genes tested in tDNA only. Green boxes indicate concordant mutations (identical mutations detected by the two platforms). Gold boxes indicate discordant mutations (different mutations reported by each platform in the same gene). Purple boxes represent partially concordant mutations (concordant and discordant mutations reported by the two platforms in the same gene). Red boxes indicate mutations detected in ctDNA only. Blue boxes indicate mutations that were found in tDNA only.

We found that 97 of the 170 patients (57.1%) had one (or more) mutations in one (or more) DDR gene(s) detected in either ctDNA and/or tDNA samples; 81 patients (47.6%) had mutations in at least one of the genes in the 6-gene subset (*ATM, APC, ARID1A, BRCA1, BRCA2* or *CDK12*). A total of 70 patients (41.1%) had mutations in *BRCA1, BRCA2* and/or *ATM* (the 3-gene subset) detected in ctDNA and/or tDNA (Figure 2), and 47 patients (27.6%) had ctDNA and/or tDNA mutations in *BRCA1* and/or *BRCA2* (2-gene subset) (Figure 1 and Table 3). The most frequently mutated DDR genes in the study HNSCC population were *BRCA2* and *ARID1A*, both mutated in 17.6% of the patients tested by either tDNA and/or ctDNA. *ATM* and *BRCA1* followed, with mutations identified in 13.5% and 10% of patients, respectively.

In total, 139 patients underwent tDNA testing. All genes in the 18-gene panel were included in tDNA testing: 66 of the patients tested (47.5%) had at least one tDNA mutation in the 18-gene panel; 55 patients (39.5%) had tDNA mutations in the 6-gene subset; 34 (24.4%) and 25 (17.9%) patients had tDNA mutations in the 3-gene and 2-gene subsets, respectively (Figure 1 and Table 3).

Out of the 18 DDR genes tested for mutations in tDNA, 16 were found to be mutated in one or more patients. Mutations in *PPP2R2A* and *RAD51C* were not detected in any patients. The most frequently mutated DDR genes, on a per patient basis, in tDNA were *BRCA2* (21 patients), *ARID1A* (12 patients), *APC* (10 patients), *CDK12* (11 patients) and *MLL3* (10 patients), respectively (Table 3). The most frequently altered gene in the tDNA analysis overall was *BRCA2*, with 46 mutations in 21 patients. The gene with the highest number of alterations in a single patient was *MLL3*, with 4.2 mutations detected in tDNA. Remarkably, one patient had 9 mutations in *BRCA2* and 9 mutations in *FANCL* gene in the tDNA analysis (Figure 1 and Table 3).

In total, 146 patients underwent ctDNA testing: 54 of these patients (37.0%) had at least one ctDNA mutation in the total gene panel assessed by the chosen platform; 34 of the patients who underwent ctDNA testing had ctDNA mutations in the 3-gene subset, and 22 of the patients who underwent ctDNA testing had ctDNA mutations in the 2-gene subset (Table 3).

All six DDR genes included in the panel (*BRCA1, BRCA2, ATM, APC, ARID1A* and *CDK12*) were found to be altered in at least one patient. The most frequently mutated DDR genes in ctDNA were *ARID1A* (19 patients), *ATM* (15 patients), *BRCA2* (14 patients) and *BRCA1* (13 patients) (Table 3). The most frequently altered gene in the ctDNA analysis was *ARID1A* with 23 mutations in 19 patients.

For the 115 patients with both tDNA and ctDNA results available, concordance of mutations among the six DDR genes common to both assays, per patient, is depicted in the oncoprint (Figure 2A). About 4.1% of patients had mutations that were concordant, 4.1% had partial concordance and 5.2% were discordant. Close to half (44.3%) of patients who underwent tDNA and ctDNA testing had only tDNA mutations, and 32% of patients had only ctDNA mutations. The mutations in the genes analyzed by FoundationOne only, per patient, are depicted in part B of the oncoprint (Figure 2B).

3.3. Pathogenic and Presumed Pathogenic Mutations

Pathogenic or presumed pathogenic mutations, as depicted in FM and G360 reports and described as "deleterious" or "inactivating," were reported in a total of 30 of the 170 study patients (17.6%) in ctDNA and/or tDNA: 16 of the 139 (11.5%) patients for whom tDNA samples were tested were found to have pathogenic or presumed pathogenic mutations, and 18 of the 146 (12.3%) for whom ctDNA samples were tested were identified as having such mutations in DDR genes. Only 4 of the 30 patients had pathogenic mutations identified in both tDNA and ctDNA, with a significant 40% of the patients being identified exclusively by ctDNA testing (Table 3).

3.4. Targetable Mutations

FM and G360 reported availability of off-label clinical protocols with PARP inhibitors for pathogenic mutations in *BRCA1*, *BRCA2*, *ATM* and, more recently, in *PALB2*, *ARID1A* and *CDK12*. Therefore, pathogenic or presumed pathogenic mutations in these genes were deemed "targetable" with PARP inhibitors in this study. Based on the information provided by FM and G360, 27 patients (15.9%) of the study patients would be eligible for off-label therapy with a PARP inhibitor, with 13 patients (9.3% of the tDNA tested patients) and 17 patients (11.6% of the ctDNA tested patients) being potential candidates (Table 4). *ATM* was the DDR gene with the highest number of pathogenic mutations reported in 11 patients (6.4% of the 170 patients tested by ctDNA and/or tDNA); 9 of the 11 patients were identified by ctDNA testing. *BRCA1* and *ARID1A* followed, with 6 and 5 patients, respectively, identified with targetable mutations, with the majority of patients identified again by ctDNA testing (5 and 3 patients, respectively) (Table 4).

Table 4. Prevalence of Clinically Significant and Targetable Mutations.

	tDNA	ctDNA	Both	Off-Label Clinical Protocol with PARP Inhibitors
BRCA1	3	5	2	FM, G360
BRCA2	3	1	0	FM, G360
ATM	2	8 [1]	0	FM, G360
ARID1A	3	2 [1]	1	G360
CDK12	1	1	0	G360
APC	2 [2]	1	1	None
PALB2	1	-	-	FM
MLL3	1	-	-	None

Occurrences are listed as number of patients with one or more mutations in a gene, rather than total number of mutations encountered for each gene. [1] One additional pathogenic mutation was reported in *BRCA1* ctDNA in the same patient who is listed under *BRCA1*. [2] One additional pathogenic mutation was reported in *BRCA2* tDNA in the same patient who is listed under *BRCA2*. ctDNA, circulating tumor DNA; FM, FoundationOne Medicine; G360, Guardant 360; tDNA, tumor tissue DNA.

3.5. Prevalence of DDR Gene Mutations across Demographic Groups

Patients were deemed as either positive or negative for mutated DDR genes in the 18-gene panel (all genes) or for ctDNA, tDNA or either (ctDNA and/or tDNA) in each of the subsets. No significant association was found between patients with mutated DDR genes in the 18-gene panel and age, gender, race, smoking status, alcohol use or stage at diagnosis. Patients with mutated DDR genes within the 3-gene subset in ctDNA and in either/both tDNA and/or ctDNA were statistically more likely to be older than the median patient age of 60 years (p values of 0.04 and 0.050, respectively). No other associations with age, gender, race, smoking status, alcohol use or stage at diagnosis were found in any of the other subsets.

Patients with DDR gene mutations detected in ctDNA and/or tDNA were associated with HNSCC subsite (p = 0.02) in the 18-gene panel analysis. Laryngeal primaries, specifically, had a higher presence of DDR gene mutations detected in this gene set detected in ctDNA (p = 0.02), tDNA (p = 0.06) or via in ctDNA and/or tDNA method (p = 0.01). Oropharyngeal primaries correlated with a lower prevalence of DDR gene mutations in patients detected in tDNA (p = 0.06) and in tDNA and/or ctDNA (p = 0.01). Statistical significance of the lower prevalence of patients with DDR gene mutations in oropharyngeal cancers was preserved in the 6-gene subset analysis (p = 0.04 for tDNA, and p = 0.01 for tDNA and/or ctDNA), in the 3-gene subset analysis (p = 0.01 for tDNA, p = 0.054 for ctDNA; and p < 0.01 for tDNA and/or ctDNA) and in the 2-gene subset analysis (p = 0.02 for tDNA, and p = 0.03 for tDNA and/or ctDNA). The 3-gene subset analysis showed an association in which patients with DDR gene mutations detected via tDNA and/or ctDNA were more likely to have more advanced disease at time of diagnosis with respect to advanced cancer stage (I–IV) (p = 0.06), N stage (N0 to N3) (p = 0.02) and within stage IV disease (between groups A, B and C) ($p = 0.03$). N stage also correlated significantly with the prevalence of patients with ctDNA mutations ($p = 0.02$).

Patients treated with chemotherapy, radiotherapy or both before collection of ctDNA had a significantly higher presence of DDR gene mutations in ctDNA ($p < 0.01$). Data also indicated an increased prevalence of mutations in tDNA and/or ctDNA in patients treated before tDNA collection ($p = 0.03$).

3.6. HPV and Smoking Status and the Prevalence of DDR Genes Mutations

HPV and/or p16 testing was available for 123 (72.35%) patients. HPV and/or p16 were negative in 65 patients (52.84% of those tested) and positive in 58 patients (47.15% of those tested). Positive HPV and/or p16 tumors were associated with increased probability to be alive at the end of the study ($p < 0.01$) and with tendency for better OS measured from the time of diagnosis ($p = 0.06$). No significant correlation between HPV status and presence of a DDR gene mutation on a per patient basis were discovered in the 18-gene analysis. In the 6-gene subset, however, patients without mutations in tDNA and/or ctDNA were found to be more likely to have HPV-positive disease ($p = 0.04$).

Information about smoking status was available for all patients included in the study: 48 of the 170 patients (28.2%) were never-smokers, and 122 patients (71.8%) were ever-smokers. A nearly significant lower presence of ctDNA DDR gene mutations was found in non-smokers compared with ever-smokers ($p = 0.06$) in the 3-gene subset analysis. Non-smokers had a nearly significant better chance to be alive at the end of the study ($p = 0.058$) and a significantly better OS measured from the time of diagnosis ($p = 0.03$) when compared to ever-smokers.

3.7. Survival Analysis

All patients had at least 6 months of follow up after the last sample collection for NGS. Median follow-up time was 615.5 days from the time of diagnosis and 232.5 days from the time of ctDNA testing. Median survival from the time of diagnosis was 820 days (95% CI 752 to 1140 days) and 372 days (95% CI 262 to 416 days) from the time of ctDNA testing. At last visit, 35.8% of patients had no evidence of disease, 28.4% had recurrent or progressive loco–regional disease, and 35.8% had metastatic disease (Table 2). Overall, patients with mutations in DDR genes had poorer prognosis (Table 5 and Figure 3).

Table 5. Correlation of Mutated DDR Genes with Survival Outcomes.

Survival Start Time Point	Overall Survival Univariate Analysis			Overall Survival Adjusted Analysis			1-Year OS	2-Year OS	Survival Last Visit
	HR	95% CI	*p* Value	HR	95% CI	*p* Value	*p* Values		
18-Gene Subset									
tDNA									
tDNA collection	0.91	0.57–1.45	0.68				0.14	0.20	0.71
Diagnosis	0.81	0.51–1.30	0.38						
tDNA and/or ctDNA				-	-	-			
tDNA collection	1.20	0.74–1.94	0.46				0.67	0.75	0.52
ctDNA collection	1.38	0.83–2.29	0.41						
Diagnosis	0.94	0.62–1.44	0.78						
6-Gene Subset									
tDNA									
tDNA collection	1.24	0.77–1.97	0.38				0.46	0.85	0.25
Diagnosis	1.24	0.78–1.98	0.36						
ctDNA									
ctDNA collection	1.81	1.15–2.85	*0.01*	1.62	0.99–2.65	*0.053*	0.10	*<0.01*	*0.04*
Diagnosis	1.38	0.88–2.15	0.16						
tDNA and/or ctDNA									
tDNA collection	1.68	1.03–2.73	*0.04*				0.40	0.21	*0.01*
ctDNA collection	1.56	0.99–2.46	*0.053*						
Diagnosis	1.29	0.85–1.96	0.23						

Table 5. Cont.

Survival Start Time Point	Overall Survival Univariate Analysis			Overall Survival Adjusted Analysis			1-Year OS	2-Year OS	Survival Last Visit
	HR	95% CI	p Value	HR	95% CI	p Value	p Values		
3-Gene Subset									
tDNA									
tDNA collection	1.09	0.63–1.86	0.77				0.42	0.77	0.92
Diagnosis	1.08	0.63–1.84	0.78						
ctDNA									
ctDNA collection	2.04	1.26–3.31	<u>*<0.01*</u>	1.85	1.10–3.12	***0.02***	0.07	<u>*0.01*</u>	<u>*0.01*</u>
Diagnosis	1.99	1.23–3.22	***0.01***						
tDNA and/or ctDNA									
tDNA collection	1.55	0.96–2.49	<u>*0.07*</u>				0.87	0.16	0.10
ctDNA collection	1.73	1.09–2.74	***0.02***						
Diagnosis	1.43	0.94–2.19	0.10						
2-Gene Subset									
tDNA									
tDNA collection	0.99	0.53–1.85	0.97				0.82	0.93	0.64
Diagnosis	0.94	0.50–1.74	0.83						
ctDNA									
ctDNA collection	1.77	1.00–3.12	***0.04***	1.82	0.99–3.38	<u>*0.06*</u>	0.15	<u>*0.04*</u>	0.15
Diagnosis	1.80	1.01–3.21	***0.04***						
tDNA and/or ctDNA									
tDNA collection	1.37	0.82–2.29	0.22				0.89	0.36	0.68
ctDNA collection	1.38	0.83–2.29	0.21						
Diagnosis	1.25	0.77–2.03	0.36						

Results with $p < 0.05$ are bolded in italics; results with $0.05 < p < 0.10$ are italicized and underlined. Abbreviations: CI, Confidence interval; ctDNA, circulating tumor DNA; HR, hazard ratio; tDNA, tumor tissue DNA.

3.8. Prognostic Value of Presence of ctDNA Mutations in DDR Genes

Patients without ctDNA DDR gene mutations in the 6-gene subset or in the 3-gene subset were significantly more likely to be alive at the end of the study ($p = 0.04$, and $p = 0.01$, respectively). Similarly, patients without ctDNA mutations specifically in BRCA2 or in APC genes were more likely to be alive at the end of the study ($p = 0.01$, and $p = 0.01$, respectively). Patients with ctDNA mutations in DDR genes in the 6-gene and in the 3-gene subsets were more likely to have a more advanced cancer status at the last visit ($p = 0.03$, and $p = 0.01$, respectively). Presence of mutated DDR genes in ctDNA was also associated with significantly worse 2-year survival ($p < 0.01$).

Patients with ctDNA DDR gene mutations had significantly worse overall survival measured from the time of ctDNA collection ($p = 0.01$) (Figure 3a). This relationship remained statistically significant in a Cox proportional hazards regression model when adjusted for age, tobacco use, tumor site, nodal stage at diagnosis and previous treatment with combined chemoradiation therapy in a multivariate analysis model ($p = 0.053$) (Table 6). Similar associations with overall survival were found in studies for patients with ctDNA DDR gene mutations in 3-gene and 2-gene subsets in the univariate ($p < 0.01$, and $p = 0.04$, respectively) and in the multivariate ($p = 0.02$, and $p = 0.04$, respectively) analyses (Tables 5 and 6 and Figure 3c,e). Association with overall survival measured from the time of diagnosis was statistically significant for patients with ctDNA mutations in the 3-gene and 2-gene analysis ($p < 0.01$, and $p = 0.04$, respectively) (Table 5 and Figure 3f).

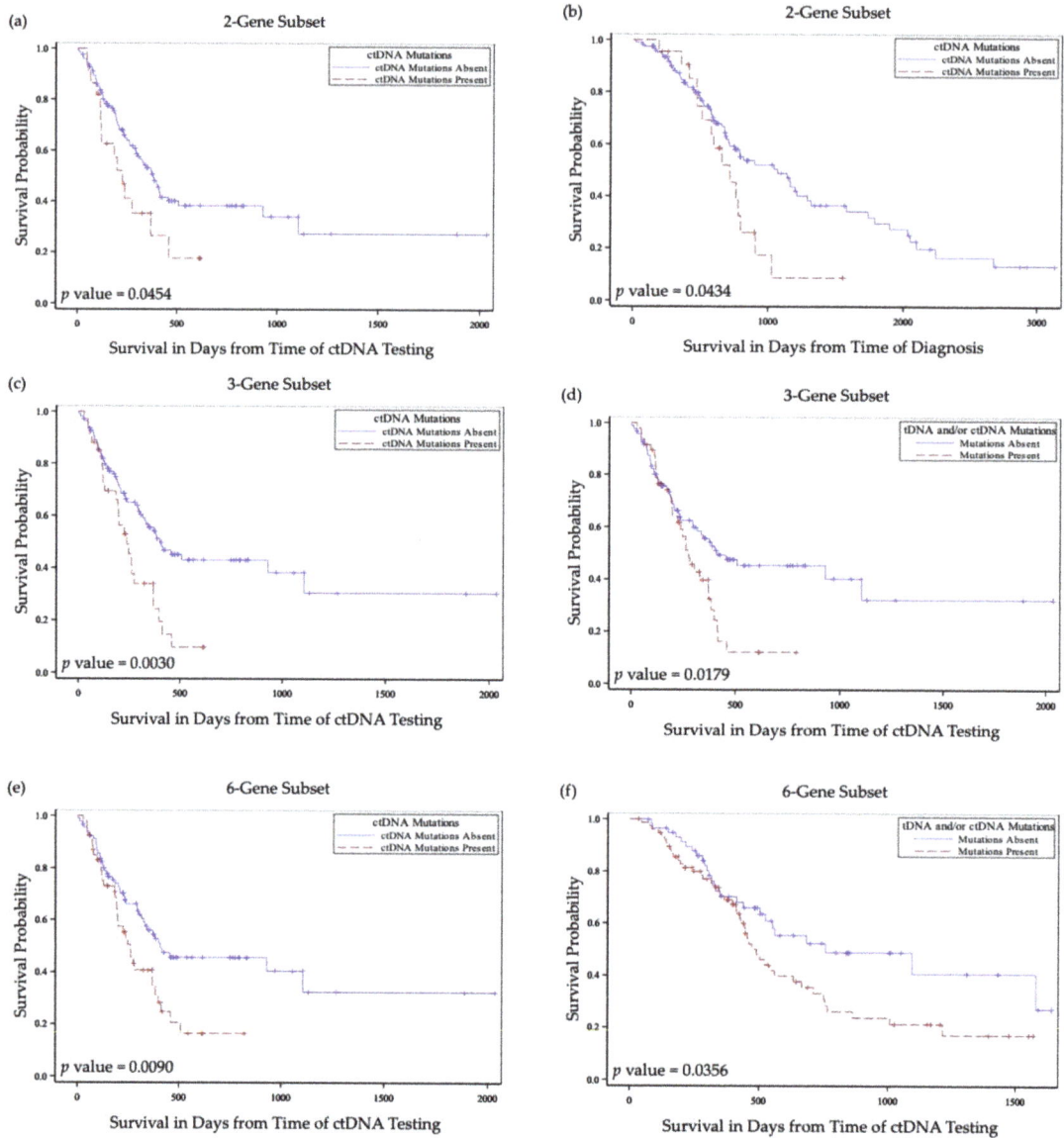

Figure 3. Kaplan–Meier curves depicting survival differences in patients with DDR gene mutations in comparison to those without DDR gene mutations. (**a**) Survival from time of ctDNA testing in patients with vs. without DDR genes mutations in ctDNA in the 2-gene subset. (**b**) Survival from time of diagnosis in patients with vs. without DDR genes mutations in ctDNA in the 2-gene subset. (**c**) Survival from time of ctDNA testing in patients with vs. without DDR genes mutations in ctDNA in the 3-gene subset. (**d**) Survival from time of ctDNA testing in patients with vs. without DDR genes mutations in tDNA and/or ctDNA in the 3-gene subset. (**e**) Survival from time of ctDNA testing in patients with vs. without DDR genes mutations in ctDNA in the 6-gene subset. (**f**) Survival from time of ctDNA testing in patients with vs. without DDR genes mutations in tDNA and/or ctDNA in the 6-gene subset. ctDNA, circulating tumor DNA; tDNA, tumor tissue DNA; blue solid lines indicate survival curves for patients without mutations in any of the selected gene panel; red dashed lines indicate survival curves for patients with at least one mutation in any of the selected gene panel.

Table 6. Results from Adjusted Cox Proportional Hazard Regression Models of Impact of the Presence of ctDNA Mutations on Overall Survival.

	6-Gene Analysis			3-Gene Analysis			2-Gene Analysis		
	HR	95% CI	*p* Value	HR	95% CI	*p* Value	HR	95% CI	*p* Value
ctDNA mutations	1.62	(0.99–2.65)	*0.053*	1.85	(1.10–3.12)	*0.020*	1.87	(1.02–3.43)	*0.042*
	p value for Adjusted Variables			*p* value for Adjusted Variables			*p* value for Adjusted Variables		
Age Below 60 Years Old (*yes* vs. *no*)	0.65			0.70			0.64		
Smoking (*never* vs. *ever*)	0.41			0.54			0.55		
N Stage (*N0 vs N1, N2, N3*)	0.33			0.49			0.31		
Subsite (*OP* vs. *OC, Pharynx, Other*)	*0.02*			*0.02*			*0.04*		
CRT Prior to ctDNA Test (*yes* vs. *no*)	*<0.01*			*<0.01*			*<0.01*		

Analyses with *p* < 0.05 are bolded in italics and underlined; results with 0.05 < *p* < 0.10 are italicized and underlined. Abbreviations: CI, Confidence interval; ctDNA, circulating tumor DNA; HR, hazard ratio; CI, hazard ratio confidence interval; CS, chi-squared analysis; N/A, non-applicable; CRT, combined chemotherapy and radiation therapy; OC, oral cavity; OP, oropharynx.

3.9. Prognostic Value of Presence of tDNA Mutations in DDR Genes

A patients' possession of tDNA DDR gene mutations showed no significant prognostic value when analyzed for correlation with disease status at the end of the study, survival at 1 or 2 year(s) or with overall survival. tDNA DDR gene mutations present specifically in APC or in CDK12 genes were associated with decreased likelihood to be alive at the end of the study ($p = 0.01$, and $p = 0.01$, respectively).

3.10. Prognostic Value of Presence of tDNA and/or ctDNA Mutations in DDR Genes

Patients with mutations in one or more DDR genes in the 6-gene and 3-gene subsets detected in tDNA and/or ctDNA were significantly more likely to have a greater extent of disease at last visit ($p < 0.01$, and $p = 0.01$, respectively) (Table 5). In the 6-gene subset analysis, patients with mutated DDR genes had significantly decreased overall survival measured from the time of ctDNA collection ($p = 0.053$) or from the time of tDNA collection ($p = 0.04$) (Figure 3b) and did not reach significance when measured from the time of diagnosis ($p = 0.07$) (Table 5). For the 3-gene subset analysis, patients with mutations in tDNA and/or ctDNA were also found to have decreased overall survival when measured from the time of ctDNA collection ($p = 0.02$) (Figure 3d) and did not reach significance when measured from the time of tDNA collection ($p = 0.07$).

Mutations present in APC or CDK12 genes, individually, were again associated with decreased likelihood to be alive at the end of the study ($p = 0.01$, and $p = 0.01$, respectively) when measured in tDNA and/or ctDNA. Interestingly, mutations in ARID1A as well as in MLL3 were associated with improved chance to be alive at the end of the study when measured in tDNA ($p = 0.04$, and $p = 0.06$, respectively) or in both tDNA and/or ctDNA for MLL3 gene ($p = 0.053$).

4. Discussion

This study is a single-institution retrospective analysis examining the prevalence, prognostic and potential therapeutic implications of DDR gene mutations in tDNA and ctDNA in a dedicated cohort of HNSCC patients. To the authors' knowledge, this study is the first to elucidate the significance and the role of the genomic profile of DDR genes in the HNSCC when evaluated by both tDNA and ctDNA analysis, alone, or in combination.

The selection of the 18 genes chosen for this study was based on literature review of genes' roles and importance in DDR pathways as well as on inclusion as biomarkers in clinical studies [17]. A subset was created for further analysis based on the testing profile available for both tDNA and ctDNA (6-gene subset). Creation of other subsets was based on potential clinical therapeutic utility, with 2-gene subset and 3-gene subset reflecting the gene biomarkers utilized for approval of PARP inhibitors in the management of breast, ovarian, pancreatic and prostate cancers. Variants of unknown significance were not excluded from data related to prevalence, analysis of demographics or prognostic associations. The decision to include these mutations was based on the notion that there was insufficient scientific data to dismiss them and that their clinical significance may become apparent in the future. However, variants of unknown significance were excluded from the reporting of the genes identified as potential targetable mutations in current clinical protocols.

The population studied in this analysis is consistent with a standard HNSCC population in terms of age, gender, race, smoking status and prevalence of HPV driven disease. A previous study on a fraction of patients in this group (75 of the 170 patients) has demonstrated a prevalence of mutations in *TP53, CDKN2A, TERT, BRCA2* and *NOTCH1* similar to other reported populations [3,15,17,24,25]. Conventional prognostication tools, including those related to HPV or smoking-driven diseases held true in this analysis. Non-smokers and those with HPV/p16 positivity had a significantly better overall survival and were more likely to be alive at the end of the study.

Data presented in this analysis demonstrates a higher than previously reported prevalence of DDR gene mutations in HNSCC. In this analysis, 47.4% had at least one tDNA mutation and 37% had at least one ctDNA mutation in the selected gene profile. *BRCA2* and *ARID1A* were the two DDR genes with the highest prevalence in our HNSCC population: both mutated in 17.6% of the patients tested in either tDNA and/or ctDNA. *ATM* and *BRCA1* were the next most common and were found to be mutated in 13.5% and 10% of patients, respectively. Other studies have reported a lower frequency of such mutations. For example, one such study reported 6% for *BRCA1* and 7% for *BRCA2*. It should be noted that such studies utilized only tumor tissue for NGS evaluation [6,26–29].

When variants of unknown significance and mutations thought to not influence gene function were excluded, pathogenic or presumed pathogenic mutations in DDR genes were reported in 29 of the 170 study patients (17%). A total of 11.5% of tDNA samples and 12.3% of ctDNA samples were found to have such mutations. These results compare well with the DDR gene mutation profile reported by other studies. For example, Heeke et al. studied genes involved in homologous recombination across multiple tumor types with the most frequently mutated genes overlapping with our study (*ARID1A, BRCA2, BRCA1*). Overall, pathogenic mutations in genes involved in homologous recombination were found in 17.6% of the 17,566 tumors tested and 6.8% of a total of 206 head and neck tumors [26]. With a variation in the selection of the less frequently mutated genes and with the addition of ctDNA testing, this study has significantly increased the percentage of theoretically actionable mutations in the HNSCC, to 17%. Addition of ctDNA to this report increased the yield of NGS by nearly two-fold when compared to tDNA testing, alone. Concordance results also supported the use of both NGS analysis methods in combination. Concordance was limited in the DDR genes analyzed, and, in more than 90% of the patients, each method brought complimentary information, increasing the yield to identify patients for precision oncology treatments. It is noteworthy that the DDR gene with the highest incidence of targetable mutations in this study is *ATM*, with pathogenic mutations reported in 6.4% of the 170 patients tested for NGS and with 9 of the 11 patients being identified by ctDNA testing. Next, *BRCA1* was identified with targetable mutations in 6 patients, with majority of patients identified again by ctDNA testing, and *ARID1A* in 5 patients.

This analysis demonstrated that several groups were predisposed to DDR gene mutations. For example, patients older than the median (60 years) were more likely to have mutations in *ATM, BRCA1* and/or *BRCA2* (the 3-gene subset) detected in ctDNA or in ctDNA and/or tDNA. Certain HNSCC subsites were more likely to have mutations in DDR genes (laryngeal primaries) and others less likely (oropharyngeal) when tested in tDNA or ctDNA or both. Analysis of the gene subsets also showed decreased prevalence of DDR gene mutations in oropharyngeal cancer. Patients with more advanced disease stage (stages I to IV), and those with more advanced stage IV disease (between groups A, B and C) were more likely to have mutations in *ATM*, *BRCA1* and/or *BRCA2* (the 3-gene subset) detected via tDNA and/or ctDNA. N stage (N0 to N3) also correlated significantly with the prevalence of ctDNA mutations in the 3-gene subset analysis. Patients treated with chemotherapy, radiotherapy or both prior to collection of their genetic samples were more likely to have DDR gene mutations in ctDNA or in samples collected by either method. To the authors' knowledge, it is the first time that these demographic correlations were identified in the study of DDR genomic profile in HNSCC, and comparative studies are not available for validation.

The 6-gene subset analysis in this study demonstrated a significantly lower prevalence of mutations in tDNA and/or ctDNA DDR genes in HPV-positive disease. All other subset analyses in tDNA and/or ctDNA support these findings, without reaching statistical significance. These results are further supported by other data in this report. Non-smokers vs. ever-smokers were also less likely to have gene mutations in the 3-gene subset analysis. In addition, given that fewer mutated DDR genes (such as in HPV-positive patients and in non-smokers) were found to be associated with improved survival, it is congruent with the HPV mutation results. This is in agreement with studies that have demonstrated increased expression (i.e., increased presence of functional copies) of DNA repair genes in HPV-positive HNSCC [30]. Two other studies reporting results from genomic cohorts originating from the University of Chicago and University of Michigan (120 and 34 patients, respectively) described that mutations in DDR genes and Fanconi Anemia genes (a spectrum that contains important overlapping genes), respectively, were more frequently associated with HPV positivity [27,31]. Differences in definition of HPV phenotype, in NGS techniques and in DDR gene panel selection could account for the discordant results. Additional effects of confounding variables, such as smoking status, age, stage of disease and previous treatment(s) could further complicate the relationship between HPV status and gene mutations.

Presence of mutated DDR genes was found to be a compelling indicator of poor prognosis. Strong statistically significant correlations were noted between the presence of DDR gene mutations and decreased overall survival when measured from the time of genetic sample collection or from time of diagnosis in ctDNA (in all subsets) and in tDNA and/or ctDNA in selected subsets (Table 3). The relationship between ctDNA DDR mutations and overall survival remained statistically significant in a Cox proportional hazards regression model when adjusted for age, tobacco use, tumor site, nodal stage at diagnosis and previous treatment with combined chemoradiation therapy in all subsets. No similar correlation was found between tDNA mutations in DDR genes and prognosis. Existing literature suggests that expression of certain DDR genes, including *BRCA1* and *BRCA2*, is associated with increased survival in HNSCC patients as the preservation of efficient repair mechanisms maintains genomic stability [32]. Similarly, another study has listed *BRCA1* expression, alone, to be indicative of survival in HNSCC [30]. As another indicator of poor prognosis, patients with DDR gene mutations were significantly more likely to have more advanced disease burden at the time of the last visit, as measured in ctDNA and in both tDNA and/or ctDNA in the 6-gene and 3-gene subsets.

Overall, statistically significant associations between the presence of mutated DDR genes and demographic variables and/or survival were more frequently identified in ctDNA rather than in tDNA. This possibly reflects differences in sampling and in NGS techniques. Challenges in tissue sample acquisition and appraisal, including availability and tumor heterogeneity, are universal to tDNA studies. Likewise, studies regarding ctDNA have uncovered that liquid biopsies do not reflect the complete mutation profile of the tumor, either, and such studies have noted increased sensitivity with increased burden of disease [15,33]. It is also feasible that differences in sequencing results between samples are also reflective of the different time points at which the samples were collected (ctDNA studies were typically performed after tDNA studies in this cohort) and, therefore, may be impacted by tumor progression, interim treatments, etc. Differences between the FoundationOne and Guardant360 sequencing techniques may affect the concordance of DDR gene mutation results and, therefore, the correlation with different clinical variables.

The high prevalence of DDR gene mutations in this cohort detected in ctDNA samples, tDNA samples or both is of considerable clinical interest, as mutations in these genes are potential targets for novel cancer treatments, including PARP inhibitors. FoundationOne and Guardant360 report off-label clinical protocols with PARP inhibitors for pathogenic or presumed pathogenic mutations in *BRCA1*, *BRCA2*, *ATM* and, more recently, in *PALB2*, *ARID1A* and *CDK12*. No off-label clinical protocols with PARP inhibitors were reported for mutations in *APC* or *MLL3*; therefore, patients with such mutations were not included here. A total of 15.9% of the 170 study patients would be eligible for off-label PARP1 inhibitor clinical protocols, with 9.3% of tDNA-tested patients and 11.6 % of ctDNA-tested patients being potential candidates. These frequencies rival reported frequency of these mutations in breast (15.6%), ovarian (20.0%), prostate (14.1%) and pancreatic cancers (15.4%) for which PARP inhibitors are currently FDA approved therapeutics [26].

Notably, this report emphasizes the utility of ctDNA testing by demonstrating improved sensitivity in the identification of patients who might benefit from targeted drug therapy. Only 3 of the 27 patients identified with presumed targetable mutations for PARP inhibitors were identified in both tDNA and ctDNA, with more than half (14) of the patients being identified exclusively by ctDNA testing. These results support efforts made in the field of precision oncology to revolutionize the treatment of HNSCC, with consideration for targeted, mutation-guided clinical protocols with single agent PARP inhibitors. Review of the literature revealed only one study that evaluated efficacy of a single agent PARP inhibitor, Olaparib, in a limited number of pre-operative HNSCC cases. In this study, Olaparib was used with or without cisplatin or durvalumab. The report concluded that mutations in DDR genes were associated with sensitivity to Olaparib in HNSCC, as has previously been demonstrated in other malignancies [34]. Additional ongoing clinical trials for treatment of HNSCC with PARP inhibitors rely on combination therapy in which chemotherapy and/or radiotherapy are used to sensitize tumors to PARP inhibitors. Such studies find basis in pre-clinical trials in which synergy was noted between PARP inhibitors and more conventional therapies [35]. These studies and others highlight the tolerability and effectivity of PARP inhibitors in HNSCC but are all in small cohorts, and none uses NGS to guide therapy [21–23]. The strong correlation of the presence of DDR gene mutations with poor survival in this study raises the possibility that NGS-guided treatment with PARP inhibitors in HNSCC might lead to improvement in survival in select patients.

This is among the largest cohorts of patients with HNSCC in whom tDNA mutations were studied and is the only report in which DDR gene mutations were analyzed in a relatively large HNSCC population by ctDNA, alone, or in combination with tDNA. Findings from this report support further use of ctDNA analysis to predict prognosis and to increase sensitivity in the detection of targetable mutations and underscore further investigations into PARP inhibitors for the treatment of HNSCC. This report has a number of limitations. Data was collected from a single institution and geographic area. Furthermore, dependence on the electronic medical record, self-reported data (for smoking and alcohol use) and utilization of commercially available NGS platforms with differences in technical approaches introduced error that could not be corrected. Finally, this correlative data does not imply causation, therefore limiting the number and types of conclusions that can be drawn.

Future Directions

This study notably demonstrates both the high prevalence of DDR gene mutations in HNSCC and the poor prognosis associated with such mutations. The increased prevalence of DDR gene mutations measured in this study was the result of combining tDNA with ctDNA testing. The low overall concordance between tDNA and ctDNA samples, and the significant contribution of ctDNA testing to the number of identified mutations targetable with PARP inhibitors, supports using the combination of the two methods in future clinical practice to raise the sensitivity of genetic testing. These results are expected to urge the advancement of clinical research with NGS-guided use of PARP inhibitors in the treatment of HNSCC, rather than the non-targeted combination with other treatment modalities, which is currently the only approach to PARP inhibitors utilization in the management of HNSCC. The indisputable association of ctDNA mutations in DDR genes with poor prognosis and survival in HNSCC further supports the acceleration of investigating PARP inhibitors in the management of HNSCC with the future goal to improve survival in this group of patients with notable poor prognosis. Expansion of the DDR gene panel to be tested for mutations should be considered in the future.

5. Conclusions

Despite the benefits of NGS in the management of many malignancies, the mutational landscape of HNSCC remains largely undescribed. This study is the largest cohort to date to analyze the genomic landscape in both blood and tumor tissue in patients with HNSCC and reports a high prevalence of DDR gene mutations in this tumor type. Utilizing both ctDNA and tDNA analysis, the incidence of targetable mutations in this HNSCC cohort was found comparable with other cancers such as breast, ovarian, prostate and pancreatic cancers for which PARP inhibitors are now standard of care. For the first time, the addition of ctDNA analysis contributed to the identification of an increased incidence of DDR gene mutations in patients older than 60 years, in laryngeal primaries, in patients with advanced stage at diagnosis and in patients with tumors previously treated with chemotherapy and/or radiotherapy, while the incidence was found significantly decreased in oropharyngeal cancer and in HPV-positive patients. Patients with DDR gene mutations in ctDNA rather than tDNA had significantly worse prognoses, with more advanced disease burden at the end of the study and with decreased overall survival in univariate analysis and in Cox proportional hazard regression models adjusted for statistically and/or clinically significant variables. These results are expected to prompt further clinical investigations with NGS-guided PARP inhibitors for the treatment of HNSCC.

Author Contributions: Conceptualization, M.P., W.Z., C.M.F., U.T., T.L.J., R.B.D.J. and K.M.B.; Methodology, H.L.W., M.P., R.B.D.J., A.T.F. and K.M.B.; investigation, H.L.W., K.M.B., A.T.F., A.A., A.H.S., M.P., K.S., R.M.P. and J.W.L.; formal analysis, R.B.D.J.; data curation, M.P., A.A., H.L.W., K.M.B. and A.T.F.; writing—original draft preparation, K.M.B., A.T.F., M.J.P. and M.P.; writing—review and editing, K.M.B., A.T.F., M.P., A.H.S., A.A., K.S., J.W.L., C.M.F., R.M.P. and M.J.P. visualization, K.M.B., A.T.F. and M.P.; supervision, M.P., T.L.J., W.Z. and C.M.F. All authors have read and agreed to the published version of the manuscript.

Funding: Biostatistical and bioinformatics services were supported by the Comprehensive Cancer Center of Wake Forest University National Cancer Institute Cancer Center Support Grant P30CA012197. Cristina M. Furdui and Mercedes Porosnicu's effort was partly supported by NIH/NCI U01 CA215848.

Institutional Review Board Statement: The study was conducted according to the guidelines of the Declaration of Helsinki and approved by the Wake Forest School of Medicine Institutional Review Board (IRB00057787).

Informed Consent Statement: Patient consent was waived in this retrospective study, as the research involved no risk for participants, and waiving consent did not adversely affect the subjects. Furthermore, all data was completely deidentified from time of its collection from the electronic medical record.

Data Availability Statement: The datasets analyzed are available from the corresponding author upon request.

Conflicts of Interest: The authors declare no conflict of interest. No outsider funding source contributed to this research and therefore there was no conflict of interest from a funding source.

References

1. Hoesli, R.C.; Ludwig, M.L.; Michmerhuizen, N.L.; Rosko, A.J.; Spector, M.E.; Brenner, J.C.; Birkeland, A.C. Genomic sequencing and precision medicine in head and neck cancers. *Eur. J. Surg. Oncol.* **2017**, *43*, 884–892. [CrossRef]
2. Agrawal, N.; Frederick, M.J.; Pickering, C.R.; Bettegowda, C.; Chang, K.; Li, R.J.; Fakhry, C.; Xie, T.-X.; Zhang, J.; Wang, J. Exome sequencing of head and neck squamous cell carcinoma reveals inactivating mutations in NOTCH1. *Science* **2011**, *333*, 1154–1157. [CrossRef] [PubMed]
3. Stransky, N.; Egloff, A.M.; Tward, A.D.; Kostic, A.D.; Cibulskis, K.; Sivachenko, A.; Kryukov, G.V.; Lawrence, M.S.; Sougnez, C.; McKenna, A. The mutational landscape of head and neck squamous cell carcinoma. *Science* **2011**, *333*, 1157–1160. [CrossRef] [PubMed]
4. Alsahafi, E.; Begg, K.; Amelio, I.; Raulf, N.; Lucarelli, P.; Sauter, T.; Tavassoli, M. Clinical update on head and neck cancer: Molecular biology and ongoing challenges. *Cell Death Dis.* **2019**, *10*, 1–17. [CrossRef]
5. Suh, Y.; Amelio, I.; Urbano, T.G.; Tavassoli, M. Clinical update on cancer: Molecular oncology of head and neck cancer. *Cell Death Dis.* **2014**, *5*, e1018. [CrossRef]
6. Lawrence, M.S.; Sougnez, C.; Lichtenstein, L.; Cibulskis, K.; Lander, E.; Gabriel, S.B.; Getz, G.; Ally, A.; Balasundaram, M.; Birol, I. Comprehensive genomic characterization of head and neck squamous cell carcinomas. *Nature* **2015**, *517*, 576–582.
7. Kim, M.P.; Lozano, G. Mutant p53 partners in crime. *Cell Death Differ.* **2018**, *25*, 161–168. [CrossRef]
8. Kang, H.; Kiess, A.; Chung, C.H. Emerging biomarkers in head and neck cancer in the era of genomics. *Nat. Rev. Clin. Oncol.* **2015**, *12*, 11. [CrossRef] [PubMed]
9. Gipson, B.J.; Robbins, H.A.; Fakhry, C.; D'Souza, G. Sensitivity and specificity of oral HPV detection for HPV-positive head and neck cancer. *Oral Oncol.* **2018**, *77*, 52–56. [CrossRef]
10. Nemajerova, A.; Amelio, I.; Gebel, J.; Dötsch, V.; Melino, G.; Moll, U.M. Non-oncogenic roles of TAp73: From multiciliogenesis to metabolism. *Cell Death Differ.* **2018**, *25*, 144–153. [CrossRef] [PubMed]
11. Rothenberg, S.M.; Ellisen, L.W. The molecular pathogenesis of head and neck squamous cell carcinoma. *J. Clin. Investig.* **2012**, *122*, 1951–1957. [CrossRef] [PubMed]
12. Si, H.; Lu, H.; Yang, X.; Mattox, A.; Jang, M.; Bian, Y.; Sano, E.; Viadiu, H.; Yan, B.; Yau, C. TNF-α modulates genome-wide redistribution of ΔNp63α/TAp73 and NF-κB cREL interactive binding on TP53 and AP-1 motifs to promote an oncogenic gene program in squamous cancer. *Oncogene* **2016**, *35*, 5781–5794. [CrossRef]
13. Castellanos, M.R.; Pan, Q. Novel p53 therapies for head and neck cancer. *World J. Otorhinolaryngol. Neck Surg.* **2016**, *2*, 68–75. [CrossRef]
14. Johnson, F.M.; Janku, F.; Lee, J.J.; Schmitz, D.; Streefkerk, H.; Frederick, M. Single-Arm Study of Bimiralisib in Head and Neck Squamous Cell Carcinoma (HNSCC) Patients (pts) Harboring NOTCH1 Loss of Function (LOF) Mutations. 2020. Available online: https://ascopubs.org/doi/abs/10.1200/JCO.2020.38.15_suppl.TPS6590 (accessed on 24 March 2021).
15. Wilson, H.L.; D'Agostino, R.B., Jr.; Meegalla, N.; Petro, R.; Commander, S.; Topaloglu, U.; Zhang, W.; Porosnicu, M. The Prognostic and Therapeutic Value of the Mutational Profile of Blood and Tumor Tissue in Head and Neck Squamous Cell Carcinoma. *Oncologist* **2020**. Available online: https://theoncologist.onlinelibrary.wiley.com/doi/pdfdirect/10.1002/onco.13573 (accessed on 24 March 2021). [CrossRef]
16. Pommier, Y.; O'Connor, M.J.; De Bono, J. Laying a trap to kill cancer cells: PARP inhibitors and their mechanisms of action. *Sci. Transl. Med.* **2016**, *8*, 362ps17. [CrossRef]
17. Nichols, A.C.; Yoo, J.; Palma, D.A.; Fung, K.; Franklin, J.H.; Koropatnick, J.; Mymryk, J.S.; Batada, N.N.; Barrett, J.W. Frequent mutations in TP53 and CDKN2A found by next-generation sequencing of head and neck cancer cell lines. *Arch. Otolaryngol. Neck Surg.* **2012**, *138*, 732–739. [CrossRef]
18. Rodríguez, A.; D'Andrea, A. Fanconi anemia pathway. *Curr. Biol.* **2017**, *27*, R986–R988. [CrossRef] [PubMed]
19. de Bono, J.; Mateo, J.; Fizazi, K.; Saad, F.; Shore, N.; Sandhu, S.; Chi, K.N.; Sartor, O.; Agarwal, N.; Olmos, D.; et al. Olaparib for Metastatic Castration-Resistant Prostate Cancer. *N. Engl. J. Med.* **2020**, *382*, 2091–2102. [CrossRef]
20. Lombardi, A.J.; Hoskins, E.E.; Foglesong, G.D.; Wikenheiser-Brokamp, K.A.; Wiesmüller, L.; Hanenberg, H.; Andreassen, P.R.; Jacobs, A.J.; Olson, S.B.; Keeble, W.W. Acquisition of relative interstrand crosslinker resistance and PARP inhibitor sensitivity in fanconi anemia head and neck cancers. *Clin. Cancer Res.* **2015**, *21*, 1962–1972. [CrossRef] [PubMed]
21. Karam, S.D.; Reddy, K.; Blatchford, P.J.; Waxweiler, T.; DeLouize, A.M.; Oweida, A.; Somerset, H.; Marshall, C.; Young, C.; Davies, K.D. Final report of a phase I trial of olaparib with cetuximab and radiation for heavy smoker patients with locally advanced head and neck cancer. *Clin. Cancer Res.* **2018**, *24*, 4949–4959. [CrossRef] [PubMed]
22. De Haan, R.; Van Werkhoven, E.; Van Den Heuvel, M.M.; Peulen, H.M.U.; Sonke, G.S.; Elkhuizen, P.; Van Den Brekel, M.W.M.; Tesselaar, M.E.T.; Vens, C.; Schellens, J.H.M. Study protocols of three parallel phase 1 trials combining radical radiotherapy with the PARP inhibitor olaparib. *BMC Cancer* **2019**, *19*, 901. [CrossRef]
23. Jelinek, M.J.; Foster, N.R.; Zoroufy, A.J.; Schwartz, G.K.; Munster, P.N.; Seiwert, T.Y.; de Souza, J.A.; Vokes, E.E. A phase I trial adding poly (ADP-ribose) polymerase inhibitor veliparib to induction carboplatin-paclitaxel in patients with head and neck squamous cell carcinoma: Alliance A091101. *Oral Oncol.* **2021**, *114*, 105171. [CrossRef] [PubMed]
24. Schwaederle, M.; Chattopadhyay, R.; Kato, S.; Fanta, P.T.; Banks, K.C.; Choi, I.S.; Piccioni, D.E.; Ikeda, S.; Talasaz, A.; Lanman, R.B. Genomic alterations in circulating tumor DNA from diverse cancer patients identified by next-generation sequencing. *Cancer Res.* **2017**, *77*, 5419–5427. [CrossRef]

25. Dubot, C.; Bernard, V.; Sablin, M.P.; Vacher, S.; Chemlali, W.; Schnitzler, A.; Pierron, G.; Rais, K.A.; Bessoltane, N.; Jeannot, E. Comprehensive genomic profiling of head and neck squamous cell carcinoma reveals FGFR1 amplifications and tumour genomic alterations burden as prognostic biomarkers of survival. *Eur. J. Cancer* **2018**, *91*, 47–55. [CrossRef]
26. Heeke, A.L.; Pishvaian, M.J.; Lynce, F.; Xiu, J.; Brody, J.R.; Chen, W.-J.; Baker, T.M.; Marshall, J.L.; Isaacs, C. Prevalence of homologous recombination–related gene mutations across multiple cancer types. *JCO Precis. Oncol.* **2018**, *2*, 1–13. [CrossRef]
27. Seiwert, T.Y.; Zuo, Z.; Keck, M.K.; Khattri, A.; Pedamallu, C.S.; Stricker, T.; Brown, C.; Pugh, T.J.; Stojanov, P.; Cho, J. Integrative and comparative genomic analysis of HPV-positive and HPV-negative head and neck squamous cell carcinomas. *Clin. Cancer Res.* **2015**, *21*, 632–641. [CrossRef] [PubMed]
28. Chung, C.H.; Guthrie, V.B.; Masica, D.L.; Tokheim, C.; Kang, H.; Richmon, J.; Agrawal, N.; Fakhry, C.; Quon, H.; Subramaniam, R.M. Genomic alterations in head and neck squamous cell carcinoma determined by cancer gene-targeted sequencing. *Ann. Oncol.* **2015**, *26*, 1216–1223. [CrossRef]
29. Aung, K.L.; Siu, L.L. Genomically personalized therapy in head and neck cancer. *Cancers Head Neck* **2016**, *1*, 1–10. [CrossRef]
30. Holcomb, A.J.; Brown, L.; Tawfik, O.; Madan, R.; Shnayder, Y.; Thomas, S.M.; Wallace, N.A. DNA repair gene expression is increased in HPV positive head and neck squamous cell carcinomas. *Virology* **2020**, *548*, 174–181. [CrossRef] [PubMed]
31. Qin, T.; Zhang, Y.; Zarins, K.R.; Jones, T.R.; Virani, S.; Peterson, L.A.; McHugh, J.B.; Chepeha, D.; Wolf, G.T.; Rozek, L.S. Expressed HNSCC variants by HPV-status in a well-characterized Michigan cohort. *Sci. Rep.* **2018**, *8*, 1–11. [CrossRef] [PubMed]
32. Bold, I.T.; Specht, A.-K.; Droste, C.F.; Zielinski, A.; Meyer, F.; Clauditz, T.S.; Münscher, A.; Werner, S.; Rothkamm, K.; Petersen, C. DNA Damage Response during Replication Correlates with CIN70 Score and Determines Survival in HNSCC Patients. *Cancers* **2021**, *13*, 1194. [CrossRef] [PubMed]
33. Galot, R.; van Marcke, C.; Helaers, R.; Mendola, A.; Goebbels, R.-M.; Caignet, X.; Ambroise, J.; Wittouck, K.; Vikkula, M.; Limaye, N. Liquid biopsy for mutational profiling of locoregional recurrent and/or metastatic head and neck squamous cell carcinoma. *Oral Oncol.* **2020**, *104*, 104631. [CrossRef] [PubMed]
34. Psyrri, A.; Papaxoinis, G.; Gavrielatou, N.; Gkotzamanidou, M.; Economopoulou, P.; Kotsantis, I.; Spathis, A.; Anastasiou, M.; Gkolfinopoulos, S.; Nifora, M. Molecular Correlates of Response to Preoperative Olaparib Alone or with Cisplatin or with Durvalumab in Head and Neck Squamous Cell Carcinoma (HNSCC): A Hellenic Cooperative Oncology Group Study. 2020. Available online: https://ascopubs.org/doi/abs/10.1200/JCO.2020.38.15_suppl.6556 (accessed on 24 March 2021).
35. Yasukawa, M.; Fujihara, H.; Fujimori, H.; Kawaguchi, K.; Yamada, H.; Nakayama, R.; Yamamoto, N.; Kishi, Y.; Hamada, Y.; Masutani, M. Synergetic effects of PARP inhibitor AZD2281 and cisplatin in oral squamous cell carcinoma in vitro and in vivo. *Int. J. Mol. Sci.* **2016**, *17*, 272. [CrossRef] [PubMed]

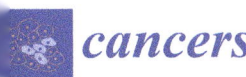

Article

A Laboratory-Friendly CTC Identification: Comparable Double-Immunocytochemistry with Triple-Immunofluorescence

Raed Sulaiman [1], Pradip De [2,3], Jennifer C. Aske [2], Xiaoqian Lin [2], Adam Dale [2], Ethan Vaselaar [2], Nischal Koirala [2], Cheryl Ageton [4], Kris Gaster [5], Joshua Plorde [6], Benjamin Solomon [7], Bradley Thaemert [8], Paul Meyer [9], Luis Rojas Espaillat [10], David Starks [10] and Nandini Dey [2,3,*]

1. Physicians Laboratory, Department of Pathology, Avera McKennan Hospital & University Health Center, Sioux Falls, SD 57105, USA; raed.sulaiman@plpath.org
2. Translational Oncology Laboratory, Avera Research Institute, Sioux Falls, SD 57105, USA; pradip.de@avera.org (P.D.); jennifer.aske@avera.org (J.C.A.); xiaoqian.lin@avera.org (X.L.); adam.dale@avera.org (A.D.); ethan.vaselaar@avera.org (E.V.); nischal.koirala@avera.org (N.K.)
3. Department of Internal Medicine, University of South Dakota SSOM, USD, Sioux Falls, SD 57105, USA
4. Department of Research Oncology, Clinical Research, Sioux Falls, SD 57105, USA; cheryl.ageton@avera.org
5. Avera Cancer Institute, Avera McKennan Hospital, Sioux Falls, SD 57105, USA; kris.gaster@avera.org
6. Diagnostic Radiology, Interventional Radiology, and Radiology, Avera Medical Group Radiology, Sioux Falls, SD 57105, USA; joshua.plorde@avera.org
7. Hematology and Oncology, Avera Medical Group Oncology & Hematology, Sioux Falls, SD 57105, USA; benjamin.solomon@avera.org
8. Bariatrics, Surgery, and General Surgery, Surgical Institute of South Dakota, Sioux Falls, SD 57105, USA; bradley.thaemert@avera.org
9. Cardiovascular/Thoracic Surgery, Surgery North Central Heart, A Division of Avera Heart Hospital, Sioux Falls, SD 57105, USA; pmeyer@ncheart.com
10. Department of Gynecologic Oncology, Avera Cancer Institute, Sioux Falls, SD 57105, USA; luis.rojasespaillat@avera.org (L.R.E.); david.starks@avera.org (D.S.)
* Correspondence: nandini.dey@avera.org

Citation: Sulaiman, R.; De, P.; Aske, J.C.; Lin, X.; Dale, A.; Vaselaar, E.; Koirala, N.; Ageton, C.; Gaster, K.; Plorde, J.; et al. A Laboratory-Friendly CTC Identification: Comparable Double-Immunocytochemistry with Triple-Immunofluorescence. *Cancers* **2022**, *14*, 2871. https://doi.org/10.3390/cancers14122871

Academic Editor: Riccardo Fodde

Received: 25 May 2022
Accepted: 5 June 2022
Published: 10 June 2022

Publisher's Note: MDPI stays neutral with regard to jurisdictional claims in published maps and institutional affiliations.

Copyright: © 2022 by the authors. Licensee MDPI, Basel, Switzerland. This article is an open access article distributed under the terms and conditions of the Creative Commons Attribution (CC BY) license (https://creativecommons.org/licenses/by/4.0/).

Simple Summary: Tumor cells that circulate in the peripheral blood of patients with solid tumors are called circulating tumor cells. Since the source of circulating tumor cells are from primary cancer sites, metastatic sites, and/or a disseminated tumor cell pool, these cells have clinical significance. The circulating tumor cells offer a rare glimpse of the evolution of the tumor and its response/resistance to treatment in a real-time non-invasive manner. Although the clinical relevance of circulating tumor cells is undeniable, the routine use of these cells remains limited due to the elusive nature of the cells, which demands highly sophisticated and costly instrumentation. We presented a specific and sensitive laboratory-friendly *parallel double-detection format* method for the simultaneous isolation and identification of circulating tumor cells from peripheral blood of 91 consented and enrolled patients with tumors of the lung, endometrium, ovary, esophagus, prostate, and liver. Our user-friendly cost-effective circulating tumor cells detection technique has the potency to facilitate the routine use of circulating tumor cells detection even in community-based cancer centers for prognosis, before and after surgery, which will provide a unique opportunity to move cancer diagnostics forward.

Abstract: The source of circulating tumor cells (CTC) in the peripheral blood of patients with solid tumors are from primary cancer, metastatic sites, and a disseminated tumor cell pool. As 90% of cancer-related deaths are caused by metastatic progression and/or resistance-associated treatment failure, the above fact justifies the undeniable predictive and prognostic value of identifying CTC in the bloodstream at stages of the disease progression and resistance to treatment. Yet enumeration of CTC remains far from a standard routine procedure either for post-surgery follow-ups or ongoing adjuvant therapy. The most compelling explanation for this paradox is the absence of a convenient, laboratory-friendly, and cost-effective method to determine CTC. We presented a specific and sensitive laboratory-friendly *parallel double-detection format* method for the simultaneous isolation and identification of CTC from peripheral blood of 91 consented and enrolled patients with various malignant solid tumors of the lung, endometrium, ovary, esophagus, prostate, and liver. Using a pressure-guided method, we used the size-based isolation to capture CTC on a commercially available microfilter. CTC identification was carried out by two expression marker-based independent staining methods, double-immunocytochemistry parallel to standard triple-immunofluorescence. The choice of markers included specific markers for epithelial cells, EpCAM and CK8,18,19, and exclusion markers for WBC, CD45. We tested the method's specificity based on the validation of the staining method, which included positive and negative spiked samples, blood from the healthy age-matched donor, healthy age-matched leucopaks, and blood from metastatic patients. Our user-friendly cost-effective CTC detection technique may facilitate the regular use of CTC detection even in community-based cancer centers for prognosis, before and after surgery.

Keywords: CTC; immunocytochemistry; *parallel double-detection*; laboratory-friendly

1. Introduction

Circulating tumor cells (CTCs) are rare and heterogeneous cellular components circulating in the peripheral blood of patients with solid tumors [1] and are considered one of the fundamental elements of the blood-based biopsy. As the source of CTCs in the bloodstream has been known to be from primary cancer sites, secondary metastatic sites, and/or a disseminated tumor cell pool, the predictive [2] and prognostic [2,3] values of CTC have been established in most solid tumors including prostate [4], hepatocellular [5], breast [6–8], colorectal [9,10] melanoma [11], head and neck [12], bladder [13], testicular [14], and gastric cancers [15] in both localized and metastatic clinical settings [1]. The prognostic and therapeutic implications of CTC phenotype detection based on epithelial–mesenchymal transition markers in the first-line chemotherapy of HER2-negative metastatic breast cancers indicated the role of CTCs in the management of the disease [16]. CTC enumeration has also proven its potential to improve the management of cancers in several other ways. The value of real-time longitudinal CTC fluctuations can provide the opportunity for (1) treatment intensification in patients with a poor prognosis or (2) de-escalation in patients with a good prognosis. CTC as an endpoint has the potential to evaluate the efficacy of treatment alongside the molecular characteristics of CTCs, which provides their theranostic value [3]. The utility of CTCs as a multifunctional biomarker focusing on their potential as pharmacodynamic endpoints either directly via the molecular characterization of specific markers or indirectly through CTC enumeration has been reported [17].

In spite of the well-recognized clinical validity and utility [18] of enumerating CTC in nonmetastatic and metastatic cancers [3], the determination of CTC as a routine strategic procedure is yet to be incorporated into standard clinical practice for the management of the disease [17]. Studies involving the treatment based on (1) CTC count, (2) CTC variations, and/or (3) the molecular characteristics of CTCs were sometimes inconclusive or are still ongoing [3]. One of the reasons CTC determination does not serve as a routine standard liquid biopsy in patients with solid tumors has been identified as the lack of much-needed improvement in the method to test CTC [19]. We need user-friendly, cost-effective, yet reproducible methods to determine CTC routinely for diagnostic (especially with germline mutation or predisposition), predictive, and prognostic purposes across different cancer centers, including community-based hospitals.

CTCs are a promising yet challenging tumor biomarker to detect. The road-block is a methodological issue, as a clinically dependable enumeration of CTC is still limited to primarily established resource-rich, comprehensive centers employing sophisticated instrumentation. Here we presented a low-cost, specific, sensitive, and fail-safe laboratory-friendly method for simultaneous isolation and identification of CTC from 91 consented and enrolled patients with various solid tumors, including lung, endometrial, ovarian, esophageal, prostate, and liver cancers.

2. Methods

2.1. Cell Lines and Reagents

Cell lines from endometrial, ovarian, breast, and lung cancers (AN3CA, Cat # HTB-111; RL-95-2, cat # CRL-1671; OVCAR3, cat # HTB-161; MCF7, cat # HTB-22; HCC1975, cat # CRL-5908 and NCI-H441 cat # CRM-HTB-174), human uterine fibroblasts (HUF; Primary Uterine Fibroblasts, Cat # PCS-460-010), and HUVEC cells were procured from ATCC (cat # PCS-100-013) and were cultured according to the standard cell culture procedures as per ATCC recommendations. Leucopak, PBMC (peripheral blood mononuclear cells) were procured from Lonza (Lonza Group Ltd., Basel, Switzerland). The CellSieve enumeration kit with either DAPI/CK-FITC/EpCAM-PE/CD45-Cy5 or DAPI/CK-FITC/CD31-PE/CD45-Cy5 was procured from Creatv Microtech.

2.2. Patients & Blood Collection

All experimental protocols were approved by the institutional and/or licensing committee/s. The informed consent(s) was obtained from all subjects and/or their legal guardian(s). Informed (IRB approved: Protocol Number Study: 2017.053-100399_ExVivo001) consents for obtaining the peripheral blood were obtained from 91 enrolled patients with various solid tumors, including lung, endometrial, ovarian, esophageal, prostate, and liver cancers. All methods were carried out in accordance with relevant guidelines and regulations. Blood samples were collected in commercially available CellSave collection tubes (Menarini Silicon Biosystems, Bologna, Italy) [20]. We included samples from patients with solid tumors at any stage/grade of the disease undergoing surgery/biopsy with or without pre-treatment/history of any previous carcinoma. We did not include any bone-marrow transplant patients or patients with liquid tumors.

2.3. Isolation and Enrichment of CTCs

The isolation and size-based enrichment of CTCs from blood was achieved by (CellSieve™; Creatv Microtech, Potomac, MD, USA) using precision, high-porosity lithographic microfilters (high capture efficiency precision CellSieve™ microfilters of biocompatible polymer with dense, uniform pores) [21–23]. Size-based filtration was carried out to eliminate red blood cells differentially and most white blood cells from whole blood, retaining larger cells on the surface of the filter [24] using a syringe pump (KD Scientific Legato 110 CMT; Analytical West, Inc., Lebanon, PA, USA) assembled with filter holder assembly (Creatv Microtech; Potomac, MD, USA).

2.4. Identification of CTCs by Double-Immunocytochemistry Assay

We seamlessly coupled the isolation and enumeration of CTC by double-immunocyto chemistry staining. The entire procedure of the $CK8,18^+/CD45^-$ (staining for CK8,18 positivity and CD45 negativity) double immunocytochemistry (ICC×2), from permeabilization to counterstaining, was carried out on a microfilter installed in the syringe pump. The isolated cells on the microfilter were permeabilized by a dual endogenous enzyme blocking buffer with 0.3% hydrogen peroxide-containing sodium azide and levamisole (DAKO; EnVision®+ Dual Link System-HRP (DAB+). Code K4065). Following washing with TBST, pH 7.1, the microfilter was incubated for 1 h at room temperature in 600–700 microliters of a mixture of 1:6000 diluted mouse mAb cytokeratin 8 and 18 (B22.1 & B23.1) (Cell Marque™ Tissue Diagnostic, Millipore-Sigma; Cat. Number: 818M-90) and 1:800 diluted rabbit mAb CD45 (Cell Signaling Technology; D9M8I XP; Catalog # 13917) primary antibodies. Following washing (×3) with TBST, pH 7.1, the microfilter was incubated for 35–40 min at room temperature in 200–300 microliters of a 1:1 mixture of secondary rabbit-Ab-AP-Polymer (Abcam DoubleStain IHC Kit: M&R on human tissue (DAB and AP/Red) Cat. # ab210059) and secondary mouse-Ab-HRP-Polymer (Abcam DoubleStain IHC Kit: M&R on human tissue (DAB and AP/Red) Cat. # ab210059) under light-protected conditions. We used DAKO 10× wash buffer (pH 7.6) (DAKO Wash Buffer 10×; Code S300685-2C) supplied as a 1 L concentrated Tris-buffered saline solution (10×)

containing Tween 20, pH 7.6 (±0.1) for washing. Following washing (×3) with DAKO wash buffer, the color was developed using DAB (3,3'-diaminobenzidine chromogen) reagents, DAB substrate buffer pH 7.5, and DAB+ chromogen (DAKO; EnVision®+ Dual Link System-HRP (DAB+) Code K4065). The chromogenic reaction was stopped by washing (×1) in DD water. DAB color was monitored under a microscope following washes (×3) in DAKO washing buffer. The chromogenic reaction of the alkaline-phosphatase was prepared using permanent Red-Substrate, permanent Red-Activator, and permanent Red-Chromogen (Abcam; Ab210059). Then, 200–300 microliters of the reconstituted final solution were used for incubation (×2) for 20 min. Following washing (×3) with DD water, the cells were counterstained (×2) with filtered DAKO hematoxylin (DAKO; Code S3302) for 10–15 min. Hematoxylin color was developed by incubating the microfilter for 3 min each time and washing using 30 mL of DD water. The air-dried membrane was mounted in a resin-based permanent non-aqueous mounting media (Richard Allan Scientific Mounting Media (Thermo Fisher Scientific: Catalog # 4111TS-TS). For ICC×2, pictures were taken at 40× objective of Olympus BX43 Microscope using cellSens 1.18 LIFE SCIENCE IMAGING SOFTWARE (OLYMPUS CORPORATION).

2.5. Parallel Identification of CTCs by Triple-Immunofluorescence Assay to Validate ICC×2

CellSieve enumeration kit from Creatv Microtech was used for CTC detection employing standard triple immunofluorescent (IF×3) staining [21–23] with certain modifications. In short, 7.5 mL whole blood and 7.5 mL fixation buffer were mixed gently in a 50 mL conical tube and incubated for 15 min at room temperature. The filter holder containing the membrane with a 7-micron pore size was assembled during this incubation period. KD scientific Legato 110 syringe pump was used to draw fluid through the filter ('push' program; 60% force) to move PBS up through the filter to pre-wet it. Next, the fixed blood sample was applied to the filter and pulled through. As per the manufacturer's protocol, we used a kit with CK8,18,19-FITC, EpCAM-PE, and CD45-Cy5 for the staining of CTCs. The images were acquired using Olympus cellSens 1.18 LIFE SCIENCE IMAGING SOFTWARE (OLYMPUS CORPORATION). We used the principle of $CD45^-/CK8,18,19^+/EpCAM^+/DAPI$ for our immuno-fluorescence method. DAPI was used for the evaluation of the nuclear size and morphology. In all the photomicrographs of figures (Figures 1–5), we indicate the measurement of the nuclear diameters.

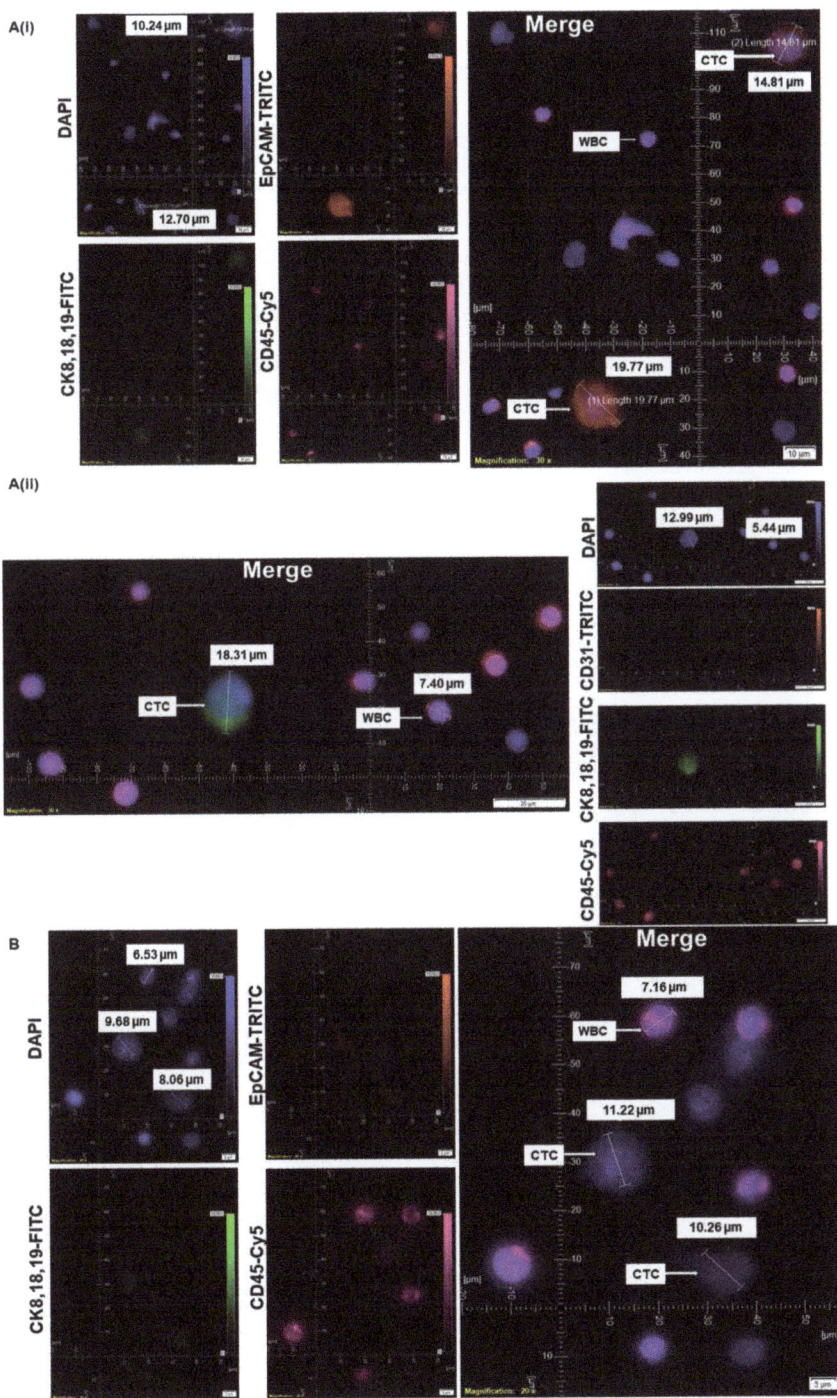

Figure 1. *Cont.*

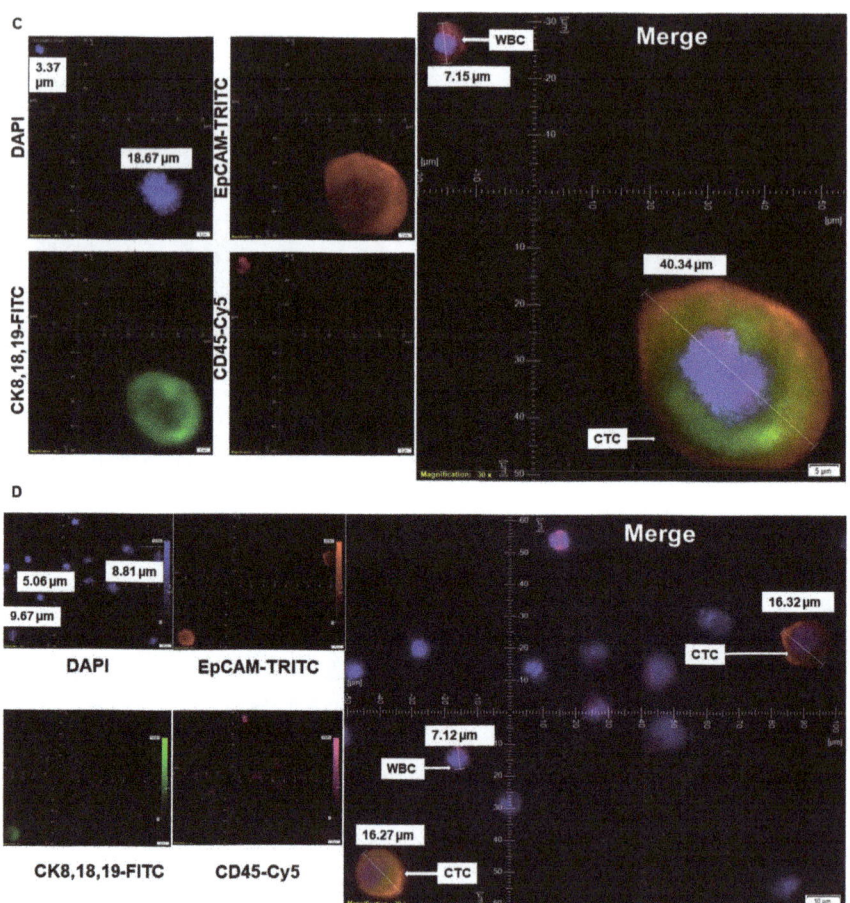

Figure 1. Standardization and validation of CTC by IF×3 using breast, ovarian, and lung cancer cell lines: Patients' blood samples spiked with titrating number (1000 cells, 750 cells, 375 cells, 250 cells/100 cells) of cell lines of different solid tumors using. Pictures were taken at 60× oil objective of an Olympus IX71 Microscope with DAPI/FITC/TRITC/CY5 filter sets. (**A**): MCF7 cells (750 cells/375 cells per 7.5 mL of patient's blood) were used for spiking blood samples, and cells were captured on a microfilter and stained with a CellSieve enumeration kit (Creatv Microtech) with either DAPI/CK-FITC/EpCAM-PE/CD45-Cy5 (**Ai**) or DAPI/CK-FITC/CD31 PE/CD45-Cy5 (**Aii**). (**B**): OVCAR3 cells (100 cells per 7.5 mL of patient's blood) were used for spiking blood samples, and cells were captured on a microfilter and stained with cell sieve enumeration kit (Creatv MicroTech) with DAPI/CK-FITC/EpCAM-PE/CD45-Cy5. (**C**): HCC1975 cells (1000 cells per 7.5 mL of patient's blood) were used for spiking blood samples, and cells were captured on a microfilter and stained with cell sieve enumeration kit (Creatv Microtech) with DAPI/CK-FITC/EpCAM-PE/CD45-Cy5. (**D**): NCI-H441 cells (250 cells per 7.5 mL of patient's blood) were used for spiking blood samples, and cells were captured on a microfilter and stained with cell sieve enumeration kit (Creatv Microtech) with DAPI/CK-FITC/EpCAM-PE/CD45-Cy5. The magnification, scale bar, and digital reticle are represented for each photomicrograph. Fluorescence images from DAPI, FITC, TRITC, and Cy5 channels were separated as pictures with a color bar. The fluorescence-photomicrographs presented the diameters (μm) of CTC and a representative WBC and their respective DAPI stained nucleus.

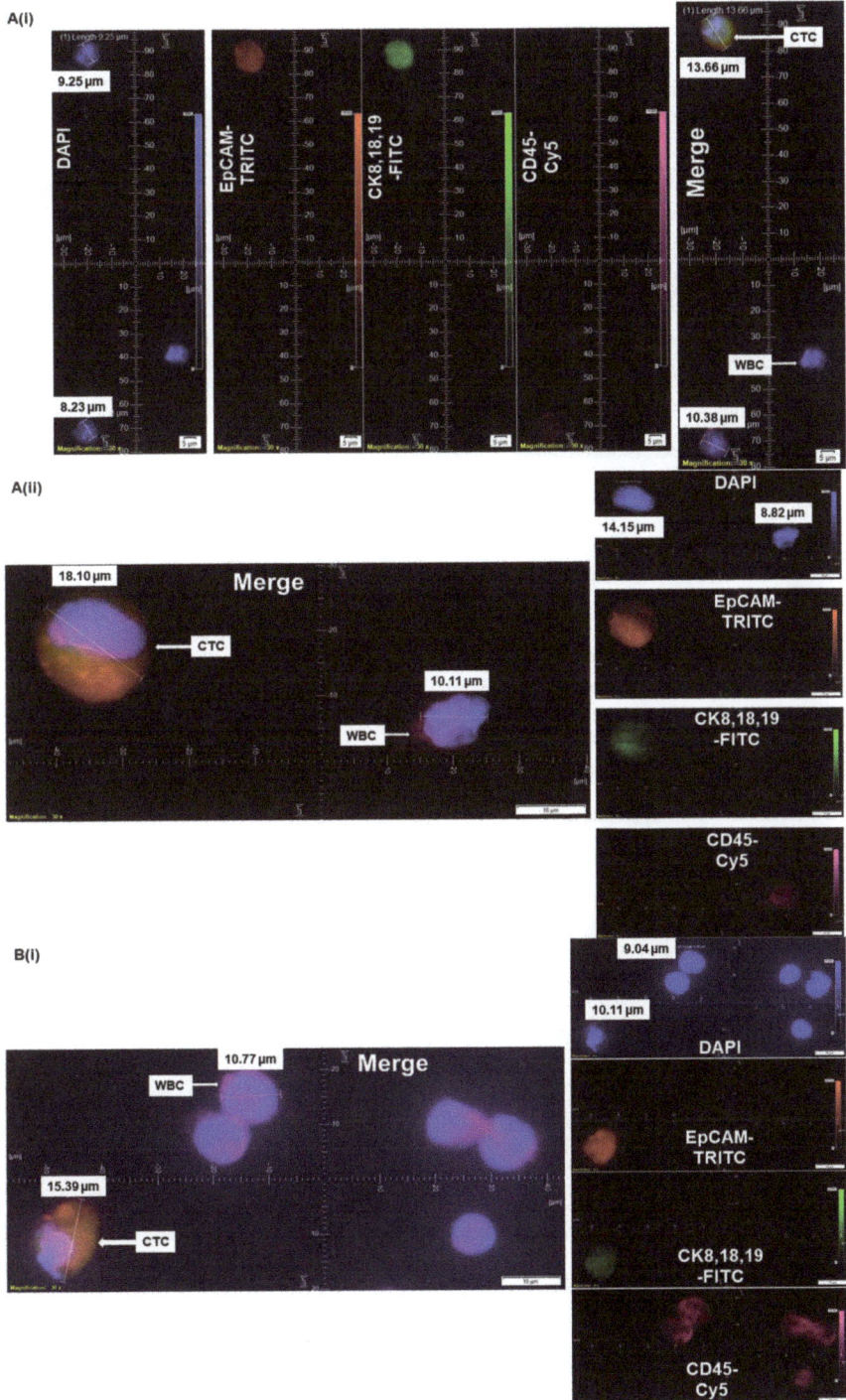

Figure 2. *Cont.*

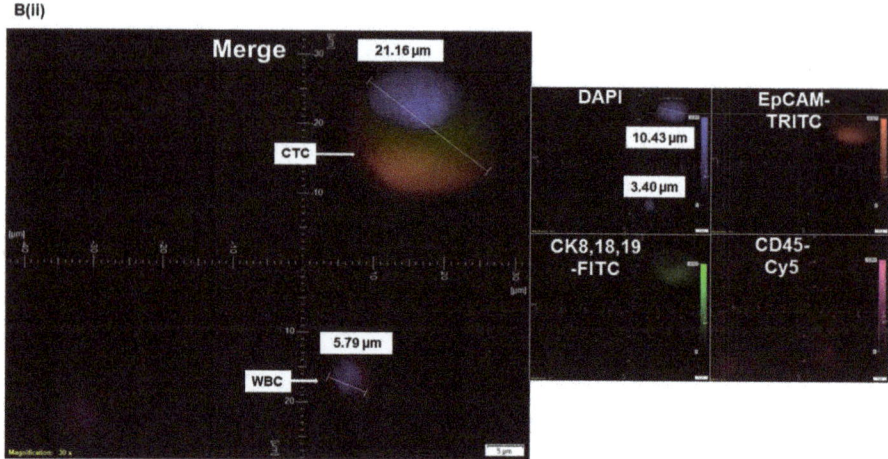

Figure 2. Validation spectrum of CTC by IF×3 using blood from patients with different clinical statuses and samples of origin: CTC from blood samples from patients with (**A**) clinical status, nonmetastatic (**Ai**) and metastatic (**Aii**) in endometrial cancers, and (**B**) samples of origin, during a biopsy from a patient with metastatic liver cancer (**Bi**) and during surgical resection of the tumor in lung cancers (**Bii**) are presented. The magnification, scale bar, and digital reticle are presented for each photomicrograph. Fluorescence images from DAPI, FITC, TRITC, and Cy5 channels were separated as pictures with a color bar. The fluorescence-photomicrographs presented the diameters (µm) of CTC and a representative WBC and their respective DAPI stained nucleus.

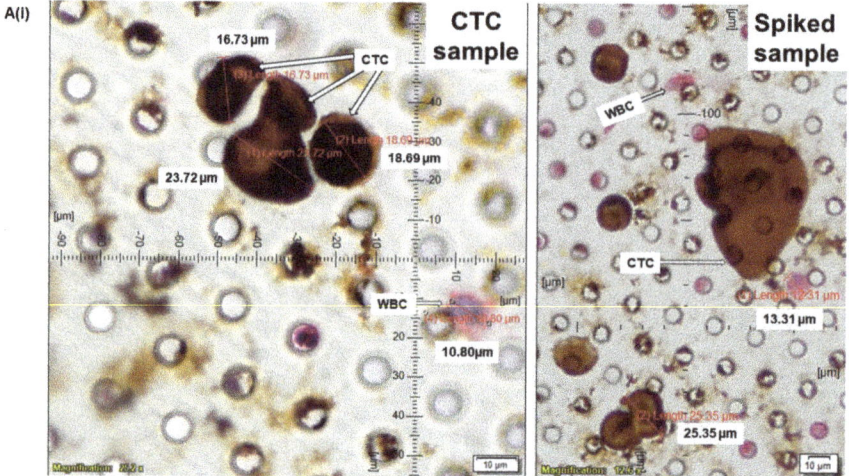

Figure 3. *Cont.*

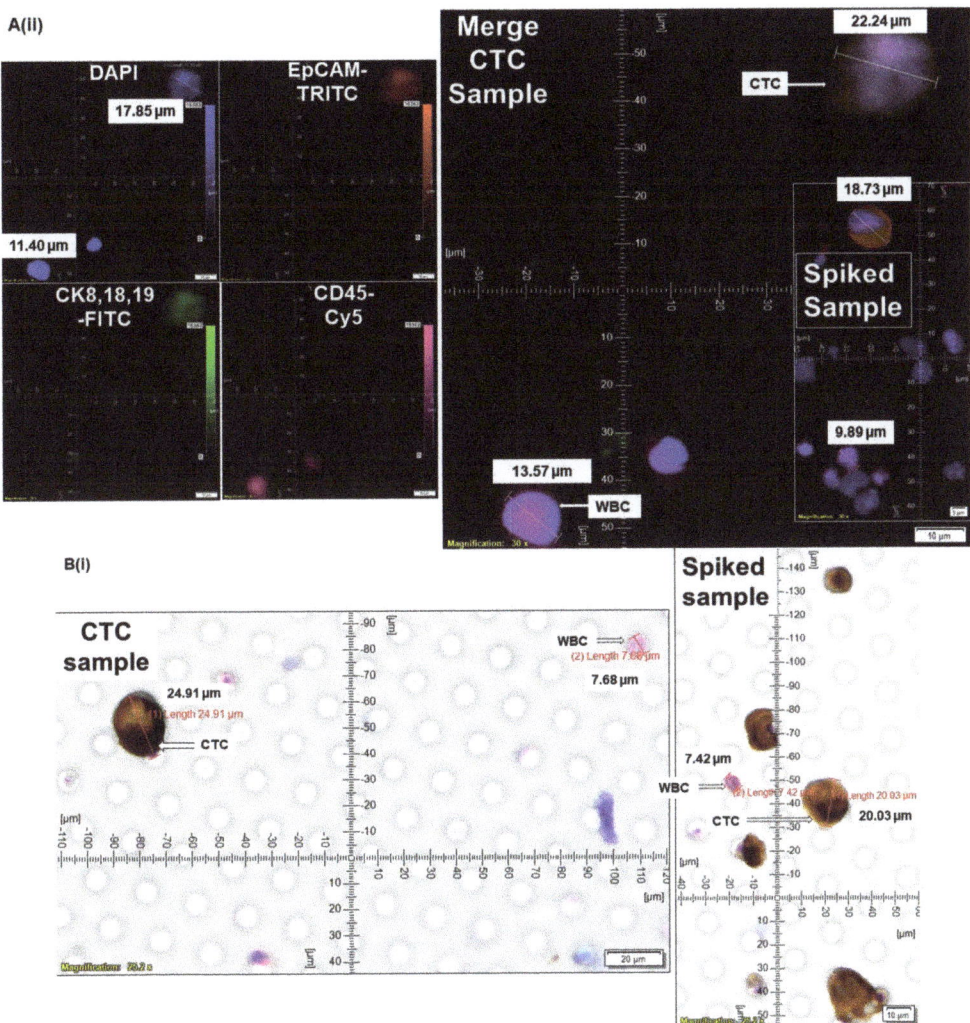

Figure 3. *Cont.*

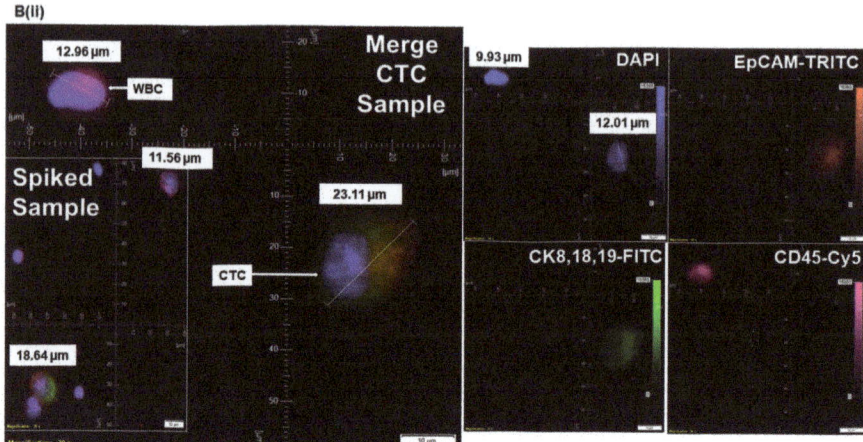

Figure 3. Standardization and validation of CTC by ICC×2 in reference to spiked IF×3 in endometrial and ovarian cancers: CTCs were captured from blood samples from patients with endometrial (**A**) and ovarian (**B**) tumors and enumerated using ICC×2 (**Ai,Bi**) in reference to IF×3 (**Aii,Bii**). Blood samples were spiked (Spiked samples) with titrating numbers (250 cells/100 cells) of NCI-H441 cells separately for both ICC×2 and IF×3. For IF×3, pictures were taken at 60× oil objective of an Olympus IX71 Microscope with DAPI/FITC/TRITC/CY5 filter sets. For ICC×2, pictures were taken at 40× objective of an Olympus BX43 Microscope. The magnification, scale bar, and digital reticle are represented for each photomicrograph. Fluorescence images from DAPI, FITC, TRITC, and Cy5 channels were separated as pictures with a color bar. The fluorescence-photomicrographs presented the diameters (μm) of CTC and a representative WBC and their respective DAPI stained nucleus. The immunocytochemistry-photomicrographs are presented with a scale bar, magnification information, digital reticule, as well as the diameters (μm) of CTC and a representative WBC.

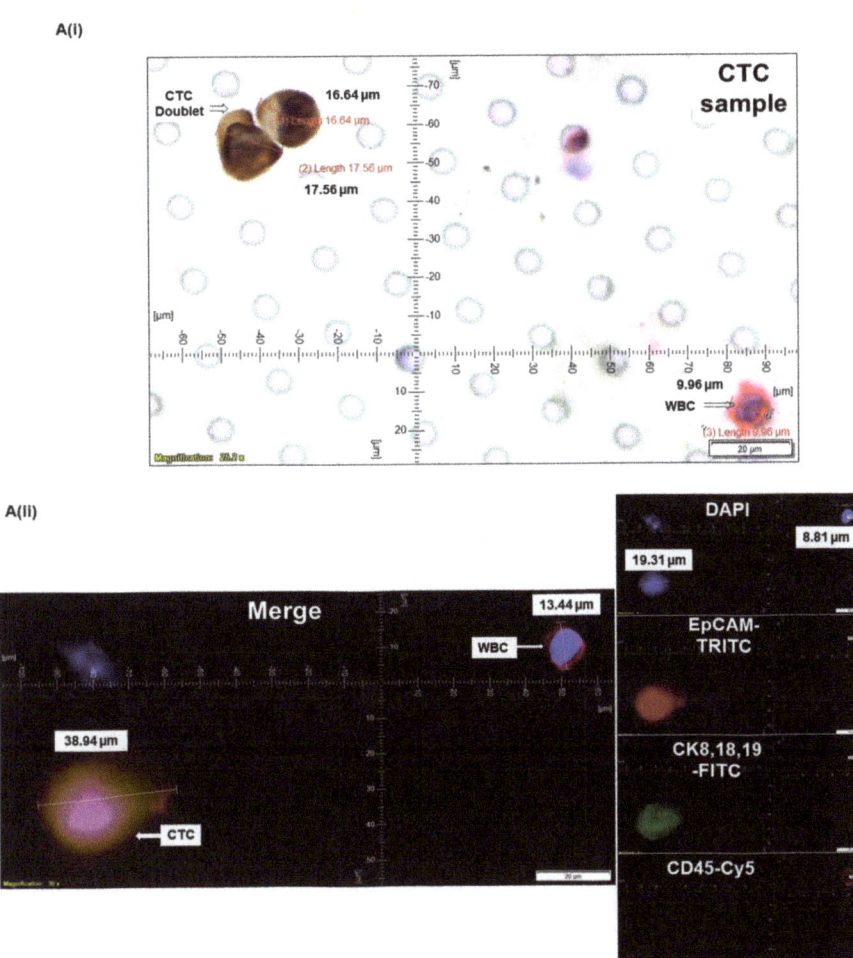

Figure 4. *Cont.*

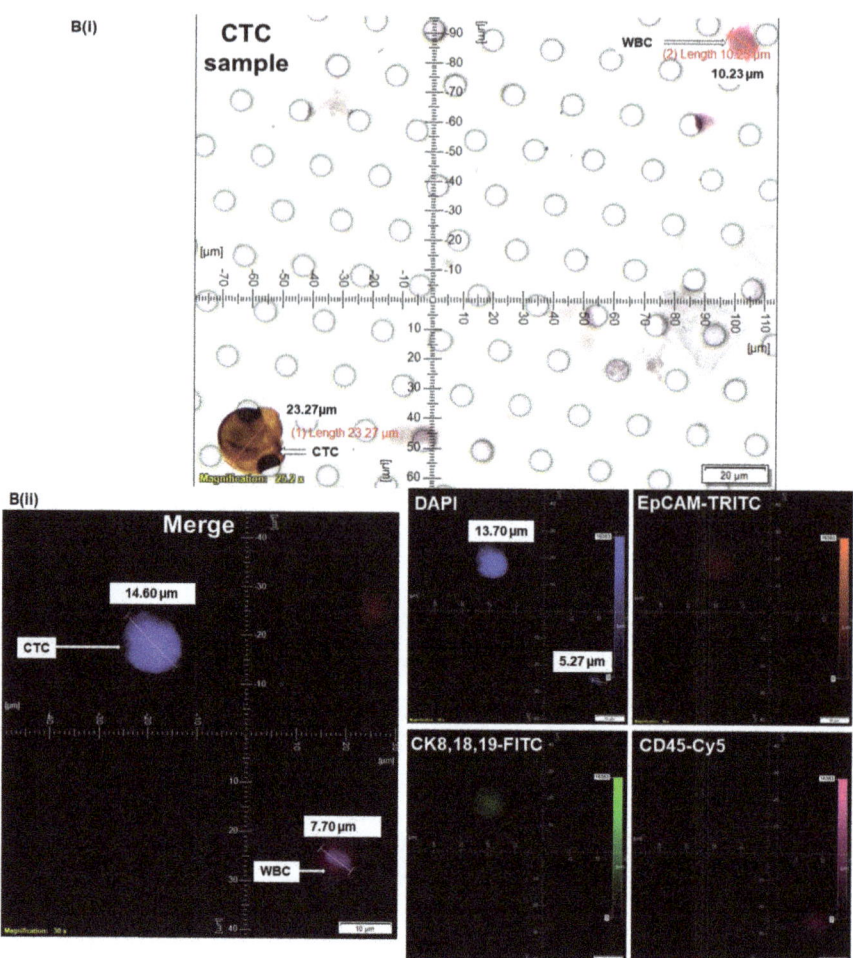

Figure 4. Determining CTC by ICC×2 in endometrial and ovarian cancers: CTCs were captured from blood samples from patients with endometrial (**A**) and ovarian (**B**) tumors and enumerated using ICC×2 (**Ai,Bi**). Blood samples were spiked (Spiked samples) with titrating number (250 cells/100 cells) of NCI-H441 cells separately for ICC×2. Corresponding CTC enumeration by IF×3 (**Aii,Bii**) is presented. For IF×3, pictures were taken at 60× oil objective of an Olympus IX71 Microscope with DAPI/FITC/TRITC/CY5 filter sets. For ICC×2, pictures were taken at 40× objective of an Olympus BX43 Microscope. The magnification, scale bar, and digital reticle are represented for each photomicrograph. Fluorescence images from DAPI, FITC, TRITC, and Cy5 channels were separated as pictures with a color bar. The fluorescence-photomicrographs presented the diameters (μm) of CTC and a representative WBC and their respective DAPI stained nucleus. The immunocytochemistry-photomicrographs are presented with a scale bar, magnification information, digital reticule, as well as the diameters (μm) of CTC and a representative WBC.

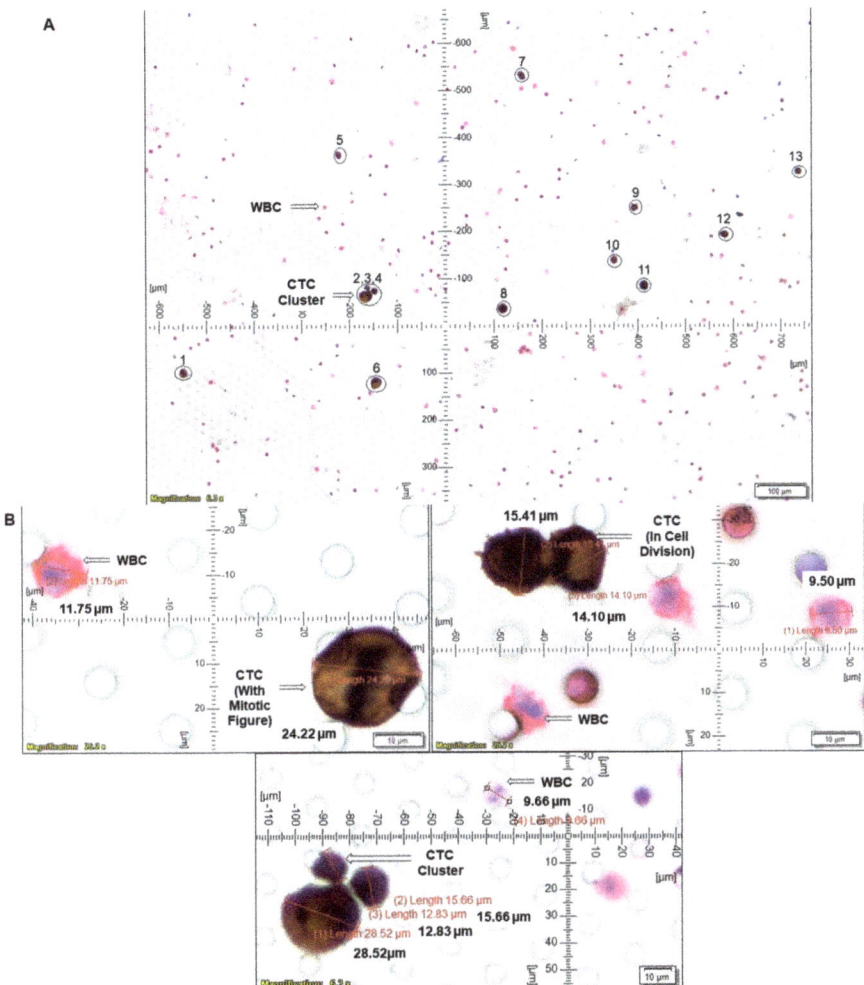

Figure 5. Clinical relevance of determination of the number of CTCs using a single case study: we determined CTC by ICC×2 from the blood of a patient with grade 2 stage I endometrial cancer: CTCs were captured from blood samples from the patient and enumerated using ICC×2 (**A,B**). Blood samples were spiked (Spiked samples) with titrating number (250 cells/100 cells) of NCI-H441 cells separately for ICC×2. For ICC×2, pictures were taken at 40× objective of an Olympus BX43 Microscope. The magnification, scale bar, and digital reticle are represented for each photomicrograph. We recorded up to 100 CTCs in the 7.5 mL of the blood with 13 CTCs in a single microscopic field (**A**) and mitotic CTCs with a mitotic figure and a cluster of 3 CTCs (**B**). The immunocytochemistry-photomicrographs presented with a scale bar, magnification information, digital reticule, as well as the diameters (μm) of CTC and a representative WBC.

2.6. Validation of CTC Assays by Double Immuno-Cytochemistry Assay and Parallel Triple Immunofluorescence Assays

Parallel identification of CTCs by triple-immunofluorescence assay was performed to validate ICC×2. Spike samples of tumor cell lines from endometrial, ovarian, breast, and lung cancers were used. The cell lines were prefixed, and the number of cells in the sample was titrated down (100 cells per spike) to test the sensitivity. The specificity was tested using epithelial cancer cell lines compared to CD31-positive HUVEC cells or normal Human Uterine Fibroblasts (HUF). Leucopak, PBMC, and blood (age-matched) from otherwise healthy persons were used to test the absence of CTC in normal individuals. The test samples were run parallel to spiked samples each time as an internal positive control. The background autofluorescence for all five channels (Microscope Olympus IX71 with DAPI/FITC/TRITC/CY5 filter sets) was tested in both CTC samples as well as spiked samples. The test samples were stained similarly except without the cocktail of primary antibody-conjugate(s). We used the same blood sample twice and separately spiked it with NCI-H441 and HUVEC cells to test the cross-reactivity between epithelial cells and endothelial cells in the peripheral blood. The spiked blood samples were stained with CD31 Kit (containing antibody cocktail for CK 8,18,19/CD45/CD31; specific for detecting endothelial cells) and EpCAM Kit (having antibody cocktail for CK 8,18,19/CD45/EpCAM; specific for detecting epithelial cells). Pictures were taken at 60× oil objective of an Olympus IX71 Microscope with DAPI/FITC/TRITC/CY5 filter sets. The image was acquired using Olympus cellSens 1.18 LIFE SCIENCE IMAGING SOFTWARE (OLYMPUS CORPORATION). The validation of the double-immunocytochemistry assay was based on a parallel validation of the triple immunofluorescence assays in the same blood samples. We used tumor cells from different organ-type cancers for validation. The expression of proteins (CK $8,18,19^+$/EpCAM$^+$/CD45$^-$/SMA$^-$/CD31$^-$) was simultaneously and independently tested using immunocytochemistry, immunofluorescence, and flow cytometry. Once validated, we ran blood samples by immunocytochemistry and immunofluorescence. Out of our 91 blood samples used for the study, we determined CTC by immunofluorescence in 89 blood samples and by immunocytochemistry in 47 blood samples. We used both immunofluorescence and immunocytochemistry methods in 44 blood samples for the concordance study. Each time a blood sample was run (immunocytochemistry and immunofluorescence), we simultaneously ran a tumor cell line, NCI-H441, with it as a positive control. A presentative picture of the NCI-H441 tumor cell line (CK $8,18,19^+$/EpCAM$^+$/CD45$^-$/DAPI) as positive control is presented in the figures (Figures 2 and 3).

3. Results

A total of 91 patients were enrolled in the study (informed consent), and their blood samples were received for standardization and detection of CTC (Table 1). Table 2 presents the background characteristics of the patients. Table 3 presents patients' pre-treatment status at surgery and history of other cancers. Among the blood samples received from 71 patients with endometrial carcinomas (used for the standardization and testing of CTC), we observed endometrioid carcinoma (invasive and non-invasive) as the predominant pathologic subtypes of the disease. The rest of the subtypes included carcinosarcoma and mixed endometrial adenocarcinomas. Among the blood samples received from 11 patients with ovarian carcinomas (used for the standardization and testing of CTC), we observed serous carcinoma (low and high grades) as the predominant pathologic subtypes of the disease. The rest of the subtypes included ovarian adenocarcinoma, adult granulosa cell tumors, ovarian mucinous cystadenoma, and appendiceal mucinous neoplasms. The different pathological subtypes of the lung disease in patients from whom we received our blood samples included squamous cell carcinoma, well-differentiated neuroendocrine tumors, and invasive adenocarcinomas. Our study included 48% of patients with Grade 1 disease, out of which blood samples of 6 patients were used for standardization and 38 were used for CTC-testing. Sixteen percent of the total patients had Grade 2 disease, out of which blood samples of 4 patients were used for standardization, and 11 were used for CTC-testing. Eighteen percent of the total patients had Grade 3 disease, out of which blood samples of 3 patients were used for standardization, and 14 were used for CTC-testing. We first standardized CTC detection by IF×3 by standard triple-immunofluorescence protocol [21–23] using blood from patients' samples spiked with several tumor cell lines, breast, lung, endometrial and ovarian cancers (Figure 1). A total of 15 blood samples from patients with cancer of different organ types were used for standardization (IF×3 and ICC×2). In addition to the blood from patients' samples, parallel blood samples from age-matched healthy individuals' leucopaks and PBMCs were used for standardization and testing auto-fluorescence. Once IF×3 was standardized, we validated our novel procedure of ICC×2-based CTC determination using standard IF×3.

Table 1. Stage-wise distribution of patients' blood samples used for the standardization and testing of CTCs, with tumors from each pathology.

Stages of Patients with Different Tumors (Endometrial, Ovary, Lung, Esophageal, Prostate, and Liver)	Total Percentage of Patients' Blood Used for the Study (%, n = 91)	Number of Blood Samples Used for CTC Standardization (n = 91)	Number of Blood Samples Used for CTC Testing (n = 91)	Percentage of Patients with Positive CTC (IF and/or ICC) (%)
Stage I	63%	6	51	45%
Stage II	5%	1	4	50%
Stage III	14%	3	10	30%
Stage IV (Metastatic)	10%	4	5	100%
Tumors from Each Organ Type				
Tumors from Each Pathology	Endometrial	Ovary	Lung	Esophageal	Prostate	Liver
Stage I	54	3	0	0	0	0
Stage II	2	1	2	0	0	0
Stage III	9	3	0	1	0	0
Stage IV (Metastatic)	3	2	1	0	2	1

Table 2. Pathology parameters of organ type (endometrial, ovarian, lung, prostate, liver, and esophageal) tumors used for the study (LVI = Lymphovascular Invasion; MI = Myometrial Invasion; MSI = Microsatellite Instability; NA = Not Applicable; ND = Not Determined; NAV = Not Available).

| De-Identified Patient Code | Pathological Parameters of Tumor Samples from Patients with Endometrial Cancer | | | | | | |
	Tumor Type-Histological	TMN	Grade	Stage	LVI	MI (%)	MSI
CTC-EC-691	Endometrioid adenocarcinoma	pT2 pN0	1	II	Present	25	NAV
CTC-EC-702	Endometrioid adenocarcinoma	pT1a N0 (sn)	1	IA	Absent	14	NAV
CTC-EC-713	Endometrioid adenocarcinoma	pT1a N0 (sn)	1	IA	Absent	15	NAV
CTC-EC-724	Endometrioid adenocarcinoma	pT1b N1a	1	IIIC1	Present	95	NAV
CTC-EC-735	Endometrioid adenocarcinoma	pT1a pN0 (i+) pMX	2	IA	Present	46	NAV
CTC-EC-746	Endometrioid adenocarcinoma	pT1a pN0	3	IA	Present	29	NAV
CTC-EC-757	Endometrioid adenocarcinoma	pT1a pNX	1	IA	Absent	0	NAV
CTC-EC-768	Endometrioid adenocarcinoma	pT1a pN0	1	IA	Absent	11	NAV
CTC-EC-779	Endometrioid adenocarcinoma	pT1b N1a	1	IIIC1	Present	67	NAV

Table 2. Cont.

De-Identified Patient Code	Pathological Parameters of Tumor Samples from Patients with Endometrial Cancer						
	Tumor Type-Histological	TMN	Grade	Stage	LVI	MI (%)	MSI
CTC-EC-7810	High grade papillary serous carcinoma	pT3b pNX	3	IIIB	Absent	100	NAV
CTC-EC-7911	Endometrioid adenocarcinoma	pT1a NX	1	IA	Absent	9	NAV
CTC-EC-8012	Endometrioid adenocarcinoma	pT1apN0(sn)	1	IA	Absent	14	NAV
CTC-EC-8113	Endometrioid adenocarcinoma	pT1a pN0 (sn)	1	IA	Absent	14	NAV
CTC-EC-8214	Extensive mutlifocal complex hyperplasia with atypia	NA	ND	I	ND	ND	NAV
CTC-EC-8315	Residual carcinosarcoma	pT1a pN0	ND	IA	Absent	26	NAV
CTC-EC-8416	Endometrioid adenocarcinoma	pT1a pNX	1	I	Absent	28	NAV
CTC-EC-8517	Endometrioid adenocarcinoma	pT2 NX	2	II	Present	87	NAV
CTC-EC-8618	Carcinosarcoma	pT2 N1mi	3	IIIC1	Present	72	Stable
CTC-EC-8719	Endometrioid adenocarcinoma	pT1a pN0sn	1	IA	Absent	0	NAV
CTC-EC-8820	Endometrioid adenocarcinoma	pT1a pN0sn	1	IA	Absent	0	High
CTC-EC-8921	Carcinosarcoma with high grade serous carcinoma and rhabdomyosarcomatous differentiation	pT1a N1mi	3	IIIC1	Absent	38	Stable
CTC-EC-9022	Endometrioid adenocarcinoma (metastatic)	pT3b pNX pM1	3	IV	Absent	50	Stable
CTC-EC-9223	Endometrioid adenocarcinoma	pT1a N0	2	IA	Absent	44	NAV
CTC-EC-9324	Benign endometrial polyp	NA	NA	NA	NA	NA	NAV
CTC-EC-9525	Endometrioid adenocarcinoma with squamous cell differentiation	pT1a N0	1	IA	Absent	0	NAV
CTC-EC-9626	Endometrioid adenocarcinoma	pT1a N0	1	I	Absent	0	NAV
CTC-EC-9727	Endometrioid adenocarcinoma	pT1a pN0	1	IA	ND	25	NAV
CTC-EC-9828	Endometrioid adenocarcinoma	pT1a N0(i+)	1	I	Absent	17	NAV
CTC-EC-9929	Endometrioid adenocarcinoma	pT1b N0	3	IB	Absent	95	NAV
CTC-EC-10030	Benign endometrial polyp	NA	NA	NA	NA	NA	NAV
CTC-EC-10131	Endometrioid adenocarcinoma	pT1a N0	2	I	Absent	11	High
CTC-EC-10232	Endometrioid adenocarcinoma	pT1a N0	1	IA	Absent	29	NAV
CTC-EC-10333	Endometrioid adenocarcinoma	pT1a (sn) pN0 pMX	3	IA	Absent	43	NAV
CTC-EC-10434	Endometrioid adenocarcinoma	pT1a N0	1	IA	Present (?)	36	NAV
CTC-EC-10535	Complex atypical hyperplasia	NA	NA	NA	NA	NA	NAV
CTC-EC-10636	Endometrioid adenocarcinoma	pT1a N0	1	IA	Absent	17	NAV

Table 2. *Cont.*

De-Identified Patient Code	Pathological Parameters of Tumor Samples from Patients with Endometrial Cancer						
	Tumor Type-Histological	TMN	Grade	Stage	LVI	MI (%)	MSI
CTC-EC-10737	Endometrioid adenocarcinoma	pT1a N0	1	IA	Absent	34	NAV
CTC-EC-10838	Endometrioid adenocarcinoma	pT1a (sn) N0	1	IA	Absent	13	NAV
CTC-EC-10939	Endometrioid adenocarcinoma	pT1a	2	IA	Present	25	NAV
CTC-EC-11040	Endometrioid adenocarcinoma	pT1a N0	1	IA	Absent	6	NAV
CTC-EC-11141	Endometrioid adenocarcinoma	pT1a pN0	3	IA	Absent	37	NAV
CTC-EC-11242	Endometrioid adenocarcinoma	pT1a (sn) N0	1	IA	Absent	35	NAV
CTC-EC-11343	Endometrioid adenocarcinoma	pT1a N0	1	IA	Absent	< 50%	NAV
CTC-EC-11444	Endometrioid adenocarcinoma	pT1b N0	3	IB	Absent	90	NAV
CTC-EC-11545	Endometrioid adenocarcinoma	pT1a pN0 (i+) (sn)	2	IA	Absent	15	NAV
CTC-EC-11646	Endometrioid adenocarcinoma	pT1a N0	2	IA	Absent	32	NAV
CTC-EC-11747	Endometrioid adenocarcinoma	pT1a N0	2	IA	Absent	8	High
CTC-EC-11848	High-grade serous endometrial adenocarcinoma	pT1a N2mi	3	IIIC2	Present	46	NAV
CTC-EC-11949	Endometrioid adenocarcinoma	pT1a sn N0	1	IA	Absent	0	NAV
CTC-EC-12050	Endometrioid adenocarcinoma	pT1b sn N1a	2	IIIC1	Present	57	NAV
CTC-EC-12151	Endometrioid adenocarcinoma	pT1a pN0 (sn)	1	IA	Absent	22	NAV
CTC-EC-12252	Endometrioid adenocarcinoma	pT1a (sn) pN0	1	IA	Absent	19	High
CTC-EC-12353	Endometrioid adenocarcinoma	pT1a pN0	1	IA	Absent	30	NAV
CTC-EC-12454	Endometrioid adenocarcinoma	pT1a pN0 (sn)	1	IA	Absent	38	NAV
CTC-EC-12555	Endometrioid adenocarcinoma	pT1a pN0	1	IA	Absent	0	NAV
CTC-EC-12656	Endometrioid carcinoma	pT1a pNX pMX	1	IA	Absent	0	NAV
CTC-EC-12757	Endometrioid adenocarcinoma	pT1a (sn) pN0	1	IA	Absent	41	NAV
CTC-EC-12858	Endometrioid adenocarcinoma	pT1a N0	1	IA	Absent	23	NAV
CTC-EC-12959	High-grade serous endometrial adenocarcinoma	pT2 (sn) N2mi	3	IIIC2	Present	87	NAV
CTC-EC-13060	Mixed cell adenocarcinoma, (50% high-grade serous, 50% clear cell)	pT1a N0 M1	3	IVB	Absent	0	NAV
CTC-EC-13161	High-grade serous endometrial adenocarcinoma	pT3a (sn) pN0 (i+)	3	IVB	Present	0	NAV

Table 2. Cont.

De-Identified Patient Code	Pathological Parameters of Tumor Samples from Patients with Endometrial Cancer						
	Tumor Type-Histological	TMN	Grade	Stage	LVI	MI (%)	MSI
CTC-EC-13262	Uterine carcinosarcoma	pT1a pN0	ND	IA	Absent	13	NAV
CTC-EC-13363	Mixed cell adenocarcinoma, (10% high-grade serous carcinoma, 90% endometrioid)	pT1a pN0 (sn)	3	IA	Absent	13	NAV
CTC-EC-13464	Endometrioid adenocarcinoma	pT1a (sn) N0	2	IA	Absent	6	NAV
CTC-EC-13565	Mixed cell adenocarcinoma, (90% high-grade serous, 10% endometrioid adenocarcinoma)	pT1a N0	3	IA	Absent	38	NAV
CTC-EC-13866	Endometrioid adenocarcinoma	pT1b N0(sn)	1	IB	Absent	64	High
CTC-EC-14067	Endometrioid adenocarcinoma	pT1a pNX	1	IA	Absent	35	NAV
CTC-EC-14268	Endometrioid adenocarcinoma	pT1a (sn) N0	2	IA	Absent	10	NAV
CTC-EC-14369	Endometrioid adenocarcinoma	pT1a pN1mi (sn)	1	IIIC1	Absent	46	NAV
CTC-EC-14570	Endometrioid adenocarcinoma	pT1a pN0 (sn)	2	I	Absent	25	NAV
CTC-EC-14771	Carcinosarcoma (predominantly endometrioid adenocarcinoma)	pT1a (sn) pN0i+	3	IA	Present	48	NAV
De-Identified Patient Code	Pathological Parameters of Tumor Samples from Patients with Ovarian Cancer						
	Tumor Type—Histological	TMN	Grade	Stage	LVI	MSI	
CTC-OC-911	Adenocarcinoma consistent with history of ovarian carcinoma	ND	ND	IIIC/IV	NA	Stable	
CTC-OC-942	Serous carcinoma	(y)pT3c pNX pMX	1	IIIC	Present	ND	
CTC-OC-1363	Adult granulosa cell tumor	pT1a NX	NA	IA	Absent	NAV	
CTC-OC-1374	Low grade serous carcinoma with abundant psammoma bodies (omentum)	ND	1	IIIA2	NA	Stable	
CTC-OC-1395	High-grade serous carcinoma	pT3b pN0	3	IIB	Absent	NAV	
CTC-OC-1416	Ovarian mucinous cystadenoma	NA	NA	NA	Absent	NAV	
CTC-OC-1447	Low grade serous borderline tumor with psammoma bodies	(m) pT3a pNX	1	IIIA	NA	NAV	
CTC-OC-1468	Simple cyst with giant cell reaction in the cyst wall	NA	NA	NA	Absent	NAV	
CTC-OC-1489	Low-grade appendiceal mucinous neoplasm	pT4b pN0 pM1b	1	IVA	Absent	NAV	
CTC-OC-14910	Low-grade serous carcinoma	pT1b pNX	1	IB	Absent	NAV	
CTC-OC-15011	Mucinous borderline tumor	pT1a	NA	1A	NA	NAV	

Table 2. *Cont.*

De-Identified Patient Code	Pathological Parameters of Tumor Samples from Patients with Lung Cancer					
	Tumor Type—Histological	TMN	Grade	Stage	LVI	MSI
CTC-LC-W201	Moderately differentiated keratinizing squamous cell carcinoma	pT1c NX	2	IVC	Present	NAV
CTC-LC-W212	Well differentiated neuroendocrine tumor (typical carcinoid)	pT1b pN0	1	ND	Absent	NAV
CTC-LC-W223	Invasive moderately differentiated adenocarcinoma, multifocal	pT3 N0	2	IIB	Absent	NAV
CTC-LC-W234	Necrotizing granulomatous inflammation	NA	NA	NA	NA	NAV
CTC-LC-W245	Squamous cell carcinoma, moderately differentiated	pT3 N0 M0	2	IIB	Absent	NAV
De-Identified Patient Code	Pathological Parameters of Tumor Samples from Patients with Liver Neoplasm					
	Tumor Type—Histological	TMN	Grade	Stage	LVI	MSI
CTC-LivC-R11	Metastatic squamous cell carcinoma	NA	NA	NA	NA	Stable
De-Identified Patient Code	Pathological Parameters of Tumor Samples from Patients with Prostate Cancer					
	Tumor Type-Histological	TMN	Grade	Stage	LVI	MSI
CTC-PC-M11	Poorly differentiated adenocarcinoma	T3b N0 MX	3	IVB	Absent	NAV
CTC-PC-M22	Metastatic adenocarcinoma of prostate	NA	NA	IVB	NA	Stable
De-Identified Patient Code	Pathological Parameters of Tumor Samples from Patients with Esophageal Cancer					
	Tumor Type—Histological	TMN	Grade	Stage	LVI	MSI
CTC-EsoC-G11	Esophageal adenocarcinoma	ypT3 N0	2	III	Present	NAV

Table 3. Demographics of the patients whose blood samples were used for the study (F = Female; M = Male; BMI = Body Mass Index).

De-Identified Patient Code	Patient Demographics of Tumor Samples: Patients with Endometrial Cancer			
	Age at Surgery (Years)	Sex	BMI	History of Other Cancers/Pre-Treatment Status at Surgery
CTC-EC-691	65	F	41.3	None
CTC-EC-702	84	F	25.2	None
CTC-EC-713	79	F	41	None
CTC-EC-724	61	F	37.8	None
CTC-EC-735	64	F	41.2	None
CTC-EC-746	81	F	29	None
CTC-EC-757	49	F	44	None
CTC-EC-768	65	F	37.3	None
CTC-EC-779	60	F	28	None
CTC-EC-7810	68	F	34.9	None
CTC-EC-7911	56	F	60.1	None

Table 3. Cont.

De-Identified Patient Code	Patient Demographics of Tumor Samples: Patients with Endometrial Cancer			
	Age at Surgery (Years)	Sex	BMI	History of Other Cancers/Pre-Treatment Status at Surgery
CTC-EC-8012	76	F	30.1	History of breast cancer treated with chemotherapy approx. 40 years prior to diagnosis.
CTC-EC-8113	49	F	42.8	None
CTC-EC-8214	50	F	49.2	None
CTC-EC-8315	64	F	42.8	History of breast ductal carcinoma in situ two years prior to diagnosis, treated with anastrozole.
CTC-EC-8416	65	F	39.8	None
CTC-EC-8517	72	F	28.1	None
CTC-EC-8618	68	F	47	None
CTC-EC-8719	52	F	44.2	None
CTC-EC-8820	59	F	34.7	None
CTC-EC-8921	63	F	32.2	None
CTC-EC-9022	83	F	36.6	None
CTC-EC-9223	77	F	40.7	None
CTC-EC-9324	55	F	36.4	None
CTC-EC-9525	71	F	41.4	None
CTC-EC-9626	79	F	37.9	History of basal cell carcinoma of the skin. No chemo-treatment.
CTC-EC-9727	70	F	23.5	None
CTC-EC-9828	63	F	33.3	None
CTC-EC-9929	65	F	29.9	None
CTC-EC-10030	58	F	52.2	None
CTC-EC-10131	62	F	21.9	None
CTC-EC-10232	68	F	30.5	None
CTC-EC-10333	56	F	31.5	None
CTC-EC-10434	65	F	31.7	History of thyroid cancer
CTC-EC-10535	57	F	33.5	None
CTC-EC-10636	74	F	33.9	None
CTC-EC-10737	43	F	43.2	None
CTC-EC-10838	65	F	34.4	None
CTC-EC-10939	66	F	52	None
CTC-EC-11040	79	F	40.8	None
CTC-EC-11141	77	F	39.8	None
CTC-EC-11242	66	F	51.3	None
CTC-EC-11343	74	F	33.4	History of skin cancer
CTC-EC-11444	62	F	33.3	None
CTC-EC-11545	65	F	32.9	None
CTC-EC-11646	65	F	33.6	None
CTC-EC-11747	46	F	38.4	None

Table 3. Cont.

De-Identified Patient Code	Patient Demographics of Tumor Samples: Patients with Endometrial Cancer			
	Age at Surgery (Years)	Sex	BMI	History of Other Cancers/Pre-Treatment Status at Surgery
CTC-EC-11848 *	56	F	26.4	None
CTC-EC-11949	65	F	29.7	None
CTC-EC-12050	46	F	44.3	None
CTC-EC-12151	44	F	34.9	None
CTC-EC-12252	68	F	41.1	None
CTC-EC-12353	79	F	49.2	None
CTC-EC-12454	68	F	30.9	None
CTC-EC-12555	60	F	38.4	History of astrocytoma
CTC-EC-12656	62	F	43.9	None
CTC-EC-12757	71	F	35.6	None
CTC-EC-12858	71	F	53.3	None
CTC-EC-12959	67	F	44.3	None
CTC-EC-13060	84	F	35.5	None
CTC-EC-13161	59	F	35.2	None
CTC-EC-13262	68	F	33.1	None
CTC-EC-13363	62	F	31.8	None
CTC-EC-13464	75	F	26.9	History of skin cancer
CTC-EC-13565	60	F	62.7	None
CTC-EC-13866	70	F	35.2	None
CTC-EC-14067	71	F	48.1	None
CTC-EC-14268	73	F	37.4	None
CTC-EC-14369	68	F	31.6	None
CTC-EC-14570	74	F	34.3	None
CTC-EC-14771	53	F	27	None
De-Identified Patient Code	Patient Demographics of Tumor Samples: Patients with Ovarian Cancer			
	Age at Surgery	Sex	BMI	History of Other Cancers/Pre-Treatment Status at Surgery
CTC-OC-911	62	F	21.1	Heavily pre-treated with multiple chemotherapeutic agents
CTC-OC-942	58	F	28.9	None
CTC-OC-1363	52	F	32.3	None
CTC-OC-1374	58	F	42	None
CTC-OC-1395	62	F	28.3	None
CTC-OC-1416	44	F	28.5	None
CTC-OC-1447	64	F	47.3	None
CTC-OC-1468	79	F	25.3	History of Diffuse Large B-Cell Lymphoma treated with RCHOP
CTC-OC-1489	78	F	26.3	None
CTC-OC-14910	82	F	30.4	None
CTC-OC-15011	19	F	35.6	None

Table 3. Cont.

De-Identified Patient Code	Patient Demographics of Tumor Samples: Patients with Lung Cancer			
	Age at Surgery	Sex	BMI	History of Other Cancers/Pre-Treatment Status at Surgery
CTC-LC-W201	53	M	18.7	History of squamous cell carcinoma of lower lip treated with surgery
CTC-LC-W212	54	F	25.3	History of breast cancer
CTC-LC-W223	70	F	34.6	None
CTC-LC-W234	50	F	38.8	None
CTC-LC-W245	73	M	25.7	None
De-Identified Patient Code	Patient Demographics of Tumor Samples: Patients with Liver Cancer			
	Age at Surgery	Sex	BMI	History of Other Cancers/Pre-Treatment Status at Surgery
CTC-LivC-R11	66	M	29.9	None
De-Identified Patient Code	Patient Demographics of Tumor Samples: Patients with Prostate Cancer			
	Age at Surgery	Sex	BMI	History of Other Cancers/Pre-Treatment Status at Surgery
CTC-PC-M11	69	M	44.3	None
CTC-PC-M22	79	M	31	None
De-Identified Patient Code	Patient Demographics of Tumor Samples: Patients with Esophageal Cancer			
	Age at Surgery	Sex	BMI	History of Other Cancers/Pre-Treatment Status at Surgery
CTC-EsoC-G11	66	M	41.2	None

* Patient with African-American ethnicity.

3.1. Standardization and Validation of CTC by IF×3 Using Breast, Ovarian, and Lung Cancer Cell Lines

Patients' blood samples were spiked with titrating numbers (1000 cells, 750 cells, 375 cells, 250 cells/100 cells) of MCF7, OVCAR3, HCC1975, and NCI-H441 tumor cell lines. The captured MCF7 cells, which were used to spike blood samples, were stained with either DAPI/CK-FITC/EpCAM-PE/CD45-Cy5 or DAPI/CK-FITC/CD31-PE/CD45-Cy5. When stained with DAPI/CK-FITC/EpCAM-PE/CD45-Cy5, the MCF7 cells were found to have a proportionately higher diameter (size 15–17 µm) bearing the typical salt-pepper nuclear morphology in a DAPI stain. The cytoplasm of the cells was positive for CK, 8,18,19, and EpCAM. When stained using the DAPI/CK-FITC/CD31-PE/CD45-Cy5 kit, the MCF7 cells were CK8,18,19$^+$/CD31$^-$/CD45$^-$/DAPI$^+$ (Figure 1(Aii)) as compared with CK8,18,19$^+$/EpCAM$^+$/CD45$^-$/DAPI$^+$ when stained using the DAPI/CK-FITC/EpCAM-PE/CD45-Cy5 antibodies (Figure 1(Ai)). A similar pattern of stains (CK8,18,19$^+$/EpCAM$^+$/CD45$^-$/DAPI$^+$) was observed for OVCAR3 (Figure 1B), HCC1975 (Figure 1C), and NCI-H441 (Figure 1D) cells using the DAPI/CK-FITC/EpCAM-PE/CD45-Cy5 antibodies. Since we did not have the confocal images, we could identify the plasma-membrane EpCAM positivity of a tumor cell depending on the orientation of the cell on the microfilter as shown in HCC1975 (Figure 1C) and NCI-H441 (Figure 1D) cells using the DAPI/CK-FITC/EpCAM-PE/CD45-Cy5 antibodies. All cell lines were found as negative for CD45-Cy5 for both sets of antibody cocktails.

3.2. Validation Spectrum of CTC by IF×3 Using Blood from Patients with Different Clinical Statuses, and Sample Origin

We validated CTC by IF×3 from a spectrum of blood from patients with different (Figure 2A) clinical status, Grade 1, Stage IA nonmetastatic endometrial cancers (pT1a pN0)

(Figure 2(Ai)) and Grade 3, Stage IVB metastatic (pT3a N0 M1) (Figure 2(Aii)) in endometrial cancers, and (B) samples of origin, including biopsy sample from a liver lesion in metastatic squamous cell carcinoma (Figure 2(Bi)) and during surgical resection of Grade 1 (pT1b N0) tumor in lung cancers (Figure 2(Bii)) using the DAPI/CK-FITC/EpCAM-PE/CD45-Cy5 antibody cocktail. We used blood from the patients with metastatic disease as an internal positive control for the presence of CTC. Confirming the standard IF×3 protocol, we observed that CTCs in each of the above-mentioned samples were more than 15–20 micron in size with an evident pathological/morphological nuclear characteristic of a tumor cell (a nuclear/cytosol ratio > 50%) by DAPI and were $CK8,18,19^+/EpCAM^+/CD45^-/DAPI^+$ when stained using the DAPI/CK-FITC/EpCAM-PE/CD45-Cy5 antibodies.

3.3. Standardization and Validation of CTC by ICC×2 in Reference to Spiked IF×3 in Endometrial and Ovarian Cancers

Having confirmed the determination of CTC by IF×3 in a spectrum of blood samples, we standardized the CTC by ICC×2 ($CK8,18^+/CD45^-$). We validated ICC×2 with spiked control using parallel IF×3 and ICC×2 procedures in the same blood sample in endometrial and ovarian cancers (Figure 3). As presented before, CTCs were captured from blood samples from patients with endometrial (Figure 3A) and ovarian (Figure 3B) tumors and enumerated using ICC×2 (Figure 3(Ai,Bi)) in reference to IF×3 (Figure 3(Aii,Bii)). Blood samples were spiked (Spiked samples) with titrating numbers (250 cells/100 cells) of NCI-H441 cells separately for both ICC×2 and IF×3. Both CTC and spiked samples exhibited a similar pattern of cell size and staining pattern ($CK8,18^+/CD45^-$) by ICC×2, which was comparable to the corresponding IF×3 staining patterns. We observed a cluster of CTCs with different diameters similar to the spiked samples of NCI-H441 (Figure 3(Ai)). CTCs were characterized and distinguished by their diameter(s), nuclear morphology (a nuclear/cytosol ratio >50%), and $CK8,18^+/CD45^-$ staining. In contrast, WBCs were smaller in size (9–15 µm) with their characteristics of nuclear morphology and $CK8,18^-/CD45^+$ staining.

3.4. Determining CTC by ICC×2 in Endometrial and Ovarian Cancers

Having established ICC×2 staining validated using parallel IF×3 spiked with tumor cell lines in blood samples of different solid tumors, we finally tested the method for the determination of CTC by ICC×2 and validated it with corresponding CTC determination by IF×3. CTCs were captured from blood samples from patients with Grade 1 Stage IA (pT1a pN0 (sn)) endometrial (Figure 4A) and Grade 1 Stage IVA (pTIVb pN0 pM1b) ovarian (Figure 4B) tumors and enumerated using ICC×2 (Figure 4(Ai,Bi)). In line with the earlier results, the CTC in ICC×2 were $CK8,18^+/CD45^-$ while the WBCs were $CK8,18^-/CD45^+$ in ICC×2, which matched with the IF×3 validation samples where CTCs were larger in diameter (>15–20 µM) with $CK8,18,19^+/EpCAM^+/CD45^-/DAPI^+$ while WBCs were smaller in diameter (9–15 µm) with $CK8,18,19^-/EpCAM^-/CD45^+/DAPI^+$ (Figure 4(Aii,Bii)).

Table 1 shows that our study included 63% of patients with Stage I disease, out of which blood samples of 6 patients were used for standardization and 51 were used for CTC-testing. Five percent of the total patients had Stage II disease, out of which a blood sample of one patient was used for standardization, and four were used for CTC-testing. Fourteen percent of the total patients had Stage III disease, out of which blood samples of 3 patients were used for standardization, and 10 were used for CTC-testing. Ten percent of our enrolled patients had Stage IV metastatic disease, out of which blood samples of four patients were used for standardization while the remaining five were used for CTC-testing. Although the percentage of CTC-positive patients with Stage I, Stage II, and Stage III diseases were 45%, 50%, and 30%, respectively, the percentage of CTC-positive patients rose to 100% in the blood of patients with Stage IV metastatic diseases. We tested the sensitivity of the ICC method by titrating the number of spiked cells; 25 cells/test, 50 cells/test, and 100 cells/test. The recovery was >50% for 25 cells/test, >60% for 50 cells/test, and >65% for 100 cells/test. The specificity was tested by $CD45^-/CK8,18,19^+/EpCAM^+/DAPI$ stain for nuclear size and morphology. We also used cell lines from cancer of different organ types, namely endometrial, ovarian, breast, and lung. We also used the commercially available CD31-kit to demonstrate the fact that CTC/tumor cells are CD31 negative (Figure 1) and to rule out a false positive. We used blood from donors, leucopaks, and PBMCs for the control.

Table 1 shows 45% CTC positivity in patients with Stage I disease. However, a detailed interrogation of the result revealed that the high percentage (45%) was obtained because we calculated the "presence of CTC" recorded in a "yes-or-no format." Importantly, we observed that out of 54 patients (those we tested for CTC) with Stage I endometrial disease, 28 patients were CTC-negative, and 26 were CTC-positive. Out of 26 CTC-positive patients, 77% (20/26) had <1–3 CTCs.

We could not determine any statistically significant correlation between grades and the number of CTC as the numbers of patients with high-grade tumors in our study cohort were significantly lower than the numbers of patients with low-grade tumors. Table 4 presents the Grade-wise distribution of patients' blood samples used for the standardization and testing of CTCs, along with tumors from each pathology.

Table 4. Grade-wise distribution of patients' blood samples used for the standardization and testing of CTCs, along with tumors from each pathology.

Grades of Patients with Different Tumors (Endometrial, Ovary, Lung, Esophageal, Prostate, and Liver)	Total Percentage of Patients' Blood Used for the Study (%)	Number of Blood Samples Used for CTC Standardization	Number of Blood Samples Used for CTC Testing	Percentage of Patients with Positive CTC (IF and/or ICC) (%)
G1	47%	5	38	50%
G2	18%	4	12	58%
G3	20%	2	16	69%
Tumors from Each Organ Type				
Tumors from Each Pathology	Endometrial	Ovary	Lung	Esophageal	Prostate	Liver
G1	37	5	1	0	0	NA
G2	12	0	3	1	0	NA
G3	16	1	0	0	1	NA

However, we observed an interesting association between the presence of CTC and the high grade/stage of the disease. Out of a total of nine patients with Stage IV/Metastatic disease, blood samples from three patients were used for standardization. Of six patients whose blood samples were used for CTC detection, 100% tested positive for CTCs. With regard to High-Grade (Grade 3) patients, we had a total of 18 patients with Grade 3 disease. Of these patients, blood samples from two patients were used for standardization. Of the remaining 16 patients, a 69% CTC positivity (11/16) was observed. There were four patients who were diagnosed with both Grade 3 and Stage IV/Metastatic disease. The blood samples from one of these patients were used for standardization; out of the remaining three patients with both Grade3 and Stage IV/Metastatic disease, 100% were tested and were found to have CTCs.

Since the CTC expression varied depending on the Stage and the Grade of the disease, we did not consider the median or average expression values across all; we stratified patients with CTC positivity according to the Stage and the most common histology type, endometrioid adenocarcinoma.

However, we determined the rate of detection of CTC in endometrial cancers. In endometrial cancers, the detection rate was 55% (35/64). The rate of detection can be explained by the fact that 75% (48/64) of our CTC-tested patients were Stage I.

We also tested the CTC detection rate in the most common histological type of endometrial cancer, endometrioid adenocarcinoma. Out of 64 patient samples tested for

CTC, 42 patients had endometrioid adenocarcinoma (Out of 42, 86% were Stage I; 36/42), and the CTC detection rate was 60% (25/42). Out of 25, 80% had Stage I disease (20/25). Interestingly, 76% (19/25) presented with 1–3 CTCs counts; out of these 19, 79% had Stage I disease (15/19).

We tested the clinical relevance of a high number of CTCs in a single case study. The presence of >100 CTCs (Figure 5) was observed at the surgery in a patient with Grade 2, stage IA endometrioid adenocarcinoma, 6% MI, and absence of lymphovascular invasion, absence of LN Status as well as Uterine Serosa and Cervical Stroma involvement. We observed 13 CTCs in a microscopic field with mitotic figures as well as 3-cell CTC clusters. The patient received four fractions of HDR vaginal cuff brachytherapy. The patient came in for surveillance, and a lesion was observed. Biopsy demonstrated recurrent endometrioid adenocarcinoma. A CT scan of the chest, abdomen, and pelvis revealed an area of poorly defined but somewhat mass-like enhancement in the region of the right vaginal cuff suspicious of disease recurrence. There were no other changes concerning additional metastatic disease elsewhere. The patient had an event within 6 months of the date of surgery.

4. Discussion

Our method of detection of CTC followed the standard CTC determination criteria including, (1) negative reactivity to immune cell marker (CD45), (2) positive reactivity to cytokeratin 8, 18, 19, (3) positive reactivity to EpCAM surface marker, and (4) morphologic characteristics [25]. Our method of determining CTC by ICC×2 gave us a *parallel double-detection format* (ICC×2 and IF×3) for a foolproof test with a higher confidence level in terms of specificity and sensitivity. We observed a concordance close to 80% in our cohort. We carried out the IF and ICC evaluation of CTC independent/without knowledge of the final pathology findings of these specimens; however, such findings were incorporated after completing our IF/ICC of CTC data collections. The sensitivity of our method of employing *a parallel double-detection format* was also tested in the built-in nature of our patient cohort. Close to 65% of our blood samples for CTC detection (standardization and testing) were samples drawn from patients with Grades 1 and 2 diseases. Table 1 showed that 68% of our blood samples for CTC detection (standardization and testing) were samples drawn from patients with Stage I and II diseases, wherein we were able to detect the presence of CTC (Table 1). Interestingly, 45% and 50% of patients with Stage I and II diseases tested positive for CTC, respectively, indicating the strength of the method and the format of determination. *Our testing format can thus be utilized in monitoring the progression of the disease post-surgery or in an adjuvant setting, providing a valuable indicator of the metastatic potential* via *longitudinal CTC detection*. As expected, 100% of our patients with Stage IV metastatic disease tested positive for CTC, which can be viewed as a positive control within a disease population. Thus, our method is built on strong validation data, including internal validation, technical validation, and disease-population-based positive and negative validation controls. We also tested CTC in blood samples from patients undergoing both biopsies and surgeries.

Studies reported the feasibility of detection of CTCs using isolation by size-based Epithelial/Trophoblastic Tumor cells (ISET®) filters and stain by May–Grünwald–Giemsa in conjunction with identification criteria of nuclear irregularity, negative reactivity to immune cell marker as well as endothelial cell markers, and presentation of visible cytoplasm [26]. To test the negativity of CTC for CD31 in IF×3, we used the additional staining kit for DAPI/CK-FITC/CD31-PE/CD45-Cy5. HUVEC (positive control for CD31 and negative control EpCAM) and NCI-H441 (positive control for EpCAM and negative control for CD31) cells as validation controls. We used spiked HUVEC cells to represent the cross-reactivity of the probable endothelial cells in the blood. CK8,18,19$^-$/EpCAM$^-$/CD45$^+$/DAPI$^+$ WBCs were CK8,18,19$^-$/CD31$^-$/CD45$^+$/DAPI$^+$. CK8,18,19$^+$/EpCAM$^+$/CD45$^-$/DAPI$^+$ NCI-H441 cells were CK8,18,19$^+$/CD31$^-$/CD45$^-$/DAPI$^+$. HUVEC cells were CK8,18,19$^{\pm}$/CD31$^+$/CD45$^-$/DAPI$^+$.

Our *parallel double-detection format* for CTC determination is efficient as it can be ready for pathological evaluation within the standard working hours of one day. The procedure is laboratory friendly and requires basic equipment and microscopes, and can be carried out with a standard grad-school laboratory setup compared with the FDA-approved CellSearch semi-automated CTC detection system or the CTC detection sensitivity of ISET [26] or using an immunomagnetic enrichment [25]. Hence, the method is cost-effective, and the cost of the consumables per 7.5 mL blood sample can be estimated at around $500 only. Thus our method can be performed at a comprehensive cancer center as well as at a community-based small cancer hospital with limited resources. Since we did not compare the method with the rest of the available methods for CTC enumeration, the data for the comparison are currently unavailable. Yet the method has its niche and edge for the above reasons. Although our *parallel double-detection format* for the determination of CTC is limited to at least 16 mL of blood, the method compensates the volume of blood for the sensitivity and specificity of CTC. However, the main trade-off for this method is its limited capacity to scale in a demanding, high-throughput situation.

One of the established pathological parameters associated with the prognosis is the presence or absence of LVSI (Lympho-Vascular Space Invasion). Our method of CTC determination will quickly provide a unique opportunity to interrogate CTC's role as a more sensitive risk factor vis-à-vis standard pathological parameters like LVSI in the context of particular histology, grades, and Stage of the disease. This might provide an opportunity to study wherein CTC can be used preoperatively (after malignant solid tumors are diagnosed on biopsies) as risk stratification for sentinel lymph nodes (SLN).

Cell-free (cf) circulating tumor (ct) derived DNA is released from tumor cells into the circulation and is often detected as part of routine liquid biopsy compared to CTC for clinical decision making. The ctDNA is used as (1) direct detection of early-stage cancers, (2) a marker for the detection of minimum residual disease, (3) an important tool to provide prognostic information, and (4) as an indicator of drug response in non-invasive liquid biopsies [27]. However, the critical challenge of this type of liquid biopsy has been in the detection/characterization of small amounts of ctDNA in large populations of cfDNA, as these analyses need to distinguish ctDNA alterations from cfDNA variants related to clonal hematopoiesis [28]. Blood-based deep-sequencing often encounters concerns about detection and misclassification of white blood cell (WBC)-derived variants in cfDNA associated with clonal hematopoiesis, especially in older patients [29,30]. In fact, Hu et al. reported a false-positive plasma genotyping due to clonal hematopoiesis where most JAK2 mutations, some TP53 mutations, and rare KRAS mutations detected in cfDNA were derived from clonal hematopoiesis instead of the tumor as mutations detected in plasma, particularly in genes mutated in clonal hematopoiesis, which might not represent the true tumor genotype, the study concluded [31]. The detection of non-tumor-derived clonal hematopoietic mutations (TP53, DNMT3A, etc.) has been reported as a source of the biological background noise of ctDNA detection that could lead to an inappropriate therapeutic decision.

The power of a longitudinal CTC, which enables serial assessments at multiple time points along a patient's journey, during or after surgery/treatment, is undeniable. However, a recent article by Vasseur et al. delineated the limitations of using CTC data in routine clinical practice [3]. In the view of currently published or ongoing trials assessing the clinical utility of CTCs [3], it can be recognized that there exist challenges in the enumeration and phenotyping of CTC [19]. The limitations of CTCs in clinical practice are (1) the low detection rate with currently available techniques [3] and (2) the need for a costly comprehensive laboratory setup. Cost-effectiveness, yet specific, sensitive, and fail-safe nature of our laboratory friendly method of CTC enumeration will potentially support prospective studies with uniform and standardized definitions of CTCs that are urgently needed [17] to evaluate the full potential of CTCs not only as prognostic, predictive, and intermediate endpoint markers but also as PD biomarkers in the future. We are currently assessing the expression of PD-L1 in CTC, which may be helpful in considering the use of

PD-1 inhibitors in clinical practice. The limitation of our platform is built in its development in a community-based cancer center; the platform is not yet tested in a prospective clinical trial. To this end, we are also actively pursuing customization of the antibody cocktail to profile the cancer-specific cell surface protein molecules (e.g., CA125) for future studies.

The strength of our method is built in its inherent development in a community-based cancer center; the method is cost-effective, time-sensitive, laboratory-friendly, and needs a single full-time employee. To this end, we tested the clinical relevance of our method in a case study. We reported on a stage I patient with >100 CTCs at surgery (with 13 CTCs in a single microscopic field; Figure 5). The patient with endometrioid adenocarcinoma had no apparent pathological features indicative of high risk for recurrence. Unfortunately, she presented with an adverse event within 6 months of surgery, strongly indicating the prognostic significance of CTC as reported in the earlier studies in different organ type cancers.

5. Conclusions

The need for easy detection of CTC is undeniable. Our user-friendly and cost-effective detection method provided an opportunity to incorporate CTC detection as a companion entity with the standard diagnostic and monitoring tests in clinics. The power of the method can be tested as a single-point and multi-point longitudinal mode in a clinical setting at the baseline, during, and after a treatment regimen. The baseline evaluation of CTC can be helpful for patient stratification, while longitudinal CTC evaluation during and after treatment can be useful for monitoring treatment response and early indicators of disease progression/drug resistance, respectively. The study presented in the MS is part of a patent application (United States Patent and Trademark Office; Application number 16/875,910.

Author Contributions: R.S., pathologist, provided the confirmatory evaluation of CTC for the triple-immunofluorescence and double-immunocytochemistry stains; P.D., senior scientist, helped in writing the MS.; J.C.A., laboratory supervisor, standardized and performed triple IF stain.; X.L. research assistant lead, standardized, and performed double ICC.; A.D., research associate, obtained consent from patients and provided technical assistance in record keeping.; E.V. obtained consent from patients and provided technical assistance in record keeping; C.A., Clinical Research Manager, helped in training and IRB process.; N.K. offered technical assistance; K.G. Assistant Vice President of Oncology Strategic Initiatives, provided insight into the overall logistical management of the study; J.P., Physician, provided insight into liver biopsy corresponding to the blood samples; B.S., physician, provided insight into prostate tumors corresponding to the blood samples; B.T., surgeon, provided insight into esophageal tumors corresponding to the blood samples; P.M., surgeon, provided insight into lung tumors corresponding to the blood samples.; L.R.E., surgeon, provided clinical insight into endometrial and ovarian tumors corresponding to the blood samples.; D.S., surgeon, provided clinical insight into endometrial and ovarian tumors corresponding to the blood samples.; N.D., senior scientist, conceptualized and supervised the study, wrote the MS and analyzed the data. All authors have read and agreed to the published version of the manuscript.

Funding: The entire study was funded by Avera Cancer Institute. This research received no external funding.

Institutional Review Board Statement: Our data has been obtained from patients' blood samples pertaining to a study protocol approved by the Institutional Review Board. All experimental protocols were approved by the institutional and/or licensing committee/s. The informed consent(s) was obtained from all subjects and/or their legal guardian(s). Informed (IRB approved: Protocol Number Study: 2017.053-100399_ExVivo001) consents for obtaining the peripheral blood were obtained from 91 enrolled patients with various solid tumors, including lung, endometrial, ovarian, esophageal, prostate, and liver cancers. All methods were carried out in accordance with relevant guidelines and regulations.

Informed Consent Statement: All the patients who participated in the study protocol (duly approved by the IRB) have given informed consent.

Data Availability Statement: We have not used any publicly available data. All data presented in the MS is obtained from the patient samples following informed consent from the patient with proper IRB approval.

Acknowledgments: We acknowledge Avera Cancer Institute for funding the entire study. We acknowledge every patient and their family for their participation in the ex vivo study at the Avera Cancer Institute.

Conflicts of Interest: The authors declare no conflict of interest.

References

1. Rossi, E.; Fabbri, F. CTCs 2020: Great Expectations or Unreasonable Dreams. *Cells* **2019**, *8*, 989. [CrossRef] [PubMed]
2. Paoletti, C.; Hayes, D.F. Circulating Tumor Cells. *Adv. Exp. Med. Biol.* **2016**, *882*, 235–258. [CrossRef] [PubMed]
3. Vasseur, A.; Kiavue, N.; Bidard, F.C.; Pierga, J.Y.; Cabel, L. Clinical utility of circulating tumor cells: An update. *Mol. Oncol.* **2021**, *15*, 1647–1666. [CrossRef]
4. Bastos, D.A.; Antonarakis, E.S. CTC-derived AR-V7 detection as a prognostic and predictive biomarker in advanced prostate cancer. *Expert Rev. Mol. Diagn.* **2018**, *18*, 155–163. [CrossRef] [PubMed]
5. Hu, B.; Yang, X.R.; Xu, Y.; Sun, Y.F.; Sun, C.; Guo, W.; Zhang, X.; Wang, W.M.; Qiu, S.J.; Zhou, J.; et al. Systemic immune-inflammation index predicts prognosis of patients after curative resection for hepatocellular carcinoma. *Clin. Cancer Res.* **2014**, *20*, 6212–6222. [CrossRef]
6. Xie, N.; Hu, Z.; Tian, C.; Xiao, H.; Liu, L.; Yang, X.; Li, J.; Wu, H.; Lu, J.; Gao, J.; et al. In Vivo Detection of CTC and CTC Plakoglobin Status Helps Predict Prognosis in Patients with Metastatic Breast Cancer. *Pathol. Oncol. Res. POR* **2020**, *26*, 2435–2442. [CrossRef]
7. Pineiro, R.; Martinez-Pena, I.; Lopez-Lopez, R. Relevance of CTC Clusters in Breast Cancer Metastasis. *Adv. Exp. Med. Biol.* **2020**, *1220*, 93–115. [CrossRef]
8. Bidard, F.C.; Proudhon, C.; Pierga, J.Y. Circulating tumor cells in breast cancer. *Mol. Oncol.* **2016**, *10*, 418–430. [CrossRef]
9. Pickhardt, P.J.; Correale, L.; Hassan, C. Positive Predictive Value for Colorectal Lesions at CT Colonography: Analysis of Factors Impacting Results in a Large Screening Cohort. *AJR. Am. J. Roentgenol.* **2019**, *213*, W1–W8. [CrossRef]
10. Nanduri, L.K.; Hissa, B.; Weitz, J.; Scholch, S.; Bork, U. The prognostic role of circulating tumor cells in colorectal cancer. *Expert Rev. Anticancer Ther.* **2019**, *19*, 1077–1088. [CrossRef]
11. Hoshimoto, S.; Shingai, T.; Morton, D.L.; Kuo, C.; Faries, M.B.; Chong, K.; Elashoff, D.; Wang, H.J.; Elashoff, R.M.; Hoon, D.S. Association between circulating tumor cells and prognosis in patients with Stage III melanoma with sentinel lymph node metastasis in a phase III international multicenter trial. *J. Clin. Oncol.* **2012**, *30*, 3819–3826. [CrossRef] [PubMed]
12. Inhestern, J.; Oertel, K.; Stemmann, V.; Schmalenberg, H.; Dietz, A.; Rotter, N.; Veit, J.; Gorner, M.; Sudhoff, H.; Junghanss, C.; et al. Prognostic Role of Circulating Tumor Cells during Induction Chemotherapy Followed by Curative Surgery Combined with Postoperative Radiotherapy in Patients with Locally Advanced Oral and Oropharyngeal Squamous Cell Cancer. *PLoS ONE* **2015**, *10*, e0132901. [CrossRef] [PubMed]
13. Gazzaniga, P.; Gradilone, A.; de Berardinis, E.; Busetto, G.M.; Raimondi, C.; Gandini, O.; Nicolazzo, C.; Petracca, A.; Vincenzi, B.; Farcomeni, A.; et al. Prognostic value of circulating tumor cells in nonmuscle invasive bladder cancer: A CellSearch analysis. *Ann. Oncol.* **2012**, *23*, 2352–2356. [CrossRef] [PubMed]
14. Nastaly, P.; Honecker, F.; Pantel, K.; Riethdorf, S. Detection of Circulating Tumor Cells (CTCs) in Patients with Testicular Germ Cell Tumors. *Methods Mol. Biol.* **2021**, *2195*, 245–261. [CrossRef] [PubMed]
15. Arigami, T.; Uenosono, Y.; Yanagita, S.; Okubo, K.; Kijima, T.; Matsushita, D.; Amatatsu, M.; Kurahara, H.; Maemura, K.; Natsugoe, S. Clinical significance of circulating tumor cells in blood from patients with gastric cancer. *Ann. Gastroenterol. Surg.* **2017**, *1*, 60–68. [CrossRef]
16. Guan, X.; Ma, F.; Li, C.; Wu, S.; Hu, S.; Huang, J.; Sun, X.; Wang, J.; Luo, Y.; Cai, R.; et al. The prognostic and therapeutic implications of circulating tumor cell phenotype detection based on epithelial-mesenchymal transition markers in the first-line chemotherapy of HER2-negative metastatic breast cancer. *Cancer Commun.* **2019**, *39*, 1. [CrossRef]
17. Yap, T.A.; Lorente, D.; Omlin, A.; Olmos, D.; de Bono, J.S. Circulating tumor cells: A multifunctional biomarker. *Clin. Cancer Res.* **2014**, *20*, 2553–2568. [CrossRef]
18. Cabel, L.; Proudhon, C.; Gortais, H.; Loirat, D.; Coussy, F.; Pierga, J.Y.; Bidard, F.C. Circulating tumor cells: Clinical validity and utility. *Int. J. Clin. Oncol.* **2017**, *22*, 421–430. [CrossRef]
19. Coumans, F.A.; Ligthart, S.T.; Uhr, J.W.; Terstappen, L.W. Challenges in the enumeration and phenotyping of CTC. *Clin. Cancer Res.* **2012**, *18*, 5711–5718. [CrossRef]
20. Stefansson, S.; Adams, D.L.; Ershler, W.B.; Le, H.; Ho, D.H. A cell transportation solution that preserves live circulating tumor cells in patient blood samples. *BMC Cancer* **2016**, *16*, 300. [CrossRef]
21. Adams, D.L.; Zhu, P.; Makarova, O.V.; Martin, S.S.; Charpentier, M.; Chumsri, S.; Li, S.; Amstutz, P.; Tang, C.M. The systematic study of circulating tumor cell isolation using lithographic microfilters. *RSC Adv.* **2014**, *9*, 4334–4342. [CrossRef] [PubMed]

22. Adams, D.L.; Stefansson, S.; Haudenschild, C.; Martin, S.S.; Charpentier, M.; Chumsri, S.; Cristofanilli, M.; Tang, C.M.; Alpaugh, R.K. Cytometric characterization of circulating tumor cells captured by microfiltration and their correlation to the CellSearch((R)) CTC test. *Cytom. Part A J. Int. Soc. Anal. Cytol.* **2015**, *87*, 137–144. [CrossRef] [PubMed]
23. Adams, D.L.; Martin, S.S.; Alpaugh, R.K.; Charpentier, M.; Tsai, S.; Bergan, R.C.; Ogden, I.M.; Catalona, W.; Chumsri, S.; Tang, C.M.; et al. Circulating giant macrophages as a potential biomarker of solid tumors. *Proc. Natl. Acad. Sci. USA* **2014**, *111*, 3514–3519. [CrossRef] [PubMed]
24. Tang, C.M.; Zhu, P.; Li, S.; Makarova, O.V.; Amstutz, P.T.; Adams, D.L. Filtration and Analysis of Circulating Cancer Associated Cells from the Blood of Cancer Patients. *Methods Mol. Biol.* **2017**, *1572*, 511–524. [CrossRef] [PubMed]
25. Witzig, T.E.; Bossy, B.; Kimlinger, T.; Roche, P.C.; Ingle, J.N.; Grant, C.; Donohue, J.; Suman, V.J.; Harrington, D.; Torre-Bueno, J.; et al. Detection of circulating cytokeratin-positive cells in the blood of breast cancer patients using immunomagnetic enrichment and digital microscopy. *Clin. Cancer Res.* **2002**, *8*, 1085–1091.
26. Kamal, M.; Leslie, M.; Horton, C.; Hills, N.; Davis, R.; Nguyen, R.; Razaq, M.; Moxley, K.; Hofman, P.; Zhang, R.; et al. Cytopathologic identification of circulating tumor cells (CTCs) in breast cancer: Application of size-based enrichment. *Clin. Diagn. Pathol.* **2019**, *4*. [CrossRef]
27. Phallen, J.; Sausen, M.; Adleff, V.; Leal, A.; Hruban, C.; White, J.; Anagnostou, V.; Fiksel, J.; Cristiano, S.; Papp, E.; et al. Direct detection of early-stage cancers using circulating tumor DNA. *Sci. Transl. Med.* **2017**, *9*. [CrossRef]
28. Leal, A.; van Grieken, N.C.T.; Palsgrove, D.N.; Phallen, J.; Medina, J.E.; Hruban, C.; Broeckaert, M.A.M.; Anagnostou, V.; Adleff, V.; Bruhm, D.C.; et al. White blood cell and cell-free DNA analyses for detection of residual disease in gastric cancer. *Nat. Commun.* **2020**, *11*, 525. [CrossRef]
29. Xie, M.; Lu, C.; Wang, J.; McLellan, M.D.; Johnson, K.J.; Wendl, M.C.; McMichael, J.F.; Schmidt, H.K.; Yellapantula, V.; Miller, C.A.; et al. Age-related mutations associated with clonal hematopoietic expansion and malignancies. *Nat. Med.* **2014**, *20*, 1472–1478. [CrossRef]
30. Jaiswal, S.; Fontanillas, P.; Flannick, J.; Manning, A.; Grauman, P.V.; Mar, B.G.; Lindsley, R.C.; Mermel, C.H.; Burtt, N.; Chavez, A.; et al. Age-related clonal hematopoiesis associated with adverse outcomes. *N. Engl. J. Med.* **2014**, *371*, 2488–2498. [CrossRef]
31. Hu, Y.; Ulrich, B.C.; Supplee, J.; Kuang, Y.; Lizotte, P.H.; Feeney, N.B.; Guibert, N.M.; Awad, M.M.; Wong, K.K.; Janne, P.A.; et al. False-Positive Plasma Genotyping Due to Clonal Hematopoiesis. *Clin. Cancer Res.* **2018**, *24*, 4437–4443. [CrossRef] [PubMed]

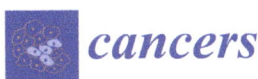

Brief Report

A Highly Sensitive Next-Generation Sequencing-Based Genotyping Platform for *EGFR* Mutations in Plasma from Non-Small Cell Lung Cancer Patients

Jung-Young Shin [1], Jeong-Oh Kim [1], Mi-Ran Lee [1], Seo Ree Kim [2], Kyongmin Sarah Beck [3] and Jin Hyoung Kang [1,2,*]

[1] Laboratory of Medical Oncology, Cancer Research Institute, College of Medicine, The Catholic University of Korea, Seoul 06591, Korea; bearjy@catholic.ac.kr (J.-Y.S.); kjo9713@catholic.ac.kr (J.-O.K.); miran13@catholic.ac.kr (M.-R.L.)
[2] Department of Medical Oncology, Seoul St. Mary's Hospital, The Catholic University of Korea, Seoul 06591, Korea; 21300424@cmcnu.or.kr
[3] Department of Radiology, Seoul St. Mary's Hospital, The Catholic University of Korea, Seoul 06591, Korea; sallahbar@catholic.ac.kr
* Correspondence: oncologykang@naver.com; Tel.: +82-2-2258-6043; Fax: +82-2-594-6043

Received: 26 September 2020; Accepted: 26 November 2020; Published: 30 November 2020

Simple Summary: In this study, Sel-Cap^{TM}, a next-generation sequencing (NGS)-based genotyping platform, showed high sensitivity for detection of *epidermal growth factor receptor* (*EGFR*) gene mutations in plasma samples collected from 185 patients with non-small cell lung cancer (NSCLC). In the early-stage NSCLC, Sel-Cap liquid biopsy was able to detect more than half the *EGFR* mutations, which were detected in tumor tissue (sensitivity: 50% and 78% for Ex19del and L858R respectively, with tumor results as the references), while the conventional NGS could not detect any. Sel-Cap liquid biopsy was particularly sensitive for resistant mutation T790M (sensitivity: 88%). In addition, we conducted a retrospective study to monitor T790M using Sel-Cap in 34 patients who progressed on first-line tyrosine kinase inhibitors (EGFR-TKIs). The study suggested that the first appearance of T790M in plasma, ranging from at treatment baseline to over three years post-EGFR-TKI initiation, may be useful for prediction of disease progression (around 5 months in advance).

Abstract: Sel-Cap^{TM}, a digital enrichment next-generation sequencing (NGS)-based cancer panel, was assessed for detection of *epidermal growth factor receptor* (*EGFR*) gene mutations in plasma for non-small cell lung cancer (NSCLC), and for application in monitoring *EGFR* resistance mutation T790M in plasma following first-line EGFR-tyrosine kinase inhibitor (EGFR-TKI) treatment. Using Sel-Cap, we genotyped plasma samples collected from 185 patients for mutations Ex19del, L858R, and T790M, and compared results to those of PNAclamp^{TM} tumor biopsy (reference method, a peptide nucleic acid-mediated polymerase chain reaction clamping) and two other NGS liquid biopsies. Over two-thirds of activating mutations (Ex19del and L858R), previously confirmed by PNAclamp, were detected by Sel-Cap, which is 4–5 times more sensitive than NGS liquid biopsy. Sel-Cap showed particularly high sensitivity for T790M (88%) and for early-stage plasma samples. The relationship between initial T790M detection in plasma and progression-free survival (PFS) following first-line EGFR-TKIs was evaluated in 34 patients. Patients with T790M detected at treatment initiation (±3 months) had significantly shorter PFS than patients where T790M was first detected >3 months post treatment initiation (median PFS: 5.9 vs. 26.5 months; $p < 0.0001$). However, time from T790M detection to disease progression was not significantly different between the two groups (median around 5 months). In conclusion, Sel-Cap is a highly sensitive platform for *EGFR* mutations in plasma, and the timing of the first appearance of T790M in plasma, determined via highly sensitive liquid biopsies, may be useful for prediction of disease progression of NSCLC, around 5 months in advance.

Keywords: *EGFR* mutation; EGFR-TKI; cfDNA; NGS; liquid biopsy; digital enrichment

1. Introduction

Nearly one in every five cancer deaths worldwide is caused by lung cancer (World Health Organization Report on Cancer, 2020, https://apps.who.int/iris/rest/bitstreams/1267643/retrieve). Non-small cell lung cancer (NSCLC) makes up the vast majority of all lung cancer cases, and approximately three-quarters of NSCLC patients are diagnosed at advanced-stage. Currently, the first-line systemic treatment for advanced-stage NSCLC is targeted therapy for those who bear driver oncogene mutations in tumor, for example, epidermal growth factor receptor (EGFR) tyrosine kinase inhibitors (TKIs) for patients with drug-activating mutations in the *EGFR* gene [1].

Exon 19 deletion (Ex19del) and exon 21 L858R are the most frequent *EGFR*-activating mutations, and the secondary gatekeeper mutation T790M, which can result from long-term exposure to first-line EGFR-TKIs, is one of the primary causes for acquired EGFR-TKI resistance [2]. During re-biopsy, T790M is found in over half of the tumor samples taken from EGFR-TKI-resistant patients [3]; however, tumor re-biopsy is usually performed post tumor relapse, and is often not feasible in clinical situations such as those involving patients in poor physical condition and/or with hardly accessible target lesions.

Cell-free DNA (cfDNA) refers to all nucleic acid fragments circulating in blood; in cancer patients, 0.01% to 90% cfDNA may consist of tumor-derived DNA [4]. Several detection techniques for *EGFR* mutations in plasma-derived cfDNA have been developed as non-invasive alternatives to tumor *EGFR* genotyping [5], such as cobas® EGFR mutation test v2, BEAMing-PCR (BEAM refers to Beads, Emulsions, Amplification and Magnetics) PCR [6], ARMS-PCR (ARMS refers to Amplification Refractory Mutation System), and ddPCR™ (dd refers to Droplet Digital). These techniques are characterized by quantitative results and a short turnaround time, but are limited to pre-defined mutations, and the sensitivity needs improvement, particularly in early-stage disease [7].

Sel-Cap lung cancer panel (hereinafter referred to as Sel-Cap) is a next-generation sequencing (NGS)-based oncogene genotyping platform, equipped with a pre-sequencing mutation-enrichment feature [8] (limit of detection: 0.01–0.05%, limit of detection is defined as the percentage of mutation copies that must be present in the specimen for a mutation to be identified). The primary objective of this study was to evaluate Sel-Cap's capacity for detecting *EGFR* mutations (Ex19del, L858R, and T790M) in plasma-derived cfDNA, by comparing it to other commonly used genotyping platforms such as peptide nucleic acid clamping (PNAclamp; currently, the most popular platform in Korea) in tumor, as well as conventional NGS (which is a non-commercialized mutation panel based on the commonly used NGS technique) and an NGS-based cancer panel in plasma. In addition, to explore Sel-Cap's potential application in monitoring for *EGFR* resistance mutation T790M in plasma to predict resistance to first-line EGFR-TKI treatments, a retrospective longitudinal study was carried out in patients who exhibited this resistance.

2. Materials and Methods

2.1. Study Population

Plasma samples used in this study were collected from patients histologically diagnosed with NSCLC (adenocarcinoma) between January 2011 and January 2019 in Seoul St. Mary's Hospital. All samples were stored by Seoul St. Mary's Hospital biobank. Before sample collection for the biobank, all the patients provided a written informed consent for the possible use of their samples in the future research.

In this study, only samples which had been previously genotyped by PNAclamp *EGFR* mutation detection kit ver.2 (PNAC-3002, Panagene, Daejeon, Korea) were included. This study was approved by the institutional review board (IRB) in Seoul St. Mary's Hospital (No. KC17TNSI0184), and was performed in accordance with the national laws, regulations, and good clinical practice (GCP) guidelines for patient data protection.

2.2. Sample Preparation

To prepare plasma samples, patients' blood was drawn into ethylenediaminetetraacetic acid (EDTA) tubes, and was immediately centrifuged at 1200× *g* at 4 °C for 15 min. The supernatant was then transferred to 1.5 mL sterile Eppendorf tubes, and centrifuged at 13,000× *g* at 4 °C for 10 min [9]. The separated plasma was stored at −80 °C until use.

cfDNA was extracted from plasma samples using a DNeasy Blood and Tissue Kit (Qiagen, Hilden, Germany) according to the manufacturer's instructions. The concentration of cfDNA was quantified using a Qubit^{TM} dsDNA HS Assay Kit (ds refers to double strand, HS refers to High-Sensitivity) with Qubit^{TM} 2.0 Fluorometer (Life Technologies, Carlsbad, CA, USA). The purity of cfDNA was evaluated with a NanoDrop ND-1000 Spectrophotometer (Thermo Fisher Scientific, Waltham, MA, USA), and only samples with an A260/A280 ratio of 1.8–2.0 passed quality control. The cfDNA was then end-repaired and size selection was performed, followed by adenylation of the 3′ end [10].

2.3. EGFR Mutation Detection Platforms

In this study, four different platforms were used for *EGFR* mutation detection, and all procedures were carried out in accordance with the manufacturer's instructions. PNAclamp, the standard diagnostic method for *EGFR* tumor biopsy in the hospital, was used as a reference, and the methodology was described in detail, previously [11]. The limit of detection of PNAclamp was determined to be >0.1%. In addition, a conventional NGS panel (Ion AmpliSeq™ Cancer Hotspot Panel, Life Technologies, Carlsbad, CA, USA), a 30-gene NGS lung cancer panel (Theragen, Suwon, Korea), and a Sel-Cap lung cancer panel (SeaSun Biomaterials, Daejeon, Korea) were used for comparison in plasma samples in two separate studies. The mutation detection cut-off value was 0.1% for Sel-Cap, and 1% for the conventional NGS and 2% for the 30-gene NGS lung cancer panel. The cut-off value was determined to be the average minimum variant allelic frequency that could be reliably detected (variant allelic frequency: percentage of mutant reads over total reads at one locus). Mutations in exon 18–20 were genotyped (Exon 18: L718Q, G719X; Exon 19: deletion; Exon 20: insertion, T790M, and S768I; Exon 21: L844V, L858R, L861Q).

2.4. Sel-Cap Mutation Enrichment PCR

In enrichment polymerase chain reaction (PCR), wild-type-specific blockers were used to preferentially hybridize with wild-type alleles and reduce the background wild-type sequence amplification, which therefore resulted in enrichment of mutant PCR fragments. The assay used 30 ng of cfDNA and was performed according to the manufacturer's protocol (SeaSun Biomaterials, Daejeon, Korea). In addition, to improve the performance of NGS, nonspecific PCR products (mainly primer dimers) were removed by Agencourt AMPure XP beads (Beckman Coulter, Vienna, Austria) using a 1:1 DNA-to-bead ratio.

2.5. NGS Library Preparation

Sequencing library preparation PCR was performed using the following: 2 μL of purified PCR product from mutation enrichment PCR amplification as the template, *EGFR* Insight 2× Seq Lib Pep Premix (SeaSun Biomaterials, Daejeon, Korea), and barcoded primer pairs. For the library preparation PCR, multiple indexing adapters were ligated to the ends of DNA fragments, and DNA fragments with specific adapters were amplified. Any unwanted short fragments were removed with Agencourt AMPure XP beads (Beckman Coulter, Brea, CA, USA) using a 1:1 DNA-to-bead ratio. The insert size of the library was detected on an Agilent 2100 Bioanalyzer (Agilent Technologies, Inc., Santa Clara, CA, USA), and effective concentration of the library was accurately quantified using a Qubit™ 2.0 Fluorometer (Life Technologies, Carlsbad, CA, USA).

2.6. Monitoring EGFR T790M in Plasma for EGFR-TKI Treatment

To explore the application of Sel-Cap in monitoring plasma *EGFR* resistance mutation T790M to predict resistance to first-line EGFR-TKIs, a retrospective inspection was conducted on the serial plasma samples collected from patients with advanced disease who (1) were treated with first/second-generation EGFR-TKIs (gefitinib, erlotinib, or afatinib) and (2) had already developed disease progression (PD). Progression-free survival (PFS) was defined as the interval between EGFR-TKI initiation and PD. Tumor response was assessed by imaging techniques (such as computed tomography and magnetic resonance imaging) and determined based on the Response Evaluation Criteria in Solid Tumors (RECIST) version 1.1 [12].

2.7. Statistical Analyses

The diagnostic performance of liquid biopsies was evaluated based on sensitivity, specificity, accuracy, and Kappa coefficient, with the PNAclamp tumor biopsy serving as the reference. Sensitivity was calculated as the percentage of positive diagnoses (*EGFR* mutations) by test platform vs. by reference platform. Specificity was calculated as the percentage of negative diagnoses (*EGFR* wild-type) by test platform vs. by reference platform. Accuracy was calculated as the percentage of positive plus negative diagnoses by test platform vs. by reference platform. A Kappa coefficient, a statistical measure used to assess agreement between platforms, between 0.6 and 0.8 is generally regarded as "substantial agreement", while a Kappa coefficient over 0.8 is generally regarded as "almost perfect agreement". Statistical analyses were performed using the SPSS (version 22.0) program (IBM Corporation, Armonk, NY, USA).

3. Results

3.1. Study Population

The CONSORT flow diagram is presented in Figure 1. We identified 250 eligible patients whose tumor samples were available and previously genotyped for *EGFR* mutations by PNAclamp, and 185 of those patients had plasma samples available. The median age of the 185 patients at diagnosis was 64 years old, and the ratio of male to female was about 4 to 5. Nearly half of the patients (57.3%) were in TNM stage III/IV (TNM: a globally standardized cancer staging system, T: primary tumor, N: regional lymph node, M: distant metastasis).

Three separate studies were conducted to evaluate Sel-Cap liquid biopsy, using plasma samples collected from 185 different patients. In the first study, plasma samples from 61 patients were tested for Ex19del and L858R by both Sel-Cap and conventional NGS (T790M was not tested because these patients' PNAclamp tumor biopsies did not include T790M); in the second study, plasma samples from all 185 patients were genotyped for Ex19del, L858R, and T790M by Sel-Cap, and in the third study, plasma samples were collected from 21 patients after they had developed resistance to first-line EGFR-TKIs and genotyped using both Sel-Cap and the NGS cancer panel. Finally, for the retrospective longitudinal T790M monitoring study, out of the patients with T790M-positive plasmas who progressed on first-line EGFR-TKIs, 34 eligible patients were identified and divided into two groups (early T790M detection and late T790M detection, based on the first time T790M was detected in plasma). Patients in the late T790M detection group all had serial plasma samples taken every 3–6 months along with a tumor response evaluation by imaging.

3.2. Sel-Cap Showed High Sensitivity for EGFR Mutations in Plasma

In the first study, the diagnostic performance of Sel-Cap liquid biopsy and a conventional NGS liquid biopsy in 61 patients, looking at Ex19del and L858R, is presented in Table 1 (with the PNAclamp tumor biopsy as the reference). The sensitivity of Sel-Cap liquid biopsy (75% for Ex19del and 65% for L858R) is 4–5 times higher than that of NGS (17% for Ex19del and 13% for L858R). When the results were stratified by disease stage, NGS showed a low sensitivity for Ex19del and L858R (36% and 22%, respectively) in advanced-stage disease, and was unable to detect any mutations in early-stage disease, while Sel-Cap showed good sensitivity in advanced-stage (72% and 78% for Ex19del and L858R, respectively) and early-stage (78% and 50%, respectively) plasma samples (Figure 2).

Although it is not the primary objective of this study, Sel-Cap was also evaluated for tumor biopsy and showed almost perfect agreement (Kappa coefficient = 1.00 and 0.96 for Ex19del and L858R, respectively) with PNAclamp tumor biopsy (Table S1).

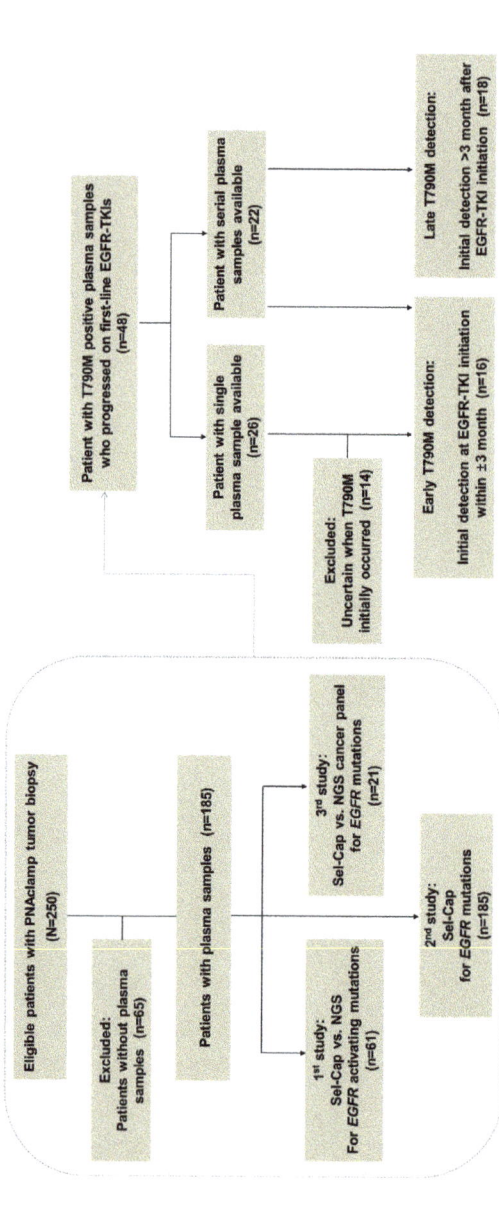

Figure 1. CONSORT flow diagram for the present study. NGS, next-generation sequencing; EGFR-TKI, epidermal growth factor receptor-tyrosine kinase inhibitor.

Table 1. Diagnostic performance of Sel-Cap and conventional NGS liquid biopsies for two EGFR activating mutations in NSCLC patients (n = 61), with paired PNAclamp tumor biopsy as the reference.

		Ex19del						L858R					
		Sel-Cap			NGS			Sel-Cap			NGS		
		Mutant	Wild	Total	Mutant	Wild	Total	Mutant	Wild	Total	Mutant	Wild	Total
PNAclamp	Mutant	15	5	20	3	15	18	11	6	17	2	14	16
	Wild	2	39	41	1	42	43	0	44	44	0	45	45
	Total	17	44	61	4	57	61	11	50	61	2	59	61
Sensitivity	(95% CI)	75%			17%			65%			13%		
		(53–89%)			(6–39%)			(41–83%)			(3–36%)		
Specificity	(95% CI)	95%			98%			100%			100%		
		(84–99%)			(88–100%)			(92–100%)			(92–100%)		
Accuracy	(95% CI)	89%			74%			90%			77%		
		(78–94%)			(62–83%)			(80–95%)			(65–86%)		
Kappa	(95% CI)	0.73			0.19			0.73			0.17		
		(0.54–0.92)			(−0.16–0.53)			(0.52–0.93)			(−0.21–0.55)		

95% CI, 95% confident interval.

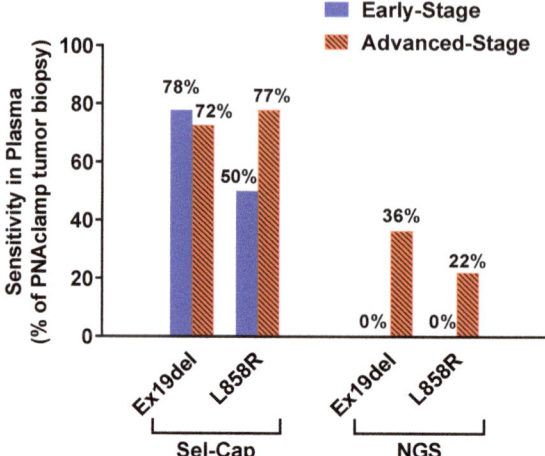

Figure 2. Comparison of sensitivity between Sel-Cap and conventional NGS liquid biopsies for two *EGFR*-activating mutations in NSCLC patients (n = 61, Table 1), stratified by disease stage (n = 30 and 31 for early-stage and advanced-stage, respectively). Sensitivity was calculated against paired PNAclamp tumor biopsy.

In the second study, the concordance between genotyping results from Sel-Cap liquid biopsy and PNAclamp tumor biopsy in 185 patients is presented in Table 2. The sensitivity for Ex19del, L858R, and T790M are 72%, 67%, and 88%, respectively. The concordance data for T790M was only calculated in 85 (out of 185) patients whose tumor samples were tested for T790M by PNAclamp, and plasma and tumor samples were collected within an interval of less than 30 days, because if there is a large time interval between plasma and tumor sample collection, the sensitivity of Sel-Cap may have been overestimated due to the occurrence of acquired T790M mutation.

Table 2. Diagnostic performance of Sel-Cap liquid biopsy for three *EGFR* mutations in NSCLC patients (n = 185), regardless of disease stage, with PNAclamp tumor biopsy as the reference.

Sel-Cap		Ex19del			L858R			T790M [a]		
		Mutant	Wild	Total	Mutant	Wild	Total	Mutant	Wild	Total
	Mutant	50	19	69	24	12	36	7	14	21
PNAclamp	Wild	1	115	116	3	146	149	1	63	64
	Total	51	134	185	27	158	185	8	77	85
Sensitivity	(95% CI)	72%	(61–82%)		67%	(50–80%)		88%	(53–98%)	
Specificity	(95% CI)	99%	(95–100%)		98%	(94–99%)		82%	(72–89%)	
Accuracy	(95% CI)	89%	(84–93%)		92%	(87–95%)		82%	(73–89%)	
Kappa	(95% CI)	0.76	(0.65–0.86)		0.71	(0.57–0.85)		0.40	(0.13–0.68)	

[a] Only patients with time interval between tumor and plasma sample collection < 30 days (because T790M is an acquired mutation) and patients who were previously tested by PNAclamp tumor biopsy for T790M were included for data analyses (n = 85).

In the third study, plasma samples collected from first-line EGFR-TKI-resistant patients (n = 21) were genotyped by Sel-Cap and NGS cancer panel (Table 3). Sel-Cap discovered three times more T790M-positive plasma samples (n = 12) than NGS cancer panel (n = 4), and two plasma samples were determined to be T790M-positive by both methods.

Table 3. Concordance between two NGS-based lipid biopsy platforms for *EGFR* mutations in NSCLC patients (n = 21), post development of resistance to first-line EGFR-TKIs.

No.	EGFR-TKI	Tumor	Plasma	
		PNAclamp	NGS Cancer Panel	Sel-Cap
1	Erlotinib	Ex19del [a]	Ex19del	Ex19del, T790M [d]
2	Erlotinib	Ex19del [a]	Wild	T790M [d]
3	Erlotinib	L858R [a]	L858R, T790M [d]	Wild
4	Erlotinib	Ex19del [a]	Wild	T790M [d]
5	Erlotinib	Ex19del [a]	Ex19del [d]	Wild
6	Gefitinib	Ex19del, T790M [a]	Wild	Wild
7	Gefitinib	Ex19del [a]	Ex19del, T790M	Ex19del, T790M
8	Afatinib	Ex19del [a]	Wild	Wild
9	Afatinib	Ex19del [a]	Ex19del	Ex19del, T790M [d]
10	Gefitinib	L858R, T790M [b]	L858R, T790M [d]	L858R
11	Gefitinib	Ex19del, T790M [b]	Wild	Wild
12	Afatinib	Ex19del [b]	Ex19del	Ex19del, T790M [d]
13	Erlotinib	T790M [c]	Wild	Wild
14	Erlotinib	T790M [c]	Wild	Wild
15	Erlotinib	L858R, T790M [c]	L858R	L858R, T790M [d]
16	Erlotinib	Ex19del, T790M [c]	Ex19del	Ex19del
17	Erlotinib	Ex19del, T790M [c]	Wild	Ex19del, T790M [d]
18	Erlotinib	Ex19del, T790M [c]	Ex19del	Ex19del, T790M [d]
19	Gefitinib	Ex19del, T790M [c]	Wild	Ex19del, T790M [d]
20	Gefinitib	Ex19del, T790M [c]	Wild	Ex19del, T790M [d]
21	Gefinitib	L858R, T790M [c]	L858R, T790M	L858R, T790M

[a] No.1–9: tumor samples collected before first-line EGFR-TKI initiation. [b] No.10–12: tumor samples collected before PD diagnosis. [c] No.13–21: tumor samples collected before second-line EGFR-TKI osimertinib initiation. [d] Underlined text indicates disconcordant results between Sel-Cap and NGS cancer panel.

3.3. Timing of First T790M Detection in Plasma is Critical for PFS of First-Line EGFR-TKIs

Forty-eight patients who developed drug resistance to first-line EGFR-TKIs (gefitinib, erlotinib, or afatinib) and had T790M-positive plasma samples were identified (Figure 1), and 26 patients had single-point plasma samples while the rest of the 22 patients had serial plasma samples which were collected every 3 months along with a tumor response evaluation by imaging techniques (the actual sampling time varied between patients). In the study to clarify the relationship between the timing of first T790M detection and PFS, single-point T790M-positive plasma samples that did not clearly show whether the mutation was detected for the first time were excluded (n = 14). The clinical characteristics of included patients (n = 34) are shown in Table S2.

The PFS following first-line EGFR-TKI treatment, and the intervals between the first T790M detection and PD, are shown in Figure 3. The PFS is significantly longer in patients where initial detection of T790M was >3 months after treatment initiation (late T790M detection), compared to patients where initial T790M detection was within ±3 months of treatment initiation (early T790M detection): the median PFS is 26.5 (range: 11.6–50.2) months vs. 5.9 (range: 1.2–24.1) months, respectively (Logrank test: hazard ratio [HR] = 4.2, 95% confidence interval [CI]: 1.7–10.6, $p < 0.0001$). In addition, the median interval between the first T790M detection and PD is 3.6 (range: 0–18.6) months for the late T790M detection group vs. 5.8 (range: 1.2–24.2) months for the early T790M detection group, which is not significantly different ($p = 0.27$). Acquired resistance to EGFR-TKI is clinically determined at least 6 months after treatment using diagnostic imaging, but T790M can be detected in plasma 2–3 months before diagnosis of acquired resistance; therefore, a cutoff at 3 months post-EGFR-TKI initiation was used in this study. The timeline plots of these patients are shown in Figure S1.

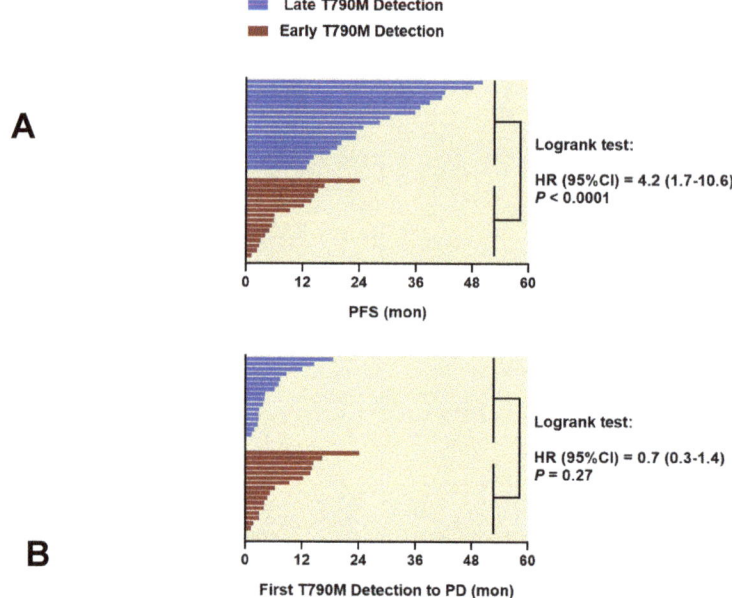

Figure 3. In patients treated by first-line EGFR-TKIs, (**A**) progression-free survival (PFS, interval between treatment initiation and disease progression) was significantly longer in the late T790M detection group (n = 18; first T790M detection: >3 months after treatment initiation) than in the early T790M detection group (n = 16; first T790M detection: at treatment initiation ± 3 months); (**B**) however, the interval between first T790M detection and disease progression was not significantly different between the two groups. *p*-values were obtained by Logrank test.

4. Discussion

In this study, we evaluated the Sel-Cap lung cancer panel, an NGS-based genotyping platform for the detection of *EGFR* mutations in patients with NSCLC, and we focused specifically on its diagnostic performance while serving as a liquid biopsy platform. To do so, Sel-Cap was compared to a standard tumor biopsy (PNAclamp) and two other liquid biopsy platforms (conventional NGS and NGS-based cancer panel) using plasma samples collected from 185 patients.

PNAclamp is currently the most popular diagnostic platform for *EGFR* mutations in Korea. In this study, PNAclamp tumor biopsy is used as the reference for all liquid biopsies. In the first study, Sel-Cap was compared to conventional NGS for detecting *EGFR*-activating mutations in 61 plasma samples. Sel-Cap showed 4–5 times higher sensitivity than NGS in plasma (75% vs. 17% for Ex19del, and 65% vs. 13% for L858R). The second study consisted of a larger sample size (n = 185) and was consistent with the first study: Sel-Cap detected over two-thirds of *EGFR*-activating mutations that were detected by PNAclamp in tumor (sensitivity: 72% for Ex19del and 67% for L858R). Sel-Cap showed very high sensitivity (88%) for *EGFR* resistance mutation T790M in plasma samples, and among the 85 plasma samples tested, Sel-Cap identified 14 more T790M-positive samples which the PNAclamp tumor biopsy was unable to detect.

Our recently published work evaluating a popular liquid biopsy cobas® EGFR mutation test v2 (cobas v2) shows that its sensitivity for *EGFR* mutations is NSCLC stage-dependent [13]. In advanced-stage disease, the sensitivity of cobas v2 liquid biopsy is satisfactory for Ex19del (over 80%) but falls short in L858R and T790M (both are below 40%); furthermore, in early-stage disease, cobas v2 shows disappointingly low sensitivity [13]. In the current study, which looked at 61 plasma samples, the sensitivity of Sel-Cap liquid biopsy for both Ex19del and L858R was high, not only in advanced-stage disease (>70%), but it also showed much higher sensitivity than cobas v2 in early-stage disease (78% vs. 13% for Ex19del, and 50% vs. 0% for L858R). Although Sel-Cap and cobas v2 were not compared directly, both of the studies used an established tumor biopsy for reference (PNAclamp and cobas v2 tumor biopsy, respectively. Our previous study showed that the Kappa co-efficient of the two tumor biopsies was 0.82, indicating almost perfect agreement [13]); therefore, this indirect comparison is reasonably justifiable. In the future, the clinical significance of *EGFR* mutations detected in plasma at early-stage should be studied, and may be particularly valuable in clarifying the connection between *EGFR* mutations in plasma and the risk of tumor relapse, especially considering tumor *EGFR* mutation status-associated EGFR protein expression is a significant risk factor for tumor relapse in early-stage NSCLC [14,15]. Finally, in the 21 plasma samples collected from advanced-stage patients who developed drug resistance to first-line EGFR-TKIs, Sel-Cap detected three times more T790M-positive plasma samples than a different NGS-based cancer panel.

To the best of our knowledge, the sensitivity of Sel-Cap liquid biopsy is the highest among all liquid biopsy platforms on record for *EGFR* mutations in early-stage NSCLC, and Sel-Cap shows one of the highest sensitivities for overall disease stage, which is comparable to ddPCR, currently regarded as the most sensitive liquid biopsy to date [16,17]. The high sensitivity of Sel-Cap for liquid biopsy is attributed to its mutation-enrichment feature. NGS-based cancer panels usually require PCR amplification of regions of interest prior to sequencing, however, the amplification of low copy number mutations tends to be exponentially less efficient than that of the wild-type allele, often leading to selective negativity of the mutations (PCR bias) [18]. In order to solve the problem, Sel-Cap assay uses wild-type-specific blockers to suppress the amplification of wild-type alleles and thus can preferentially amplify mutant alleles. In addition to the high sensitivity, another clinically meaningful advantage of Sel-Cap liquid biopsy is that less plasma (0.7–0.8 mL) is required for each test compared to other platforms (2–10 mL).

For some of the patients in the study, T790M mutation was detected in plasma by Sel-Cap even at what is considered the baseline for first-line EGFR-TKIs (treatment initiation within ±3 months). Our study did not calculate the portion of T790M-positive patients among all EGFR-TKI-naïve patients, but previous studies estimate that T790M can be found in around 2% of *EGFR*-activating mutation-positive EGFR-TKI-naïve plasma samples [19] and frozen tumor samples [20]; however, the percentage can be much higher (>40%) in FFPE tumor samples, likely due to higher incidence of false positives [20]. This disadvantage (false positivity) of *EGFR* testing using FFPE tumor also suggests that if liquid biopsy sensitivity can rival that of tumor biopsy, it may become a good surrogate for tissue *EGFR* testing [21], since it usually shows low false positivity.

It is estimated that nearly half of first-line EGFR-TKI-treated patients may acquire the T790M mutation after long-term treatment [3], which is in line with the T790M-positive rate observed in the 21 post-PD plasma samples in our study. Before liquid biopsy platforms were available, the conventional T790M detection was conducted through tumor re-biopsy after disease progression, and the prognostic value of T790M diagnosis was very limited [22]. In recent years, an increasing number of studies on monitoring T790M in plasma have been conducted [17,19,23–26]. In our study, excluding those who were already T790M-positive at treatment baseline (early T790M detection group), the median time for the initial detection of T790M in plasma (in late T790M detection group) was 23.4 months (ranging from 5.5 to 38.2 months) post-EGFR-TKI initiation, which is similar to the results reported in a recently published monitoring study [23]. Interestingly, regardless of whether T790M is initially detected at baseline or after long-term treatment, the time to PD post-T790M detection was not significantly different (median time ~5 months). Several previous studies conducted similar longitudinal monitoring for T790M in NSCLC patients who had tumor progression on EGFR-TKI treatments [19,24]. In their studies, 40–70% of the patients showed initial T790M detection in plasma at the time of PD or after. For those whose T790M first appeared before PD diagnosis, the time between the detection and PD was typically 2–3 months. Our study shows that Sel-Cap can not only detect T790M before PD for the vast majority of patients (16/18 patients, according to the late T790M detection group), but it can also predict PD at least 2–3 months earlier than an ordinary liquid biopsy, and therefore could increase the time window for physicians to plan the next treatment and monitoring programs.

In addition, our study emphasized that monitoring programs should be individualized. For instance, because the patients with T790M detected at baseline tend to develop drug resistance to first-line EGFR-TKIs much faster than those who have T790M detected >3 months later, a monitoring program with more frequent intervals may be needed for patients with baseline T790M. On the other hand, in patients without baseline T790M, since the longitudinal monitoring period for initial T790M detection varies vastly, for those who continuously respond to first-line EGFR-TKIs, longer monitoring intervals between liquid biopsies can be considered to ease the financial burden of testing. More importantly, in future studies, the risk factors for the occurrence of T790M in plasma should be investigated and considered [27] so that monitoring of T790M by liquid biopsy may become more efficient. Previous studies found that T790M was more prevalent in metastatic tumors than primary tumors in NSCLC patients [28], and tumor size was positively and significantly correlated with cfDNA level in ovarian cancer [29] and melanoma [30]. Our team is currently looking for correlations between primary and/or metastatic tumor size, *EGFR* mutations in plasma, and disease progression.

This study has several limitations. First, in the study with 185 plasma samples (the third study), the sensitivity of Sel-Cap was not stratified by disease stage because this information was not known for all of the samples. Second, all the patients included in the retrospective monitoring study had at least one T790M-positive plasma sample and developed disease progression on first-line EGFR-TKI treatments, and the study did not include samples collected from those who might have missed diagnosis of T790M due to single sampling, or from those who were still responding to first-line EGFR-TKI treatments. A prospective study is needed to validate the clinical application of Sel-Cap for prediction of disease progression, compared to the standard imaging diagnostic techniques. Third, in this real-world study, the plasma sampling for the longitudinal monitoring of T790M did not strictly follow a schedule; in some patients, the actual T790M detection time in plasma could have been a few months earlier.

Sensitive and reliable genotyping platforms are the premise of successful lung cancer target therapy. Ideally, such platforms should also be non-invasive, fast, and affordable. So far, our study has generated encouraging results for the application of Sel-Cap, a highly sensitive digital enrichment NGS liquid biopsy for NSCLC. With the increasing discovery of other EGFR-TKI resistance mechanisms besides T790M (for example, *EGFR* mutation copy number [26] and c-met overexpression [31]) and with the increasing understanding of other factors influencing the detection of T790M in plasma-derived cfDNA, we may be able to predict the occurrence of drug-resistance more accurately and determine the optimal time to switch to the third-generation EGFR-TKIs. We foresee that regular monitoring for *EGFR* mutations with sensitive liquid biopsy platforms, such as Sel-Cap, may become the standard of practice in the future precision medicine for NSCLC.

5. Conclusions

In this study conducted using plasma samples collected from 185 NSCLC patients, Sel-Cap, a digital enrichment NGS-based lung cancer panel, shows very high sensitivity for *EGFR* mutations in cfDNA, even in early-stage disease. The application of Sel-Cap liquid biopsy in a retrospective, longitudinal monitoring study suggests that highly sensitive platforms for *EGFR* resistance mutation T790M in plasma may allow for prediction of disease progression around 5 months in advance, unlike tumor re-biopsy or less sensitive liquid biopsy, where the T790M is often detected after disease progression.

Supplementary Materials: The following are available online at http://www.mdpi.com/2072-6694/12/12/3579/s1, Figure S1: Timeline plots showing intervals between EGFR-TKI initiation, first T790M detection, and disease progression in patients (n = 34) who developed drug resistance to first-line EGFR-TKI treatments. Table S1: Diagnostic performance of Sel-Cap and NGS tumor biopsies for two EGFR activating mutations in NSCLC patients (n = 61), with paired PNAclamp tumor biopsy as the reference. Table S2: Clinical characteristics of patients included in the retrospective longitudinal monitoring study (n = 34).

Author Contributions: J.H.K. and J.-Y.S. conceptualized the study; S.R.K. and K.S.B. collected the patients' data; J.-O.K., J.-Y.S., and M.-R.L. conducted the experiments; J.H.K. and J.-Y.S. did the data analyses; J.H.K. and J.-Y.S. wrote the manuscript. All authors reviewed and revised the manuscript. J.H.K. approved the final version. All authors have read and agreed to the published version of the manuscript.

Funding: This work was supported by the Industrial Strategic Technology Development Program—Korea Post-Genome Project (10067810, The development of kit for screening of cancer-related target genes with high sensitivity in the liquid biopsy) funded by the Ministry of Trade, Industry & Energy (MOTIE, Korea).

Acknowledgments: We appreciate Jin Medical Science Service for language help.

Conflicts of Interest: Jin Hyoung Kang has acted as an advisor for Merck, MSD, Ono/BMS, AstraZeneca, Eli Lilly, and Yuhan, has received research funding from Ono, AstraZeneca, Böehringer Ingelheim, Yuhan, and Daichi Sankyo, and has acted as a speaker for Pfizer, Roche, Merck, and Böehringer Ingelheim. All the other authors declare no conflict of interest.

References

1. Hirsch, F.R.; Scagliotti, G.V.; Mulshine, J.L.; Kwon, R.; Curran, W.J., Jr.; Wu, Y.L.; Paz-Ares, L. Lung cancer: Current therapies and new targeted treatments. *Lancet* **2017**, *389*, 299–311. [CrossRef]
2. Morgillo, F.; Della Corte, C.M.; Fasano, M.; Ciardiello, F. Mechanisms of resistance to EGFR-targeted drugs: Lung cancer. *ESMO Open* **2016**, *1*, e000060. [CrossRef] [PubMed]
3. Ma, C.; Wei, S.; Song, Y. T790M and acquired resistance of EGFR TKI: A literature review of clinical reports. *J. Thorac. Dis.* **2011**, *3*, 10–18. [CrossRef] [PubMed]
4. Diaz, L.A., Jr.; Bardelli, A. Liquid biopsies: Genotyping circulating tumor DNA. *J. Clin. Oncol.* **2014**, *32*, 579–586. [CrossRef] [PubMed]
5. Stewart, C.M.; Tsui, D.W.Y. Circulating cell-free DNA for non-invasive cancer management. *Cancer Genet.* **2018**, *228–229*, 169–179. [CrossRef]
6. Garcia, J.; Wozny, A.S.; Geiger, F.; Delherme, A.; Barthelemy, D.; Merle, P.; Tissot, C.; Jones, F.S.; Johnson, C.; Xing, X.; et al. Profiling of circulating tumor DNA in plasma of non-small cell lung cancer patients, monitoring of epidermal growth factor receptor p.T790M mutated allelic fraction using beads, emulsion, amplification, and magnetics companion assay and evaluation in future application in mimicking circulating tumor cells. *Cancer Med.* **2019**, *8*, 3685–3697. [CrossRef]
7. Xue, V.W.; Wong, C.S.C.; Cho, W.C.S. Early detection and monitoring of cancer in liquid biopsy: Advances and challenges. *Expert Rev. Mol. Diagn.* **2019**, *19*, 273–276. [CrossRef]
8. Lee, B.; Lee, B.; Han, G.; Kwon, M.J.; Han, J.; Choi, Y.L. KRAS Mutation Detection in Non-small Cell Lung Cancer Using a Peptide Nucleic Acid-Mediated Polymerase Chain Reaction Clamping Method and Comparative Validation with Next-Generation Sequencing. *Korean J. Pathol.* **2014**, *48*, 100–107. [CrossRef]
9. Xue, V.W.; Ng, S.S.M.; Leung, W.W.; Ma, B.B.Y.; Cho, W.C.S.; Au, T.C.C.; Yu, A.C.S.; Tsang, H.F.A.; Wong, S.C.C. The Effect of Centrifugal Force in Quantification of Colorectal Cancer-Related mRNA in Plasma Using Targeted Sequencing. *Front. Genet.* **2018**, *9*, 165. [CrossRef]
10. Mouliere, F.; Robert, B.; Arnau Peyrotte, E.; Del Rio, M.; Ychou, M.; Molina, F.; Gongora, C.; Thierry, A.R. High fragmentation characterizes tumour-derived circulating DNA. *PLoS ONE* **2011**, *6*, e23418. [CrossRef]
11. Kim, H.J.; Lee, K.Y.; Kim, Y.C.; Kim, K.S.; Lee, S.Y.; Jang, T.W.; Lee, M.K.; Shin, K.C.; Lee, G.H.; Lee, J.C.; et al. Detection and comparison of peptide nucleic acid-mediated real-time polymerase chain reaction clamping and direct gene sequencing for epidermal growth factor receptor mutations in patients with non-small cell lung cancer. *Lung Cancer* **2012**, *75*, 321–325. [CrossRef] [PubMed]
12. Eisenhauer, E.A.; Therasse, P.; Bogaerts, J.; Schwartz, L.H.; Sargent, D.; Ford, R.; Dancey, J.; Arbuck, S.; Gwyther, S.; Mooney, M.; et al. New response evaluation criteria in solid tumours: Revised RECIST guideline (version 1.1). *Eur. J. Cancer* **2009**, *45*, 228–247. [CrossRef] [PubMed]
13. Kim, J.O.; Shin, J.Y.; Kim, S.R.; Shin, K.S.; Kim, J.; Kim, M.Y.; Lee, M.R.; Kim, Y.; Kim, M.; Hong, S.H.; et al. Evaluation of Two EGFR Mutation Tests on Tumor and Plasma from Patients with Non-Small Cell Lung Cancer. *Cancers* **2020**, *12*, 785. [CrossRef] [PubMed]
14. Traynor, A.M.; Weigel, T.L.; Oettel, K.R.; Yang, D.T.; Zhang, C.; Kim, K.; Salgia, R.; Iida, M.; Brand, T.M.; Hoang, T.; et al. Nuclear EGFR protein expression predicts poor survival in early stage non-small cell lung cancer. *Lung Cancer* **2013**, *81*, 138–141. [CrossRef]

15. Douillard, J.Y.; Pirker, R.; O'Byrne, K.J.; Kerr, K.M.; Storkel, S.; von Heydebreck, A.; Grote, H.J.; Celik, I.; Shepherd, F.A. Relationship between EGFR expression, EGFR mutation status, and the efficacy of chemotherapy plus cetuximab in FLEX study patients with advanced non-small-cell lung cancer. *J. Thorac. Oncol.* **2014**, *9*, 717–724. [CrossRef]
16. Li, C.; He, Q.; Liang, H.; Cheng, B.; Li, J.; Xiong, S.; Zhao, Y.; Guo, M.; Liu, Z.; He, J.; et al. Diagnostic Accuracy of Droplet Digital PCR and Amplification Refractory Mutation System PCR for Detecting EGFR Mutation in Cell-Free DNA of Lung Cancer: A Meta-Analysis. *Front. Oncol.* **2020**, *10*, 290. [CrossRef]
17. Lee, J.Y.; Qing, X.; Xiumin, W.; Yali, B.; Chi, S.; Bak, S.H.; Lee, H.Y.; Sun, J.M.; Lee, S.H.; Ahn, J.S.; et al. Longitudinal monitoring of EGFR mutations in plasma predicts outcomes of NSCLC patients treated with EGFR TKIs: Korean Lung Cancer Consortium (KLCC-12-02). *Oncotarget* **2016**, *7*, 6984–6993. [CrossRef]
18. Kebschull, J.M.; Zador, A.M. Sources of PCR-induced distortions in high-throughput sequencing data sets. *Nucleic Acids Res.* **2015**, *43*, e143. [CrossRef]
19. Usui, K.; Yokoyama, T.; Naka, G.; Ishida, H.; Kishi, K.; Uemura, K.; Ohashi, Y.; Kunitoh, H. Plasma ctDNA monitoring during epidermal growth factor receptor (EGFR)-tyrosine kinase inhibitor treatment in patients with EGFR-mutant non-small cell lung cancer (JP-CLEAR trial). *Jpn. J. Clin. Oncol.* **2019**, *49*, 554–558. [CrossRef]
20. Ye, X.; Zhu, Z.Z.; Zhong, L.; Lu, Y.; Sun, Y.; Yin, X.; Yang, Z.; Zhu, G.; Ji, Q. High T790M detection rate in TKI-naive NSCLC with EGFR sensitive mutation: Truth or artifact? *J. Thorac. Oncol.* **2013**, *8*, 1118–1120. [CrossRef]
21. Goldman, J.W.; Noor, Z.S.; Remon, J.; Besse, B.; Rosenfeld, N. Are liquid biopsies a surrogate for tissue EGFR testing? *Ann. Oncol.* **2018**, *29*, i38–i46. [CrossRef] [PubMed]
22. Ichihara, E.; Hotta, K.; Kubo, T.; Higashionna, T.; Ninomiya, K.; Ohashi, K.; Tabata, M.; Maeda, Y.; Kiura, K. Clinical significance of repeat rebiopsy in detecting the EGFR T790M secondary mutation in patients with non-small cell lung cancer. *Oncotarget* **2018**, *9*, 29525–29531. [CrossRef] [PubMed]
23. Dal Maso, A.; Lorenzi, M.; Roca, E.; Pilotto, S.; Macerelli, M.; Polo, V.; Cecere, F.L.; Del Conte, A.; Nardo, G.; Buoro, V.; et al. Clinical Features and Progression Pattern of Acquired T790M-positive Compared with T790M-negative EGFR Mutant Non-small-cell Lung Cancer: Catching Tumor and Clinical Heterogeneity Over Time Through Liquid Biopsy. *Clin. Lung Cancer* **2020**, *21*, 1–14.e13. [CrossRef] [PubMed]
24. Sueoka-Aragane, N.; Katakami, N.; Satouchi, M.; Yokota, S.; Aoe, K.; Iwanaga, K.; Otsuka, K.; Morita, S.; Kimura, S.; Negoro, S.; et al. Monitoring EGFR T790M with plasma DNA from lung cancer patients in a prospective observational study. *Cancer Sci.* **2016**, *107*, 162–167. [CrossRef] [PubMed]
25. Zheng, D.; Ye, X.; Zhang, M.Z.; Sun, Y.; Wang, J.Y.; Ni, J.; Zhang, H.P.; Zhang, L.; Luo, J.; Zhang, J.; et al. Plasma EGFR T790M ctDNA status is associated with clinical outcome in advanced NSCLC patients with acquired EGFR-TKI resistance. *Sci. Rep.* **2016**, *6*, 20913. [CrossRef] [PubMed]
26. Iwama, E.; Sakai, K.; Hidaka, N.; Inoue, K.; Fujii, A.; Nakagaki, N.; Ota, K.; Toyozawa, R.; Azuma, K.; Nakatomi, K.; et al. Longitudinal monitoring of somatic genetic alterations in circulating cell-free DNA during treatment with epidermal growth factor receptor-tyrosine kinase inhibitors. *Cancer* **2020**, *126*, 219–227. [CrossRef]
27. Ouyang, W.; Yu, J.; Huang, Z.; Chen, G.; Liu, Y.; Liao, Z.; Zeng, W.; Zhang, J.; Xie, C. Risk factors of acquired T790M mutation in patients with epidermal growth factor receptor-mutated advanced non-small cell lung cancer. *J. Cancer* **2020**, *11*, 2060–2067. [CrossRef]
28. Huang, Y.H.; Hsu, K.H.; Tseng, J.S.; Chen, K.C.; Hsu, C.H.; Su, K.Y.; Chen, J.J.W.; Chen, H.W.; Yu, S.L.; Yang, T.Y.; et al. The Association of Acquired T790M Mutation with Clinical Characteristics after Resistance to First-Line Epidermal Growth Factor Receptor Tyrosine Kinase Inhibitor in Lung Adenocarcinoma. *Cancer Res. Treat.* **2018**, *50*, 1294–1303. [CrossRef]
29. Wang, X.; Wang, L.; Su, Y.; Yue, Z.; Xing, T.; Zhao, W.; Zhao, Q.; Duan, C.; Huang, C.; Zhang, D.; et al. Plasma cell-free DNA quantification is highly correlated to tumor burden in children with neuroblastoma. *Cancer Med.* **2018**. [CrossRef]
30. Valpione, S.; Gremel, G.; Mundra, P.; Middlehurst, P.; Galvani, E.; Girotti, M.R.; Lee, R.J.; Garner, G.; Dhomen, N.; Lorigan, P.C.; et al. Plasma total cell-free DNA (cfDNA) is a surrogate biomarker for tumour burden and a prognostic biomarker for survival in metastatic melanoma patients. *Eur. J. Cancer* **2018**, *88*, 1–9. [CrossRef]

31. Bylicki, O.; Paleiron, N.; Assie, J.B.; Chouaid, C. Targeting the MET-Signaling Pathway in Non-Small-Cell Lung Cancer: Evidence to Date. *OncoTargets Ther.* **2020**, *13*, 5691–5706. [CrossRef] [PubMed]

Publisher's Note: MDPI stays neutral with regard to jurisdictional claims in published maps and institutional affiliations.

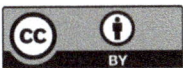

© 2020 by the authors. Licensee MDPI, Basel, Switzerland. This article is an open access article distributed under the terms and conditions of the Creative Commons Attribution (CC BY) license (http://creativecommons.org/licenses/by/4.0/).

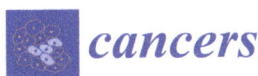

Brief Report

Evaluation of Two *EGFR* Mutation Tests on Tumor and Plasma from Patients with Non-Small Cell Lung Cancer

Jeong-Oh Kim [1], Jung-Young Shin [1], Seo Ree Kim [2], Kab Soo Shin [2], Joori Kim [2], Min-Young Kim [1], Mi-Ran Lee [1], Yonggoo Kim [3], Myungshin Kim [3], Sook Hee Hong [2] and Jin Hyoung Kang [1,2,*]

- [1] Laboratory of Medical Oncology, Cancer Research Institute, College of Medicine, The Catholic University of Korea, Seoul 06591, Korea; kjo9713@catholic.ac.kr (J.-O.K.); bearjy@catholic.ac.kr (J.-Y.S.); kiminy414@catholic.ac.kr (M.-Y.K.); miran13@catholic.ac.kr (M.-R.L.)
- [2] Department of Medical Oncology, Seoul St. Mary's Hospital, The Catholic University of Korea, Seoul 06591, Korea; seoreek@gmail.com (S.R.K.); agx002@naver.com (K.S.S.); jooriworld@gmail.com (J.K.); ssuki76@catholic.ac.kr (S.H.H.)
- [3] Department of Laboratory Medicine, Seoul St. Mary's Hospital, The Catholic University of Korea, Seoul 06591, Korea; yonggoo@catholic.ac.kr (Y.K.); microkim@catholic.ac.kr (M.K.)
- * Correspondence: oncologykang@naver.com; Tel.: +82-2-2258-6043

Received: 1 March 2020; Accepted: 24 March 2020; Published: 26 March 2020

Abstract: Epidermal growth factor receptor (*EGFR*) mutation testing is essential for individualized treatment using tyrosine kinase inhibitors. We evaluated two *EGFR* mutation tests, cobas v2 and PANAMutyper, for detection of *EGFR* activating mutations Ex19del, L858R, and T790M in tumor tissue and plasma from 244 non-small cell lung cancer (NSCLC) patients. The Kappa coefficient (95% CI) between the tests was 0.82 (0.74–0.92) in tumor samples (suggesting almost perfect agreement) and 0.69 (0.54–0.84) in plasma (suggesting substantial agreement). In plasma samples, both tests showed low to moderate sensitivity depending on disease stage but high diagnostic precision (86%–100%) in all disease stages (sensitivity: percentage of mutations in tumors that are also detected in plasma; precision: percentage of mutations in plasma which are also detected in tumors). Among the 244 patients, those previously diagnosed as T790M carriers who received osimertinib treatment showed dramatically better clinical outcomes than T790M carriers without osimertinib treatment. Taken together, our study supports interchangeable use of cobas v2 and PANAMutyper in tumor and plasma *EGFR* testing. Both tests have high diagnostic precision in plasma but are particularly valuable in late-stage disease. Our clinical data in T790M carriers strongly support the clinical benefits of osimertinib treatment guided by both *EGFR* mutation tests.

Keywords: circulating free DNA; liquid biopsy; epidermal growth factor receptor; tyrosine kinase inhibitor; osimertinib

1. Introduction

The introduction of tyrosine kinase inhibitors (TKIs) for non-small cell lung cancer (NSCLC) has greatly improved treatment outcomes in patients with epidermal growth factor receptor (*EGFR*) mutations [1–3]. The importance of *EGFR* mutation testing in TKI treatment is well-recognized [4], and its cost-effectiveness has been established in many countries [5–7]. Inaccurate *EGFR* mutation tests may cause marked loss of quality-adjusted life-years [8]. Direct sequencing of tumor DNA is the gold standard diagnostic method for detecting *EGFR* mutations, but clinical utility is limited due to its high cost, long turnaround time, and low sensitivity (limit of detection >20%; limit of detection is defined as the percentage of tumor cells that must be present in the specimen for a mutation to be identified [4]). New *EGFR* mutation tests such as real-time polymerase chain reaction (RT-PCR), amplification refractory mutation system (ARMS), peptide nucleic acid (PNA)-based PCR, and droplet digital PCR (dd-PCR) provide reliable, quick test results with high sensitivity (limit of detection: 0.01%–1%) and have therefore gained currency in clinical settings [9]. Meanwhile, due to the difficulty in obtaining sufficient amounts of tumor tissue and repeat tumor biopsy, there is a growing trend of testing *EGFR* mutations using liquid biopsy.

The objective of this study was to evaluate the concordance of two commercial *EGFR* mutation tests: an RT-PCR method cobas EGFR mutation test v2 (cobas v2) and a PNA-based PCR method PANAMutyper R EGFR (PANAMutyper) in tumor tissue and plasma from NSCLC patients. The cobas v2 was initially approved by the US Food Drug Administration, and the PANAMutyper was initially approved by the Korea Ministry of Food and Drug Safety. The PANAMutyper test combines PNA-based PCR clamping (PNAClamp) with multiplex fluorescence melting curve analysis (PANA S-Melting) using a fluorescence-labeled PNA probe, which allows detection of 47 hotspot mutations between *EGFR* exon 18 and exon 21 [10]. While evaluating the concordance of the tests, we particularly focused on the performance of the tests in plasma samples and in a subgroup of patients with diagnosis of *EGFR* T790M mutation (An acquired TKI resistance-related *EGFR* gatekeeper mutation, which substitutes a threonine with a methionine at position 790 of exon 20).

2. Materials and Methods

2.1. Study Population

Electronic medical records (EMRs) were used to identify eligible patients histologically diagnosed with NSCLC between January 2013 and April 2019 with tumor tissue or plasma sample stored at the Seoul St. Mary's Hospital Biobank. When multiple samples were available from the same patient, samples from the first biopsy were used for testing. Almost all of the eligible patients had been tested for *EGFR* mutations using PNA-based PCR clamping [11] (PNAClamp, Daejeon, Korea) before. For patients treated with osimertinib (Tagrisso, formerly AZD9291; AstraZeneca, Macclesfield, UK), samples from the latest biopsy before osimertinib treatment initiation were used. The research plan of the current study was approved by the Institutional Review Board (IRB) of Seoul at St. Mary's Hospital (KC17DESI0147). At the time of sample collection, all patients provided a biobank-written informed consent form for the possible use of their samples in future research.

2.2. EGFR Mutation Tests

Tumor samples were collected and prepared as formalin-fixed, paraffin-embedded sides. Tumor DNA was extracted using a Maxwell 16 FFPE Tissue LEV DNA Purification Kit (Promega, Madison, WI, USA) for PANAMutyper tests (PANAGENE, Daejeon, Korea) and using a cobas DNA Sample Preparation Kit (Roche Molecular Systems, Pleasanton, CA, USA) for cobas v2 tests. Plasma was prepared by the Seoul St. Mary's Hospital Biobank and stored at −70 °C. For this study, plasma samples were used to separate the supernatant for circulating free DNA (cfDNA) extraction. The cfDNA was extracted using QIAamp Circulating Nucleic Acid Kit (Qiagen, Hilden, Germany) and cobas cfDNA Sample Preparation Kit (Roche Molecular Systems, Pleasanton, CA, USA). Only DNA samples that passed qualitative and quantitative quality control (according to the kit manufacturers' protocols) were used for *EGFR* mutation tests.

For PANAMutyper test, 5 µL DNA was added to 20 µL polymerase chain reaction (PCR) reagent (a mixture of 19 µL of peptide nucleic acid (PNA) probe and 1 µL of Taq DNA polymerase). PCR was carried out using the CFX96 Real-Time PCR Detection System (Bio-Rad, Hercules, CA, USA). The PCR-generated melting curves and the genotype of each sample were determined according to the specific fluorescence and melting temperature (Tm) of the melting curves. For cobas v2 test, DNA concentrations were set to 2 ng/µL and detected using a defined workflow channel in a cobas v2 4800 analyzer (Roche Molecular Systems, Pleasanton, CA, USA). Mutation analysis of cobas v2 was performed by Roche Korea using an algorithm specific to the cfDNA test. Both analyses were performed according to the manufacturers' protocols.

2.3. Data Analyses

The concordance of the *EGFR* mutation tests was evaluated with cobas v2 as the reference using (1) positive percentage agreement (PPA) or sensitivity (the percentage of mutations in cobas v2 that is also detected in PANAMutyper); (2) negative percentage agreement (NPA) or specificity (the percentage of wild-type determined by cobas v2 that is also determined by PANAMutyper); (3) overall percentage of agreement (OPA) or accuracy (the percentage of wild-type plus mutations in cobas v2 that are also detected in PANAMutyper); and (4) Kappa coefficient (a statistical measure used to assess agreement between observers that provides more information than OPA because it takes into account chance agreement). A Kappa coefficient between 0.6 and 0.8 is generally regarded as "substantial agreement", and a Kappa coefficient over 0.8 is generally regarded as "almost perfect agreement" [12]. Diagnostic precision in plasma was evaluated to indicate the percentage of mutations detected in plasma that were also detected in tumors. Tumor response was assessed by imaging techniques (such as computed tomography and magnetic resonance imaging) and determined based on the Response Evaluation Criteria in Solid Tumors (RECIST) 1.1 [13]. Survival time was defined as the period between osimertinib treatment initiation (or biopsy for patients who did not receive osimertinib) and the last follow-up (the study was closed on December 28 2019). All statistical analyses were performed with SPSS v.21 software (IBM SPSS, Armonk, NY, USA), and p value < 0.05 was considered statistically significant.

3. Results

3.1. Patients

A total of 244 eligible patients were identified (Figure 1). The ratio of male to female was 1.24:1, the median age was 66 years (range 29–85 years), and 133 were non-smokers (55%). Nearly half of the patients (51%) were in TNM stage III/IV (TNM: cancer staging system; T: primary tumor; N: lymph node; M: distant metastasis), and three-quarters of the patients had lung adenocarcinoma (76%). Nineteen tests from 17 patients were determined to be invalid (tests were invalid if samples failed to pass qualitative and quantitative quality control); 13 patients had invalid PANAMutyper test results (all from blood samples); 6 patients had invalid cobas v2 tests (5 from tumor samples and 1 from blood sample). These patients were excluded from data analyses. Considering the large sample size, both tests were considered successful in generating valid results.

Of the 227 patients with valid test results, the clinical characteristics of patients with *EGFR* wild-type were demographically different from those with *EGFR* activating mutations (Table 1). The median age of the wild-type group was five years older than that of the mutant group, and there were significantly less females, more smokers, and more squamous cell cancer in the wild-type group than the mutant group ($p < 0.001$ for all comparisons).

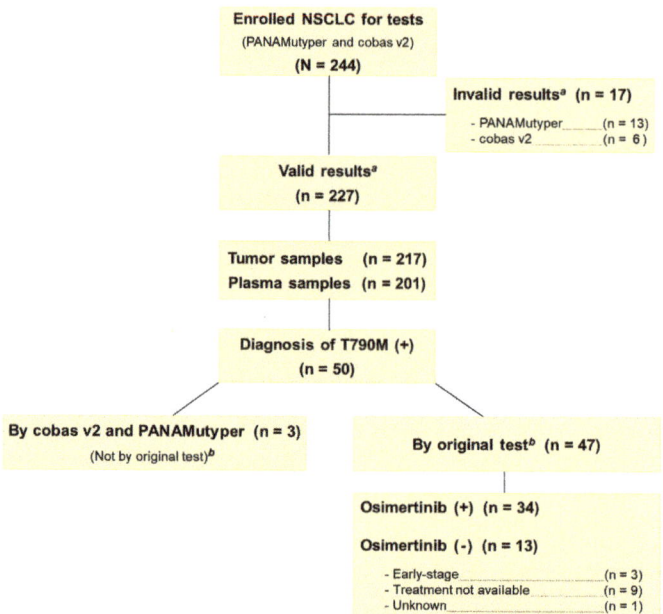

Figure 1. Consort diagram and study flowchart. [a] Tests were considered valid only if samples failed to pass qualitative and quantitative quality control. [b] Original test was peptic nucleic acid (PNA) clamping test.

Table 1. Characteristics of patients (n = 227) with valid *EGFR* test results using two mutation tests.

Patient Demographics (Wild vs. Mutant)	PANAMutyper Test Result			cobas v2 Test Result		
	Wild (n = 130)	Mutant (n = 97)	*p* value	Wild (n = 143)	Mutant (n = 84)	*p* Value
Age [a]						
Median y (range)	68 (44–85)	63 (35–83)	$p < 0.001$	68 (44–85)	63 (35–83)	$p < 0.001$
Sex [b]						
Male	89 (39%)	36 (16%)	$p < 0.001$	99 (44%)	26 (12%)	$p < 0.001$
Female	41 (18%)	61 (27%)		44 (19%)	58 (26%)	
Smoking history [b]						
Never	57 (25%)	68 (30%)		61 (27%)	64 (28%)	
Former	57 (25%)	24 (11%)	$p < 0.001$	66 (29%)	15 (6.6%)	$p < 0.001$
Current	16 (7.0%)	5 (2.2%)		16 (7.0%)	5 (2.2%)	
Histology [b]						
Adenocarcinoma	83 (37%)	91 (40%)		90 (40%)	84 (37%)	
Squamous	45 (20%)	6 (2.6%)	$p < 0.001$	51 (23%)	0	$p < 0.001$
Large cell	2 (0.9%)	0		2 (0.9%)	0	
TNM stage [b,c]						
I	48 (21%)	33 (15%)		53 (23%)	28 (12%)	
II	22 (9.7%)	9 (4.0%)	$p = 0.644$	23 (10%)	8 (3.5%)	$p = 0.491$
III	29 (13%)	11 (4.8%)		34 (15%)	6 (2.6%)	
IV	31 (14%)	44 (19%)		33 (15%)	42 (19%)	

[a] Independent *t*-test for *EGFR* wild vs. *EGFR* mutant groups diagnosed by the same assay. [b] Chi-square test for *EGFR* wild vs. *EGFR* mutant groups diagnosed by the same assay. [c] TNM stage was determined at the sample collection (TNM: cancer staging system; T: primary tumor; N: lymph node; M: distant metastasis).

3.2. Concordance between Two Tests in Tumor and in Plasma

The concordant and discordant *EGFR* mutation test results in tumor tissue are shown in Table 2. In tumor tissue, the mutation detection rate was 43% by PANAMutyper and 37% by cobas v2. When cobas v2 was used as the reference for PANAMutyper, sensitivity (PPA) was 94%, specificity (NPA) was 90%, and accuracy (OPA) was 91%. Kappa coefficient was 0.82, indicating almost perfect agreement between tests in tumor samples.

In plasma, the mutation detection rate was 15% by PANAMutyper and 14% by cobas v2. For PANAMutyper, sensitivity (PPA) was 72%, NPA was 96%, and OPA was 93%. Kappa coefficient of the tests was 0.69, indicating a substantial agreement in plasma.

Table 2. Concordance of two *EGFR* mutation tests in tumor tissue and plasma samples.

Test Results (Reference: cobas v2)	Tumor Tissue (n = 217)	Plasma (n = 201)
Concordant Results		
Both Wild	123 (57%)	165 (82%)
Both Mutant	75 (35%)	21 (10%)
Ex19del	17 (8.5%)	11 (5.5%)
L858R	14 (6.5%)	3 (1.4%)
T790M	1 (0.5%)	2 (1.0%)
L858R+T790M	30 (14%)	3 (1.5%)
Ex19del+T790M	13 (6.0%)	2 (1.0%)
Discordant Result		
P_Mutant/c_Wild [a]	14 (6.5%)	7 (3.5%)
c_Mutant/P_Wild [b]	1 (0.5%)	6 (3.0%)
Different Mutant	4 (1.8%)	2 (1.0%)
Test Evaluation		
Sensitivity (PPA) [c] (95% CI)	94% (86%–97%)	72% (54%–85%)
Specificity (NPA) [c] (95% CI)	90% (84%–94%)	96% (92%–98%)
Accuracy (OPA) [c] (95% CI)	91% (87%–94%)	93% (88%–95%)
Kappa Coefficient (95% CI)	0.82 (0.74–0.92)	0.69 (0.54–0.84)

[a] P_Mutant/c_Wild: PANAMutyper result is mutant but cobas v2 result is wild; [b] c_Mutant/P_Wild: cobas v2 result is mutant but PANAMutyper result is wild; [c] Calculation with cobas v2 as reference; EGFR, epidermal growth factor receptor; OPA, overall percentage agreement; PPA, positive percentage agreement; NPA, negative percentage agreement.

3.3. Concordance of Test Results between Tumor Tissue and Plasma

The *EGFR* mutation test results between tumor tissue and plasma were compared. For subjects with early-stage disease (stage I/II), only a small portion (0%–20%) of mutations found in tumor samples were also detected in plasma by PANAMutyper and cobas v2. Contrastingly, for subjects with advanced-stage disease (stage III/IV), test sensitivity (PPA) in plasma (with results in tumor samples as references) was markedly higher: around one-third of L858R and T790M and more than two-thirds of Ex19del in tumor can be detected in plasma (Figure 2A). For all disease stages, diagnostic precision for the three mutations in plasma (with results in tumor samples as references) was 100% by PANAMutyper and 86%–100% by cobas v2 (Figure 2B).

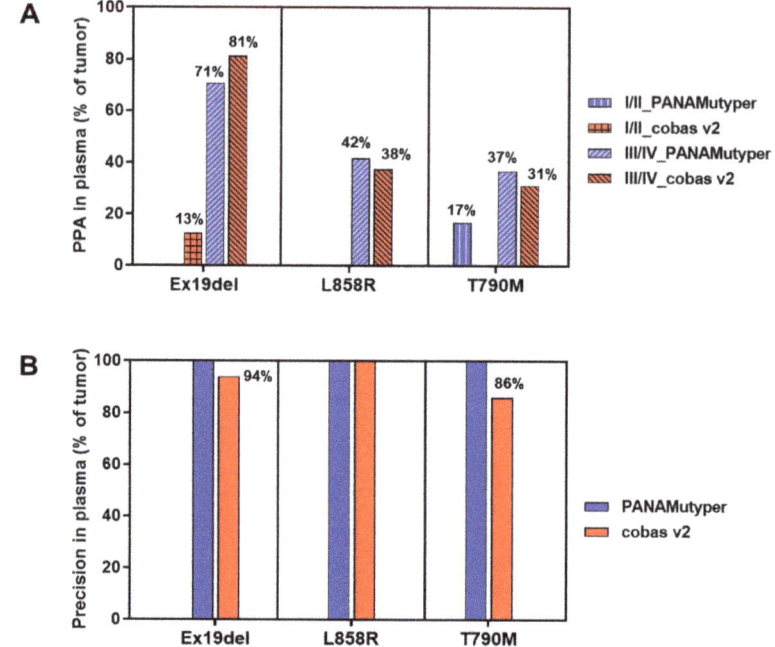

Figure 2. Detection of three *EGFR* mutations in plasma samples. (**A**) PPA of the two tests in plasma, stratified by disease stage. PPA is calculated as percentage of mutations detected in tumor that are also detected in plasma. (**B**) Precision of the two tests in plasma for all disease stages. Precision is calculated as the percentage of mutations detected in plasma that are also detected in tumor. PPA, positive percentage agreement; EGFR, epidermal growth factor receptor.

3.4. Re-Analyses of Discordant Results

Test results from 19 tumor samples were discordant between PANAMutyper and cobas v2 tests. These were compared to the original test results obtained using PNA clamping (Table 3). Ten tumor sample results were consistent between cobas v2 and PNA clamping, including nine wild-types and one Ex19del+T790M. Six tumor sample results were consistent between PANAMutyper and PNA clamping, including three L858R, one Ex19dels, one Ex19del+T790M, and one L858R+T790M. Two tumor sample results differed on all three tests. We attempted to verify the discordant results using dd-PCR. However, only six tumor samples had sufficient tissue for DNA extraction: four test results were in agreement with PANAMutyper, and two were in agreement with cobas v2.

Table 3. Reanalysis of discordance between PANAMutyper and cobas v2 tests.

No	TNM Stage	PANAMutyper	Cobas v2	PNA Clamping	dd-PCR
1	IIa	Ex19del	Wild	Ex19del	-
2	Ib	Ex19del	Wild	Wild	-
3	Ia	Ex20ins	Wild	Wild	-
4	IIIa	G719S	Wild	Wild	-
5	IIa	G719S	Wild	Wild	-
6	IIIb	G719S+T790M	Wild	Wild	-
7	IIIb	L858R	Wild	Wild	Wild
8	Ib	L858R	Wild	Wild	-
9	IIIb	L858R	Wild	Wild	L858R
10	Ia	L858R	Wild	L858R [a]	-
11	IV	L858R	Wild	L858R [a]	-
12	IV	L858R	Wild	L858R	L858R
13	IIIa	T790M	Wild	Ex20 Gln787Gln [b]	-
14	Ia	T790M	Wild	Wild	-
15	IV	L858R+T790M	T790M	L858R+T790M	L858R+T790M
16	Ia	G719C+S768I+T790M	G719X+S768I	-	-
17	IV	Ex19del	Ex19del+T790M	Ex19del+T790M	Ex19del+T790M
18	IV	Ex19del+T790M	Ex19del	Ex19del+T790M	Ex19del+T790M
19	IV	Wild	Ex19del	T790M	-

Underlined results indicate concordance with PANAMutyper, and framed results indicate concordance with cobas v2. [a] PNA clamping result is L858R or L861Q; [b] Synonymous mutation, c.2361G>A.

3.5. Test Results in Patients with T790M Mutation

Of the 227 patients with valid test results, 47 patients were identified as T790M carriers by original PNA clamping test. These patients provided 46 tumor and 23 plasma samples (Figure 3). The concordance of PANAMutyper and cobas v2 results from this subgroup was evaluated using PPA only because all patients were diagnosed as *EGFR* mutants by the original PNA clamping test, and Kappa coefficient is inappropriate for skewed tests. The PPA (95% CI) of PANAMutyper was 91% (79%–97%) in tumor samples and 82% (52%–95%) in plasma. Among the 47 previously identified T790M carriers, 34 patients received osimertinib treatment. These 34 patients were at TNM stage IV and heavily treated at the time of osimertinib initiation (having previously received 3–10 lines of treatment). Of these patients, objective tumor response (complete response or partial response) was achieved in 74% (n = 25) of patients, and disease control was achieved in 88% (n = 30) of patients (Figure 3A). On the other hand, 16 patients were diagnosed with *EGFR* T790M mutation from the tumor samples by both PANAMutyper and cobas v2 but did not receive osimertinib treatment, including three patients who had early-stage disease without progression and 13 patients with late stage disease. Eight late-stage patients received tumor response evaluation, only one had stable disease, and the others showed progression. Six patients died, and seven patients were lost to follow-up (Figure 3B).

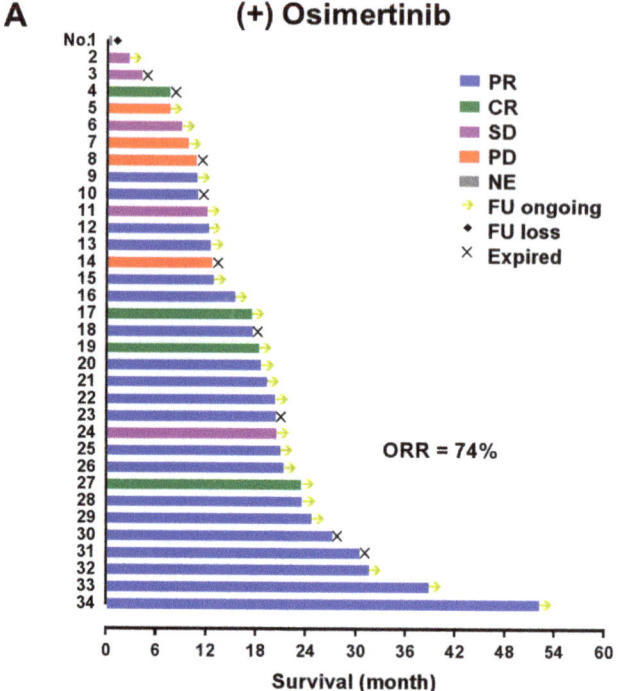

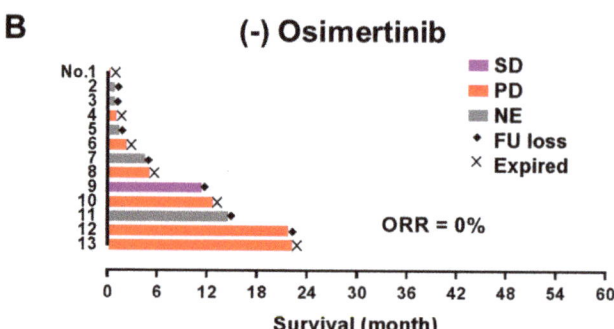

Figure 3. Survival and the best tumor response in patients with *EGFR* T790M mutation. (**A**) Patients who received osimertinib following development of drug resistance and T790M detection. All patients had previously received 3–10 lines of treatment, and osimertinib was used based on detection of T790M mutation using the PNA clamping test. (**B**) Patients with late-stage disease who were diagnosed with T790M mutation (by PNA clamping test: n = 10; by PANAMutyper and cobas v2: n = 3) but did not receive osimertinib. Arrows indicate ongoing follow-up; diamonds indicate loss to follow-up. PR, partial response; CR, complete response; SD, stable disease; PD, progressive disease; NE, not evaluated; FU loss, loss to follow-up; ORR, objective response rate.

4. Discussion

This study is the first to compare PANAMutyper and cobas v2, two popular commercial *EGFR* mutation tests in Korea, for testing in both tumor and plasma samples from NSCLC patients. A large sample size of 244 patients was obtained, including 191 patients with paired samples (tumor and plasma). Results of the current study provide evidence that the two tests are equally accurate and can be used interchangeably.

A meta-analysis published in 2015 included over 30,000 NSCLC patients to create a "global *EGFR* mutMap" for global *EGFR* mutation frequency [14]. This study demonstrated that the overall *EGFR* mutation frequency is much higher in the Asia-Pacific area (47%) compared to Europe and America (15%–25%) and reported that the frequency in Korea is 43% (20%–56%), which is close to our result of 43% by PANAMutyper and 37% by cobas v2.

We observed significant demographic differences between those diagnosed with *EGFR* wild-type and those with *EGFR* mutations (Table 1). Consistent with previous reports [15–17], those with *EGFR* mutations were more likely to be female or non-smokers. In addition, patients without *EGFR* mutations were about five years older than those with *EGFR* mutations. This is probably because we included patients with squamous NSCLC who are less likely to have *EGFR* mutation but tend to be older than those with non-squamous NSCLC [18].

In this study, the two *EGFR* mutation tests were concordant in more than 90% of tumor and plasma samples (Table 2). The Kappa coefficient, a robust measurement for test agreement [12], showed that the two tests were in almost perfect agreement in tumors and in substantial agreement in plasma. Our results support use of the two tests interchangeably for *EGFR* activating mutation diagnosis in tumor samples.

The PNA-based PCR technology used by PANAMutyper has a lower limit of detection (>0.1%) [10] than the RT-PCR technology used by cobas v2 (>1%, according to cobas v2 label: https://www.accessdata.fda.gov/cdrh_docs/pdf12/P120019S007c.pdf). The difference in limit of detection between the two tests may explain why most of the inconsistent results (14 out of 19 samples) formed the same pattern: diagnosis of wild-type by cobas v2 but mutant by PANAMutyper (Table 3). Retesting these samples with a more sensitive method (such as dd-PCR) may validate the results. Unfortunately, only six of the discordant tumor samples had sufficient tissue remaining for dd-PCR retests, meaning that the sample size is too small to draw a conclusion for validation.

In the current study, the *EGFR* mutation detection rate in plasma was considerably low in early-stage cancer (stage I/II), similar to reports by other studies [19,20]. However, in late-stage cancer (stage III/IV), the two tests were able to detect over two-thirds of Ex19del and one-third of L858R and T790M mutations in tumors using plasma samples (Figure 2). Plasma detection rates by cobas v2 were consistent with a previous study [9].

Notably, despite a much lower detection rate in plasma than tumor, the diagnostic precision of both tests was very high (100% for PANAMutyper, 86%–100% for cobas v2). Therefore, although the current efficacy of osimertinib has only been established in patients with T790M-positive results in tumor, but not in patients with T790M-positive results only in plasma (according to cobas v2 label), the very high T790M diagnostic precision of both tests in plasma suggests that patients with T790M-positive plasma findings almost certainly have the mutation in tumor tissue also. Therefore, T790M-positive results in plasma should be considered sufficient evidence to initiate osimertinib treatment. Indeed, the latest guideline published by the International Association for the Study of Lung Cancer (IASLC) [21] and lung cancer education book published by the American Society of Clinical Oncology [4] place a higher priority on liquid biopsy over tumor biopsy in patients with progressive or recurrent disease.

In the subgroup of patients with previously diagnosed T790M mutation, PANAMutyper and cobas v2 tests were equally effective in identifying T790M mutation. Our real-world data in Figure 3 indicates that patients with T790M mutation respond favorably to osimertinib, with an impressive objective response rate of 74%. Contrastingly, those who did not receive osimertinib treatment showed very poor clinical prognosis and follow-up; for the most part, these patients were not treated by osimertinib because T790M mutations were diagnosed before osimertinib was approved or reimbursed through insurance in Korea (Figure 1). Although these osimertinib efficacy data are not from a randomized controlled study, they are consistent with a recently published phase III trial [3] and clearly show that osimertinib treatment, if guided by a reliable *EGFR* T790M mutation test, may lead to fundamentally superior clinical outcomes.

5. Conclusions

Two commercial *EGFR* mutation tests approved in Korea, cobas v2 and PANAMutyper, show highly concordant test results in both tumor and plasma samples from NSCLC patients. Although both tests show low sensitivity in plasma in early-stage disease, their high diagnostic precision in plasma make them attractive screening tools for identifying TKI treatment-feasible patients. Our study shows that around one-third or two-thirds (depending on the mutation) of the TKI treatment-feasible patients with late-stage NSCLC can be identified using liquid biopsy with both tests. Our real-world data reinforce the important role of reliable *EGFR* T790M mutation tests in guiding third-generation TKI treatments.

Author Contributions: J.H.K., J.-O.K., J.-Y.S. conceptualized the study; S.R.K., K.S.S., J.K. collected the patients' data; S.H.H., Y.K., M.K. instructed the methodology; J.-O.K., J.-Y.S., M.-Y.K., M.-R.L. conducted the experiments; J.H.K., J.-O.K., J.-Y.S. did the data analyses; J.H.K., J.-O.K., J.-Y.S. wrote the manuscript. J.H.K. approved the final version. All authors have read and agreed to the published version of the manuscript.

Funding: This research was funded by AstraZeneca Korea.

Acknowledgments: We appreciate Jin Medical Science Service for language help.

Conflicts of Interest: The authors declare no conflicts of interest.

References

1. Hsu, W.H.; Yang, J.C.; Mok, T.S.; Loong, H.H. Overview of current systemic management of EGFR-mutant NSCLC. *Ann. Oncol.* **2018**, *29*, i3–i9. [CrossRef]
2. Mok, T.S.; Cheng, Y.; Zhou, X.; Lee, K.H.; Nakagawa, K.; Niho, S.; Lee, M.; Linke, R.; Rosell, R.; Corral, J.; et al. Improvement in Overall Survival in a Randomized Study That Compared Dacomitinib With Gefitinib in Patients With Advanced Non-Small-Cell Lung Cancer and EGFR-Activating Mutations. *J. Clin. Oncol.* **2018**, *36*, 2244–2250. [CrossRef] [PubMed]
3. Soria, J.C.; Ohe, Y.; Vansteenkiste, J.; Reungwetwattana, T.; Chewaskulyong, B.; Lee, K.H.; Dechaphunkul, A.; Imamura, F.; Nogami, N.; Kurata, T.; et al. Osimertinib in Untreated EGFR-Mutated Advanced Non-Small-Cell Lung Cancer. *N. Engl. J. Med.* **2018**, *378*, 113–125. [CrossRef] [PubMed]
4. Pennell, N.A.; Arcila, M.E.; Gandara, D.R.; West, H. Biomarker Testing for Patients With Advanced Non-Small Cell Lung Cancer: Real-World Issues and Tough Choices. *Am. Soc. Clin. Oncol. Educ. Book* **2019**, *39*, 531–542. [CrossRef]
5. Lim, E.A.; Lee, H.; Bae, E.; Lim, J.; Shin, Y.K.; Choi, S.E. Economic Evaluation of Companion Diagnostic Testing for EGFR Mutations and First-Line Targeted Therapy in Advanced Non-Small Cell Lung Cancer Patients in South Korea. *PLoS ONE* **2016**, *11*, e0160155. [CrossRef]
6. Arrieta, O.; Anaya, P.; Morales-Oyarvide, V.; Ramirez-Tirado, L.A.; Polanco, A.C. Cost-effectiveness analysis of EGFR mutation testing in patients with non-small cell lung cancer (NSCLC) with gefitinib or carboplatin-paclitaxel. *Eur. J. Health Econ.* **2016**, *17*, 855–863. [CrossRef]
7. Narita, Y.; Matsushima, Y.; Shiroiwa, T.; Chiba, K.; Nakanishi, Y.; Kurokawa, T.; Urushihara, H. Cost-effectiveness analysis of EGFR mutation testing and gefitinib as first-line therapy for non-small cell lung cancer. *Lung Cancer* **2015**, *90*, 71–77. [CrossRef]
8. Cheng, M.M.; Palma, J.F.; Scudder, S.; Poulios, N.; Liesenfeld, O. The Clinical and Economic Impact of Inaccurate EGFR Mutation Tests in the Treatment of Metastatic Non-Small Cell Lung Cancer. *J. Pers. Med.* **2017**, *7*, 5. [CrossRef]
9. Thress, K.S.; Brant, R.; Carr, T.H.; Dearden, S.; Jenkins, S.; Brown, H.; Hammett, T.; Cantarini, M.; Barrett, J.C. EGFR mutation detection in ctDNA from NSCLC patient plasma: A cross-platform comparison of leading technologies to support the clinical development of AZD9291. *Lung Cancer* **2015**, *90*, 509–515. [CrossRef]
10. Han, J.Y.; Choi, J.J.; Kim, J.Y.; Han, Y.L.; Lee, G.K. PNA clamping-assisted fluorescence melting curve analysis for detecting EGFR and KRAS mutations in the circulating tumor DNA of patients with advanced non-small cell lung cancer. *BMC Cancer* **2016**, *16*, 627. [CrossRef]

11. Choi, S.Y.; Kim, H.W.; Jeon, S.H.; Kim, B.N.; Kang, N.; Yeo, C.D.; Park, C.K.; Kim, Y.K.; Lee, Y.H.; Lee, K.Y.; et al. Comparison of PANAMutyper and PNAClamp for Detecting KRAS Mutations from Patients With Malignant Pleural Effusion. *In Vivo* **2019**, *33*, 945–954. [CrossRef] [PubMed]
12. Viera, A.J.; Garrett, J.M. Understanding interobserver agreement: The kappa statistic. *Fam. Med.* **2005**, *37*, 360–363. [PubMed]
13. Eisenhauer, E.A.; Therasse, P.; Bogaerts, J.; Schwartz, L.H.; Sargent, D.; Ford, R.; Dancey, J.; Arbuck, S.; Gwyther, S.; Mooney, M.; et al. New response evaluation criteria in solid tumours: Revised RECIST guideline (version 1.1). *Eur. J. Cancer* **2009**, *45*, 228–247. [CrossRef] [PubMed]
14. Midha, A.; Dearden, S.; McCormack, R. EGFR mutation incidence in non-small-cell lung cancer of adenocarcinoma histology: A systematic review and global map by ethnicity (mutMapII). *Am. J. Cancer Res.* **2015**, *5*, 2892–2911.
15. Jazieh, A.R.; Jaafar, H.; Jaloudi, M.; Mustafa, R.S.; Rasul, K.; Zekri, J.; Bamefleh, H.; Gasmelseed, A. Patterns of epidermal growth factor receptor mutation in non-small-cell lung cancers in the Gulf region. *Mol. Clin. Oncol.* **2015**, *3*, 1371–1374. [CrossRef]
16. Chang, Q.; Zhang, Y.; Xu, J.; Zhong, R.; Qiang, H.; Zhang, B.; Han, B.; Qian, J.; Chu, T. First-line pemetrexed/carboplatin or cisplatin/bevacizumab compared with paclitaxel/carboplatin/bevacizumab in patients with advanced non-squamous non-small cell lung cancer with wild-type driver genes: A real-world study in China. *Thorac. Cancer* **2019**, *10*, 1043–1050. [CrossRef]
17. Chang, W.Y.; Wu, Y.L.; Su, P.L.; Yang, S.C.; Lin, C.C.; Su, W.C. The impact of EGFR mutations on the incidence and survival of stages I to III NSCLC patients with subsequent brain metastasis. *PLoS ONE* **2018**, *13*, e0192161. [CrossRef]
18. Tas, F.; Ciftci, R.; Kilic, L.; Karabulut, S. Age is a prognostic factor affecting survival in lung cancer patients. *Oncol. Lett.* **2013**, *6*, 1507–1513. [CrossRef]
19. Takai, E.; Totoki, Y.; Nakamura, H.; Morizane, C.; Nara, S.; Hama, N.; Suzuki, M.; Furukawa, E.; Kato, M.; Hayashi, H.; et al. Clinical utility of circulating tumor DNA for molecular assessment in pancreatic cancer. *Sci. Rep.* **2015**, *5*, 18425. [CrossRef]
20. Chen, K.Z.; Lou, F.; Yang, F.; Zhang, J.B.; Ye, H.; Chen, W.; Guan, T.; Zhao, M.Y.; Su, X.X.; Shi, R.; et al. Circulating Tumor DNA Detection in Early-Stage Non-Small Cell Lung Cancer Patients by Targeted Sequencing. *Sci. Rep.* **2016**, *6*, 31985. [CrossRef]
21. Lindeman, N.I.; Cagle, P.T.; Aisner, D.L.; Arcila, M.E.; Beasley, M.B.; Bernicker, E.H.; Colasacco, C.; Dacic, S.; Hirsch, F.R.; Kerr, K.; et al. Updated Molecular Testing Guideline for the Selection of Lung Cancer Patients for Treatment With Targeted Tyrosine Kinase Inhibitors: Guideline From the College of American Pathologists, the International Association for the Study of Lung Cancer, and the Association for Molecular Pathology. *J. Thorac. Oncol.* **2018**, *13*, 323–358. [CrossRef] [PubMed]

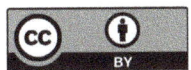

© 2020 by the authors. Licensee MDPI, Basel, Switzerland. This article is an open access article distributed under the terms and conditions of the Creative Commons Attribution (CC BY) license (http://creativecommons.org/licenses/by/4.0/).

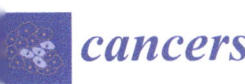

Review

Bête Noire of Chemotherapy and Targeted Therapy: CAF-Mediated Resistance

Pradip De [1], Jennifer Aske [1], Raed Sulaiman [2] and Nandini Dey [1,*]

[1] Translational Oncology Laboratory, Avera Cancer Institute, Sioux Falls, SD 57105, USA; pradip.de@avera.org (P.D.); jennifer.aske@avera.org (J.A.)
[2] Department of Pathology, Avera McKennan Hospital, Sioux Falls, SD 57105, USA; raed.sulaiman@plpath.org
* Correspondence: nandini.dey@avera.org

Citation: De, P.; Aske, J.; Sulaiman, R.; Dey, N. Bête Noire of Chemotherapy and Targeted Therapy: CAF-Mediated Resistance. *Cancers* 2022, *14*, 1519. https://doi.org/10.3390/cancers14061519

Academic Editor: Catherine Tomasetto

Received: 11 February 2022
Accepted: 14 March 2022
Published: 16 March 2022

Publisher's Note: MDPI stays neutral with regard to jurisdictional claims in published maps and institutional affiliations.

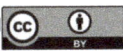

Copyright: © 2022 by the authors. Licensee MDPI, Basel, Switzerland. This article is an open access article distributed under the terms and conditions of the Creative Commons Attribution (CC BY) license (https://creativecommons.org/licenses/by/4.0/).

Simple Summary: Tumor cells struggle to survive following treatment. The struggle ends in either of two ways. The drug combination used for the treatment blocks the proliferation of tumor cells and initiates apoptosis of cells, which is a win for the patient, or tumor cells resist the effect of the drug combination used for the treatment and continue to evade the effect of anti-tumor drugs, which is a *bête noire* of therapy. Cancer-associated fibroblasts are the most abundant non-transformed element of the microenvironment in solid tumors. Tumor cells play a direct role in establishing the cancer-associated fibroblasts' population in its microenvironment. Since cancer-associated fibroblasts are activated by tumor cells, cancer-associated fibroblasts show unconditional servitude to tumor cells in their effort to resist treatment. Thus, cancer-associated fibroblasts, as the critical or indispensable component of resistance to the treatment, are one of the most logical targets within tumors that eventually progress despite therapy. We evaluate the participatory role of cancer-associated fibroblasts in the development of drug resistance in solid tumors. In the future, we will establish the specific mode of action of cancer-associated fibroblasts in solid tumors, paving the way for cancer-associated-fibroblast-inclusive personalized therapy.

Abstract: In tumor cells' struggle for survival following therapy, they resist treatment. Resistance to therapy is the outcome of well-planned, highly efficient adaptive strategies initiated and utilized by these transformed tumor cells. Cancer cells undergo several reprogramming events towards adapting this opportunistic behavior, leading them to gain specific survival advantages. The strategy involves changes within the transformed tumors cells as well as in their neighboring non-transformed extra-tumoral support system, the tumor microenvironment (TME). Cancer-Associated Fibroblasts (CAFs) are one of the components of the TME that is used by tumor cells to achieve resistance to therapy. CAFs are diverse in origin and are the most abundant non-transformed element of the microenvironment in solid tumors. Cells of an established tumor initially play a direct role in the establishment of the CAF population for its own microenvironment. Like their origin, CAFs are also diverse in their functions in catering to the pro-tumor microenvironment. Once instituted, CAFs interact in unison with both tumor cells and all other components of the TME towards the progression of the disease and the worst outcome. One of the many functions of CAFs in influencing the outcome of the disease is their participation in the development of resistance to treatment. CAFs resist therapy in solid tumors. A tumor–CAF relationship is initiated by tumor cells to exploit host stroma in favor of tumor progression. CAFs in concert with tumor cells and other components of the TME are abettors of resistance to treatment. Thus, this liaison between CAFs and tumor cells is a *bête noire* of therapy. Here, we portray a comprehensive picture of the modes and functions of CAFs in conjunction with their role in orchestrating the development of resistance to different chemotherapies and targeted therapies in solid tumors. We investigate the various functions of CAFs in various solid tumors in light of their dialogue with tumor cells and the two components of the TME, the immune component, and the vascular component. Acknowledgment of the irrefutable role of CAFs in the development of treatment resistance will impact our future strategies and ability to design improved therapies inclusive of CAFs. Finally, we discuss the future implications of this understanding from a therapeutic standpoint and in light of currently ongoing and completed CAF-based NIH clinical trials.

Keywords: cancer-associated fibroblasts; resistance; chemotherapy; targeted therapy

1. Introduction

Cancer-associated fibroblasts (CAFs) within the tumor microenvironment (TME) are non-transformed, tumor-cell-activated heterogeneous populations of cells having multiple origins and functions [1,2]. Detailed descriptions of the origin, functions, interactions with tumor cells, and heterogeneity of CAFs were previously provided by us elsewhere [3,4]. CAFs are activated by tumor cells in their favor. Once activated in an established tumor, CAFs act as crucial supporters of tumor growth, progression, and response to treatment.

The functions of CAFs in an established tumor include the following: (1) ECM (extra-cellular matrix) remodeling via collagenolysis to promote invasion and EMT (endothelial–mesenchymal transition); (2) increasing tissue stiffness to initiate angiogenic resistance and immune suppression; (3) induction of tumor angiogenesis; (4) secretomic induction of EMT by TGFbeta; (5) increasing secretomic factors of tumor-promoting or immune-suppressing ligands such as hepatocyte growth factor; fibroblast growth factors 1 and 2; stromal cell-derived factor 1 (SDF1/CXCL12); chemokine (C-C motif) ligands (CCL) 2, 5, 7, and 16; interleukin 6/8; and platelet derived growth factor; (6) metabolic reversal of reverse Warburg effect (non-glycolysis in tumor cells, glycolysis in stroma cells) and 'lactate shuttle' effect; (7) immune evasion via activation of M2 macrophages (CD163 positive); (8) inhibition of apoptosis in tumor cells; (9) activation of many of pro-proliferative tumor cell signaling; (10) immune reprogramming and antigen presentation; (11) adaptation to oxidative stress and hypoxic response; (12) promotion of stemness-promoting signals; (13) promotion of metastasis-associated phenotypes; (14) attenuation of drug response [1,5–18].

The range of functions of CAFs is comprehensive, and the actions of CAFs are contextual. The interactions of CAFs with tumor cells and TME components change with the evolution of the tumor, its metastatic progression, and its response to therapy. In summary, the functions of CAFs are structured to assist and promote tumor cells via direct and indirect interactions. Thus, CAFs form a centralized communication network within the TME that favors tumor cell growth, metastasis, and resistance to drug treatment [19]. The versatility of the functions of CAFs' make them abettors of drug resistance and identifies them as prospective anti-tumor therapy targets [20,21]. Here, we investigate the role of CAFs in the development of resistance to chemotherapy and targeted therapy. We seek to evaluate whether co-targeting CAFs will have a participatory benefit towards managing the burden of resistance. We discuss the opportunity that CAFs present to improve and evolve the management of the disease from a tumor-centric approach to a *tumor–CAF-centric approach*.

2. CAF Heterogeneity and Resistance to Chemotherapy in Solid Tumors

2.1. CAF Heterogeneity

CAFs are heterogeneous in terms of their origin in different organ-type cancers, as well as in the progression of the disease. The heterogeneous subpopulations of CAFs, such as myoblastic CAFs (myCAFs) and inflammatory CAFs (iCAFs), have been extensively studied in fibroinflammatory PDAC disease characterized by dense and highly proliferating desmoplastic stroma. In fact, Li et al. identified genes associated with the differentiation of myCAFs and iCAFs [22–24]. Adipose-derived MSCs (AD-MSCs) have been shown to possess a high multilineage potential and self-renewal capacity and were reported as the CAF sources in PDAC by Miyazaki et al. [24]. Their study identified that AD-MSCs could differentiate into distinct CAF subtypes, myCAFs and iCAFs, depending on the different co-culture conditions in vitro. The diverse functions of iCAFs and myCAFs have also been reported in cholangiocarcinoma; breast cancers; prostate, head, and neck squamous cell carcinoma; and bladder and colon cancers. The diversity of CAF subpopulations was also recently reported to promote the growth of cholangiocarcinoma, wherein hepatic stellate cells (HSC) are the primary cause of CAF differentiation into myCAFs and iCAFs [25]. The hyaluronan synthase 2 myCAFs, but not type I collagen-expressing myCAFs, promoted tumor progression, while HGF-expressing iCAFs enhanced tumor growth via tumor-expressed MET, thereby directly linking CAFs to tumor cells. Another subset of CAFs, FAP+CAFs, were identified by Kieffer et al. in breast cancers that mediated immunosuppression and immunotherapy resistance via a positive feedback loop between specific CAF-S1 clusters and Tregs [26]. In prostate cancer, a differential mode of activation of iCAFs and myCAFs has been reported [27]. IL-1a/ELF3/YAP pathways are involved in iCAF differentiation, while TGF-beta1 induces myCAFs. One of the ways CAFs classically interact with the tumor cell EMT function was reported by Goulet et al. in bladder cancer, where IL-6 cytokine was found to be highly expressed in iCAFs, and its receptor IL-6R was found on RT4 bladder cancer cells [28]. Perhaps the most intriguing functional heterogeneity of CAFs was reported by Pan et al. in PDAC-CAF-exhibited organ-specific metastatic potential leading to different levels of heterogeneity of CAFs in different metastatic niches [29]. Several cell signaling pathways have been reported to be involved in the functioning of iCAFs and myCAFs, including the Hedgehog pathway [30]; Wnt pathway [31]; integrin a11B1 signaling [32]; cMET-HGF pathway [25]; IL-6 signaling [28]; EMT signaling via transcription factors SNAIL1, TWIST1, and ZEB1 [28]; and IL1B-mediated crosstalk [33]. Recently, Steele et al. reported that the Hedgehog pathway acts in a paracrine manner in PDAC, with ligands secreted by tumor cells signaling to stromal CAFs. The Hedgehog pathway activation is higher in PDPN+ alphaSMA+ myCAFs compared with iCAFs, and its inhibition impairs tumor growth by altering the fibroblast compartment in PDAC. Hedgehog pathway inhibition resulted in a reduction in myCAF numbers and a significant expansion of iCAFs, leading to an increase in the iCAF/myCAF ratio. As iCAFs are a source of inflammatory signals, the authors observed an increase in iCAFs upon Hedgehog inhibition, which correlated with changes in immune infiltration (significantly decreased CD8+ T cells and increased CD4+ T cells and CD25+CD4+ T cells; abundant FOXP3+ regulatory T cells) that are consistent with a more immunosuppressive pancreatic cancer microenvironment. The paracrine activation differentially elevated myCAFs compared with iCAFs, leading to favorable alterations of cytotoxic T cells and Tregs, causing increased immunosuppression [30]. Wnt signaling in CAFs represents a non-cell-autonomous mechanism for colon cancer progression [31]. Mose et al. reported Sfrp1 epithelial–mesenchymal transition phenotype induction in tumor cells without affecting tumor-intrinsic Wnt signaling, suggesting involvement of non-immune stromal cells. Low levels of Wnt signals induced the iCAF subtype, which in co-culture with organoids induced EMT, whereas high levels induced contractile myCAFs to attenuate the EMT phenotype.

The tumors with (1) an accumulation of stromal CAFs, (2) the presence of fibrotic stroma, (3) a high expression level of stroma signature genes, or (4) a high tumor/stroma ratio in the primary tumor are associated with poor prognosis in various cancers, including colon, gastric, esophagus, breast, NSCLC (non-small cell lung cancer), and liver cancers [34–40]. It is understood that chemotherapy's limited effect (benefit) and the progression or recurrence of disease through therapy in many solid tumors are attributed to the development of resistance within tumor cells in support of the stroma. As a dominant component of tumor stroma, CAFs interact with both a tumor cell and the TME. The versatility of CAF functions and their several modes of interaction with tumor cells and all components of stroma (ECM and cells of the TME) indicate that a metastasis or progression of disease following treatment is aided and abetted by CAFs. Once a therapy-resistive circuitry is established between tumor cells and the CAFs of the stroma, tumor-centric therapy alone essentially becomes insufficient. Figure 1 presents the distribution pattern of the types of resistance to chemotherapy based on specific mediators of CAF functions in solid tumors. The four types of mediators of action employed by CAFs to orchestrate the development of resistance to chemotherapy are presented in the cartoon. The most common mode of interaction is a paracrine, wherein CAFs signal to either tumor cells or other components of the TME via characteristic secretomes. In addition to the involvement of characteristic secretomes, exosomal cargos delivering different miRNAs that target various cell signaling proteins are common mediators of CAFs. The paracrine mode of action of CAFs is the predominant form of action, represented by six types of organ tumors (organ tumors are indicated by their respective ribbon colors, as presented in the figure legends). CAF crosstalk with tumor cells, and the TME occurs via exosomal cargo, imparting resistance to four organ cancers. The extracellular vesicle, secretome, and autocrine or paracrine modes are much less involved in the modes of action (Figure 1). The sizes of the boxes indicate the number of studies in each box. Among resistance to different types of chemotherapies, cisplatin resistance has been found to be very common, which is involved in both paracrine and exosomal cargo modes of action (the shapes in the inset indicate the types of resistances in different tumors).

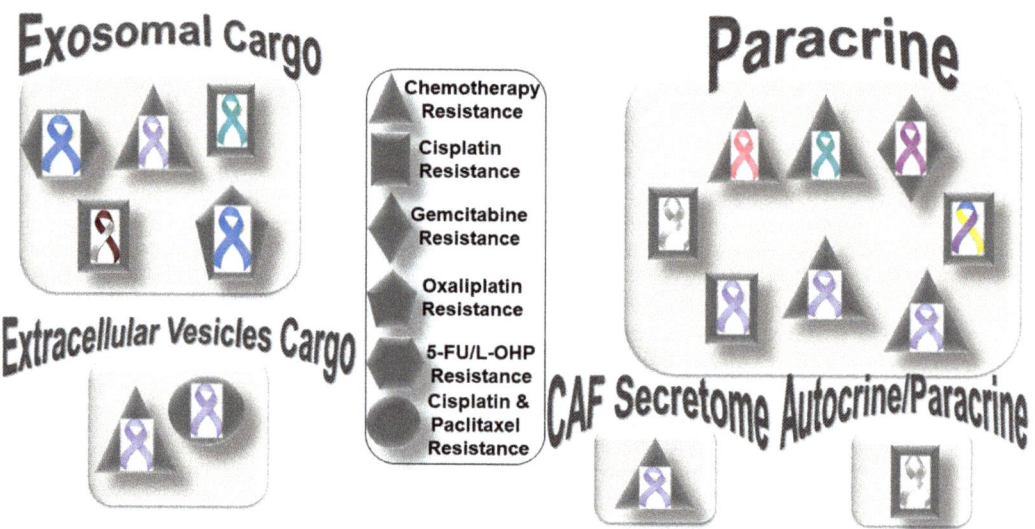

Figure 1. Distribution pattern of types of resistance to chemotherapy based on specific mediators of CAF functions in solid tumors: The four mediators employed by CAFs to orchestrate the development of resistance to chemotherapy are presented in the cartoon. The most common mode of interaction is paracrine, wherein CAFs signal to either tumor cells or other components of the TME via characteristic secretome. In addition to the involvement of the characteristic secretome, exosomal cargos delivering different miRNAs that target various cell signaling proteins are common mediators of CAF actions. Among different organ cancers, gastric cancers have been reported to be the most common tumors in which CAFs are involved in the development of resistance to chemotherapy. The sizes of the boxes indicate the number of studies in each box. The shapes indicate the types of resistance in different tumors (inset). L-OHP is a new derivative of oxaliplatin; 5-FU is fluorouracil. Organ tumors are indicated by their respective ribbon colors. Head and neck cancer: white and burgundy; stomach cancer: periwinkle blue; colon cancer: dark blue; ovarian cancer: teal; lung cancer: white or pearl; breast cancer: pink; pancreatic cancer: purple; bladder cancer: blue, yellow, and purple.

Among the different types of solid tumors, gastric cancers have been reported to be the most common tumors exhibiting CAF-mediated resistance to chemotherapy, which involve paracrine, exosomal cargo, extracellular vesicle, and secretomic modes of action. Secretion of IL-11 from CAFs activated the IL-11/IL-11R/gp130/JAK/STAT3/Bcl antiapoptosis signaling pathway in gastric cancer cells. Thus, CAF-derived IL-11 secretion caused resistance to chemotherapy regimens in gastric cancers [41]. In another study, CAF-induced activation of the JAK-STAT signaling has been proposed to confer chemoresistance in gastric cancer cells, while interleukin-6 (IL-6) was identified as a CAF-specific secretory protein that protects gastric cancer cells via paracrine signaling. Interestingly, clinical data have shown that IL-6 was differentially expressed in the stromal portion of cancer tissues, while IL-6 upregulation was positively correlated with poor responsiveness to chemotherapy [42]. In line with the above facts, several CAF-targeting agents have been tested in experimental models, as reviewed elsewhere [43]. Resistance to conventional chemotherapeutics in gastric cancers has been reported to be mediated by CAF-derived extracellular vesicles [44]. Annexin A6 initiated network formation and drug resistance within the ECM via activation of beta1 integrin-FAK-YAP signaling. Annexin A6 within CAF extracellular vesicles has been shown to stimulate FAK-YAP signaling by stabilizing beta1 integrin at the cell surface of gastric cancer cells, which subsequently induces drug resistance. In addition to extracellular vesicles, CAFs also communicate via exosomal cargos, which carry miRNAs and mediate resistance to specific chemotherapeutic agents, as presented in the following section.

2.2. CAFs and Specific Resistance to Cisplatin

Reports of CAF-mediated development of cisplatin resistance are more prevalent than any other chemotherapy agent. In certain solid tumors, the mechanism involved intracellular pathway signaling such as JNK or NF-κB, adhesion molecules such as annexin A3, or specific proteins such as plasminogen activator inhibitor-1. In lung cancers, CAFs have been reported to express a higher level of annexin A3 (ANXA3) than normal fibroblasts. The crosstalk was demonstrated using CAF-CM (CAF-conditioned media) incubation, which increased the ANXA3 level in lung cancer cells, which subsequently enhanced cisplatin resistance by inhibiting cisplatin-induced apoptosis involving ANXA3/JNK signaling [45]. In lung adenocarcinoma, cisplatin resistance was associated with the expression of SMAalpha expression [46]. In their study, Masuda et al. demonstrated that the inhibition of plasminogen activator inhibitor-1 increased the chemotherapeutic effect in lung cancer through suppressing the myofibroblast characteristics of CAFs. CAF-derived IL-8 promoted chemoresistance to cisplatin in gastric cancer via NF-κB activation and ABCB1 upregulation [47]. In bladder cancers, stromal CAFs enhanced cisplatin resistance via stimulating IGF-1/ERbeta/Bcl-2 signaling, wherein CAFs regulated ERbeta expression through IGF-1/AKT/c-Jun signaling following c-Jun phosphorylation and promoted ESR2 gene transcription [48]. In other cancers, exosomal cargo carried miRNA to mediate the CAFs' effect. In ovarian cancer, CAF-mediated cisplatin resistance was reported to involve CAF-derived exosomes, which overexpressed miR-98-5p [49]. In immunocompromised mice, miR-98-5p targeted CDKN1A to inhibit CDKN1A expression and promoted cisplatin resistance by virtue of cell cycle progression. In head and neck cancer, cisplatin resistance is perpetrated by CAF-derived exosomal miR-196a targeting CDKN1B and ING6 [50]. Whether the nature of CAF mediators of cisplatin resistance is organ-specific or not needs to be concluded with more data in this field. From the current literature, it is evident that exosomal miRNA predominantly mediates platinum-based chemotherapy resistance (cisplatin and oxaliplatin), with a few exceptions such as tamoxifen resistance in breast [51] and radioresistance in colorectal cancers [52,53]. In the context of resistance to radiotherapy, CAFs are highly radio-resistant, even at high doses of radiation. CAFs resist apoptosis signals following radiation and become senescent, producing a distinct combination of immunoregulatory molecules. Hence, acquired radio resistance has been associated with CAF function [54,55]. A recent minireview summarized findings on the interactions between CAF, ionizing radiation, and immune cells in the tumor microenvironment [56]. Targeting CAFs, regulatory T cells, and tumor-associated macrophages in combination radio–immunotherapies has been reported to improve cancer treatment [57]. Future studies will also need to clarify the functional segregation of the two modes of events and whether it exists in the development of CAF-mediated resistance in solid tumors.

2.3. CAFs and Specific Resistance to Paclitaxel

CAF-mediated resistance to paclitaxel was reported in ovarian cancers. In ovarian cancers, the lipoma-preferred partner gene has been reported to mediate CAF–endothelial cell crosstalk in signaling chemoresistance [58]. CAFs upregulated the lipoma-preferred partner gene in microvascular endothelial cells via calcium-dependent signaling, and lipoma-preferred partner expression levels in intratumoral microvascular endothelial cells correlated with survival and chemoresistance in patients. Lipoma-preferred partners upregulated focal adhesion and stress fiber formation to promote endothelial cell motility and permeability. Experimental suppression of lipoma-preferred partners improved paclitaxel delivery to cancer cells by decreasing intratumoral microvessel leakiness.

2.4. CAFs and Specific Resistance to a Combination of Cisplatin and Paclitaxel

Specific resistance to a combination of cisplatin and paclitaxel aided by CAFs is encountered in gastric cancers. Exosomal miR-522 suppressed ferroptosis and promoted acquired chemoresistance (decreased chemosensitivity) by targeting ALOX15 and blocking lipid–ROS accumulation involving the intercellular pathway. Both cisplatin and paclitaxel treatment promoted miR-522 secretion from CAFs by activating the USP7/hnRNPA1 axis, leading to ALOX15 suppression and decreased lipid–ROS accumulation in gastric cancer cells [59].

2.5. CAFs and Specific Resistance to Oxaliplatin

CAFs orchestrate oxaliplatin resistance in colorectal cancers [60]. Colorectal cancer-associated lncRNA is transferred from CAFs to the cancer cells via exosomes, where it suppresses colorectal cancer (CRC) cell apoptosis, confers chemoresistance, and activates the Wnt/beta-catenin pathway. Long-non-coding RNA interacts directly with mRNA stabilizing protein (human antigen R) to increase beta-catenin mRNA and protein levels. Specific resistance to 5-FU/L-OHP (oxaliplatin) has been reported in colorectal cancers. In colorectal cancers, chemotherapy resistance was attributed to CAF-secreted exosomes [61]. A direct transfer of exosomes to colorectal tumor cells led to a significant increase in miR-92a-3p levels in cancer cells. An increased expression of miR-92a-3p activated the Wnt/beta-catenin pathway and inhibited mitochondrial apoptosis by directly inhibiting FBXW7 and MOAP1, contributing to stemness, EMT, metastasis, and 5-FU/L-OHP resistance.

2.6. CAFs and Specific Resistance to Gemcitabine

CAF-mediated resistance to gemcitabine involves CAF-derived SDF-1. SDF-1 stimulated malignant progression and gemcitabine resistance in pancreatic cancer due to paracrine induction of SATB-1 within tumor cells. SDF-1-mediated upregulation of SATB-1 expression in tumor cells contributed to the maintenance of CAF properties, forming a reciprocal feedback loop involving the SDF-1/SATB-1 pathway [62]. It is apparent from the results of the above studies that mediators of CAFs in the development of resistance to different chemotherapeutics are specific not only to organ cancers but also the particular drug. In an ideal world, we should be searching for an organ-specific blood-based marker that can correlate or indicate CAF-mediated development of resistance to chemotherapy.

3. CAFs and Resistance to Targeted Therapy in Solid Tumors

CAF-mediated resistance to targeted therapy in solid tumors can be categorized into (1) specific resistance to hormone-receptor-targeted anti-cancer drugs and (2) specific resistance to non-hormonal pathway-targeted anti-cancer drugs (Figure 2). One characteristic feature of this type of resistance is the lack of mediation via miRNA compared to resistance to chemotherapy. The only exception to this characteristic is a novel subset of CD63+ CAFs that mediated resistance to tamoxifen in breast cancers via exosomal miR-22 [51]. CD63+ CAFs have been reported to secrete miR-22-rich exosomes, which act through its targets, ERalpha and PTEN, to confer tamoxifen resistance in breast cancer cells. The details of the development of resistance to hormone receptor-targeted anti-cancer drugs mediated by CAFs in breast cancers have been reviewed elsewhere [63]. CAFs have been involved in mediating anti-androgen resistance in prostate cancers in a paracrine manner. Zhang et al. identified neuregulin 1 (NRG1) in the CAF supernatant [64]. CAF-derived NRG1 promoted resistance in tumor cells through the activation of HER3 involving the NRG1/HER3 axis, proving a paracrine mechanism of anti-androgen resistance in prostate cancer. In line with the above fact, an inadequate response to second-generation anti-androgen therapy was recorded in castration-resistant patients with NRG1 activity.

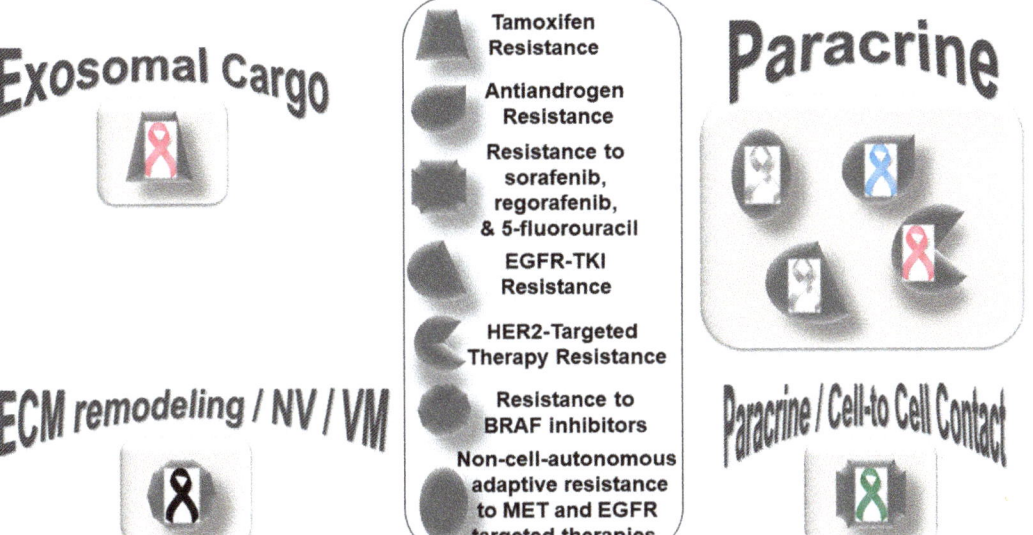

Figure 2. Distribution pattern of types of resistance to targeted therapy based on specific mediators of CAF functions in solid tumors: The four types of mediators of action employed by CAFs to orchestrate the development of resistance to targeted therapy are presented in the cartoon. The most common mode of interaction is paracrine, wherein CAFs signal to either tumor cells or other components of the TME via characteristic secretome. In addition to the involvement of characteristic secretome, exosomal cargos delivering different miRNAs that target various cell signaling proteins are common mediators of CAF action. The sizes of the boxes indicate the number of studies in each box. The shapes indicate the types of resistance in different tumors (inset). Organ tumors are indicated by their respective ribbon colors. Lung cancer: white or pearl; skin cancer: black. liver cancer: emerald green; breast cancer: pink; prostate cancer: light blue.

The role of the activation of EGFR, Wnt/beta-catenin, Hippo, TGF-beta, and JAK/STAT cascades in CAFs in relation to the chemoresistance and invasive or metastatic behavior of cancer cells [65] has strengthened the concept that CAFs should be included as a target for therapy in solid tumors. CAF-mediated resistance to non-hormonal pathway-targeted anti-cancer drugs has been observed in lung, breast, melanoma, and hepatocellular cancers. CAF-mediated non-cell-autonomous adaptive resistance to MET- and EGFR-targeted therapies in lung cancers via a metabolic shift involving paracrine crosstalk between tumor cells under drug exposure and their surrounding CAFs has been reported [66]. Apicella et al. demonstrated that with prolonged exposure to tyrosine kinase inhibitors (TKIs), EGFR- or MET-addicted cancer cells undergo a metabolic shift upregulating glycolysis and lactate production. High secreted levels of lactate stimulate CAFs to produce hepatocyte growth factor (HGF) in a nuclear factor kappa B (NFkB)-dependent manner. This HGF, in turn, activates MET-dependent signaling within cancer cells, counteracting the effects of tyrosine kinase inhibitors (TKIs). In tumor cells of lung adenocarcinoma with EGFR mutations, primary EGFR-TKI resistance was associated with high hepatocyte growth factor in CAFs [67]. Conditioned media from CAFs increased the resistance of PC-9 cells to EGFR-TKI, indicating that with the secretion of higher amounts of CAF-derived humoral factors, HGF is responsible for EGFR-TKI resistance [67]. Understandably, this kind of fail-safe metabolic reprogramming not only allows cellular resistance to the drug but also re-establishes a tumor–TME circuitry, which can also merge with the local immune signaling [68–71]. As with prostate cancers [64] and melanomas [72], CAFs have been involved in developing resistance to targeted therapies in breast cancers. CAFs participate in the HER2-targeted therapy resistance in breast cancers via the TAF/FGF5/FGFR2/c-Src/HER2 axis [73]. CAF-derived NRG1 (an HER3 ligand) causes resistance to trastuzumab [74,75], TKIs [76], and T-DM1 [77] in HER2-positive breast cancers. In the Neosphere trial, HER2-positive breast tumors with high NRG1 expression appeared to resist trastuzumab–docetaxel but not pertuzumab–trastuzumab–docetaxel [78]. Guardia et al. identified CAFs as the primary source of NRG1 in HER2-positive breast cancers. The study showed their role in mediating resistance to trastuzumab, which can be overcome by dual anti-HER2 blockade following pertuzumab–trastuzumab [78]. Recently, a study examined the value of 'pathological reactive stroma' (defined as stromal-predominant breast cancer) as a predictor for trastuzumab resistance in patients with early HER2-positive breast cancer receiving adjuvant therapy in the FinHER phase III trial, reporting an association between trastuzumab resistance and the presence of 'reactive stroma' [79]. The pathological reactive stroma and the mRNA gene signatures that reflected reactive stroma were tested in 209 HER2-positive breast cancer samples and were found to be correlated with distant disease-free survival. Interestingly, reactive stroma did not correlate with tumor-infiltrating lymphocytes. The study concluded that the 'pathological reactive stroma' in HER2-positive or ER-negative early breast cancer tumors might predict resistance to adjuvant trastuzumab therapy.

In line with the pro-tumorigenic role of 'pathological reactive stroma', CAFs are known to promote organoid tumor growth in co-culture. The paracrine crosstalk between CAFs and cancer cells regulated physiological characteristics of CAFs, which in turn imparted resistance to cancer cells. In metastatic melanomas, CAFs resist the function of BRAF inhibitors via their crosstalk with tumor cells (vascular mimicry), the ECM, and endothelial cells (neovascularization). The development of drug resistance to BRAF inhibitors is mediated via ECM reprogramming action of CAFs [19]. Recently, Liu et al. reported the activation of nuclear beta-catenin signaling in melanoma CAFs during the development of resistance to BRAF inhibitor or MEK inhibitors, underscoring the role of BRAF-inhibitor-induced CAF reprogramming in matrix remodeling and the therapeutic escape of melanoma cells [80].

CAF populations expressing FAP/ITGA11/COL1A1/CCN2 have been shown to be negatively correlated with disease-free survival in this cancer. The resistance to BRAF inhibitors is the result of CAF-mediated reprogramming of the ECM. The stiffness of the ECM caused by CAFs has been associated with integrin-dependent signaling. Fibroblast-specific production of CCN2, whose overexpression in melanomas was independent of BRAF mutational status, signals through integrins and was found to be essential for neovascularization and vasculogenic mimicry. In hepatocellular carcinomas, tumor cells resist targeted anti-cancer drugs including sorafenib, regorafenib, and 5-fluorouracil in the presence of CAFs via a direct cell–cell contact, as tested in a transwell system through paracrine signaling [81].

CAF signaling in the development of drug resistance is tumor-specific in prostate cancers and lung adenocarcinomas, as presented above. In prostate cancers, CAF-derived neuregulin 1 NRG1 promotes resistance in tumor cells by activating HER3 involving the NRG1/HER3 axis, proving a paracrine mechanism of antiandrogen resistance in a paracrine manner, as presented above [64]. In lung adenocarcinomas bearing EGFR mutations, primary EGFR-TKI resistance is mediated via hepatocyte growth factor from CAFs. CM from CAFs increased the resistance of EGFR mutant lung adenocarcinoma cell line PC-9 cells to EGFR-TKI, indicating that the secretion of higher amounts of HGF is the robust feature of EGFR-TKI-resistance-promoting CAFs [67]. The mode of action of CAFs and the nature of their involvement with respect to the tumor cells and the TME are less studied. The pattern of crosstalk is just beginning to emerge, which can define distinct therapeutic paradigms. In a recent study, Engelman's group reported three subtypes of lung CAFs that can influence the personalized treatment of non-small cell lung cancer patients. The 3 subtypes of CAFs identified in their study are (1) subtype I with HGF^{High}, FGF7$^{High/Low}$, p-SMAD2^{Low}, targeting driver, HGF-MET, and FGF7-FGFR2; (2) subtype II with HGF^{High}, FGF7^{High}, p-SMAD2^{Low}, targeting driver, and FGF7-FGFR2; and (3) subtype III with HGF^{Low}, FGF7^{Low}, and p-SMAD2^{High} [82]. They reported that specific subtypes are associated with particular functions and clinical responses. Subtype I and II CAFs function to protect cancer cells, while subtype III CAFs are involved with a better clinical response via immune cell migration with additional value in immuno-oncology. In addressing the heterogeneity of CAFs, the study systematically connected functions of subpopulations of lung CAFs to specific functions of CAFs in the context of clinical response and resistance to pathway-targeted drugs. Similar studies in the future will delineate the relationships of the mode of action of CAFs with drugs in organ-type cancers in solid tumors. Despite the different mediating actions of CAFs, it will be imperative to know how CAFs support a tumorigenic pathway in cancer cells in the face of pathway-targeted treatment that ultimately leads to the ineffectiveness of the therapy. Supplemental targeting of CAF signals opens an opportunity to improve personalized medicine and bears the promise of a better outcome.

4. Regulation of CAF Functions and Therapeutic Opportunity

4.1. CAFs as the Target within the TME

The irrefutable involvement of CAFs in the development of resistance to chemo- and targeted therapy and progression as presented above justifies the recognition of CAFs as a logical target for treatment. The interest in CAFs as a target of therapy arose from analyses of data from the conventional tumor-cell-centric view of cancer, targeting only the tumor component. The limited success of tumor-cell-centric therapies is a direct proof-of-concept that the TME bears undeniable responsibility for successful disease progression in solid tumors. From the conceptual aspect, any sequence-based therapy primarily refers to sequencing of the entire tumor tissue, which constitutes both cancer and the TME (CAFs along with immune cells and angiogenic components). Hence, the approach does not provide separate information on the subgroups, tumor cell cluster, CAF cluster, or immune cluster. Intratumoral heterogeneity contributes to the development of resistance to anti-cancer therapeutics. Thus, the heterogeneity of CAFs presents opportunities for CAF-targeted cancer therapies in precision medicine [65,83]. However, the burden of cost and management needs to be taken into account. CAFs as components of the TME have been targeted to suppress tumor growth [84]. Based on their specific surface markers and secreted molecules, Laplagne et al. reviewed the potential of targeting different aspects of CAFs, including cells inducing depletion, reprogramming, differentiation, or inhibition of their pro-tumor functions or recruitment. Several approaches involving immunotherapies, vaccines, small interfering RNA, or small molecules were developed to target components of the TME, as reviewed elsewhere [84].

CAFs are a coherent target in the TME [85]. The versatility of CAFs means they are a target for anti-tumor therapy to 'switch off' the pro-tumor stroma [20,65,86]. There are five ways to counter the CAF-mediated patronage of cancer cells, which eventually cause resistance to treatment and disrupt disease management. The strategic points to control the function of CAFs are (1) preventing the activation of CAFs by targeting or counteracting signals from tumor cells, (2) regulating the activation of CAFs by targeting the CAF population directly, (3) regulating the pro-tumorigenic signals from CAFs, (4) regulating the pro-angiogenic signals from CAFs, and (5) regulating the pro-immune evasion and anti-immune surveillance signals from CAFs (Figure 3). These potential CAF intervention points represent 'action items' to 'switch off' the pro-resistance CAFs within the tumor stroma.

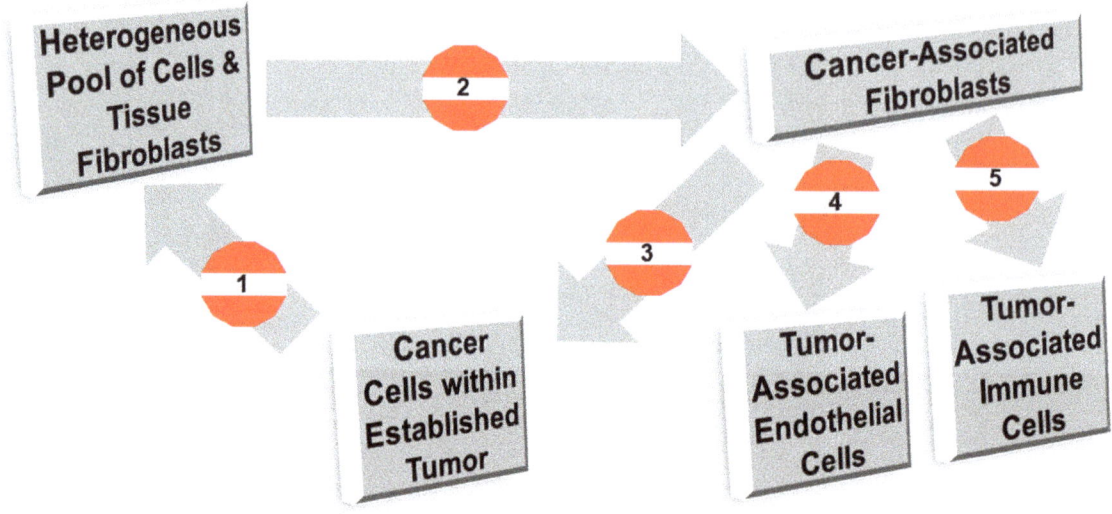

Figure 3. Strategic opportunities to regulate CAF functions in an established or progressing solid tumor. The strategic points to control the function of CAFs are (1) prevention of activation of CAFs by targeting or counteracting signals from tumor cells, (2) regulating the activation of CAFs by targeting the CAF population directly, (3) regulating the pro-tumorigenic signals from CAFs, (4) regulating the pro-angiogenic signals from CAFs, and (5) regulating the pro-immune evasion and anti-immune surveillance signals from CAFs. These strategic points represent 'action items' to 'switch off' the pro-resistance CAFs within the tumor stroma.

4.2. Stromal Normalization and CAF-Targeted Therapy in Combating Resistance to Chemotherapy and Targeted Therapy

CAFs co-operate with tumor cells to drive the progression of the disease [65–67]. The progression of the disease can be attributed to this collaboration of CAFs with tumor cells based on several factors and events, either individually or collectively, including (1) the EMT; (2) stemness; (3) response to hypoxia; (4) pro-proliferative and anti-apoptotic signals; (5) immune, metabolic, and ECM reprogramming; (6) metastasis-associated phenotypes; and (7) escape and resistance to therapy.

CAFs have been targeted using both conventional and unconventional modes of disease management in solid tumors, diagnostics, and therapeutics. Although CAFs have been identified using several markers, FAP and alpha-SMA are among the most versatile markers associated with the identification and function of CAFs [87]. FAP has been targeted in tumors for imaging and therapy using several approaches, including immunoconjugates (an antibody–maytansinoid conjugate (mAb FAP5-DM1)), CAR T cells, tumor immunotherapy, vaccines, peptide drug complexes, FAP inhibitors, and antibodies [87–89]. The depletion of FAP-positive CAFs enhanced anti-tumor immunity, as reported in several studies [90–94], proving the validity of the target. In fact, co-targeting FAP in combination with tumor-centric FAP-targeting strategies was shown to be more effective [95–97]. Anti-FAP antibody sibrotuzumab labeled with 131Iodine has been reported for the treatment of patients with metastasized FAP-positive carcinomas in a phase I dose-escalation study [98]. To test the diagnostic and prognostic value of the imaging of activated fibroblasts, Lindner et al. developed the radiotracers FAPI-01 and FAPI-02 with specific binding to human and murine FAP with a rapid and almost complete internalization [86]. The DOTA-linked compound FAPI-02 with better pharmacokinetic and biochemical properties was tested for quantitative analysis of tracer uptake in 80 patients with 28 different tumor entities (54 primary tumors and 229 metastases). Their study indicated that FAP inhibitors have a promising role as tracers for diagnostic applications in desmoplastic tumors.

CAFs have been targeted using nano or gold particles in a radio-pharmacological manner. CAFs have been reported to be explicitly targeted by nanocarriers with optimized physicochemical properties in liver cancer. Surface-modified nanocarriers with a cyclic peptide binding to the PDGFRβ or mannose-6-phosphate binding to the IGFRII effectively directed the drug to activate CAFs in vivo [99]. Gold nanoparticles measuring 20 nm in diameter inhibited CAF activation by disrupting multicellular communication between the tumor and microenvironment and altering the levels of multiple fibroblast activation or inactivation proteins, such as TGF-β1, PDGF, uPA, and TSP1, secreted by ovarian cancer cells and TME cells [100]. Passive and active strategies for the nanodelivery systems targeting CAFs for improved anti-tumor effect and tumor drug penetration have been summarized elsewhere [101,102]. The recent advancements in targeting CAFs with diagnostic and therapeutic radiopharmaceuticals by applying new radiotheranostic compounds (targeted radionuclide imaging and therapy) using clinically identified biomarkers to improve clinical outcomes are promising [103,104].

CAF targeting has also been studied in rare solid tumors with highly desmoplastic stroma in intrahepatic cholangiocarcinomas [105–107]. Mertens et al. reported that navitoclax induced apoptosis in CAFs and in myofibroblastic human hepatic stellate cells but lacked similar effects in quiescent fibroblasts or cholangiocarcinoma cells, arguing for the use of navitoclax (Bcl2/Mcl inhibitor) for destroying CAFs in the TME [108]. In desmoplastic cholangiocarcinoma, the use of light-activated nanohyperthermia has been described to modulate the tumor microenvironment [109]. A recent study employed multifunctional iron oxide nanoflowers decorated with gold nanoparticles (GIONF) as efficient nanoheaters to achieve complete tumor regression following three sessions of mild hyperthermia. CAFs were targeted via preferential uptake of GIONF. A photothermal depletion of CAFs resulted in a significant early reduction in tumor stiffness (normalized tumor stiffness) followed by tumor regression. Katsube et al. employed near-infrared photoimmunotherapy (NIR-PIT) as a novel method of cancer treatment using a highly selective monoclonal antibody (mAb)–photosensitizer conjugate against fibroblast activation protein (FAP)-targeted NIR-PIT, in which IR700 was conjugated to a FAP-specific antibody to target CAFs (CAF-targeted NIR-PIT: CAFs-PIT) [110]. The elimination of CAFs by CAFs-PIT demonstrated that the combination of 5-FU and NIR-PIT caused a 70.9% tumor reduction, while 5-FU alone achieved only a 13.3% reduction, suggesting the recovery of 5-FU sensitivity in CAF-rich esophageal tumors in experimental models.

Yet another classic example of stromal resistance mediated through CAFs is represented by PDAC (pancreatic ductal adenocarcinoma), a disease in which the five-year overall survival for pancreatic cancer is still less than 10%, despite advances in therapeutic modalities [111]. Pancreatic tumors present a highly fibrotic stroma containing activated CAFs, which create an immunosuppressive TME. CAFs secrete immunoregulatory and chemo-attractive factors, preventing tumor-reactive T-cell responses. Gorchs and Kaipe summarized different therapy strategies targeting the CAF–T cell axis, focusing on CAF-derived soluble immunosuppressive factors and chemokines to highlight the strategies that can be used to target CAFs in the context of the capability of heterogeneous CAFs to modulate functions of TILs and myeloid cells in desmoplastic pancreatic ductal adenocarcinomas (PDACs) [111]. Although the CAF-immune cell dialogue is beyond this review's scope, identifying the immunological functions of different CAF subsets (for example, inflammatory fibroblasts (iCAFs) and myofibroblasts (myCAFs)) that help tumor cells to (1) evade immune surveillance and (2) potentiate immune exhaustion may be essential for the development of an effective combinational treatment for desmoplastic solid tumors.

4.3. CAF-Mediated Immune Reprogramming

Since CAFs induce immunotherapy resistance and influence tumor immunity and immunotherapy [112,113], CAFs have been targeted using various modes in anti-cancer immunotherapy [114]. The establishment of mechanisms of CAF-mediated blockade of CD8+ cytotoxic T-cell accumulation in tumors has provided therapeutic opportunities [115]. CAFs crosstalk and co-evolve with cancer stem cells [116]. Therapeutic targeting of the manipulation of cancer stem cells [116,117] and immune-reprogramming using CAFs provides a window of opportunity beyond this review's scope. In an exceptionally aggressive and treatment-resistant human cancer, the role of dermal fibroblasts in suppressing the tumorigenesis has been documented, which are subsequently converted or activated to CAFs, which are phenotypically and epigenetically different from normal dermal fibroblasts. Flach et al. demonstrated that melanoma cells could stimulate the recruitment of fibroblasts and activate them, resulting in melanoma cell growth by providing both structural (extracellular matrix proteins) and chemical support (growth factors). Thus, CAFs collaborate with melanoma cells and resist drug therapy [118]. Kinugasa et al. demonstrated that established CAFs enhance tumor growth in vivo in B16 melanoma-bearing mice. These CAFs strongly express CD44 in the hypovascular and hypoxic areas of the TME or following treatment with angiogenesis inhibitors. CD44 expression in CAFs maintains the stemness of cancer stem and initiating cells via direct interaction and is involved in drug resistance [119]. Bellei et al. reviewed the melanoma–CAF dialogue based on TGF-beta, MAPK, Wnt/beta-catenin, and Hippo signaling [120]. It makes sense that the activation of the Wnt/beta-catenin pathway may lead to the expression of CD44 (target gene) in CAFs and signaling for the stemness-driven drug resistance of the disease.

4.4. CAF-Mediated EMT and ECM Reprogramming

The induction of stemness and EMT are two main phenotypic steps of the multi-step process of metastasis in solid tumors. It is worth mentioning that stemness and morphological transition between the epithelioid and fibroblastoid features of tumor cells are closely integrated, especially in the types of solid tumors, wherein cancer cells with fibroblastoid morphological changes exhibit increased motility and invasiveness due to decreased cell–cell adhesion, reminiscent of EMT in many solid tumors. In promoting metastasis, the silencing of DNMT1 is correlated with the enhancement of the induction of EMT and the CSC (cancer stem cells) phenotype in prostate cancer cells [121]. functional connection of CAFs in EMT via DNA methylation was presented in the study by Pistore et al. in advanced prostate cancer. The secreted factors in conditioned media from CAFs explanted from two unrelated patients were found to stimulate concurrent DNA hypo- and hypermethylation required for EMT and stemness in PC3 and DU145, indicating that CAF-released factors induce genome methylation changes required for EMT and stemness in EMT-prone cancer cells [122]. One such secreted factor from CAFs was reported to be TGF-beta in several solid tumors [123–126]. Cardenas et al. demonstrated that TGF-beta stimulated EMT and that metastasis catalyzed the global DNA hypermethylation changes in the epithelial ovarian cancer cells, while the DNMT inhibitor blocked the hypermethylation and EMT [127]. In fact, TGF blockade has been reported to improve the distribution and efficacy of therapeutics in breast carcinoma by normalizing the tumor stroma interstitial matrix by decreasing collagen I content to improve the intratumoral penetration of both a low-molecular-weight conventional chemotherapeutic drug and a nanotherapeutic Doxil [128]. CAF-induced epigenetic modification of cancer cells leading to drug resistance could be a potential way to design a CAF-targeted inclusive strategy for therapy in the future. In line with the association of CD44 expression in CAFs as discussed above, CAFs have been shown to secrete soluble factors belonging to Wnt family members and the Wnt/beta-catenin pathway. WNT16B and SFRP2 activated the canonical Wnt pathway in tumor cells and induced cytotoxic chemotherapy resistance in prostate cancer [129,130]. In colorectal cancers, chemoresistance in cancer-initiating cells was also increased by CAFs. Lotti et al. conducted a comparative analysis of matched colorectal cancer specimens from patients before and after cytotoxic treatment to demonstrate a significant increase in CAFs. Chemotherapy-treated human CAFs promoted cancer-initiating cell self-renewal via IL-17A, and IL-17A was found to be overexpressed in colorectal CAFs in response to chemotherapy, as validated directly in patient-derived specimens without culture [131]. The study directly proved that CAFs respond to therapy in favor of tumor cells and strongly supported the unmet need to include a CAF-directed therapy towards the 'normalization' of the 'resistant stroma'.

4.5. CAF-Mediated Metabolic Reprogramming and Hypoxic Response

As cancer cells biochemically reprogram their metabolism as their hallmark, they generate lactic acid from glucose or glutamine. Cancer cells export lactic acid out, preventing intracellular acidification causing increased lactate levels and an acidic pH level in the extracellular milieu [71]. Lisanti et al. reviewed metabolic coupling between mitochondria in cancer cells and catabolism in stromal fibroblasts [132]. Unlike tumor cells, CAFs are catabolic by default. CAFs donate L-lactate, ketones, glutamine, other amino acids, and fatty acids to cancer cells to metabolize via their TCA cycle and oxidative phosphorylation. This metabolic coupling explains how metabolic energy and biomass are supplied by the CAFs to cancer cells. Lisanti et al. demonstrated that catabolic metabolism and the glycolytic reprogramming in the CAFs (a loss of caveolin-1 and an increase in MCT4 in CAF) are influenced by oncogenes in epithelial cancer cells, including BRCA1-deficient breast and ovarian cancer cells, in concert with the TME [133]. Interestingly, both oncogenic activation (of RAS, NFkB, and TGF-β) and loss of the tumor suppressor (BRCA1) have comparable effects on CAF. Arguably, such a 'metabolic symbiosis' could provide an explanation for the 'fibroblast addiction' or 'metabolic parasites' in primary and metastatic tumor cells [134] and could present a target for therapy, wherein CAFs could be decoupled from tumor cells. The ensuing hypoxic environment adds yet another layer to the chemoresistance [135] due to the influence of low pH on the cytotoxicity of paclitaxel, mitoxantrone, and topotecan [136]. Hypoxia is a fact of life for cancer cells in solid tumors [137–139]. As a critical player in the development of drug resistance, it is most logical that CAFs will have a direct role in modulating drug sensitivity or action in a hypoxic environment. CAFs secrete elements of different angiogenic and immunogenic signaling pathways, including VEGF and T-cell-mediated cytotoxicity, respectively, under hypoxic conditions [140–142]. Masamune et al. reported hypoxia-induced pro-fibrogenic and pro-angiogenic responses in pancreatic stellate cells [143]. Pancreatic stellate cells expressed several angiogenic molecules, including VEGF receptors, angiopoietin-1, and Tie-2. Studying the effects of hypoxia and conditioned media of hypoxia-treated pancreatic stellate cells on cell functions and on human umbilical vein endothelial cells, Masamune et al. demonstrated that hypoxia accelerated migration, type I collagen expression, and VEGF production in pancreatic stellate cells. Conditioned media of hypoxia-treated pancreatic stellate cells induced migration of pancreatic stellate cells, which was inhibited by the anti-VEGF antibody. Conditioned media of hypoxia-treated pancreatic stellate cells, on the other hand, induced endothelial cell proliferation, migration, and angiogenesis in vitro and in vivo. In line with the above study, endothelial cells co-cultured with CAFs under hypoxia or exposed to the conditioned medium of hypoxic CAFs have been shown to sprout significantly more than the normoxic counterpart in breast cancers [144]. These data functionally connect CAF activity with the tumor angiogenesis and resistance or metastasis progression associated with tumor cell phenotypes under hypoxic conditions, strengthening the argument in favor of a CAF-inclusive treatment strategy.

4.6. CAF-Based NIH Clinical Trials

The clinical trials targeting CAFs in solid tumors are based on antagonizing CAF functions. Overall, trials can be divided into (1) reprogramming of CAFs, (2) inhibition of CAF functions, (3) targeting of CAF-mediated desmoplasia, and (4) CAF-specific immunotherapy. The details of these trials are presented elsewhere [145]. FAP proteins are some one of the common targets in the clinical trials related to CAFs. Accordingly, anti-FAP vaccination has been reported in various tumor models [146]. The other aspects of CAF-related trials involve targeting the interactions between tumor-promoting CAFs and the surrounding microenvironment and reprogramming CAFs into quiescent fibroblasts or reprogramming tumor-promoting CAFs into tumor-restraining CAFs, as presented in detail elsewhere [147].

Reviewing the CAF-associated clinical trials on the ClinicalTrials.gov site, we present 17 trials involving CAFs (Table 1). These studies have used various aspects of markers or functions of CAFs, the culture or co-culture of CAFs, testing of drug combinations targeting CAFs, or disease detection using CAF-based radiochemicals, as mentioned before. The studies ranged from observational to interventional or treatment to open-label. The primary purposes also varied from diagnostic to treatment to exploratory basic science. Most of the trials were conducted in disease conditions of advanced or malignant neoplasms of solid tumors in adults. Table 1 presents the relevant ongoing and completed trials involving CAFs posted in ClinicalTrials.gov (as of February 2022). The studies were performed in advanced or malignant neoplasms of solid tumors in adults, including hepatocellular, lung, breast, and pancreatic cancers. The observational study, NCT01549275, is among the two completed studies. This 'case-only' prospective study enrolled 105 patients with hepatocellular carcinomas. The prospective study evaluated the success rate of the primary culture of hepatocellular carcinoma cells and CAFs from the residual specimens in routine fine-needle aspiration of hepatic tumors and the potential application of this method as an additional tool for personalized treatment of patients. The primary outcome measure was to find the correlation between the growth speeds of the cultured cells and the AJCC TNM stage (7th Eds) at entering the study within a time frame of 28 days after plating of cells. The other completed study, NCT02161523, tested the impact of lung CAFs on mast cell activation in lung cancers. This prospective observational study involved fewer patients than the first, with non-small cell lung carcinomas. This study evaluated the paracrine function of CAFs and directly measured the factors in the lung TME (which includes other cells such as fibroblasts that are attributed to mast cell activation). The trial was conducted to determine whether CAF cells derived from lung tumors, together with the lung cancer cells or microvesicles derived from these cells, are able to stimulate mast cells to degranulate or release various cytokines and chemokines. CAFs were co-cultured with both lung cancer cell lines (A-549) or microvesicles derived from these cells and the human mast cell line (LAD2). The collected supernatants were used to determine degranulation and cytokine release from these mast cells as the primary outcome by measuring the levels of b-hexosaminidase (a marker for mast cells degranulation) and the cytokines levels within a time frame of 1–2 weeks.

In addition to the studies covering the functions of CAFs, studies have also been undertaken to utilize CAFs in developing resistance to chemotherapy in solid tumors in combination with tumor-centric therapy. The role of CAFs in the reprogramming of the ECM by altering the state of hyaluronic acid and the consequences for the tumor ECM and tumor vasculature have been presented in several reviews [148–150]. Hyaluronan synthase 2 has been reported to be expressed in CAFs to promote invasion in oral cancers [151]. An in vitro evaluation of simultaneous targeting of tumor cells and CAFs with a paclitaxel–hyaluronan bioconjugate was carried out in non-melanoma skin cancers by Bellei et al. [152].

Table 1. Trials involving CAFs in cancers as posted in ClinicalTrials.gov (Updated on February 2022) are represented. The 17 trials include various organ cancers in solid tumors, including breast, colorectal, prostate, lung, pancreatic, hepatocellular, ovarian, and oral carcinomas.

Clinical Trials.gov Identifier and Sponsor	Title	Recruitment Status: Study Start Date and Study Completion Date	Condition or Disease	Study Type	Enrollment	Study Design — Observational/Intervention Model:	Time Perspective and Primary Purpose
NCT 01549275; Kaohsiung Medical University Chung-Ho Memorial Hospital, Taiwan	Primary Cell Culture of Hepatic Tumorous Cells From Routine Fine-Needle Aspiration	Completed: Study Start Date; April 2010; Study Completion Date: July 2013	Hepatocellular Carcinoma	Observational	105 participants	Case-Only	Prospective
NCT 02161523; Meir Medical Center, Kfar Saba, Israel	The Impact of Lung Cancer-Derived Fibroblasts on Mast Cell Activation	Completed: Study Start Date; 1 July 2014; Study Completion Date: 1 June 2015	Lung Cancer	Observational	20 participants	Other	Prospective
NCT 03481920; PH Research, S.L. Madrid, Spain	A Pilot Trial of PEGPH20 (Pegylated Hyaluronidase) in Combination With Avelumab (Anti-PD-L1 0010718C) in Chemotherapy Resistant Pancreatic Cancer	Terminated: Study Start Date; 10 January 2018; Study Completion Date: 10 June 2019	Pancreatic Ductal Adenocarcinoma-Pancreatic Cancer; Drug: PEGylated Recombinant Human Hyaluronidase (PEGPH20) Drug: Avelumab; Early Phase 1	Intervention/treatment (Open Label)	7 participants	Single Group Assignment	Not Mentioned
NCT 03777943; University Ghent, GIHeelkunde, University Hospital, Ghent, Belgium	Role of the Peritoneal Microenvironment in the Pathogenesis and Spread of Colorectal Carcinomatosis (MMT)	Recruiting; Study Start Date; 1 November 2017; Estimated Study Completion Date: December 2020	Peritoneal Carcinomatosis	Observational: Intervention/treatment; Procedure: Sampling peritoneal tissue	50 participants	Other	Prospective
NCT 04554719; Wuhan Union Hospital, China	Clinical Application of Fibroblast Activation Protein PET/MRI for Diagnosis and Staging in Malignant Tumors	Recruiting; Study Start Date; 22 May 2020; Estimated Study Completion Date: 21 December 2022	Malignant Neoplasm	Interventional (Clinical Trial)	100 participants	Single Group Assignment: Intervention/treatment Drug: 68Ga-DOTA-FAPI Device: PET/MR Device: PET/CT	Primary Purpose: Diagnostic

157

Table 1. Cont.

Clinical Trials.gov Identifier and Sponsor	Title	Recruitment Status: Study Start Date and Study Completion Date	Condition or Disease	Study Type	Enrollment	Study Design Observational/ Intervention Model:	Time Perspective and Primary Purpose
NCT 04939610; Clovis Oncology, Inc. USA	LuMIERE: A Phase 1/2, Multicenter, Open-Label, Non-Randomized Study to Investigate Safety and Tolerability, Pharmacokinetics, Dosimetry, and Preliminary Activity of 177Lu-FAP-2286 in Patients With an Advanced Solid Tumor: A Study of 177Lu-FAP-2286 in Advanced Solid Tumors (LuMIERE)	Recruiting; Study Start Date; 14 June 2021; Estimated Study Completion Date: 1 June 2026	Solid Tumor	Intervention/treatment; Interventional (Clinical Trial); Drug: 68Ga-FAP-2286 Drug: 177Lu-FAP-2286; Phase 1 Phase 2	170 participants	Sequential Assignment /Non-Randomized	Primary Purpose: Treatment
NCT 04621435; Thomas Hope, University of California, San Francisco, Clovis Oncology, Inc. USA	Imaging of Solid Tumors Using 68Ga-FAP-2286	Recruiting; Study Start Date; 14 December 2020; Estimated Study Completion Date: 31 December 2023	Solid Tumors, Adult Metastatic Cancer	Intervention/treatment: Interventional (Clinical Trial) Drug: Gallium-68 labelled (68Ga-) FAP-2286 Procedure: Positron Emission Tomography (PET) imaging; Phase 1	65 participants	Parallel Assignment; Allocation: Non-Randomized	Primary Purpose: Diagnostic

Table 1. *Cont.*

Clinical Trials.gov Identifier and Sponsor	Title	Recruitment Status: Study Start Date and Study Completion Date	Condition or Disease	Study Design			
				Study Type	Enrollment	Observational/ Intervention Model:	Time Perspective and Primary Purpose
NCT 04459273; UCLA Jonsson Comprehensive Cancer Center, Cancer Center at the University of California Los Angeles, USA	Prospective Exploratory Study of FAPi PET/CT With Histopathology Validation in Patients With Various Cancers (FAPI PET RDRC): PET Biodistribution Study of 68Ga-FAPI-46 in Patients With Different Malignancies: An Exploratory Biodistribution Study With Histopathology Validation	Recruiting; Study Start Date; 27 August 2020; Estimated Study Completion Date: 1 July 2024	Bladder Carcinoma, Cervical Carcinoma, Cholangiocarcinoma, Hematopoietic and Lymphoid Cell Neoplasm, Hepatocellular Carcinoma, Malignant Adrenal Gland Neoplasm, Malignant Brain Neoplasm, Malignant Pleural Neoplasm, Malignant Skin Neoplasm, Malignant Solid Neoplasm, Malignant Testicular Neoplasm, Malignant Thymus Neoplasm, Neuroendocrine Neoplasm, Thyroid Gland Carcinoma, Urothelial Carcinoma	Interventional (Clinical Trial); Procedure: Computed Tomography Drug: Gallium Ga 68 FAPI-46 Procedure: Positron Emission Tomography;	30 participants	Intervention Model: Single Group Assignment; (Open Label)	Prospective Exploratory Study Primary Purpose: Basic Science
NCT 01878695; Sidney Kimmel Cancer Center at Thomas Jefferson University, USA	Pilot Study of Anti-Oxidant Supplementation With N-Acetyl Cysteine in Stage 0/I Breast Cancer (NAC)	Completed: Actual Study Start Date: 26 July 2012; Actual Study Completion Date: 14 May 2015	Stage 0/1 Breast CancerPost BiopsyPre-surgery; Drug: IV/oral N-acetyl-cysteine; Phase 1	Interventional (Clinical Trial)	13 participants	Single Group Assignment; (Open Label)	Primary Purpose: Treatment

Table 1. Cont.

Clinical Trials.gov Identifier and Sponsor	Title	Recruitment Status: Study Start Date and Study Completion Date	Condition or Disease	Study Type	Study Design Enrollment	Study Design Observational/ Intervention Model:	Time Perspective and Primary Purpose
NCT 05196334; Herlev Hospital, Herlev, Copenhagen, Denmark	Pharmacotyping of Patient-derived Pancreatic Cancer Organoids From Endoscopic Ultrasound-Guided Biopsy as a Tool for Predicting Oncological Response	1 July 2021 and 31 December 2024	Pancreatic Cancer	Observational	40 participants	Cohort	Prospective
NCT 05034146; Zhongnan Hospital of Wuhan University, Wuhan, Hubei, China	The Diagnostic Efficiency of 68Ga-FAPI PET/CT in Malignant Tumors	23 February 2021 and 28 February 2023	Fibroblast Activation Protein Inhibitor PET/CT Malignant Neoplasm	Interventional (Clinical Trial)	100 participants	Intervention Model: Single Group Assignment	Primary Purpose: Diagnostic
NCT 04504110; Peking Union Medical College Hospital; Beijing, China	A Prospective Study to Evaluate 68Ga-FAPI-04 and 18F-FDG PET/CT in Patients With Epithelial Ovarian Cancer: Compared With Histological Findings	5 August 2020 and August 2021	Epithelial Ovarian Cancer	Interventional (Clinical Trial); Phase 2	30 participants	Intervention Model: Single Group Assignment	Diagnostic
NCT 05030597; Zhongnan Hospital of Wuhan University, Wuhan, Hubei, China	Exploring the Application Value of PET Molecular Imaging Targeting FAP in Oral Squamous Cell Carcinoma	15 September 2021 and 31 December 2023	PET/CT FAPI Oral Cancer	Interventional (Clinical Trial)	100 participants	Intervention Model: Single Group Assignment	Diagnostic
NCT 05209750; The Netherlands Cancer Institute	Pilot Study of FAPI PET/CT for Locoregional (Re)Staging of Lymph Nodes in Colorectal Carcinoma	February 2022 and August 2024	Colorectal Cancer	Interventional (Clinical Trial)	30 participants	Intervention Model: Single Group Assignment	Diagnostic

Table 1. *Cont.*

Clinical Trials.gov Identifier and Sponsor	Title	Recruitment Status: Study Start Date and Study Completion Date	Condition or Disease	Study Design			
				Study Type	Enrollment	Observational/Intervention Model:	Time Perspective and Primary Purpose
NCT 02587793; Kaohsiung Medical University Chung-Ho Memorial Hospital; Taiwan	Primary Culture of Residual Specimens Obtained From Aspiration of Hepatic Tumor to Predict the Prognosis of the Patients	October 2014 and 31 July 2018	Hepatocellular Carcinoma	Observational	208 participants	Observational Model: Case-Only	Prospective
NCT 05064618; Nagoya University Hospital, Nagoya, Aich, Japan	Phase I/II Investigator-initiated Clinical Trial of MIKE-1 With Gemcitabine and Nab-Paclitaxel Combination Therapy for Unresectable Pancreatic Cancer	23 August 2021 and 30 April 2025	Pancreatic Cancer	Interventional (Clinical Trial) Phase 1 Phase 2	55 participants	Intervention Model: Sequential Assignment; Non-Randomized	Treatment
NCT 02307058; University of Miami, Florida, USA	A Phase II Randomized Trial of MRI-Guided Prostate Boosts Via Initial Lattice Stereotactic vs. Daily Moderately Hypofractionated Radiotherapy—The Miami BLaStM Trial	5 February 2015 and June 2028	Prostate Cancer	Interventional (Clinical Trial)	164 participants	Intervention Model: Parallel Assignment; Randomized	Treatment

CAFs can provide a physical and vascular barrier, depriving the tumor of TILs and protecting against chemotherapy. Hence, the 'normalization of the TME' has been proposed as a viable target of treatment, especially in solid tumors with high desmoplastic reactions such as chemotherapy-resistant advanced PDAC. The *NCT03481920* study was a pilot trial of PEGPH20 (pegylated hyaluronidase) in combination with avelumab (anti-PD-L1 MSB0010718C) in chemotherapy-resistant pancreatic cancers. The purpose of this multi-center, open-label, non-randomized early phase 1 trial (intervention–treatment) was to evaluate the pharmacodynamics, safety, and efficacy of PEGPH20 in combination with avelumab in adult patients with chemotherapy-resistant advanced or locally advanced PDAC. The study tested the hypothesis that elimination of HA (hyaluronic acid) in the pancreatic TME mediated by PEG PH20 would result in increased tumor vascularization and vessel patency, as well as stromal remodeling with increased immune infiltration. The activity of immune checkpoint inhibitors such as avelumab was facilitated by at least two mechanisms, including an increase in drug delivery and increasing immune infiltration.

Another function of CAFs within the TME is associated with EMT and mesothelial–mesenchymal transition in the context of peritoneal dissemination. Peritoneal dissemination is a frequent metastatic route for cancers of the ovary and gastrointestinal tract. Solid tumors in the abdomen, such as gastric, colorectal, and ovarian cancers, commonly disseminate via a transcoelomic route, an event associated with a poor prognosis [153]. Metastases are influenced by CAFs, a cell population that derives from different sources. CAFs are known to derive from mesothelial cells via mesothelial–mesenchymal transition during a peritoneal metastasis [154]. A type II EMT, known as mesothelial–mesenchymal transition (MMT), occurs after peritoneal damage. Myofibroblast conversion of mesothelial cells contributes to peritoneal fibrosis associated with peritoneal dialysis and post-surgical peritoneal adhesion. In a recent report, Gordillo et al. reported that MMT contributes to the generation of CAFs in locally advanced primary colorectal carcinomas [155]. In a prospective recruiting study, *NCT03777943*, the role of the peritoneal microenvironment in the pathogenesis and spread of colorectal carcinomatosis (MMT) was evaluated. The study investigated the extent and role of MMT and CAFs in the pathogenesis of colorectal peritoneal carcinomatosis. The primary outcome of the study was the analysis and sampling of peritoneal tissue via immunohistochemistry of CD44, integrins, ICAM-1, hyaluronate, and VCAM-1 (adhesion molecules); calretinin, mesothelin, WT1, cytokeratins, and E-cadherin (mesothelial markers); α-SMA, FAP, and podoplanin (CAF specific markers); and PDGF, VEGF, and other angiogenesis-related markers within 6 months after the collection of the samples from patients presenting with colorectal peritoneal carcinomatosis.

Normal residential fibroblasts become activated by tumor cells and are sources of CAFs. Fibroblast activation protein (FAP) is one of the emerging reliable markers of CAFs [1,156,157]. FAP is a transmembrane protein expressed on CAFs and has been shown to be differentially present on a number of solid tumors as a marker of CAFs. FAPs have been exploited for certain diagnostic and treatment purposes in clinical trials. Radionuclide-labeled fibroblast activation protein inhibitors (FAPI) targeting FAP as a tracer for PET imaging have been tested for targeted diagnosis and treatment of cancer. Although the function of FAP is yet to be established, imaging studies have shown that FAP could be detected with FAPI PET/CT.

The interventional open-label clinical Trial, *NCT04554719*, with a primary diagnostic purpose, studied the clinical application of FAP PET/MRI for diagnosis and staging. This prospective trial, in which 100 patients with malignant neoplasm participated, was based on the background that FAP is overexpressed in CAFs, which is closely related to tumor growth, invasion, metastasis, immunosuppression, and prognosis, while the expression level of FAP in normal tissues and organs is very low. The trial used integrated PET/MR and PET/CT with the agent 68Ga-FAPI ((gallium-68 (68Ga)–FAPI) as a new novel positron tracer and the conventional imaging agent F-18 (fluorodeoxyglucose 18F-FDG) to diagnose and stage various cancers with the aim of making up for the deficiency in FDG–PET imaging in the diagnosis and staging of certain cancers. Another clinical trial was named

NCT04621435, with a primary purpose of diagnosis based on FAP-2286, a peptidomimetic molecule that binds to FAP. The study was a single-arm prospective trial that evaluated the ability of a novel imaging agent gallium-68-labeled (68Ga-) FAP-2286 (68Ga-FAP-2286) to detect metastatic cancer in adults with solid tumors using 68Ga-FAP-2286 tracer. In contrast to the above studies, the phase 1/2 recruiting trial NCT04939610 (LuMIERE) tested 68Ga-FAP-2286 and 177Lu-FAP-2286 for the primary purpose of treatment. This multicenter, open-label, non-randomized study investigated the safety, tolerability, pharmacokinetics, dosimetry, and preliminary activity of 177Lu-FAP-2286 in 170 participating patients with advanced solid tumors. Phase 1 of the study evaluated the safety and tolerability of 177Lu-FAP-2286 and determined the recommended phase 2 dose (RP2D) in patients with advanced solid tumors. Phase 2 of the study evaluated the objective response rate (ORR) in patients with specific solid tumors. NCT04459273, a prospective exploratory trial, studied the PET biodistribution of 68Ga-FAPI-46 (FAPi PET/CT) in patients with a wide range of solid tumors. The study investigated how an imaging technique called 68Ga-FAPi-46 PET/CT can determine where and to which degree the FAPi (fibroblast activation protein inhibitor) tracer (68Ga-FAPi-46) accumulated in normal and cancer tissues in patients. The trial sought to define the biodistribution of gallium Ga 68 fibroblast activation protein inhibitor (FAPi)-46 (68Ga-FAPi-46) in normal and cancer tissues of patients with various malignancies.

CAFs are responsible for metabolic reprogramming in the TME, involving ROS in certain solid tumors [123,158]. The NCT01878695 trial, sponsored by the Sidney Kimmel Cancer Center at Thomas Jefferson University, on the contrary, plans to assess the feasibility of evaluating the effects of n-acetylcysteine on tumor cell metabolism by determining the changes in expression of caveolin -1 and MCT4 in CAFs in pre- and post-therapy breast tissue samples treated with NAC (N-acetyl derivative of the naturally occurring amino acid, L-cysteine). This interventional open-label clinical trial with a primary purpose of treatment is a pilot study of anti-oxidant supplementation with N-acetyl cysteine in stage 0/I breast cancers.

From the detailed overview of the clinical trials presented above, it is apparent that CAFs offer a reasonable target that is complementary to the tumor-centric management of the disease. CAFs and their markers offer a basic scientific, diagnostic, and complementary (companion) treatment opportunity, more so in advanced solid tumors of breast, pancreas, peritoneal, and lung carcinomatosis. One remarkable fact emerging from the current literature is the conspicuous lack of basic and translational data regarding gynecological malignancies such as ovarian and endometrial cancers. The role of the endometrial stroma in pathogenesis is known, and human endometrial stromal cells have been found to express CD90, CD10, and CD140b [159]. In situ staining of the human myometrium and endometrium demonstrated heterogeneous staining for Thy 1. Freshly derived fibroblast strains from the myometrium and endometrium showed heterogeneous Thy 1 expression [160]. In fact, the prognostic significance of the tumor/stromal ratio (TSR), which is established in several solid tumors, has also been reported in endometrial carcinoma [161]. In their first attempt to characterize the fibromyxoid stromal reaction (desmoplasia) and a lymphocytic infiltrate, Espinosa et al. sought to find out the relationship between the desmoid-type fibromatosis stromal signature and the presence of desmoplasia [162]. Although a study by Micke et al. failed to find a significant difference in the Kaplan–Meier plots of the overall survival between stroma-rich and stroma-poor groups of endometrial patients [163], Espinosa et al. demonstrated that desmoplasia correlated positively with the desmoid-type fibromatosis expression signature, and stromal signatures have significant clinicopathological associations. Considering the (1) presence of fibroblasts in the uterine stroma, (2) the role of CAFs in the neoplastic transformation and progression of the disease, and (3) the significance of the stromal signature in endometrial cancers, the inadequacy of data and lack of trials in endometrial cancers remain puzzling. The conspicuous lack of information on the role of CAFs in the development of drug resistance in endometrial tumors can be explained by (1) the absence of relevant data regarding the characterization of CAFs based on a drug resistance condition in the context of different pathological parameters, genomic alterations, and outcome data and (2) the absence of a correct model system. It is understood that a bulk of endometrial cancers are detected early, whereby patients undergo surgical resection. Drug resistance conditions in the advanced or late stages in endometrial cancers are rarely presented where the tumor tissue can be accessed surgically. The characterization of endometrial CAFs and their presentation in the context of pathological parameters, genomic alterations, and outcome data in the future will pave the pathway for developing a model to test the functions of endometrial CAFs in a drug resistance scenario. However, it should be emphasized that we are only beginning to understand the complexity of the functions of CAFs and their function-specific markers in solid tumors. The future will unveil the clinical utility of the knowledge.

5. Forward Thinking

Resistance to therapy is a pro-tumorigenic event. CAFs are employed by tumor cells to create a pro-tumorigenic microenvironment following treatment. Resistance to treatment is the outcome of a highly efficient adaptive strategy orchestrated by cancer cells via reprogramming of their default signals, which co-occurs with the reprogramming of every component of the TME in their favor, including CAFs. Such an opportunistic event allows the tumor cells to gain contextual survival and progressive metastatic advantages. Tumor–stroma co-evolution can lead to the development of drug resistance. The liaison between CAFs and tumor cells can be viewed as a *bête noire* of therapy. Thus, CAFs as the critical or indispensable components of stromal resistance to treatment are the most logical targets within a tumor that has eventually progressed despite therapy. As the roles of CAFs in several aspects of tumor progression and the development of drug resistance are unfolding, the notion of CAFs being friend or foe [164] is evolving. CAFs are neither heroes nor villains [165]. CAFs are less cause for panic but demand more urgent action, especially in scenarios involving a therapy-resistant progressing tumor. We need to know more about how CAFs form multi-faceted support systems for drug-resisting progressing tumors to exercise that knowledge in empowering the management of the disease by including CAF-directed stromal-targeting agents [166] in the arsenal of targeted therapy options.

The roles of CAFs in several common and rare tumors, as presented above, give us an idea about their role in (1) tumor progression and (2) modes of development of resistance to treatment. It has to be recognized that the heterogeneity of CAFs could be associated with better outcomes or response to therapy as opposed to their pro-tumor actions. Bhattacharjee et al. demonstrated direct CAF–tumor interactions as a tumor-promoting mechanism, mediated by myCAF-secreted hyaluronan and inflammatory-iCAF-secreted HGF [167]. The pro-tumorigenic effects seen in their study were opposed by myCAF-expressed type I collagen, which suppressed tumor growth by mechanically restraining the tumor spread. Their study directly indicated that there is a scope for the therapeutic maneuvering of CAF function in favor of the patient outcome by targeting specific signals for the tumor-promoting function of CAFs, while promoting the myCAF-expressed type I collagen. This report, similar to other articles [25], indicated the possibility of establishing therapeutically targetable CAF-subtype-specific mediators for future treatment directed towards stromal normalization of desmoplastic tumors.

The study of CAFs and their origins, markers, and functions in the development of drug resistance can be conducted in tumors of the pancreas, breasts, stomach, esophagus, colorectal, prostate, and lungs, as well as melanoma, head and neck squamous cell carcinoma, renal cell carcinoma, and cholangiocarcinomas. Understandably, CAF-inclusive clinical trials are instituted in these organ cancers via various modes of intervention [145]. In a recent review, Koustoulidou et al. presented an overview of several modes of intervention using (a) anti-FAP mAbs (b)-engineered T-cells expressing an FAP-recognizing mAb (e.g., CAR-T cells) to target FAP+ CAFs, which resulted in their immune-cell-mediated destruction and removal, (c) enzymatic breakdown of hyaluronic acid to remodel the ECM for better accessibility of drugs to immune cells with tumor parenchyma, (d) blocking of CAF activity by interleukin-6, (e) transformation of CAFs into the quiescent state by vitamin D, and (f) blocking of CAF-induced metabolic reprogramming of tumor cells [104]. Recently, organ-specific subtypes of CAFs have been identified and associated with different functions in aiding and abetting tumor cells, as reported by Engelman's group [82]. Their study will encourage others to study the organ-specific roles of subtypes of CAFs and their particular modes of action in the progression of tumors.

As we evaluate the participatory role of CAFs in the development of drug resistance in solid tumors, we will have to design a workable model to test our hypotheses; ideally on a patient-to-patient basis in the context of each patient's unique genomic alteration(s). The possibility of co-targeting CAFs and testing whether they will have a clinical benefit towards managing the burden of resistance in the future will rely on such a model system, which will accommodate tailored testing of the roles of patient-derived CAFs in the context of both tumors cells and other components of the TME. Although much effort is still needed to translate CAF-directed anti-cancer strategies from the bench to the clinic, the future will establish the specific modes of action of CAFs in particular organ-type solid tumors, paving the way for CAF-inclusive personalized therapy in solid tumors.

In summary, we will require actionable insights into the functions of CAF subtype(s) to incorporate CAF-directed therapy in clinics. Actionable information on the CAF subtypes in the context of their functions will be needed regarding (1) specific clusters associated with immunosuppression and immunotherapy resistance [26], (2) therapeutically targetable CAF-subtype-specific mediators [25], (3) the Hedgehog pathway inhibition by a smoothened antagonist, LDE225-mediated differential activation of myCAFs or iCAFs leading to alterations of cytotoxic T cells and Tregs [30], (4) IL1B blocking agents to counteract the iCAF-mediated pro-tumorigenic actions associated with tolerance to cytotoxic drugs [33], and (5) differential targeting of tumor-promoting CAF mediators while preserving the specific anti-tumor functions, for example in the way type I collagen may 'normalize' stroma from tumor-promoting to tumor-restricting phenotypes [167].

6. Take-Home Message

The undeniable subpopulation-specific functions of CAFs in tumor growth, progression, and drug or immunotherapy resistance directly provide evidence for the therapeutically targetable role of CAFs. The aim of normalization of the TME by targeting CAFs remains unmet. CAFs are heterogeneous and organ-type-specific in origin, markers, and function. Hence, the best way to develop a 'workable hypothesis' for the functions of CAFs would be to generate strictly organ-specific experimental evidence. It is imperative to know the functions of specific signals from different CAF subtypes within the TME of organ-type cancer(s). We can exploit the information for (1) targeting of the pro-normalization signals from CAFs while attenuating the pro-growth progression and immunosuppressive CAF signals and (2) identifying potential CAF markers to investigate the mechanisms underlying the roles of CAFs in the TME.

7. Conclusions

In the era of precision medicine, which offers clinicians to treat patients with genomics-guided matched drug combination(s), the cure still remains an exception and not the rule. CAF-mediated development of resistance is the bête noire of chemotherapy and targeted therapy as CAF directly supports the development of resistance. The state-of-art management of today's disease does not necessarily include a CAF-inclusive therapy. We are just beginning to appreciate that the knowledge about the CAF functions and inhibition is critical in managing the disease towards developing a CAF-inclusive therapy.

Author Contributions: The review was conceptualized and initiated by N.D. The article was written by N.D. and P.D. R.S. provided a critical evaluation of the review and pathological insight into the development of CAF-mediated resistance. The figures were made by N.D. and P.D., while J.A. prepared the library, edited the article, and helped in the writing of the manuscript. All authors have read and agreed to the published version of the manuscript.

Funding: Authors acknowledge Avera Research Institute, Sioux Falls, SD, for funding. No external funding was received.

Acknowledgments: The authors acknowledge Avera Research Institute, Sioux Falls, SD, and the Department of Internal Medicine, SSOM, USD, Sioux Falls, SD.

Conflicts of Interest: The authors declare no conflict of interest.

References

1. Biffi, G.; Tuveson, D.A. Diversity and Biology of Cancer-Associated Fibroblasts. *Physiol. Rev.* **2021**, *101*, 147–176. [CrossRef] [PubMed]
2. Park, D.; Sahai, E.; Rullan, A. SnapShot: Cancer-Associated Fibroblasts. *Cell* **2020**, *181*, 486–486.e1. [CrossRef] [PubMed]
3. De, P.; Aske, J.; Dey, N. Cancer-Associated Fibroblast Functions as a Road-Block in Cancer Therapy. *Cancers* **2021**, *13*, 5246. [CrossRef] [PubMed]
4. De, P.; Aske, J.; Dey, N. Cancer-Associated Fibroblasts in Conversation with Tumor Cells in Endometrial Cancers: A Partner in Crime. *Int. J. Mol. Sci.* **2021**, *22*, 9121. [CrossRef]
5. Yang, X.; Lin, Y.; Shi, Y.; Li, B.; Liu, W.; Yin, W.; Dang, Y.; Chu, Y.; Fan, J.; He, R. FAP Promotes Immunosuppression by Cancer-Associated Fibroblasts in the Tumor Microenvironment via STAT3-CCL2 Signaling. *Cancer Res.* **2016**, *76*, 4124–4135. [CrossRef] [PubMed]
6. Didier Meseure, K.D.A. Cancer Metabolic and immune reprogramming: The intimate interaction between cancer cells and microenviroment. *Cancer Prev. Curr. Res.* **2014**, *1*, 21–30. [CrossRef]
7. Pavlides, S.; Whitaker-Menezes, D.; Castello-Cros, R.; Flomenberg, N.; Witkiewicz, A.K.; Frank, P.G.; Casimiro, M.C.; Wang, C.; Fortina, P.; Addya, S.; et al. The reverse Warburg effect: Aerobic glycolysis in cancer associated fibroblasts and the tumor stroma. *Cell Cycle* **2009**, *8*, 3984–4001. [CrossRef]
8. Whitaker-Menezes, D.; Martinez-Outschoorn, U.E.; Lin, Z.; Ertel, A.; Flomenberg, N.; Witkiewicz, A.K.; Birbe, R.C.; Howell, A.; Pavlides, S.; Gandara, R.; et al. Evidence for a stromal-epithelial "lactate shuttle" in human tumors: MCT4 is a marker of oxidative stress in cancer-associated fibroblasts. *Cell Cycle* **2011**, *10*, 1772–1783. [CrossRef]
9. Costa, A.; Scholer-Dahirel, A.; Mechta-Grigoriou, F. The role of reactive oxygen species and metabolism on cancer cells and their microenvironment. *Semin. Cancer Biol.* **2014**, *25*, 23–32. [CrossRef]
10. Costa, A.; Kieffer, Y.; Scholer-Dahirel, A.; Pelon, F.; Bourachot, B.; Cardon, M.; Sirven, P.; Magagna, I.; Fuhrmann, L.; Bernard, C.; et al. Fibroblast Heterogeneity and Immunosuppressive Environment in Human Breast Cancer. *Cancer Cell* **2018**, *33*, 463–479.e410. [CrossRef]
11. Elyada, E.; Bolisetty, M.; Laise, P.; Flynn, W.F.; Courtois, E.T.; Burkhart, R.A.; Teinor, J.A.; Belleau, P.; Biffi, G.; Lucito, M.S.; et al. Cross-Species Single-Cell Analysis of Pancreatic Ductal Adenocarcinoma Reveals Antigen-Presenting Cancer-Associated Fibroblasts. *Cancer Discov.* **2019**, *9*, 1102–1123. [CrossRef] [PubMed]
12. Mariathasan, S.; Turley, S.J.; Nickles, D.; Castiglioni, A.; Yuen, K.; Wang, Y.; Kadel, E.E., III; Koeppen, H.; Astarita, J.L.; Cubas, R.; et al. TGFbeta attenuates tumour response to PD-L1 blockade by contributing to exclusion of T cells. *Nature* **2018**, *554*, 544–548. [CrossRef] [PubMed]
13. Monteran, L.; Erez, N. The Dark Side of Fibroblasts: Cancer-Associated Fibroblasts as Mediators of Immunosuppression in the Tumor Microenvironment. *Front. Immunol.* **2019**, *10*, 1835. [CrossRef] [PubMed]
14. Kato, T.; Noma, K.; Ohara, T.; Kashima, H.; Katsura, Y.; Sato, H.; Komoto, S.; Katsube, R.; Ninomiya, T.; Tazawa, H.; et al. Cancer-Associated Fibroblasts Affect Intratumoral CD8(+) and FoxP3(+) T Cells Via IL6 in the Tumor Microenvironment. *Clin. Cancer Res. Off. J. Am. Assoc. Cancer Res.* **2018**, *24*, 4820–4833. [CrossRef] [PubMed]
15. Ji, Z.; Tian, W.; Gao, W.; Zang, R.; Wang, H.; Yang, G. Cancer-Associated Fibroblast-Derived Interleukin-8 Promotes Ovarian Cancer Cell Stemness and Malignancy Through the Notch3-Mediated Signaling. *Front. Cell Dev. Biol.* **2021**, *9*, 684505. [CrossRef] [PubMed]
16. Su, S.; Chen, J.; Yao, H.; Liu, J.; Yu, S.; Lao, L.; Wang, M.; Luo, M.; Xing, Y.; Chen, F.; et al. CD10(+)GPR77(+) Cancer-Associated Fibroblasts Promote Cancer Formation and Chemoresistance by Sustaining Cancer Stemness. *Cell* **2018**, *172*, 841–856.e816. [CrossRef]
17. Zhang, Y.; Tang, H.; Cai, J.; Zhang, T.; Guo, J.; Feng, D.; Wang, Z. Ovarian cancer-associated fibroblasts contribute to epithelial ovarian carcinoma metastasis by promoting angiogenesis, lymphangiogenesis and tumor cell invasion. *Cancer Lett.* **2011**, *303*, 47–55. [CrossRef]
18. Yu, Y.; Xiao, C.H.; Tan, L.D.; Wang, Q.S.; Li, X.Q.; Feng, Y.M. Cancer-associated fibroblasts induce epithelial-mesenchymal transition of breast cancer cells through paracrine TGF-beta signalling. *Br. J. Cancer* **2014**, *110*, 724–732. [CrossRef]
19. Leask, A. A centralized communication network: Recent insights into the role of the cancer associated fibroblast in the development of drug resistance in tumors. *Semin. Cell Dev. Biol.* **2020**, *101*, 111–114. [CrossRef]
20. Khan, G.J.; Sun, L.; Khan, S.; Yuan, S.; Nongyue, H. Versatility of Cancer Associated Fibroblasts: Commendable Targets for Anti-tumor Therapy. *Curr. Drug Targets* **2018**, *19*, 1573–1588. [CrossRef]
21. Dzobo, K.; Dandara, C. Architecture of Cancer-Associated Fibroblasts in Tumor Microenvironment: Mapping Their Origins, Heterogeneity, and Role in Cancer Therapy Resistance. *Omics. J. Integr. Biol.* **2020**, *24*, 314–339. [CrossRef] [PubMed]

22. Li, B.; Pei, G.; Yao, J.; Ding, Q.; Jia, P.; Zhao, Z. Cell-type deconvolution analysis identifies cancer-associated myofibroblast component as a poor prognostic factor in multiple cancer types. *Oncogene* **2021**, *40*, 4686–4694. [CrossRef] [PubMed]
23. Vaish, U.; Jain, T.; Are, A.C.; Dudeja, V. Cancer-Associated Fibroblasts in Pancreatic Ductal Adenocarcinoma: An Update on Heterogeneity and Therapeutic Targeting. *Int. J. Mol. Sci.* **2021**, *22*, 3408. [CrossRef] [PubMed]
24. Miyazaki, Y.; Oda, T.; Mori, N.; Kida, Y.S. Adipose-derived mesenchymal stem cells differentiate into pancreatic cancer-associated fibroblasts In Vitro. *FEBS Open Bio* **2020**, *10*, 2268–2281. [CrossRef]
25. Affo, S.; Nair, A.; Brundu, F.; Ravichandra, A.; Bhattacharjee, S.; Matsuda, M.; Chin, L.; Filliol, A.; Wen, W.; Song, X.; et al. Promotion of cholangiocarcinoma growth by diverse cancer-associated fibroblast subpopulations. *Cancer Cell* **2021**, *39*, 866–882, Erratum in *Cancer Cell* **2021**, *39*, 883. [CrossRef]
26. Kieffer, Y.; Hocine, H.R.; Gentric, G.; Pelon, F.; Bernard, C.; Bourachot, B.; Lameiras, S.; Albergante, L.; Bonneau, C.; Guyard, A.; et al. Single-Cell Analysis Reveals Fibroblast Clusters Linked to Immunotherapy Resistance in Cancer. *Cancer Discov.* **2020**, *10*, 1330–1351. [CrossRef]
27. Tran, L.L.; Dang, T.; Thomas, R.; Rowley, D.R. ELF3 mediates IL-1alpha induced differentiation of mesenchymal stem cells to inflammatory iCAFs. *Stem Cells* **2021**, *39*, 1766–1777. [CrossRef]
28. Goulet, C.R.; Champagne, A.; Bernard, G.; Vandal, D.; Chabaud, S.; Pouliot, F.; Bolduc, S. Cancer-associated fibroblasts induce epithelial-mesenchymal transition of bladder cancer cells through paracrine IL-6 signalling. *BMC Cancer* **2019**, *19*, 137. [CrossRef]
29. Pan, X.; Zhou, J.; Xiao, Q.; Fujiwara, K.; Zhang, M.; Mo, G.; Gong, W.; Zheng, L. Cancer-associated fibroblast heterogeneity is associated with organ-specific metastasis in pancreatic ductal adenocarcinoma. *J. Hematol. Oncol.* **2021**, *14*, 184. [CrossRef]
30. Steele, N.G.; Biffi, G.; Kemp, S.B.; Zhang, Y.; Drouillard, D.; Syu, L.; Hao, Y.; Oni, T.E.; Brosnan, E.; Elyada, E.; et al. Inhibition of Hedgehog Signaling Alters Fibroblast Composition in Pancreatic Cancer. *Clin. Cancer Res. Off. J. Am. Assoc. Cancer Res.* **2021**, *27*, 2023–2037. [CrossRef]
31. Mosa, M.H.; Michels, B.E.; Menche, C.; Nicolas, A.M.; Darvishi, T.; Greten, F.R.; Farin, H.F. A Wnt-Induced Phenotypic Switch in Cancer-Associated Fibroblasts Inhibits EMT in Colorectal Cancer. *Cancer Res.* **2020**, *80*, 5569–5582. [CrossRef] [PubMed]
32. Zeltz, C.; Alam, J.; Liu, H.; Erusappan, P.M.; Hoschuetzky, H.; Molven, A.; Parajuli, H.; Cukierman, E.; Costea, D.E.; Lu, N.; et al. Alpha11beta1 Integrin is Induced in a Subset of Cancer-Associated Fibroblasts in Desmoplastic Tumor Stroma and Mediates In Vitro Cell Migration. *Cancers* **2019**, *11*, 765. [CrossRef] [PubMed]
33. Diaz-Maroto, N.G.; Garcia-Vicien, G.; Polcaro, G.; Banuls, M.; Albert, N.; Villanueva, A.; Mollevi, D.G. The Blockade of Tumoral IL1beta-Mediated Signaling in Normal Colonic Fibroblasts Sensitizes Tumor Cells to Chemotherapy and Prevents Inflammatory CAF Activation. *Int. J. Mol. Sci.* **2021**, *22*, 4960. [CrossRef] [PubMed]
34. de Kruijf, E.M.; van Nes, J.G.; van de Velde, C.J.; Putter, H.; Smit, V.T.; Liefers, G.J.; Kuppen, P.J.; Tollenaar, R.A.; Mesker, W.E. Tumor-stroma ratio in the primary tumor is a prognostic factor in early breast cancer patients, especially in triple-negative carcinoma patients. *Breast Cancer Res. Treat.* **2011**, *125*, 687–696. [CrossRef] [PubMed]
35. Lv, Z.; Cai, X.; Weng, X.; Xiao, H.; Du, C.; Cheng, J.; Zhou, L.; Xie, J.; Sun, K.; Wu, J.; et al. Tumor-stroma ratio is a prognostic factor for survival in hepatocellular carcinoma patients after liver resection or transplantation. *Surgery* **2015**, *158*, 142–150. [CrossRef] [PubMed]
36. Mesker, W.E.; Junggeburt, J.M.; Szuhai, K.; de Heer, P.; Morreau, H.; Tanke, H.J.; Tollenaar, R.A. The carcinoma-stromal ratio of colon carcinoma is an independent factor for survival compared to lymph node status and tumor stage. *Cell. Oncol. Off. J. Int. Soc. Cell. Oncol.* **2007**, *29*, 387–398. [CrossRef] [PubMed]
37. Wang, K.; Ma, W.; Wang, J.; Yu, L.; Zhang, X.; Wang, Z.; Tan, B.; Wang, N.; Bai, B.; Yang, S.; et al. Tumor-stroma ratio is an independent predictor for survival in esophageal squamous cell carcinoma. *J. Thorac. Oncol. Off. Publ. Int. Assoc. Study Lung Cancer* **2012**, *7*, 1457–1461. [CrossRef]
38. Zhang, T.; Xu, J.; Shen, H.; Dong, W.; Ni, Y.; Du, J. Tumor-stroma ratio is an independent predictor for survival in NSCLC. *Int. J. Clin. Exp. Pathol.* **2015**, *8*, 11348–11355.
39. Wu, Y.; Grabsch, H.; Ivanova, T.; Tan, I.B.; Murray, J.; Ooi, C.H.; Wright, A.I.; West, N.P.; Hutchins, G.G.; Wu, J.; et al. Comprehensive genomic meta-analysis identifies intra-tumoural stroma as a predictor of survival in patients with gastric cancer. *Gut* **2013**, *62*, 1100–1111. [CrossRef]
40. Lee, D.; Ham, I.H.; Son, S.Y.; Han, S.U.; Kim, Y.B.; Hur, H. Intratumor stromal proportion predicts aggressive phenotype of gastric signet ring cell carcinomas. *Gastric Cancer Off. J. Int. Gastric Cancer Assoc. Jpn. Gastric Cancer Assoc.* **2017**, *20*, 591–601. [CrossRef]
41. Ma, J.; Song, X.; Xu, X.; Mou, Y. Cancer-Associated Fibroblasts Promote the Chemo-resistance in Gastric Cancer through Secreting IL-11 Targeting JAK/STAT3/Bcl2 Pathway. *Cancer Res. Treat.* **2019**, *51*, 194–210. [CrossRef] [PubMed]
42. Ham, I.H.; Oh, H.J.; Jin, H.; Bae, C.A.; Jeon, S.M.; Choi, K.S.; Son, S.Y.; Han, S.U.; Brekken, R.A.; Lee, D.; et al. Targeting interleukin-6 as a strategy to overcome stroma-induced resistance to chemotherapy in gastric cancer. *Mol. Cancer* **2019**, *18*, 68. [CrossRef] [PubMed]
43. Ham, I.H.; Lee, D.; Hur, H. Role of Cancer-Associated Fibroblast in Gastric Cancer Progression and Resistance to Treatments. *J. Oncol.* **2019**, *2019*, 6270784. [CrossRef]
44. Uchihara, T.; Miyake, K.; Yonemura, A.; Komohara, Y.; Itoyama, R.; Koiwa, M.; Yasuda, T.; Arima, K.; Harada, K.; Eto, K.; et al. Extracellular Vesicles from Cancer-Associated Fibroblasts Containing Annexin A6 Induces FAK-YAP Activation by Stabilizing beta1 Integrin, Enhancing Drug Resistance. *Cancer Res.* **2020**, *80*, 3222–3235. [CrossRef] [PubMed]

45. Wang, L.; Li, X.; Ren, Y.; Geng, H.; Zhang, Q.; Cao, L.; Meng, Z.; Wu, X.; Xu, M.; Xu, K. Cancer-associated fibroblasts contribute to cisplatin resistance by modulating ANXA3 in lung cancer cells. *Cancer Sci.* **2019**, *110*, 1609–1620. [CrossRef] [PubMed]
46. Masuda, T.; Nakashima, T.; Namba, M.; Yamaguchi, K.; Sakamoto, S.; Horimasu, Y.; Miyamoto, S.; Iwamoto, H.; Fujitaka, K.; Miyata, Y.; et al. Inhibition of PAI-1 limits chemotherapy resistance in lung cancer through suppressing myofibroblast characteristics of cancer-associated fibroblasts. *J. Cell. Mol. Med.* **2019**, *23*, 2984–2994. [CrossRef] [PubMed]
47. Zhai, J.; Shen, J.; Xie, G.; Wu, J.; He, M.; Gao, L.; Zhang, Y.; Yao, X.; Shen, L. Cancer-associated fibroblasts-derived IL-8 mediates resistance to cisplatin in human gastric cancer. *Cancer Lett.* **2019**, *454*, 37–43. [CrossRef]
48. Long, X.; Xiong, W.; Zeng, X.; Qi, L.; Cai, Y.; Mo, M.; Jiang, H.; Zhu, B.; Chen, Z.; Li, Y. Cancer-associated fibroblasts promote cisplatin resistance in bladder cancer cells by increasing IGF-1/ERbeta/Bcl-2 signalling. *Cell Death Dis.* **2019**, *10*, 375. [CrossRef]
49. Guo, H.; Ha, C.; Dong, H.; Yang, Z.; Ma, Y.; Ding, Y. Cancer-associated fibroblast-derived exosomal microRNA-98-5p promotes cisplatin resistance in ovarian cancer by targeting CDKN1A. *Cancer Cell Int.* **2019**, *19*, 347. [CrossRef]
50. Qin, X.; Guo, H.; Wang, X.; Zhu, X.; Yan, M.; Wang, X.; Xu, Q.; Shi, J.; Lu, E.; Chen, W.; et al. Exosomal miR-196a derived from cancer-associated fibroblasts confers cisplatin resistance in head and neck cancer through targeting CDKN1B and ING5. *Genome Biol.* **2019**, *20*, 12. [CrossRef]
51. Gao, Y.; Li, X.; Zeng, C.; Liu, C.; Hao, Q.; Li, W.; Zhang, K.; Zhang, W.; Wang, S.; Zhao, H.; et al. CD63(+) Cancer-Associated Fibroblasts Confer Tamoxifen Resistance to Breast Cancer Cells through Exosomal miR-22. *Adv. Sci.* **2020**, *7*, 2002518. [CrossRef] [PubMed]
52. Chen, X.; Liu, J.; Zhang, Q.; Liu, B.; Cheng, Y.; Zhang, Y.; Sun, Y.; Ge, H.; Liu, Y. Exosome-mediated transfer of miR-93-5p from cancer-associated fibroblasts confer radioresistance in colorectal cancer cells by downregulating FOXA1 and upregulating TGFB3. *J. Exp. Clin. Cancer Res. CR* **2020**, *39*, 65. [CrossRef]
53. Chen, X.; Liu, Y.; Zhang, Q.; Liu, B.; Cheng, Y.; Zhang, Y.; Sun, Y.; Liu, J. Exosomal miR-590-3p derived from cancer-associated fibroblasts confers radioresistance in colorectal cancer. *Mol. Therapy Nucleic Acids* **2021**, *24*, 113–126. [CrossRef] [PubMed]
54. Zhang, H.; Hua, Y.; Jiang, Z.; Yue, J.; Shi, M.; Zhen, X.; Zhang, X.; Yang, L.; Zhou, R.; Wu, S. Cancer-associated Fibroblast-promoted LncRNA DNM3OS Confers Radioresistance by Regulating DNA Damage Response in Esophageal Squamous Cell Carcinoma. *Clin. Cancer Res. Off. J. Am. Assoc. Cancer Res.* **2019**, *25*, 1989–2000. [CrossRef] [PubMed]
55. Domogauer, J.D.; de Toledo, S.M.; Howell, R.W.; Azzam, E.I. Acquired radioresistance in cancer associated fibroblasts is concomitant with enhanced antioxidant potential and DNA repair capacity. *Cell Commun. Signal. CCS* **2021**, *19*, 30. [CrossRef]
56. Ragunathan, K.; Upfold, N.L.E.; Oksenych, V. Interaction between Fibroblasts and Immune Cells Following DNA Damage Induced by Ionizing Radiation. *Int. J. Mol. Sci.* **2020**, *21*, 8635. [CrossRef]
57. Darragh, L.B.; Oweida, A.J.; Karam, S.D. Overcoming Resistance to Combination Radiation-Immunotherapy: A Focus on Contributing Pathways Within the Tumor Microenvironment. *Front. Immunol.* **2018**, *9*, 3154. [CrossRef]
58. Leung, C.S.; Yeung, T.L.; Yip, K.P.; Wong, K.K.; Ho, S.Y.; Mangala, L.S.; Sood, A.K.; Lopez-Berestein, G.; Sheng, J.; Wong, S.T.; et al. Cancer-associated fibroblasts regulate endothelial adhesion protein LPP to promote ovarian cancer chemoresistance. *J. Clin. Investig.* **2018**, *128*, 589–606. [CrossRef]
59. Zhang, H.; Deng, T.; Liu, R.; Ning, T.; Yang, H.; Liu, D.; Zhang, Q.; Lin, D.; Ge, S.; Bai, M.; et al. CAF secreted miR-522 suppresses ferroptosis and promotes acquired chemo-resistance in gastric cancer. *Mol. Cancer* **2020**, *19*, 43. [CrossRef]
60. Deng, X.; Ruan, H.; Zhang, X.; Xu, X.; Zhu, Y.; Peng, H.; Zhang, X.; Kong, F.; Guan, M. Long noncoding RNA CCAL transferred from fibroblasts by exosomes promotes chemoresistance of colorectal cancer cells. *Int. J. Cancer* **2020**, *146*, 1700–1716. [CrossRef]
61. Hu, J.L.; Wang, W.; Lan, X.L.; Zeng, Z.C.; Liang, Y.S.; Yan, Y.R.; Song, F.Y.; Wang, F.F.; Zhu, X.H.; Liao, W.J.; et al. CAFs secreted exosomes promote metastasis and chemotherapy resistance by enhancing cell stemness and epithelial-mesenchymal transition in colorectal cancer. *Mol. Cancer* **2019**, *18*, 91. [CrossRef] [PubMed]
62. Wei, L.; Ye, H.; Li, G.; Lu, Y.; Zhou, Q.; Zheng, S.; Lin, Q.; Liu, Y.; Li, Z.; Chen, R. Correction: Cancer-associated fibroblasts promote progression and gemcitabine resistance via the SDF-1/SATB-1 pathway in pancreatic cancer. *Cell Death Dis.* **2021**, *12*, 232. [CrossRef] [PubMed]
63. Ruocco, M.R.; Avagliano, A.; Granato, G.; Imparato, V.; Masone, S.; Masullo, M.; Nasso, R.; Montagnani, S.; Arcucci, A. Involvement of Breast Cancer-Associated Fibroblasts in Tumor Development, Therapy Resistance and Evaluation of Potential Therapeutic Strategies. *Curr. Med. Chem.* **2018**, *25*, 3414–3434. [CrossRef] [PubMed]
64. Zhang, Z.; Karthaus, W.R.; Lee, Y.S.; Gao, V.R.; Wu, C.; Russo, J.W.; Liu, M.; Mota, J.M.; Abida, W.; Linton, E.; et al. Tumor Microenvironment-Derived NRG1 Promotes Antiandrogen Resistance in Prostate Cancer. *Cancer Cell* **2020**, *38*, 279–296.e279. [CrossRef]
65. Yoshida, G.J. Regulation of heterogeneous cancer-associated fibroblasts: The molecular pathology of activated signaling pathways. *J. Exp. Clin. Cancer Res. CR* **2020**, *39*, 112. [CrossRef]
66. Apicella, M.; Giannoni, E.; Fiore, S.; Ferrari, K.J.; Fernandez-Perez, D.; Isella, C.; Granchi, C.; Minutolo, F.; Sottile, A.; Comoglio, P.M.; et al. Increased Lactate Secretion by Cancer Cells Sustains Non-cell-autonomous Adaptive Resistance to MET and EGFR Targeted Therapies. *Cell Metab.* **2018**, *28*, 848–865.e846. [CrossRef]
67. Suzuki, E.; Yamazaki, S.; Naito, T.; Hashimoto, H.; Okubo, S.; Udagawa, H.; Goto, K.; Tsuboi, M.; Ochiai, A.; Ishii, G. Secretion of high amounts of hepatocyte growth factor is a characteristic feature of cancer-associated fibroblasts with EGFR-TKI resistance-promoting phenotype: A study of 18 cases of cancer-associated fibroblasts. *Pathol. Int.* **2019**, *69*, 472–480. [CrossRef]

68. Yoshida, G.J. Metabolic reprogramming: The emerging concept and associated therapeutic strategies. *J. Exp. Clin. Cancer Res. CR* **2015**, *34*, 111. [CrossRef]
69. Ippolito, L.; Morandi, A.; Taddei, M.L.; Parri, M.; Comito, G.; Iscaro, A.; Raspollini, M.R.; Magherini, F.; Rapizzi, E.; Masquelier, J.; et al. Cancer-associated fibroblasts promote prostate cancer malignancy via metabolic rewiring and mitochondrial transfer. *Oncogene* **2019**, *38*, 5339–5355. [CrossRef]
70. Gong, J.; Lin, Y.; Zhang, H.; Liu, C.; Cheng, Z.; Yang, X.; Zhang, J.; Xiao, Y.; Sang, N.; Qian, X.; et al. Reprogramming of lipid metabolism in cancer-associated fibroblasts potentiates migration of colorectal cancer cells. *Cell Death Dis.* **2020**, *11*, 267. [CrossRef]
71. Brown, T.P.; Ganapathy, V. Lactate/GPR81 signaling and proton motive force in cancer: Role in angiogenesis, immune escape, nutrition, and Warburg phenomenon. *Pharmacol. Ther.* **2020**, *206*, 107451. [CrossRef] [PubMed]
72. Capparelli, C.; Rosenbaum, S.; Berger, A.C.; Aplin, A.E. Fibroblast-derived neuregulin 1 promotes compensatory ErbB3 receptor signaling in mutant BRAF melanoma. *J. Biol. Chem.* **2015**, *290*, 24267–24277. [CrossRef] [PubMed]
73. Fernandez-Nogueira, P.; Mancino, M.; Fuster, G.; Lopez-Plana, A.; Jauregui, P.; Almendro, V.; Enreig, E.; Menendez, S.; Rojo, F.; Noguera-Castells, A.; et al. Tumor-Associated Fibroblasts Promote HER2-Targeted Therapy Resistance through FGFR2 Activation. *Clin. Cancer Res. Off. J. Am. Assoc. Cancer Res.* **2020**, *26*, 1432–1448. [CrossRef] [PubMed]
74. Motoyama, A.B.; Hynes, N.E.; Lane, H.A. The efficacy of ErbB receptor-targeted anticancer therapeutics is influenced by the availability of epidermal growth factor-related peptides. *Cancer Res.* **2002**, *62*, 3151–3158. [PubMed]
75. Watanabe, S.; Yonesaka, K.; Tanizaki, J.; Nonagase, Y.; Takegawa, N.; Haratani, K.; Kawakami, H.; Hayashi, H.; Takeda, M.; Tsurutani, J.; et al. Targeting of the HER2/HER3 signaling axis overcomes ligand-mediated resistance to trastuzumab in HER2-positive breast cancer. *Cancer Med.* **2019**, *8*, 1258–1268. [CrossRef] [PubMed]
76. Xia, W.; Petricoin, E.F., 3rd; Zhao, S.; Liu, L.; Osada, T.; Cheng, Q.; Wulfkuhle, J.D.; Gwin, W.R.; Yang, X.; Gallagher, R.I.; et al. An heregulin-EGFR-HER3 autocrine signaling axis can mediate acquired lapatinib resistance in HER2+ breast cancer models. *Breast Cancer Res. BCR* **2013**, *15*, R85. [CrossRef]
77. Phillips, G.D.; Fields, C.T.; Li, G.; Dowbenko, D.; Schaefer, G.; Miller, K.; Andre, F.; Burris, H.A., 3rd; Albain, K.S.; Harbeck, N.; et al. Dual targeting of HER2-positive cancer with trastuzumab emtansine and pertuzumab: Critical role for neuregulin blockade in antitumor response to combination therapy. *Clin. Cancer Res. Off. J. Am. Assoc. Cancer Res.* **2014**, *20*, 456–468. [CrossRef]
78. Guardia, C.; Bianchini, G.; Arpi, L.O.; Menendez, S.; Casadevall, D.; Galbardi, B.; Dugo, M.; Servitja, S.; Montero, J.C.; Soria-Jimenez, L.; et al. Preclinical and Clinical Characterization of Fibroblast-derived Neuregulin-1 on Trastuzumab and Pertuzumab Activity in HER2-positive Breast Cancer. *Clin. Cancer Res. Off. J. Am. Assoc. Cancer Res.* **2021**, *27*, 5096–5108. [CrossRef]
79. Sonnenblick, A.; Salmon-Divon, M.; Salgado, R.; Dvash, E.; Ponde, N.; Zahavi, T.; Salmon, A.; Loibl, S.; Denkert, C.; Joensuu, H.; et al. Reactive stroma and trastuzumab resistance in HER2-positive early breast cancer. *Int. J. Cancer* **2020**, *147*, 266–276. [CrossRef]
80. Liu, T.; Zhou, L.; Xiao, Y.; Andl, T.; Zhang, Y. BRAF Inhibitors Reprogram Cancer-Associated Fibroblasts to Drive Matrix Remodeling and Therapeutic Escape in Melanoma. *Cancer Res.* **2022**, *82*, 419–432. [CrossRef]
81. Liu, J.; Li, P.; Wang, L.; Li, M.; Ge, Z.; Noordam, L.; Lieshout, R.; Verstegen, M.M.A.; Ma, B.; Su, J.; et al. Cancer-Associated Fibroblasts Provide a Stromal Niche for Liver Cancer Organoids That Confers Trophic Effects and Therapy Resistance. *Cell. Mol. Gastroenterol. Hepatol.* **2021**, *11*, 407–431. [CrossRef] [PubMed]
82. Hu, H.; Piotrowska, Z.; Hare, P.J.; Chen, H.; Mulvey, H.E.; Mayfield, A.; Noeen, S.; Kattermann, K.; Greenberg, M.; Williams, A.; et al. Three subtypes of lung cancer fibroblasts define distinct therapeutic paradigms. *Cancer Cell* **2021**, *11*, 1531–1547. [CrossRef] [PubMed]
83. Kanzaki, R.; Pietras, K. Heterogeneity of cancer-associated fibroblasts: Opportunities for precision medicine. *Cancer Sci.* **2020**, *111*, 2708–2717. [CrossRef] [PubMed]
84. Laplagne, C.; Domagala, M.; Le Naour, A.; Quemerais, C.; Hamel, D.; Fournie, J.J.; Couderc, B.; Bousquet, C.; Ferrand, A.; Poupot, M. Latest Advances in Targeting the Tumor Microenvironment for Tumor Suppression. *Int. J. Mol. Sci.* **2019**, *20*, 4719. [CrossRef]
85. Pure, E.; Lo, A. Can Targeting Stroma Pave the Way to Enhanced Antitumor Immunity and Immunotherapy of Solid Tumors? *Cancer Immunol. Res.* **2016**, *4*, 269–278. [CrossRef]
86. Lindner, T.; Loktev, A.; Giesel, F.; Kratochwil, C.; Altmann, A.; Haberkorn, U. Targeting of activated fibroblasts for imaging and therapy. *EJNMMI Radiopharm. Chem.* **2019**, *4*, 16. [CrossRef]
87. Pure, E.; Blomberg, R. Pro-tumorigenic roles of fibroblast activation protein in cancer: Back to the basics. *Oncogene* **2018**, *37*, 4343–4357. [CrossRef]
88. Ostermann, E.; Garin-Chesa, P.; Heider, K.H.; Kalat, M.; Lamche, H.; Puri, C.; Kerjaschki, D.; Rettig, W.J.; Adolf, G.R. Effective immunoconjugate therapy in cancer models targeting a serine protease of tumor fibroblasts. *Clin. Cancer Res. Off. J. Am. Assoc. Cancer Res.* **2008**, *14*, 4584–4592. [CrossRef]
89. Welt, S.; Divgi, C.R.; Scott, A.M.; Garin-Chesa, P.; Finn, R.D.; Graham, M.; Carswell, E.A.; Cohen, A.; Larson, S.M.; Old, L.J.; et al. Antibody targeting in metastatic colon cancer: A phase I study of monoclonal antibody F19 against a cell-surface protein of reactive tumor stromal fibroblasts. *J. Clin. Oncol. Off. J. Am. Soc. Clin. Oncol.* **1994**, *12*, 1193–1203. [CrossRef]

90. Feig, C.; Jones, J.O.; Kraman, M.; Wells, R.J.; Deonarine, A.; Chan, D.S.; Connell, C.M.; Roberts, E.W.; Zhao, Q.; Caballero, O.L.; et al. Targeting CXCL12 from FAP-expressing carcinoma-associated fibroblasts synergizes with anti-PD-L1 immunotherapy in pancreatic cancer. *Proc. Natl. Acad. Sci. USA* **2013**, *110*, 20212–20217. [CrossRef]
91. Arnold, J.N.; Magiera, L.; Kraman, M.; Fearon, D.T. Tumoral immune suppression by macrophages expressing fibroblast activation protein-alpha and heme oxygenase-1. *Cancer Immunol. Res.* **2014**, *2*, 121–126. [CrossRef] [PubMed]
92. Kraman, M.; Bambrough, P.J.; Arnold, J.N.; Roberts, E.W.; Magiera, L.; Jones, J.O.; Gopinathan, A.; Tuveson, D.A.; Fearon, D.T. Suppression of antitumor immunity by stromal cells expressing fibroblast activation protein-alpha. *Science* **2010**, *330*, 827–830. [CrossRef] [PubMed]
93. Lo, A.; Wang, L.S.; Scholler, J.; Monslow, J.; Avery, D.; Newick, K.; O'Brien, S.; Evans, R.A.; Bajor, D.J.; Clendenin, C.; et al. Tumor-Promoting Desmoplasia Is Disrupted by Depleting FAP-Expressing Stromal Cells. *Cancer Res.* **2015**, *75*, 2800–2810. [CrossRef] [PubMed]
94. Wang, L.C.; Lo, A.; Scholler, J.; Sun, J.; Majumdar, R.S.; Kapoor, V.; Antzis, M.; Cotner, C.E.; Johnson, L.A.; Durham, A.C.; et al. Targeting fibroblast activation protein in tumor stroma with chimeric antigen receptor T cells can inhibit tumor growth and augment host immunity without severe toxicity. *Cancer Immunol. Res.* **2014**, *2*, 154–166. [CrossRef]
95. Brunker, P.; Wartha, K.; Friess, T.; Grau-Richards, S.; Waldhauer, I.; Koller, C.F.; Weiser, B.; Majety, M.; Runza, V.; Niu, H.; et al. RG7386, a Novel Tetravalent FAP-DR5 Antibody, Effectively Triggers FAP-Dependent, Avidity-Driven DR5 Hyperclustering and Tumor Cell Apoptosis. *Mol. Cancer Ther.* **2016**, *15*, 946–957. [CrossRef] [PubMed]
96. Huang, T.; Wang, H.; Chen, N.G.; Frentzen, A.; Minev, B.; Szalay, A.A. Expression of anti-VEGF antibody together with anti-EGFR or anti-FAP enhances tumor regression as a result of vaccinia virotherapy. *Mol. Ther. Oncolytics* **2015**, *2*, 15003. [CrossRef] [PubMed]
97. Zhang, Y.; Ertl, H.C. Depletion of FAP+ cells reduces immunosuppressive cells and improves metabolism and functions CD8+T cells within tumors. *Oncotarget* **2016**, *7*, 23282–23299. [CrossRef]
98. Scott, A.M.; Wiseman, G.; Welt, S.; Adjei, A.; Lee, F.T.; Hopkins, W.; Divgi, C.R.; Hanson, L.H.; Mitchell, P.; Gansen, D.N.; et al. A Phase I dose-escalation study of sibrotuzumab in patients with advanced or metastatic fibroblast activation protein-positive cancer. *Clin. Cancer Res. Off. J. Am. Assoc. Cancer Res.* **2003**, *9*, 1639–1647.
99. Kaps, L.; Schuppan, D. Targeting Cancer Associated Fibroblasts in Liver Fibrosis and Liver Cancer Using Nanocarriers. *Cells* **2020**, *9*, 2027. [CrossRef]
100. Zhang, Y.; Elechalawar, C.K.; Hossen, M.N.; Francek, E.R.; Dey, A.; Wilhelm, S.; Bhattacharya, R.; Mukherjee, P. Gold nanoparticles inhibit activation of cancer-associated fibroblasts by disrupting communication from tumor and microenvironmental cells. *Bioact. Mater.* **2021**, *6*, 326–332. [CrossRef]
101. Guo, J.; Zeng, H.; Chen, Y. Emerging Nano Drug Delivery Systems Targeting Cancer-Associated Fibroblasts for Improved Antitumor Effect and Tumor Drug Penetration. *Mol. Pharm.* **2020**, *17*, 1028–1048. [CrossRef] [PubMed]
102. Truffi, M.; Mazzucchelli, S.; Bonizzi, A.; Sorrentino, L.; Allevi, R.; Vanna, R.; Morasso, C.; Corsi, F. Nano-Strategies to Target Breast Cancer-Associated Fibroblasts: Rearranging the Tumor Microenvironment to Achieve Antitumor Efficacy. *Int. J. Mol. Sci.* **2019**, *20*, 1263. [CrossRef] [PubMed]
103. Zhuravlev, F. Theranostic radiopharmaceuticals targeting cancer-associated fibroblasts. *Curr. Radiopharm.* **2020**, *14*, 374–393. [CrossRef] [PubMed]
104. Koustoulidou, S.; Hoorens, M.W.H.; Dalm, S.U.; Mahajan, S.; Debets, R.; Seimbille, Y.; de Jong, M. Cancer-Associated Fibroblasts as Players in Cancer Development and Progression and Their Role in Targeted Radionuclide Imaging and Therapy. *Cancers* **2021**, *13*, 1100. [CrossRef] [PubMed]
105. Sirica, A.E. The role of cancer-associated myofibroblasts in intrahepatic cholangiocarcinoma. *Nat. Reviews. Gastroenterol. Hepatol.* **2011**, *9*, 44–54. [CrossRef]
106. Vaquero, J.; Aoudjehane, L.; Fouassier, L. Cancer-associated fibroblasts in cholangiocarcinoma. *Curr. Opin. Gastroenterol.* **2020**, *36*, 63–69. [CrossRef]
107. Hogdall, D.; Lewinska, M.; Andersen, J.B. Desmoplastic Tumor Microenvironment and Immunotherapy in Cholangiocarcinoma. *Trends Cancer* **2018**, *4*, 239–255. [CrossRef]
108. Mertens, J.C.; Fingas, C.D.; Christensen, J.D.; Smoot, R.L.; Bronk, S.F.; Werneburg, N.W.; Gustafson, M.P.; Dietz, A.B.; Roberts, L.R.; Sirica, A.E.; et al. Therapeutic effects of deleting cancer-associated fibroblasts in cholangiocarcinoma. *Cancer Res.* **2013**, *73*, 897–907. [CrossRef]
109. Nicolas-Boluda, A.; Vaquero, J.; Laurent, G.; Renault, G.; Bazzi, R.; Donnadieu, E.; Roux, S.; Fouassier, L.; Gazeau, F. Photothermal Depletion of Cancer-Associated Fibroblasts Normalizes Tumor Stiffness in Desmoplastic Cholangiocarcinoma. *ACS Nano* **2020**, *14*, 5738–5753. [CrossRef]
110. Katsube, R.; Noma, K.; Ohara, T.; Nishiwaki, N.; Kobayashi, T.; Komoto, S.; Sato, H.; Kashima, H.; Kato, T.; Kikuchi, S.; et al. Fibroblast activation protein targeted near infrared photoimmunotherapy (NIR PIT) overcomes therapeutic resistance in human esophageal cancer. *Sci. Rep.* **2021**, *11*, 1693. [CrossRef]
111. Gorchs, L.; Kaipe, H. Interactions between Cancer-Associated Fibroblasts and T Cells in the Pancreatic Tumor Microenvironment and the Role of Chemokines. *Cancers* **2021**, *13*, 2995. [CrossRef] [PubMed]
112. Barrett, R.L.; Pure, E. Cancer-associated fibroblasts and their influence on tumor immunity and immunotherapy. *Elife* **2020**, *9*, 7243. [CrossRef] [PubMed]

13. Yu, L.; Liu, Q.; Huo, J.; Wei, F.; Guo, W. Cancer-associated fibroblasts induce immunotherapy resistance in hepatocellular carcinoma animal model. *Cell. Mol. Biol.* **2020**, *66*, 36–40. [CrossRef] [PubMed]
14. Liu, T.; Han, C.; Wang, S.; Fang, P.; Ma, Z.; Xu, L.; Yin, R. Cancer-associated fibroblasts: An emerging target of anti-cancer immunotherapy. *J. Hematol. Oncol.* **2019**, *12*, 86. [CrossRef]
15. Freeman, P.; Mielgo, A. Cancer-Associated Fibroblast Mediated Inhibition of CD8+ Cytotoxic T Cell Accumulation in Tumours: Mechanisms and Therapeutic Opportunities. *Cancers* **2020**, *12*, 2687. [CrossRef]
16. Valcz, G.; Buzas, E.I.; Sebestyen, A.; Krenacs, T.; Szallasi, Z.; Igaz, P.; Molnar, B. Extracellular Vesicle-Based Communication May Contribute to the Co-Evolution of Cancer Stem Cells and Cancer-Associated Fibroblasts in Anti-Cancer Therapy. *Cancers* **2020**, *12*, 2324. [CrossRef]
17. Huang, T.X.; Guan, X.Y.; Fu, L. Therapeutic targeting of the crosstalk between cancer-associated fibroblasts and cancer stem cells. *Am. J. Cancer Res.* **2019**, *9*, 1889–1904.
18. Flach, E.H.; Rebecca, V.W.; Herlyn, M.; Smalley, K.S.; Anderson, A.R. Fibroblasts contribute to melanoma tumor growth and drug resistance. *Mol. Pharm.* **2011**, *8*, 2039–2049. [CrossRef]
19. Kinugasa, Y.; Matsui, T.; Takakura, N. CD44 expressed on cancer-associated fibroblasts is a functional molecule supporting the stemness and drug resistance of malignant cancer cells in the tumor microenvironment. *Stem Cells* **2014**, *32*, 145–156. [CrossRef]
20. Bellei, B.; Migliano, E.; Picardo, M. A Framework of Major Tumor-Promoting Signal Transduction Pathways Implicated in Melanoma-Fibroblast Dialogue. *Cancers* **2020**, *12*, 3400. [CrossRef]
21. Lee, E.; Wang, J.; Yumoto, K.; Jung, Y.; Cackowski, F.C.; Decker, A.M.; Li, Y.; Franceschi, R.T.; Pienta, K.J.; Taichman, R.S. DNMT1 Regulates Epithelial-Mesenchymal Transition and Cancer Stem Cells, Which Promotes Prostate Cancer Metastasis. *Neoplasia* **2016**, *18*, 553–566. [CrossRef] [PubMed]
22. Pistore, C.; Giannoni, E.; Colangelo, T.; Rizzo, F.; Magnani, E.; Muccillo, L.; Giurato, G.; Mancini, M.; Rizzo, S.; Riccardi, M.; et al. DNA methylation variations are required for epithelial-to-mesenchymal transition induced by cancer-associated fibroblasts in prostate cancer cells. *Oncogene* **2017**, *36*, 5551–5566. [CrossRef] [PubMed]
23. Cruz-Bermudez, A.; Laza-Briviesca, R.; Vicente-Blanco, R.J.; Garcia-Grande, A.; Coronado, M.J.; Laine-Menendez, S.; Alfaro, C.; Sanchez, J.C.; Franco, F.; Calvo, V.; et al. Cancer-associated fibroblasts modify lung cancer metabolism involving ROS and TGF-beta signaling. *Free Radic. Biol. Med.* **2019**, *130*, 163–173. [CrossRef] [PubMed]
24. Biffi, G.; Oni, T.E.; Spielman, B.; Hao, Y.; Elyada, E.; Park, Y.; Preall, J.; Tuveson, D.A. IL1-Induced JAK/STAT Signaling Is Antagonized by TGFbeta to Shape CAF Heterogeneity in Pancreatic Ductal Adenocarcinoma. *Cancer Discov.* **2019**, *9*, 282–301. [CrossRef]
25. Chakravarthy, A.; Khan, L.; Bensler, N.P.; Bose, P.; De Carvalho, D.D. TGF-beta-associated extracellular matrix genes link cancer-associated fibroblasts to immune evasion and immunotherapy failure. *Nat. Commun.* **2018**, *9*, 4692. [CrossRef]
26. Ishimoto, T.; Miyake, K.; Nandi, T.; Yashiro, M.; Onishi, N.; Huang, K.K.; Lin, S.J.; Kalpana, R.; Tay, S.T.; Suzuki, Y.; et al. Activation of Transforming Growth Factor Beta 1 Signaling in Gastric Cancer-associated Fibroblasts Increases Their Motility, via Expression of Rhomboid 5 Homolog 2, and Ability to Induce Invasiveness of Gastric Cancer Cells. *Gastroenterology* **2017**, *153*, 191–204.e116. [CrossRef]
27. Cardenas, H.; Vieth, E.; Lee, J.; Segar, M.; Liu, Y.; Nephew, K.P.; Matei, D. TGF-beta induces global changes in DNA methylation during the epithelial-to-mesenchymal transition in ovarian cancer cells. *Epigenetics* **2014**, *9*, 1461–1472. [CrossRef]
28. Liu, J.; Liao, S.; Diop-Frimpong, B.; Chen, W.; Goel, S.; Naxerova, K.; Ancukiewicz, M.; Boucher, Y.; Jain, R.K.; Xu, L. TGF-beta blockade improves the distribution and efficacy of therapeutics in breast carcinoma by normalizing the tumor stroma. *Proc. Natl. Acad. Sci. USA* **2012**, *109*, 16618–16623. [CrossRef]
29. Sun, Y.; Campisi, J.; Higano, C.; Beer, T.M.; Porter, P.; Coleman, I.; True, L.; Nelson, P.S. Treatment-induced damage to the tumor microenvironment promotes prostate cancer therapy resistance through WNT16B. *Nat. Med.* **2012**, *18*, 1359–1368. [CrossRef]
30. Sun, Y.; Zhu, D.; Chen, F.; Qian, M.; Wei, H.; Chen, W.; Xu, J. SFRP2 augments WNT16B signaling to promote therapeutic resistance in the damaged tumor microenvironment. *Oncogene* **2016**, *35*, 4321–4334. [CrossRef]
31. Lotti, F.; Jarrar, A.M.; Pai, R.K.; Hitomi, M.; Lathia, J.; Mace, A.; Gantt, G.A., Jr.; Sukhdeo, K.; DeVecchio, J.; Vasanji, A.; et al. Chemotherapy activates cancer-associated fibroblasts to maintain colorectal cancer-initiating cells by IL-17A. *J. Exp. Med.* **2013**, *210*, 2851–2872. [CrossRef] [PubMed]
32. Lisanti, M.P.; Martinez-Outschoorn, U.E.; Sotgia, F. Oncogenes induce the cancer-associated fibroblast phenotype: Metabolic symbiosis and "fibroblast addiction" are new therapeutic targets for drug discovery. *Cell Cycle* **2013**, *12*, 2723–2732. [CrossRef] [PubMed]
33. Martinez-Outschoorn, U.E.; Lisanti, M.P.; Sotgia, F. Catabolic cancer-associated fibroblasts transfer energy and biomass to anabolic cancer cells, fueling tumor growth. *Semin. Cancer Biol.* **2014**, *25*, 47–60. [CrossRef] [PubMed]
34. Jung, J.G.; Le, A. Targeting Metabolic Cross Talk Between Cancer Cells and Cancer-Associated Fibroblasts. *Adv. Exp. Med. Biol.* **2021**, *1311*, 205–214. [CrossRef]
35. Harrison, L.; Blackwell, K. Hypoxia and anemia: Factors in decreased sensitivity to radiation therapy and chemotherapy? *Oncologist* **2004**, *9* (Suppl. S5), 31–40. [CrossRef]
36. Vukovic, V.; Tannock, I.F. Influence of low pH on cytotoxicity of paclitaxel, mitoxantrone and topotecan. *Br. J. Cancer* **1997**, *75*, 1167–1172. [CrossRef]
37. Simon, M.C. (Ed.) *Diverse Effects of Hypoxia on Tumor Progression*; Springer: Berlin/Heidelberg, Germany, 2010; Volume 345.

138. Bertout, J.A.; Patel, S.A.; Simon, M.C. The impact of O^2 availability on human cancer. *Nat. Reviews Cancer* **2008**, *8*, 967–975. [CrossRef]
139. Keith, B.; Simon, M.C. Hypoxia-inducible factors, stem cells, and cancer. *Cell* **2007**, *129*, 465–472. [CrossRef]
140. Kugeratski, F.G.; Atkinson, S.J.; Neilson, L.J.; Lilla, S.; Knight, J.R.P.; Serneels, J.; Juin, A.; Ismail, S.; Bryant, D.M.; Markert, E.K.; et al. Hypoxic cancer-associated fibroblasts increase NCBP2-AS2/HIAR to promote endothelial sprouting through enhanced VEGF signaling. *Sci. Signal.* **2019**, *12*, 8247. [CrossRef]
141. Giaccia, A.J.; Schipani, E. Role of carcinoma-associated fibroblasts and hypoxia in tumor progression. *Curr. Top. Microbiol. Immunol.* **2010**, *345*, 31–45. [CrossRef]
142. Ziani, L.; Buart, S.; Chouaib, S.; Thiery, J. Hypoxia increases melanoma-associated fibroblasts immunosuppressive potential and inhibitory effect on T cell-mediated cytotoxicity. *Oncoimmunology* **2021**, *10*, 1950953. [CrossRef] [PubMed]
143. Masamune, A.; Kikuta, K.; Watanabe, T.; Satoh, K.; Hirota, M.; Shimosegawa, T. Hypoxia stimulates pancreatic stellate cells to induce fibrosis and angiogenesis in pancreatic cancer. *Am. J. Physiology Gastroint. Liver Physiol.* **2008**, *295*, 709–717. [CrossRef] [PubMed]
144. Kugeratski, F.G.; Hernandez, J.R.; Kalna, G.; Zanivan, S. Abstract A34: Hypoxic cancer-associated fibroblasts secrete regulators of angiogenesis: Novel potenital players revealed by MS. *Cancer Res.* **2016**, *76*. [CrossRef]
145. Ganguly, D.; Chandra, R.; Karalis, J.; Teke, M.; Aguilera, T.; Maddipati, R.; Wachsmann, M.B.; Ghersi, D.; Siravegna, G.; Zeh, H.J., 3rd; et al. Cancer-Associated Fibroblasts: Versatile Players in the Tumor Microenvironment. *Cancers* **2020**, *12*, 2652. [CrossRef]
146. Lee, J.; Fassnacht, M.; Nair, S.; Boczkowski, D.; Gilboa, E. Tumor immunotherapy targeting fibroblast activation protein, a product expressed in tumor-associated fibroblasts. *Cancer Res.* **2005**, *65*, 11156–11163. [CrossRef]
147. Sunami, Y.; Boker, V.; Kleeff, J. Targeting and Reprograming Cancer-Associated Fibroblasts and the Tumor Microenvironment in Pancreatic Cancer. *Cancers* **2021**, *13*, 697. [CrossRef]
148. Najafi, M.; Farhood, B.; Mortezaee, K. Extracellular matrix (ECM) stiffness and degradation as cancer drivers. *J. Cell. Biochem.* **2019**, *120*, 2782–2790. [CrossRef]
149. Nissen, N.I.; Karsdal, M.; Willumsen, N. Collagens and Cancer associated fibroblasts in the reactive stroma and its relation to Cancer biology. *J. Exp. Clin. Cancer Res. CR* **2019**, *38*, 115. [CrossRef]
150. McCarthy, J.B.; El-Ashry, D.; Turley, E.A. Hyaluronan, Cancer-Associated Fibroblasts and the Tumor Microenvironment in Malignant Progression. *Front. Cell Dev. Biol.* **2018**, *6*, 48. [CrossRef]
151. Zhang, Z.; Tao, D.; Zhang, P.; Liu, X.; Zhang, Y.; Cheng, J.; Yuan, H.; Liu, L.; Jiang, H. Hyaluronan synthase 2 expressed by cancer-associated fibroblasts promotes oral cancer invasion. *J. Exp. Clin. Cancer Res. CR* **2016**, *35*, 181. [CrossRef]
152. Bellei, B.; Caputo, S.; Migliano, E.; Lopez, G.; Marcaccini, V.; Cota, C.; Picardo, M. Simultaneous Targeting Tumor Cells and Cancer-Associated Fibroblasts with a Paclitaxel-Hyaluronan Bioconjugate: In Vitro Evaluation in Non-Melanoma Skin Cancer. *Biomedicines* **2021**, *9*, 597. [CrossRef] [PubMed]
153. Koopmans, T.; Rinkevich, Y. Mesothelial to mesenchyme transition as a major developmental and pathological player in trunk organs and their cavities. *Commun. Biol.* **2018**, *1*, 170. [CrossRef] [PubMed]
154. Sandoval, P.; Jimenez-Heffernan, J.A.; Rynne-Vidal, A.; Perez-Lozano, M.L.; Gilsanz, A.; Ruiz-Carpio, V.; Reyes, R.; Garcia-Bordas, J.; Stamatakis, K.; Dotor, J.; et al. Carcinoma-associated fibroblasts derive from mesothelial cells via mesothelial-to-mesenchymal transition in peritoneal metastasis. *J. Pathol.* **2013**, *231*, 517–531. [CrossRef]
155. Gordillo, C.H.; Sandoval, P.; Munoz-Hernandez, P.; Pascual-Anton, L.; Lopez-Cabrera, M.; Jimenez-Heffernan, J.A. Mesothelial-to-Mesenchymal Transition Contributes to the Generation of Carcinoma-Associated Fibroblasts in Locally Advanced Primary Colorectal Carcinomas. *Cancers* **2020**, *12*, 499. [CrossRef] [PubMed]
156. Nurmik, M.; Ullmann, P.; Rodriguez, F.; Haan, S.; Letellier, E. In search of definitions: Cancer-associated fibroblasts and their markers. *Int. J. Cancer* **2020**, *146*, 895–905. [CrossRef] [PubMed]
157. Kahounova, Z.; Kurfurstova, D.; Bouchal, J.; Kharaishvili, G.; Navratil, J.; Remsik, J.; Simeckova, S.; Student, V.; Kozubik, A.; Soucek, K. The fibroblast surface markers FAP, anti-fibroblast, and FSP are expressed by cells of epithelial origin and may be altered during epithelial-to-mesenchymal transition. *Cytometry. Part A J. Int. Soc. Anal. Cytol.* **2018**, *93*, 941–951. [CrossRef] [PubMed]
158. Hanley, C.J.; Mellone, M.; Ford, K.; Thirdborough, S.M.; Mellows, T.; Frampton, S.J.; Smith, D.M.; Harden, E.; Szyndralewiez, C.; Bullock, M.; et al. Targeting the Myofibroblastic Cancer-Associated Fibroblast Phenotype Through Inhibition of NOX4. *J. Natl. Cancer Inst.* **2018**, *110*, 109–120. [CrossRef]
159. Konrad, L.; Kortum, J.; Nabham, R.; Gronbach, J.; Dietze, R.; Oehmke, F.; Berkes, E.; Tinneberg, H.R. Composition of the Stroma in the Human Endometrium and Endometriosis. *Reprod. Sci.* **2018**, *25*, 1106–1115. [CrossRef]
160. Koumas, L.; King, A.E.; Critchley, H.O.; Kelly, R.W.; Phipps, R.P. Fibroblast heterogeneity: Existence of functionally distinct Thy 1(+) and Thy 1(-) human female reproductive tract fibroblasts. *Am. J. Pathol.* **2001**, *159*, 925–935. [CrossRef]
161. Panayiotou, H.; Orsi, N.M.; Thygesen, H.H.; Wright, A.I.; Winder, R.; Hutson, R.; Cummings, M. The prognostic significance of tumour-stroma ratio in endometrial carcinoma. *BMC Cancer* **2015**, *15*, 955. [CrossRef]
162. Espinosa, I.; Catasus, L.; D'Angelo, E.; Mozos, A.; Pedrola, N.; Bertolo, C.; Ferrer, I.; Zannoni, G.F.; West, R.B.; van de Rijn, M.; et al. Stromal signatures in endometrioid endometrial carcinomas. *Mod. Pathol.* **2014**, *27*, 631–639. [CrossRef] [PubMed]

63. Micke, P.; Strell, C.; Mattsson, J.; Martin-Bernabe, A.; Brunnstrom, H.; Huvila, J.; Sund, M.; Warnberg, F.; Ponten, F.; Glimelius, B.; et al. The prognostic impact of the tumour stroma fraction: A machine learning-based analysis in 16 human solid tumour types. *EBioMedicine* **2021**, *65*, 103269. [CrossRef] [PubMed]
64. Chen, X.; Song, E. Turning foes to friends: Targeting cancer-associated fibroblasts. *Nat. Reviews. Drug Discov.* **2019**, *18*, 99–115. [CrossRef] [PubMed]
65. Gieniec, K.A.; Butler, L.M.; Worthley, D.L.; Woods, S.L. Cancer-associated fibroblasts-heroes or villains? *Br. J. Cancer* **2019**, *121*, 293–302. [CrossRef] [PubMed]
66. Krisnawan, V.E.; Stanley, J.A.; Schwarz, J.K.; DeNardo, D.G. Tumor Microenvironment as a Regulator of Radiation Therapy: New Insights into Stromal-Mediated Radioresistance. *Cancers* **2020**, *12*, 2916. [CrossRef] [PubMed]
67. Bhattacharjee, S.; Hamberger, F.; Ravichandra, A.; Miller, M.; Nair, A.; Affo, S.; Filliol, A.; Chin, L.; Savage, T.M.; Yin, D.; et al. Tumor restriction by type I collagen opposes tumor-promoting effects of cancer-associated fibroblasts. *J. Clin. Investig.* **2021**, *131*. [CrossRef] [PubMed]

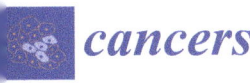

Article

Relationship between Tumor Mutational Burden, PD-L1, Patient Characteristics, and Response to Immune Checkpoint Inhibitors in Head and Neck Squamous Cell Carcinoma

Kimberly M. Burcher [1,†], Jeffrey W. Lantz [1,†], Elena Gavrila [1], Arianne Abreu [2], Jack T. Burcher [3], Andrew T. Faucheux [1], Amy Xie [1], Clayton Jackson [1], Alexander H. Song [1], Ryan T. Hughes [1], Thomas Lycan, Jr. [1], Paul M. Bunch [1], Cristina M. Furdui [1], Umit Topaloglu [1], Ralph B. D'Agostino, Jr. [1], Wei Zhang [1] and Mercedes Porosnicu [1,*]

[1] Wake Forest Baptist Medical Center, Winston-Salem, NC 27157, USA; kburcher@wakehealth.edu (K.M.B.); jwlantz@wakehealth.edu (J.W.L.); egavrila@wakehealth.edu (E.G.); afaucheu@wakehealth.edu (A.T.F.); axie@wakehealth.edu (A.X.); cwjackso@wakehealth.edu (C.J.); asong@wakehealth.edu (A.H.S.); ryhughes@wakehealth.edu (R.T.H.); tlycan@wakehealth.edu (T.L.J.); pbunch@wakehealth.edu (P.M.B.); cfurdui@wakehealth.edu (C.M.F.); Umit.Topaloglu@wakehealth.edu (U.T.); rdagosti@wakehealth.edu (R.B.D.J.); wezhang@wakehealth.edu (W.Z.)
[2] Lewisgale Medical Center, Salem, VA 24153, USA; a_abreu0419@email.campbell.edu
[3] Lake Erie College of Medicine, Bradenton, FL 34211, USA; jburcher83447@med.lecom.edu
* Correspondence: mporosni@wakehealth.edu
† These authors equally contributed to the study.

Simple Summary: Immunotherapy has prompted a dramatic change in the management of head and neck squamous cell carcinoma (HNSCC), but the percentage of patients benefiting from treatment is limited to 20% or less. The application of precision oncology to HNSCC introduces the potential for the emergence of biomarkers that may predict a response to immunotherapy and assist with the selection of patients that may benefit from treatment with an immune checkpoint inhibitors. In this retrospective study, the results of tumor mutational burden and programmed death ligand-1 measurements from HNSCC tumors were evaluated independently for their associations with demographics, risk factors, disease characteristics, survival, and response to ICI. Results of this study are expected to assist in laying the groundwork for creating a framework in which PD-L1 and TMB coexist with other variables to predict response to ICI on an individual level.

Abstract: Failure to predict response to immunotherapy (IO) limited its benefit in the treatment of head and neck squamous cell cancer (HNSCC) to 20% of patients or less. Biomarkers including tumor mutational burden (TMB) and programmed death ligand-1 (PD-L1) were evaluated as predictors of response to IO, but the results are inconsistent and with a lack of standardization of their methods. In this retrospective study, TMB and PD-L1 were measured by commercially available methodologies and were correlated to demographics, outcome, and response to PD-1 inhibitors. No correlation was found between TMB and PD-L1 levels. High TMB was associated with smoking and laryngeal primaries. PD-L1 was significantly higher in African Americans, patients with earlier stage tumors, nonsmokers, and nonethanol drinkers. Patients with high TMB fared better in univariate and multivariate survival analysis. No correlation was found between PD-L1 expression and prognosis. There was a statistically significant association between PFS and response to IO and TMB. There was no association between response to ICI and PD-L1 in this study, possibly affected by variations in the reporting method. Further studies are needed to characterize the biomarkers for IO in HNSCC, and this study supports further research into the advancement of TMB in prospective studies.

Keywords: HNSCC; TMB; immunotherapy; immune checkpoint inhibitors; PD-L1

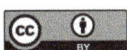

1. Introduction

Prognoses in oncology have dramatically improved with the development of immunotherapy (IO), particularly with the advent of immune checkpoint inhibitors (ICI). Antibodies to programmed death-1 (PD-1) receptor and the programmed death ligand-1 (PD-L1) are specific kinds of ICI which function by inhibiting the binding of the programmed death-1 (PD-1) receptor to PD-L1, thus allowing tumor cells to be recognized as "other" and eliminated by a patient's immune system (Figure 1) [1]. Emerging data indicate patients with HNSCC are likely to benefit from breakthroughs in ICI, presumably due to the high levels of circulating immune cells and high levels of neoantigens within these tumors (Figure 1) [2]. Clinical trials evaluating the response to ICIs in recurrent unresectable and metastatic HNSCC have shown significant improvement in overall survival (OS) when PD-1 inhibitors are utilized alone or in combination with chemotherapy [3–7].

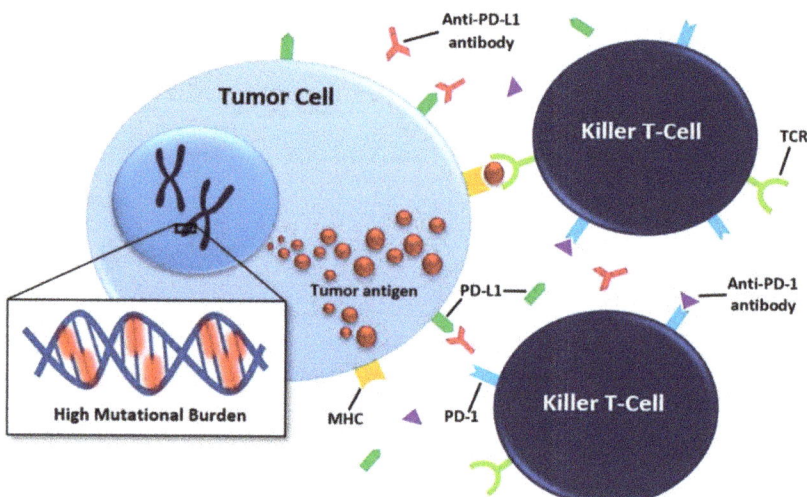

Figure 1. A brief review of the mechanism of action of PD-1/PD-L1 ICIs. Abbreviations: MHC, major histocompatibility complex; PD-1, programmed death-1; PD-L1, programmed death ligand-1; and TCR, T-cell receptor.

Despite these promising developments, fewer than 20% of HNSCC patients respond to treatment with ICI within the FDA approved setting, with the majority of patients displaying primary resistance [8]. With current clinical trials seeking to advance PD-1 ICI to curative settings, improved patient selection as a means of increasing the percentage of responders is critical, urging the development of reliable biomarkers predictive of the response to ICI. Many immune biomarkers including PD-L1 expression, tumor mutational burden (TMB), tumor immune cell infiltration, circulating immune cells, HPV, changes within the microbiome, and certain risk factors such as smoking have been suggested as predictors of HNSCC response to ICI, but the data remain in its infancy, without causative association and often with conflicting results within the literature [9]. Furthermore, there remains a limited understanding of how responses to ICI, prognosis, and each of the proposed biomarkers may be impacted by environmental factors or individual patient characteristics.

As a logical biomarker for the prediction of response to anti-PD1/PD-L1 agents, PD-L1 expression remains the only biomarker studied in prospective clinical trials in HNSCC. Studies place HNSCC amongst the malignancies with the highest frequency of PD-L1 positivity, defined as PD-L1 expression $\geq 1\%$ when measured by either tumor proportion score (TPS) or combined positive score (CPS). It has been estimated that between 57% and 82% of HNSCC patients are PD-L1 positive [5,10,11]. PD-L1 expression is often described as an inexact measurement of response to ICI with levels broadly correlating to response rates; however, it is well known that some PD-L1 negative patients do respond to ICI, and some patients with high PD-L1 levels do not [12].

Given the inconsistencies in results produced by the utilization of PD-L1 to predict response to ICI, many alternative biomarkers have been suggested. The chief prospect amongst these alternatives is TMB, a measure of the total number of coding mutations in a tumor's genome and reported in number of mutations per mega base (mut/Mb) of DNA sequenced [13]. In theory, higher TMB conveys a higher expression of tumor neoantigens, which elicit an increased antitumor immune response, conferring greater sensitivity to ICI (Figure 1) [9]. This has been proven to be the case in many malignancies, and at times, TMB has been reported to outperform PD-L1 in prediction of response; however, the data are incomplete and occasionally contradictory, and thus no consensus has been reached regarding widespread clinical use [13–25]. Although TMB has been approved for the selection of patients with cancer for IO treatment independent of tumor type [26], few data are available in HNSCC. Additionally, few studies correlate TMB to demographics or survival of HNSCC patients, and the results of studies that do attempt these correlations remain inconsistent [26,27]. The predictive power of TMB in regard to response to ICI in HNSCC also has yet to be defined. To date, there are no prospective studies regarding the use of tissue TMB as a biomarker to predict response to ICI, but retrospective analyses have successfully correlated high TMB with response to ICIs in HNSCC [9,24,27–29]. Similarly, the emerging role of circulating/blood TMB remains undefined, but preliminary results are promising [30,31].

Inconsistency in results is common in the literature regarding biomarkers such as PD-L1 and TMB. This is not exclusive to HNSCC. The variation in the assays used to measure these variables and reporting appear to be important contributors. Standardization efforts are ahead for PD-L1, with FDA approval of PD-L1 IHC 22C3 pharmDx reported as CPS, as a companion diagnostic for pembrolizumab treatment in HNSCC. Validation in clinical research and practice is ongoing. No such efforts have been undertaken for TMB, which has not yet been evaluated in prospective setting in HNSCC.

Joining the effort to lay a groundwork for the use of PD-L1 and TMB biomarkers to guide protocols regarding the use of PD-L1 ICI in HNSCC, this retrospective study correlates the level of expression of these biomarkers with demographic and outcome data in a dedicated HNSCC population. Additionally, the investigators correlate PD-L1 and TMB expression with response to PD-L1 ICI in the cohort of treated HNSCC patients. The primary objective of this study is to investigate the feasibility of continued pursuits of PD-L1 and TMB in prospective clinical trials in which ICI would be used to treat HNSCC. Importantly, the commercially available methodologies for measurement of the biomarkers were utilized.

2. Materials and Methods

This is a single-institution retrospective review of adult patients with HNSCC treated at the Wake Forest Baptist Comprehensive Cancer Center between August 2014 and October 2020 who had tumor tissue submitted for next-generation sequencing (NGS) and/or PD-L1 testing. The Wake Forest School of Medicine Institutional Review Board (IRB00057787) reviewed this study and granted approval. HNSCC patients were required to have had a valid TMB or PD-L1 test to be included in this study. Patients with cutaneous SCC or salivary gland cancers were excluded.

TMB was measured via FoundationOne (F1) testing (Foundation Medicine, Cambridge MA, USA) (F1). PD-L1 was analyzed by the standard, FDA-approved, immunohistochemistry 22C3 pharmDx kit, performed commercially by F1 and, in a small number of patients, by Mayo Clinic laboratories. PD-L1 expression was reported as a tumor proportion score (TPS) until 2019 and by the combined positive score (CPS) thereafter. PD-L1 was analyzed both as a 3-tiered and 2-tiered variable. The 3-tiered PD-L1 variable (3tPD-L1) was divided into categories similar to those in Keynote-048 and consisted of three groups: those with a PD-L1 of 0 (3tPD-L1-(0)), those with a PD-L1 between 1 and 19 (3tPD-L1-(1–19)) and those with PD-L1 greater than or equal to 20 (3tPD-L1-(20+)). Due to the low number of patients in the 3tPD-L1-(0) group, PD-L1 was also analyzed as a 2-tiered variable (2tPD-L1). In the 2tPD-L1, the 3tPD-L1-(0) and 3tPD-L1-(1–19) were grouped together and referred to as 2tPD-L1-(<20) and was compared to a group of patients with PD-L1 values greater than or equal to 20 referred to as 2tPD-L1-(20+). TMB was likewise initially divided into three categories (3-tiered-TMB) with low scores (TMB less than 6 mut/Mb), intermediate scores (TMB greater than or equal to 6 but less than 20 mut/Mb), and high scores group (TMB greater or equal to 20 mut/Mb) as recommended by F1, but, due to poor distribution across the sample population, no analysis was performed for the 3-tiered variable. Similar to PD-L1, TMB was recategorized into a 2-tiered variable, with those with TMB scored less than 6 mut/mb in the TMB-(<6) category and those with TMB of 6 or greater in the TMB-(6+) category. In instances in which PD-L1 or TMB tests were repeated, the highest resulted number was reported.

Demographic data and patient characteristics were obtained from the electronic medical record and included age (greater or less than 60 years old), sex, disease stage at diagnosis per AJCC 8th edition, HPV by PCR or p16 status, smoking status (grouped as never-smokers vs. ever-smokers, where ever-smokers were defined as former or current smokers), alcohol use, tumor subsite (oral cavity, oropharynx, larynx, hypopharynx, nasopharynx, paranasal sinuses, or unknown primary), and treatment received before tumor tissue collection (chemotherapy, radiotherapy, or both).

Outcome measures included OS measured from the time of diagnosis and from the time of tumor tissue collection. Survival at 1 and 2 years measured from the date of tumor tissue collection, survival at the end of the study, and extent/burden of disease at last visit were also included in outcome data. It should be noted that for all calculations in which the extent of disease was measured, three categories were considered. These were defined as "no evidence of disease", "localized disease", and "metastatic disease". Multivariate analysis was performed for both TMB and PD-L1 groups separately.

Treatment response was measured by CT or MRI and categorized according to RECIST v1.1. Patients with complete response (CR), partial response (PR), or stable disease (SD) for at least 6 months as best overall response (BOR) were grouped in a category called "responders". Patients who progressed through the treatment (PD) without achieving a response as above were called "nonresponders". Progression-free survival (PFS) was measured from the first day of treatment with ICI to the day of confirmed tumor progression, or to the day of death if the patient died before tumor progression was documented, or until the last visit if there was no tumor progression.

Statistical Analysis

Descriptive statistics were calculated for all variables. These included means and standard deviations for continuous measures and counts and percentages for categorical measures. TMB and PD-L1 levels were portioned into tiers as described above (TMB into 2 tiers and PD-L1 into 2 or 3 tiers). We then examined the association between categorical variables and the TMB/PD-L1 groupings using Fisher's exact test (for binary variables) and chi-square test for categorical variables with 3 or more levels. Continuous variables were compared across TMB/PD-L1 groups using t-tests (for 2 tier groups) and one-way analysis of variance models for 3tPD-L1. Time-to-event data were examined in two ways: one examining time from diagnosis until event (i.e., death) and the second examining time from testing until event. Kaplan–Meier curves were generated for examining survival distributions both overall and by TMB or PD-L1 groups. Log-rank tests were used to compare groups. Next, Cox proportional hazards regression models were fit to examine the relationship of TMB or PD-L1 groups with survival after adjusting for patient level characteristics including age, tobacco use, tumor site, stage at diagnosis, and prior treatment with combined chemoradiation therapy. Next, we evaluated treatment response to immunotherapy as BOR and PFS. Fisher's exact tests and chi-square tests (as described above) were used to determine whether PD-L1 and TMB categories were associated with the BOR treatment categories. We compared average PFS days between responders and nonresponders using a 2-sample t-test. Next, we compared PFS days by PD-L1 and TMB categories as described above using 1-way ANOVA models and PD-L1 and TMB levels (as continuous values) using Pearson correlations. Hazard ratios and corresponding 95% confidence intervals were estimated from these proportional hazard regression models. In all analyses, an alpha level of 0.05 was used to determine the significance of data. Statistical analysis system (SAS) 9.4 was used to perform all analyses in this study.

3. Results

3.1. Patient Characteristics

In total, 139 patients met inclusion criteria for this study. Of these, 128 patients had TMB results, 95 patients had PD-L1, and 92 patients had results for both metrics. The demographic and disease characteristics of the patients included in this analysis are available for review in Table 1. Age, race, and gender in this study are congruent with a standard population of patients with HNSCC.

Table 1. Characteristics of all patients included in the study.

Characteristics	TMB Patients No. (%)	PD-L1 Patients No. (%)	Characteristics	TMB Patients No. (%)	PD-L1 Patients No. (%)
Age at Diagnosis (Years)			**Primary Tumor Location**		
Median	60	61	Nasopharynx	8 (6.2)	7 (7.4)
≥60	64 (50)	50 (52.6)	Oropharynx	50 (39.1)	37 (38.9)
<60	64 (50)	45 (47.4)	Oral Cavity	33 (25.8)	23 (24.2)
			Hypopharynx	7 (5.5)	5 (5.3)
Gender			Larynx	22 (17.2)	16 (16.8)
Male	89 (69.5)	68 (71.6)	Sino-Nasal	5 (3.9)	4 (4.2)
Female	39 (30.4)	27 (28.4)	Unknown	3 (2.3)	3 (3.2)
Race			**Disease Stage at Time of Diagnosis**		
Caucasian	108 (84.4)	79 (83.2)			
African American	13 (10.2)	13 (13.7)			
Other	7 (5.4)	3 (3.1)	**Cancer Stage**		
			I	19 (14.8)	17 (17.9)
ETOH Status			II	21 (16.4)	18 (18.9)
Never	63 (49.2)	46 (48.4)	III	29 (22.7)	15 (15.8)
Former	28 (21.9)	22 (23.2)	IV	59 (46.1)	45 (47.4)
Active	37 (28.9)	27 (28.4)			
			Cancer Stage IV		
Smoking Status			IVA	39 (66.1)	29 (64.4)
Never	37 (28.9)	29 (30.5)	IVB	14 (23.7)	11 (24.4)
Former	39 (30.5)	30 (31.6)	IVC	6 (10.2)	5 (11.2)
Active	52 (40.6)	36 (37.9)			
			N Stage		
HPV and/or p16			N0	37 (28.9)	27 (28.4)
Negative	56 (43.8)	43 (45.3)	N1	29 (22.7)	20 (21.1)
Positive	40 (31.2)	29 (30.5)	N2	49 (38.3)	37 (38.9)
Not Tested	32 (25)	23 (24.2)	N3	13 (10.1)	11 (11.6)
BMI			**Tissue Source**		
<18.5	19 (14.7)	11 (11.9)	Primary Tumor	83 (65.4)	55 (60.4)
18.5–24.9	42 (32.6)	33 (35.9)	Regional Node	11 (8.7)	10 (11.0)
25–29.9	39 (30.2)	30 (32.6)	Metastatic Lesion	11 (8.7)	9 (9.9)
≥30	29 (22.5)	18 (19.6)	Recurrence	22 (17.3)	17 (18.7)

Abbreviations: BMI, body mass index; HPV, human papilloma virus; PD-L1, programmed death ligand-1; TMB, tumor mutational burden.

3.2. Prevalence of PD-L1 and TMB within the Study Population and Correlation between the Two Variables

Of the 95 patients with recorded measurements of PD-L1 expression, 80 patients (84%) had results from testing performed by F1, and 15 patients (16%) had results from testing performed by the Mayo Clinic Laboratory. PD-L1 was measured by TPS in 52 patients (55%) and by CPS in the remaining 43 patients (45%). The mean PD-L1 score was 26.41% (standard deviation 33.78). The median score was 10%. Twelve patients (13%) had 3tPD-L1-(0). In addition, 46 patients (48%) had 3tPD-L1-(1–19), and 37 patients (39%) had 3tPD-L1-(20+) (Figure 2A). The 2tPD-L1 re-distribution resulted in 58 patients (61%) in the 2tPD-L1-(<20) group and 37 patients (39%) in the 2tPD-L1-(20+) group.

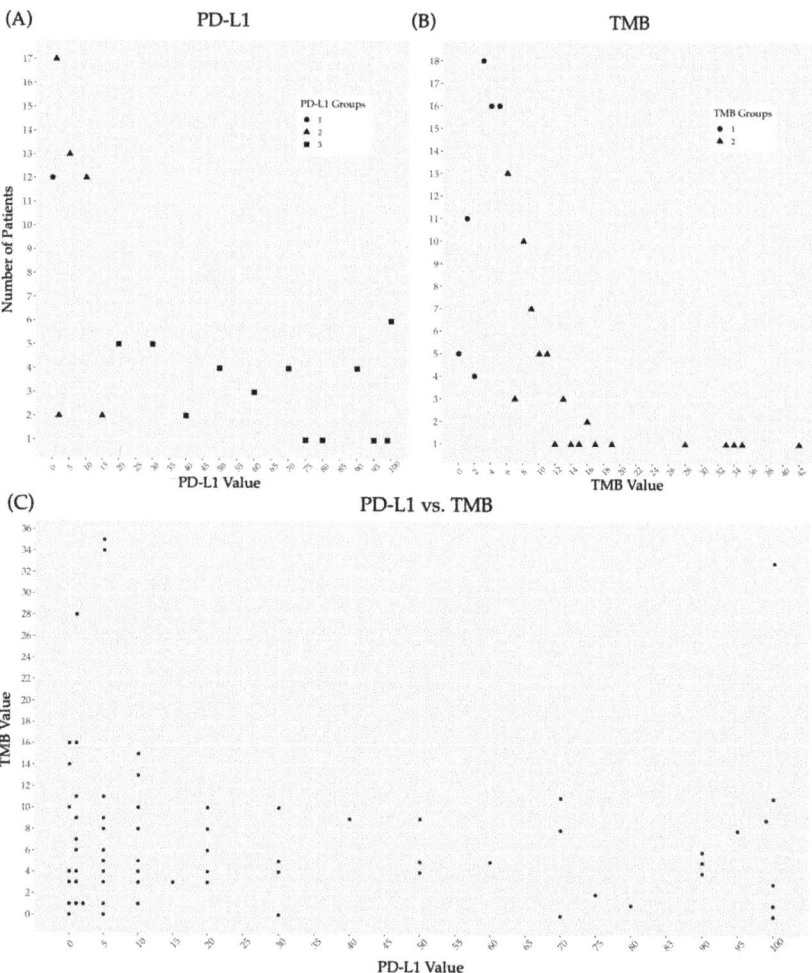

Figure 2. Distribution of continuous PD-L1 and continuous TMB and scatter plot demonstrating the relationship between each. (**A**) Distribution of PD-L1 across 3tPD-L1-(0) (group 1, circles), 3tPD-L1-(1–19) (group 2, triangles) and 3tPD-L1-(20+) (group 3, squares); (**B**) Distribution of TMB across TMB-(<6) (group 1, circles) and TMB-(6+) (group 2, triangles); (**C**) Scatter plot demonstrating the failure of PD-L1 to correlate to TMB. Abbreviations: PD-L1, programmed death ligand-1; and TMB, tumor mutational burden.

The mean TMB of the 128 patients included in TMB analysis was 6.98 mut/Mb (standard deviation 6.85), and the median was 5.0 mut/Mb. The TMB-(<6) category consisted of 70 patients (55%), and 58 patients (45%) were in the TMB-(6+) category (Figure 2B).

A total of 92 patients had both PD-L1 and TMB testing results available. Of these, 12 patients (13%) were in the 3tPD-L1-(0) category, 44 patients (48%) were in the 3tPD-L1-(1–19) category, and 35 patients (39%) were in the 3tPD-L1-(20+) category. In addition, 38 patients (42%) were in the TMB-(6+) category, and 53 patients (58%) were in the TMB-(<6) category. There were no statistically significant correlations identified between PD-L1 expression and TMB as categorical variables ($p = 0.84$) (Figure 2C).

3.3. Correlation between PD-L1 Expression and Patient Characteristics

African Americans had statistically significant higher PD-L1 expression than Caucasians, with 69.2% vs. 35.4% classified in the 2tPD-L1 $\geq$ 20 ($p = 0.04$). The analysis lost statistical significance in the three-tiered variant. There were no significant correlations identified between age or gender and 3tPD-L1 or 2tPD-L1, although it was noted that patients older than 60 and women regardless of age had a tendency toward higher PD-L1 expression. There was no significant correlation between HPV status and PD-L1, both in 2tPD-L1 ($p = 0.74$) and 3tPD-L1 ($p = 0.35$) analysis; however, in the 3tPD-L1 analysis it was noted that there were no HPV-positive patients in the 3tPD-L1-(0) category, while 18.6% of HPV-negative patients were 3tPD-L1-(0) (Table 2).

Table 2. Correlation of select demographic and patient specific data with 3-tiered-PD-L1 and 2-tiered TMB categories.

Variable		3tPD-L1 Analysis				TMB Analysis		
		No. (Row %)			p	No. (Row %)		p
		$\geq$20	1–19	0		$\geq$6	<6	
Age	<60	14 (31.1)	25 (55.6)	6 (13.3)	0.240	31 (48.4)	33 (51.6)	0.478
	$\geq$60	23 (46.0)	21 (42.0)	6 (12.0)		27 (42.2)	37 (57.8)	
Gender	Male	24 (35.3)	35 (51.5)	9 (13.2)	0.510	37 (41.6)	52 (58.4)	0.199
	Female	13 (48.1)	11 (40.7)	3 (11.1)		21 (53.8)	18 (46.2)	
Race	Caucasian	28 (35.4)	41 (51.9)	10 (12.7)	**0.046**	52 (48.1)	56 (51.9)	0.087
	AA	9 (69.2)	2 (15.4)	2 (15.4)		3 (23.1)	10 (76.9)	
HPV	+	11 (38.0)	18 (62.1)	0 (0.0)	0.354	16 (40.0)	24 (60.0)	0.804
	−	18 (41.9)	17 (39.5)	8 (18.6)		21 (37.5)	35 (62.5)	
Smoking History	Current	12 (33.3)	17 (47.2)	7 (19.4)	**0.044**	31 (59.6)	21 (40.4)	**0.029**
	Former	10 (33.3)	16 (53.3)	4 (13.3)		13 (33.3)	26 (66.7)	
	Never	15 (51.7)	13 (44.8)	1 (3.4)		14 (37.8)	23 (62.2)	
Alcohol History	Current	7 (25.9)	15 (55.6)	5 (18.5)	**0.012**	18 (48.6)	19 (51.4)	0.326
	Former	6 (27.3)	12 (54.5)	4 (18.2)		15 (53.6)	13 (46.4)	
	Never	24 (52.2)	19 (41.3)	3 (6.5)		25 (39.7)	38 (60.3)	
BMI	$\geq$30	10 (55.5)	7 (38.9)	1 (5.6)	0.072	9 (31.0)	20 (69.0)	0.071
	<30	25 (33.8)	37 (50.0)	12 (16.2)		50 (50.0)	50 (50.0)	
Previous CRT	+	15 (41.7)	16 (44.4)	5 (13.9)	0.868	23 (51.1)	22 (48.9)	0.331
	−	22 (37.3)	30 (50.8)	7 (11.9)		35 (42.2)	48 (57.8)	
Primary Tumor Location	OC	10 (43.5)	11 (47.8)	2 (8.7)	0.400	16 (48.5)	17 (51.5)	0.685
	Other	21 (36.2)	28 (48.3)	9 (15.5)		35 (44.3)	44 (55.7)	
	Laryngeal	6 (37.5)	8 (50)	2 (12.5)	0.984	16 (72.7)	6 (27.3)	**0.004**
	OTT	25 (38.5)	31 (47.7)	9 (13.8)		35 (38.9)	55 (61.1)	
	OP	15 (40.5)	16 (43.2)	6 (16.2)	0.965	15 (30.0)	35 (70.0)	**0.003**
	Other	16 (36.4)	23 (52.3)	5 (11.4)		36 (58.1)	26 (41.9)	

Table 2. Cont.

Variable		3tPD-L1 Analysis				TMB Analysis		
		No. (Row %)			p	No. (Row %)		p
		≥20	1–19	0		≥6	<6	
Stage at Diagnosis	I	10 (58.8)	7 (41.2)	0 (0.0)	0.035	7 (36.8)	12 (63.2)	0.522
	II	7 (38.9)	11 (61.1)	0 (0.0)		11 (52.4)	10 (45.5)	
	III	4 (26.7)	6 (40.0)	5 (33.3)		11 (37.9)	18 (62.1)	
	IV	16 (35.6)	22 (48.9)	7 (15.6)		29 (49.2)	30 (50.8)	
	IVA	5 (71.4)	2 (28.6)	0 (0.0)	0.802	22 (56.4)	17 (43.6)	0.146
	IVB	13 (59.1)	6 (27.3)	3 (13.6)		5 (35.7)	9 (64.3)	
	IVC	11 (68.8)	3 (18.8)	2 (12.5)		2 (33.3)	4 (66.7)	
	T0–2	20 (46.5)	23 (53.5)	0 (0.0)	*0.008*	23 (42.6)	31 (57.4)	0.864
	T3–4	17 (54.8)	2 (6.5)	12 (38.7)		39 (52.7)	35 (47.3)	
	N0	11 (40.7)	10 (37.0)	6 (19.4)	0.949	17 (45.9)	20 (54.1)	0.751
	N1	9 (45.0)	11 (55.0)	0 (0.0)		11 (37.9)	18 (62.1)	
	N2	13 (35.1)	20 (54.0)	4 (10.8)		24 (49.0)	25 (51.0)	
	N3	4 (36.3)	5 (45.5)	2 (18.2)		6 (46.2)	7 (53.8)	
	M0	34 (38.2)	43 (48.3)	12 (13.5)	0.372	54 (45.0)	66 (55.0)	0.784
	M1	3 (50.0)	3 (50.0)	0 (0.0)		4 (50.0)	4 (50.0)	

Results with $p \leq 0.05$ are bolded in italics; results with $0.05 < p < 0.10$ are italicized and underlined. 3tPD-L1, 3-tiered PD-L1; AA, African American; BMI, Body Mass Index; CRT, chemoradiotherapy; HPV, human papilloma virus; OC, oral cavity; OP, oropharyngeal; OTT, other throat tumors; PD-L1, programmed death ligand-1; and TMB, tumor mutational burden.

In the evaluation of modifiable traits, current nonsmokers had a significantly higher percentage of patients in the 3tPD-L1-(20+) category when compared with current smokers (51.7% vs. 33.3%; $p = 0.04$). The same significance held true when never-smokers were compared to ever-smokers (current and former smokers) ($p = 0.04$). Similarly, PD-L1 and alcohol use were associated in a statistically significant manner. More than half of never-drinkers (52.2%) vs. only 25.9% of drinkers were within the 3tPD-L1-(20+) category ($p = 0.01$). The statistical advantage was maintained in the 2tPD-L1 analysis ($p = 0.04$). Low PD-L1 was also noted to be associated with low BMI, but this trend did not reach significance (2tPD-L1 $p = 0.088$ and 3tPD-L1 $p = 0.07$). Exposure to radiotherapy, chemotherapy, or to chemoradiotherapy before tumor tissue collection for NGS or PD-L1 testing did not correlate with either PD-L1 analysis.

There was no correlation found between 2tPD-L1 or 3tPD-L1 expression and the primary tumor site ($p = 0.36$ and $p = 0.61$, respectively), and no trends were identified to influence further analysis.

A statistically significant correlation was found in the 3tPD-L1 analysis of the disease stage (I–IV) at diagnosis, with a higher percentage of patients with early-stage disease having 3tPD-L1-(20+) (58.8% patients with stage I disease vs. 35.6% with stage IV disease; $p = 0.04$). In particular, PD-L1 associated with tumor stage but not with nodal stage. In early tumor stages (T0–T2), 46.5% of patients were identified with 3tPD-L1-(20+) vs. only 32.7% of patients with tumor stages T3–T4, and 0% patients with early T stage vs. 23% of patients with advanced T stages were in the 3tPD-L1-(0) group ($p < 0.01$).

3.4. Correlation between TMB and Patient Characteristics

Due to the extremely low proportion of patients within TMB 20+ category (just five patients) in the three-tiered TMB variable (Figure 2B), no attempts were made to a three-tiered TMB correlative analysis. Going forward, all references are limited to the two-tiered TMB analysis. There were no significant correlations found between the TMB and age ($p = 0.48$) or gender. There was a notably higher proportion of women in the TMB-(6+) group (53.8% vs. 41.6%), but the association was not statistically significant ($p = 0.20$). Correlation of TMB with race showed that 48.1% of Caucasians vs. only 23 % of African

Americans had a TMB-(6+) ($p = 0.09$). Of note, there was no correlation between TMB and HPV status ($p = 0.80$).

Active tobacco users were significantly more likely to be in the TMB-(6+) category when compared to former and never-smokers (60% vs. 33.3% and vs. 37.8%; $p = 0.03$). There was no significant association between TMB and alcohol use. Patients with a body mass index (BMI) great than 30 were more likely to have low TMB-(<6) (69% vs. 50%), but this trend failed to meet statistical significance ($p = 0.07$). Patients with previous exposure to chemoradiotherapy (CRT) before tumor tissue collection were more likely to be in the TMB-(6+) category but this trend did not reach significance ($p = 0.09$). Exposure to treatment with radiation or chemotherapy or both prior to tissue collection was not associated with TMB.

A strongly significant correlation was found between TMB and primary tumor location ($p < 0.01$). Specifically, the patients within the TMB-(6+) category were significantly more likely to have cancers of the larynx in comparison to other locations (72.7% vs. 38.9%; $p < 0.01$) and significantly less likely to have cancers of the oropharynx as opposed to other locations (29.4% vs. 70.6%; $p < 0.01$). The stage at the time of diagnosis (I–IV) did not correlate to TMB. Similarly, there was no correlation between T stage, N stage, or M stage and TMB.

3.5. Prognostic Value of PD-L1 Expression

For all patients with PD-L1 expression data, the median follow-up time for testing was 588 days from the time of diagnosis with a median survival time of 791 days (95% CI 708 to 1199 days). Overall, 47 patients (66%) were alive at one year from diagnosis and 13 (23.2%) were alive at two years from diagnosis. Survival at one or two years was not associated with PD-L1 expression level. More than half of surviving patients (67%) had residual disease at last visit. There was no correlation between PD-L1 groups and the extent of disease at last visit.

PD-L1 expression did not correlate to survival in 2tPD-L1 or 3tPD-L1 analysis from time of tissue collection or from time of diagnosis. In the 2tPD-L1 analysis, the median survival in the 2tPD-L1-(<20) group was 521 days (95% CI 412–1008 days) and was not significantly different from median survival in the 2tPD-L1-(20+) group, 541 days (95% CI 415–666 days) ($p = 0.89$). Survival from time of diagnosis was also found to be insignificantly different between 2tPD-L1 groups where the median survival in the 2tPD-L1-(<20) group was 1044 days (95% CI 711–1292 days) and the median survival in the 2tPD-L1-(20+) group was 752 days (95% CI 504–1320 days) ($p = 0.47$). Differences in survival between 3tPD-L1 groups were similarly unimpressive in regard to time from tissue collection and diagnosis ($p = 0.95$ and $p = 0.51$, respectively). Additional information regarding correlation between PD-L1 and outcome/survival can be found in Table 3, Table 4, and Figure 3. In an adjusted Cox proportional hazard regression model, the impact of the 3t-PD-L1 variable was not related to survival when controlled for age, smoking, nodal status, subsite, and exposure to CRT ($p = 0.09$) and related to poorer OS in the two-tiered analysis ($p = 0.03$) (Tables 3 and 4). When TMB score was added to the adjusted variables above, the 2tPD-L1 more accurately could predict survival; however, this, too, did not quite reach significance ($p = 0.051$) (Table 4).

3.6. Prognostic Value of TMB

For all patients with TMB score data, the median follow-up time was 616 days from the time of cancer diagnosis with a median survival from diagnosis of 521 days (95% CI 412–1008 days). Overall, 72 patients (69.9%) were alive at one year from diagnosis, and 25 (30.86%) were alive at two years from diagnosis. At the time of the last visit, 39% of patients had no evidence of disease, 24% had recurrent or progressive locoregional disease, 12% had metastatic disease, and 25% had locoregional and metastatic disease. There was no association between disease status at last visit and TMB ($p = 0.39$).

Table 3. Association of high PD-L1 expression and TMB with survival outcomes.

Survival Start Time Point	Overall Survival Univariate Analysis for Highest Scores			Overall Survival Adjusted Analysis for Highest Scorers			1 Year OS	2 Year OS
	HR	95% CI	p value	HR	95% CI	p value	p values	
2tPD-L1								
From Time of Diagnosis	1.28	0.72–2.27	0.473	2.02	(1.06–3.86)	<u>*0.033*</u>	0.951	0.320
From Time of Sample Collection	1.05	0.57–1.97	0.888					
3tPD-L1								
From Time of Diagnosis	0.97	0.42–2.22	0.938	1.28	(0.46–3.61)	<u>*0.092*</u>	0.522	0.386
From Time of Sample Collection	0.95	0.41–2.24	0.949					
TMB								
From Time of Diagnosis	0.51	0.30–0.86	<u>*0.081*</u>	0.49	(0.27–0.90)	<u>*0.021*</u>	0.950	0.121
From Time of Sample Collection	0.63	0.37–1.06	<u>*0.014*</u>					

Results with $p < 0.05$ are bolded in italics and underlined; results with $0.05 < p < 0.10$ are italicized and underlined. Abbreviations: 3tPD-L1, 3-tiered PD-L1; 2tPD-L1, 2-tiered PD-L1; CI, confidence interval; HR, hazard ratio; PD-L1, programmed death ligand-1; OS, overall survival; and TMB, tumor mutational burden.

Table 4. Results from adjusted Cox proportional hazard regression models of impact of the presence of PD-L1 and TMB on overall survival.

	3tPD-L1			TMB			TMB and 2tPD-L1					
	HR	95% CI	p	HR	95% CI	p	PD-L1 HR	PD-L1 95% CI	PD-L1 p	TMB HR	TMB 95% CI	TMB p
Highest Scoring Groups	1.28	(0.46–3.61)	<u>*0.092*</u>	0.49	(0.27–0.90)	<u>*0.021*</u>	1.99	(1.0–3.97)	<u>*0.051*</u>	0.35	(0.16–0.76)	<u>*0.008*</u>
	p values for Adjusted Variables			p values for Adjusted Variables			p values for Adjusted Variables					
Age Below 60 Years Old (yes vs. no)	0.52			0.508			0.656					
Smoking (never vs. ever)	<u>*0.016*</u>			<u>*0.058*</u>			<u>*0.005*</u>					
N Stage (N0, N1, N2, N3)	<u>*0.003*</u>			0.709			<u>*0.007*</u>					
Subsite (OP vs. OC vs Pharynx vs. other)	0.338			0.126			0.518					
Previous CRT (yes vs. no)	<u>*0.027*</u>			<u>*0.0209*</u>			0.182					

Analyses with $p < 0.05$ are bolded in italics and underlined; results with $0.05 < p < 0.10$ are italicized and underlined; Abbreviations: 2tPD-L1, 2-tiered PD-L1; 3tPD-L1, 3-tiered PD-L1; CI, confidence interval; HR, hazard ratio; N/A, nonapplicable; CRT, combined chemotherapy and radiation therapy; PD-L1, programmed death ligand-1; and TMB, tumor mutational burden.

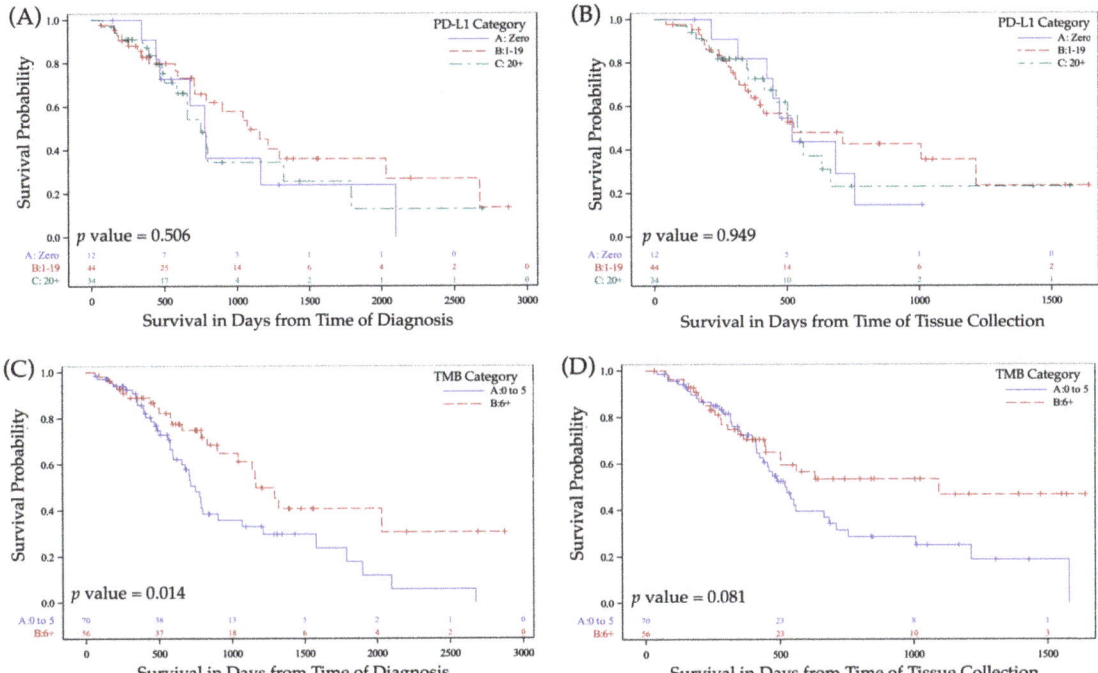

Figure 3. Kaplan–Meier curves for PD-L1 and TMB variables. (**A**) Survival from time of diagnosis in patients with 3tPD-L1-(20+) vs. 3tPD-L1-(1–19) vs. 3tPD-L1-(0); (**B**) Survival from time of tissue acquisition in patients with 3tPD-L1-(20+) vs. 3tPD-L1-(1–19) vs. 3tPD-L1-(0); (**C**) Survival from time of diagnosis in patients with TMB-(6+) vs. TMB-(<6); (**D**) Survival from time of tissue acquisition in patients with TMB-(6+) vs. TMB-(<6). Abbreviations: PD-L1, programmed death ligand-1; 3tPD-L1-(20+), PD-L1 $\geq$ 20; 3tPD-L1-(1–19), 0 < PD-L1 < 20; 3tPD-L1-(0), PD-L1=0; and TMB, tumor mutational burden; TMB-(<6), TMB less than 6; TMB-(6+), TMB greater than or equal to 6. Legend: Blue solid lines indicate survival curves for patients with TMB-(<6) or with 3tPD-L1-(0); Red dashed lines indicate survival curves for patients with TMB-(6+) or with 3tPD-L1-(1–19); Green dashed lines indicate curves for patients with 3tPD-L1-(20+) in the 3tPD-L1 analysis. Abbreviations: PD-L1, programmed death-ligand1; and TMB, tumor mutational burden.

Generally, patients within the TMB-(6+) category fared better than those within the TMB-(<6) category, but differences in survival at 1 and 2 years were not significant (Table 3). Survival from the time of diagnosis was significantly better in patients within TMB-(6+) (752 days (95% CI 599–905 days) and 1165 days (95% CI beginning at 902 with the upper limit not yet reached, $p = 0.01$). When considered from the time of tumor sample collection, survival was only marginally better in the TMB-(6+) category ($p = 0.08$). The survival significance from the time of diagnosis was upheld in an adjusted Cox proportional hazard regression model of survival controlled for PD-L1 category, age, smoking, nodal status, subsite, and previous exposure to CRT ($p = 0.02$). This remained significant in an analysis in which 2tPD-L1 was added to the analysis ($p < 0.01$) (Table 3, Table 4, and Figure 3).

3.7. Treatment with PD-L1/PD-1 Inhibitors and Correlation with PD-L1 and TMB

A total of 79 patients in this study received at least one treatment with an ICI. Treatment efficacy was able to be evaluated in 51 of these patients. Of the 28 patients that could not be evaluated, nine patients (32%) received a planned treatment with less than three administrations of a PD-L1 inhibitor in a neoadjuvant setting and were not able to be evaluated for treatment efficacy. Nineteen patients (68%) had treatment cessation before the initial scans to measure therapeutic response, due to treatment toxicity, poor tolerance, continued rapid progression of malignancy leading to complications or hospice transitions, or decision to discontinue treatment by the patient for other reasons. Of the 51 patients with measurable response, there were 27 patients who progressed, 3 patients with stable disease, 10 patients with partial response, and 11 patients with complete response. In total, 44 of the 51 patients were treated with pembolizumab, and only two patients were treated with a PD-L1 inhibitor within a clinical protocol (Supplementary Table S1). In all analyses regarding response to ICI, patients who had CR, PR, or SD with more than 6 months duration were grouped in a category referred as "responders" and were compared against patients with tumor progression referred to as "nonresponders". Amongst all 51 patients, 24 patients were categorized as responders, and 27 patients were categorized as nonresponders. Responders received an average 19.6 (range: 3–35) administrations of an ICI, while nonresponders received only 5.3 (2–9) administrations. The average PFS was 910 days for patients with CR, 388 days for patients with PR, 237 days for the patients with SD, and 109 days for patients with PD. PFS was statistically significantly longer in responders with an average of 661.7 days (185 to 1825 days) vs. nonresponders who had an average of 109 days (63–190 days) ($p < 0.01$).

Of the 51 evaluable patients, there were 36 patients with available PD-L1 expression data with 19 patients defined as responders and 17 patients as nonresponders. There were no associations found between PD-L1 level and response to treatment with ICI. When compared as a continuous variable, the mean PD-L1 was 26.4 (95% CI 9.6–43.2) in responders vs. 26.5 (95% CI 11.0–41.9) in nonresponders ($p = 0.99$). When compared as a three-tiered variable, the percentage of responders and nonresponders in the 3tPD-L1-(0) category was 10.5% and 11.6%, respectively, and 36.8% and 41.1% in the 3tPD-L1-(20+) category ($p = 0.89$). Similarly, there were no associations identified between PD-L1 and PFS in patients treated with ICIs. PFS was 208 days for 3tPD-L1-(0), 374 days for 3tPD-L1-(1–19), and 404 days for the 3tPD-L1-(20+) category ($p = 0.66$). There was no significant correlation between PD-L1 measured as a continues variable and PFS ($p = 0.62$)

There were 40 patients with available TMB data that were able to be evaluated for treatment response, with 20 patients categorized as responders and 20 patients categorized as nonresponders. There was a statistically significant association between the response to treatment with ICI and continuous TMB, with a mean TMB of 11.3 mut/Mb (95% CI 6.6 mut/Mb-16.0 mut/Mb) in responders and 4.9 mut/Mb (95% CI 3.4 mut/Mb-6.4 mut/Mb) in nonresponders ($p = 0.01$). Correlation of treatment response with TMB as a categorical variable demonstrated a similar correlation, with 12 responders (60% of the total responders) and 6 nonresponders (30% of the total responders) found within the TMB-(6+) category ($p = 0.056$). Similarly, there was a statistically significant association of TMB with PFS when analyzed as a continues variable ($p = 0.01$), and statistical significance was maintained in a categorical analysis, with PFS found to be 261.7 days in the TMB-(0–5) and 538.7 in the TMB-(6+) ($p = 0.04$).

4. Discussion

The establishment of PD-L1 ICIs has brought about a new era in the management of patients with HNSCC. Efforts in clinical research are now focused on defining strategies to increase the efficacy of PD-L1 ICIs by identifying those who are best suited to receive these therapies. PD-L1 and TMB have been the dominant targets investigated as potential biomarkers of response to ICIs, yet, especially in HNSCC, the results remain not only scarce but frequently inconsistent.

In this single-institution retrospective analysis, the PD-L1 and TMB data of 132 HN-SCC patients (95 patients with PD-L1 data, 128 patients with TMB data, and 91 patients with both PD-L1 and TMB data) were correlated with their demographics, survival and, when appropriate, response to ICI. This study population is consistent with a standard HNSCC population in terms of age, gender, race, smoking, and HPV status (Table 1). Conventional prognostication tools held true in this analysis. Smoking, as well as advanced nodal stage were associated with worse survival in a multivariate analysis (Table 4). Both

PD-L1 and TMB were measured with standardized, commercially available methods. To the authors' knowledge, this is one of few studies involving a comprehensive analysis of both TMB and PD-L1 in a dedicated HNSCC population, utilizing universally available, standardized measurements of each variable. Published studies present frequently conflicting results, most likely affected by variations in the utilized assays, as well as variations in the thresholds used to define results.

The median PD-L1 score in this study was 10%, and 87% of patients with PD-L1 data expressed PD-L1 positivity (PD-L1 expression ≥ 1). This proportion of PD-L1 positive disease is slightly higher than previous HNSCC cohorts analyzed in the literature where studies have demonstrated positivity rates between 57% and 82% [5,10,11]. It was thought that earlier disease stage might account for this finding, as significantly more patients in this study who were diagnosed at an earlier stage (overall and with respect to T stage alone) were found to have higher PD-L1 expression (Table 2), and there was a relative surplus of early-stage patients in the study cohort in comparison to the predominance of recurrent/metastatic disease in cohorts from the literature.

PD-L1 was evaluated as both a three-tiered and two-tiered variable. The tier cutoff points of the 3tPD-L1 variable were influenced by the KEYNOTE-048 study [32]. Although the three tiered approach had the considerable advantage of distinguishing PD-L1 negative disease (3tPD-L1-(0)), an important category in the decision tree guiding therapy in the current standard first line management of metastatic/recurrent HNSCC, the distribution of the patients in the resultant groups were dissimilar. In an attempt to help offset the bias introduced by the lack of uniformity in the methods used to measure PD-L1 expression (TPS vs. CPS) and the low number of patients in the 3tPD-L1-(0) group, the decision was made to combine the lower two categories into a single group, thereby generating the two-tiered variable (2tPD-L1). Ultimately, there were more significant associations between the 3tPD-L1 variable and demographic data, thus illustrating the importance of distinguishing PD-L1 positivity from PD-L1 negativity in HNSCC.

The median TMB analyzed was 5 mut/Mb, consistent with other reports [33]. Although the split of TMB between groups was based on Foundation Medicine guideline, the groups would be similar for a threshold based on median TMB, with 70 patients in the TMB-(<6) group and 58 patients in the TMB-(6+) group. Similar to the reports in HNSCC [27,28] and in other malignancies [24,33,34], this study demonstrated that there was no significant relationship between PD-L1 and TMB, reflecting the dynamic interactions between the two variables.

This study is the first to demonstrate an association between higher PD-L1 expression and the African American race. This held true in both the 2tPD-L1 and the 3tPD-L1 analysis. Notably, the 3tPD-L1 analysis also correlated Caucasian race to lower PD-L1 in a statistically significant manner. Conversely, a higher proportion of Caucasians had high TMB-(6+) than African Americans (48.1% vs. 23%), although this higher proportion was not statistically significant.

A study of The Cancer Genome Atlas (TCGA) HNSCC population did not find any significant correlation between TMB and race or gender but did identify a statistically significant association between high TMB and age above 60 [34]. This finding was confirmed by other reports on the same public TCGA HNSCC database [35] as well as in another study involving 100,000 human cancer genomes in which many malignancies were considered [33]. Such correlations of TMB or PD-L1 with age were not identified in this study.

Female gender was the only category in this analysis to show a trend toward both higher PD-L1 expression (48% of females vs. 35.3% of males were in the 3tPD-L1-(20+) group) and higher TMB (53.8% of females vs. 41.6% of males were in the TMB-(6+) group). This trend did not reach statistical significance possibly due to the inherent lower number of females inflicted by this type of cancer and subsequently being included in our analysis. Similar association of PD-L1 overexpression with female gender was reported by two studies in patients with oral cavity SCC [36,37], while a retrospective study of patients with oropharyngeal HNSCC reported no significant difference in age and gender and PD-L1 expression [38].

Smokers were found to have both a lower level of PD-L1 expression and higher TMB, compared with never-smokers or former smokers. This TMB finding is further supported by two other recent reports. One such project was dedicated to a population size similar to this study [28] and another analyzed the TCGA-HNSCC [34]. Our study additionally demonstrated an association between alcohol consumption and lower PD-L1 expression. A review of the literature revealed two studies, focused on oral cavity SCC on this topic (a meta-analysis [36] and a smaller retrospective study of 55 patients [39]) which found a similar significant relationship between low-PD-L1 with alcohol consumption.

There are no consensus data regarding HPV status in association with PD-L1 and TMB. Previous studies in HNSCC concerning patients treated with surgery and adjuvant CRT [40] and those with oropharyngeal primaries [41] reported a significant correlation of PD-L1 expression with p16 status. Conversely, another study regarding patients with oropharyngeal SCC did not identify any significant difference in PD-L1 expression between HPV positive and negative tumors [38]. Similarly, there are conflicting data in the literature concerning the relationship between HPV/p16 and TMB. Some studies have shown that high TMB was associated with HPV negative disease [28,42], and others have demonstrated no significant correlation between the two variables [34]. There was no significant association between HPV and PD-L1 or TMB in this study. It was noted, however, that more patients with HPV negative disease were in the 3tPD-L1-(0) group (18.5% of patients), and no patients with 3tPD-L1-(0) had HPV positive disease. Although these findings did not reach significance, they support the theory that the relationships between PD-L1, TMB, and immune cell infiltration are more complicated and the immune pathways that assist in response are influenced by many components of the tumor microenvironment including HPV status, alcohol use, and/or tobacco use [42].

In this cohort, a trend that did not reach statistical significance suggested that BMI greater than 30 was associated with high PD-L1 and low TMB. Interestingly, reports in 976 patients with diverse tumors treated with PD-1/PD-L1 inhibitors showed that the response to treatment was significantly higher in overweight/obese patients compared to nonoverweight patients [43].

In concordance with two other reports on patients with HNSCC [34,44], this study found that TMB was associated with tumor location in a statistically significant way. The proportion of patients with laryngeal tumors was significantly increased, and oropharyngeal cancer decreased, in the TMB-(6+) group when compared to patients with any other throat tumor location. No correlation of PD-L1 with tumor location was identified.

Advanced cancer stage (I–IV) and advanced T stage (T3–T4 vs. T0–T2) were associated with low PD-L1 in this analysis. Of the 12 patients with PD-L1(0), seven patients had T4, and five patients had T3 tumors (Table 4). This finding is supported by a meta-analysis in patients with oral cavity SCC [36] but diverges from a study in oropharyngeal cancer [38]. Furthermore, in a review of a TCGA HNSCC population, Zhang et al. reported an association of advanced clinical stage and large tumor size with TMB rather than with PD-L1 [42]. This correlation was not identified in our study.

PD-L1 did not correlate with survival at 1 or 2 years or with OS in univariate analysis (Table 3). In the multivariate survival analysis of the 2tPD-L1 variable, 2tPD-L1-(20+) predicted worse survival comparative with 2tPD-L1-(0–19). Previous studies have found the same, including one meta-analysis and two retrospective reviews, all addressing oral cavity SCC patients [36,37,45]. Another meta-analysis in HNSCC and a study in oropharyngeal SCC patients reported no association of PDL1 expression with survival [38,46]. Conversely, three retrospective reviews of HNSCC patients reported the association of PD-L1 expression with improved OS [40,47–49].

TMB significantly correlated with OS measured from the time of diagnosis (Table 3). This significance was maintained in a Cox proportional hazards regression model when adjusted for age, tobacco use, tumor site, nodal stage at diagnosis, previous treatment with chemotherapy, radiation or combined chemoradiation therapy, and PD-L1 level in a multivariate analysis model (Table 4). Similar with PD-L1, the literature reports are controversial regarding TMB's association with survival. This is not surprising given the expected influences of disease characteristics, treatment, biopsy sites, and the variability in measurement techniques. Additionally, the finding that those in the higher TMB group had a better response to PD-L1 ICI in combination with the facts that a high proportion of our patient population had TMB-(6+) and were treated with PD-L1 ICI, most likely influenced survival in this study. Reports in the literature support the correlation between high TMB and improved OS, including the reports of univariate and multivariate survival of patients with oral cavity squamous cell cancer treated with surgery as their primary intervention [50]. Conversely, a multicenter retrospective study of patients treated with definitive CRT found a significant correlation of TMB with poor survival [51]. Finally, a study of 10,000 patients from TCGA with different tumors showed an association of TMB with response to IO but not with OS [25].

A total of 79 patients in this study received at least one treatment with an ICI, of which 51 patients were evaluable for treatment response. It should be noted that the percentage of responders in this study is higher than previously reported in the literature (26.5%), with a particularly high percentage of patients with CR (13.9%). This finding might be correlated with the fact that almost half of these patients (5 out of 11 patients) were treated with other therapeutic interventions that might have potentiate immune response to ICIs (palliative radiotherapy (three patients), combined palliative chemotherapy (one patient), and concurrent definitive chemoradiotherapy for a second head and neck cancer primary (one patient)) (Supplementary Table S1). One patient with metastatic HNSCC who achieved a durable CR (1875 days to date, with no recurrence) after just three administrations of a PD-1 inhibitor will be presented in a separate publication. Of the 51 patients with evaluable response, 40 patients had TMB results, and 36 patients had PD-L1 results. There was a statistically significant association between the response to treatment with ICI and continuous TMB score with a mean TMB of 11.2 in responders and 4.9 in nonresponders ($p = 0.01$). Evaluation as a categorical variable demonstrated that 66.6% of the responders and 33.3% of the nonresponders were within the high TMB (6+) category ($p = 0.055$). Furthermore, TMB corelated significantly with PFS in both categorical and continuous analysis. There are other published reports supporting TMB as a possible predictor of response to ICIs. In a retrospective analysis of 126 HNSCC patients treated with anti-PD-1/PD-L1 agents, TMB was found to be significantly higher among responders (21.3 vs. 8.2 mut/MB, $p < 0.01$) [28]. The study of a cohort from KEYNOTE-012 sought to characterize this further and demonstrated that TMB was predictive of response to pembrolizumab in HPV negative patients but not in HPV positive patients [29]. Finally, though the role of circulating/blood TMB has yet to be defined, retrospective studies in HNSCC have a linked response to ICI with circulating/blood TMB $\geq$ 16 mut/Mb [45,47].

There was no association between response to treatment with ICI or PFS and PD-L1 level analyzed as a categorical ($p = 0.66$ and $p = 0.89$, respectively) or continuous variable ($p = 0.62$ and $p = 0.99$, respectively). In this study, PD-L1 values were measured by both TPS (55% of patients) and CPS (45% of patients), and due to the small sample size, no attempts were made to separate the analysis of PD-L1 by the reporting technique and correlate each of these distinct groups with PFS or response to treatment with ICI. It should be noted that the literature suggests that such an analysis could yield a different result; KEYNOTE-040 and -048 reported PD-L1 by CPS and demonstrated a significant correlation between PD-L1 and response to ICI [10,52,53], but CHECKMATE-141 failed to show a significant correlation between tumor response to Nivolumab and PD-L1 overexpression when PD-L1 was reported by TPS [5].

In summary, this study reported significant association of high PD-L1 expression with the African American race, nonsmoking and nonalcohol use, with early clinical cancer stage and early tumor stage, and with poor survival in a multivariate analysis. No predictive value for PFS or for BOR to ICIs was identified in the PD-L1 analysis. High TMB was reported to be significantly associated with smoking, tumor location in the larynx, and survival in both univariate and a multivariate analysis, as well as with PFS and BOR to ICIs.

Notably, this study comprehensively analyzed both PD-L1 and TMB in a dedicated HNSCC cohort. The utilization of standardized, commercially available methodologies is another unique feature among reports in HNSCC, encouraging the reproducibility and building of a consistent database. A direct comparison between TMB and PD-L1 results was not employed due to the variation of PD-L1 reporting (TPS and CPS) triggered by the more recent approval by the FDA of CPS as a companion diagnostic. The other limitations of this study include the retrospective nature of the review and a limited sample size, especially in the analysis regarding response to ICI.

Future Directions

Furthermore, additional studies are needed to generate the necessary context and framework of standardized variables aimed to predict response of HNSCC to IO in general and to ICIs in particular. The standardization of assays is the next step in assisting with the creation of consistent results and the development of thresholds for high and low scoring groups that are both sensitive and specific in HNSCC for further predictive analysis. The recent availability of TMB as a circulating biomarker that bypasses the need for tissue procurement and allows a dynamic assessment makes it a more attractive biomarker. The association of TMB with prognosis and response to ICI presented by this study and others warrants further attention and prompts the advancement of TMB in future prospective clinical studies of ICIs, with the ultimate goal of becoming a companion diagnostic for recommendation of ICIs in HNSCC.

5. Conclusions

ICIs have changed the landscape of the treatment of HNSCC. Regardless, less than 20% of the treated patients benefit from these novel therapeutics, prompting urgent studies to help identify predictors of response and improve patient selection. This study has demonstrated the utility of TMB as a prognostic variable and predictive marker of response to ICI. In addition, the study pointed to the significant association of high TMB with active tobacco use and with primary tumor location in the larynx. High PD-L1 values were associated with the African American race, high T stage, high overall disease stage, non-/ex-smokers, and non-/ex-drinkers. More information is needed to create a framework in which PD-L1 and TMB co-exist with other variables to predict response to ICI on an in-dividual level. Nonetheless, the existing data for each of these independent variables are promising in the world of precision oncology, and the results of the current study argue for the advancement of TMB in prospective research.

Supplementary Materials: The following are available online at https://www.mdpi.com/article/10.3390/cancers13225733/s1, Table S1: Characterization of Patients who Received Immunotherapy.

Author Contributions: Conceptualization, M.P., W.Z., R.B.D.J., K.M.B., C.M.F., and U.T.; methodology, M.P., R.B.D.J., K.M.B., R.T.H., T.L.J., and P.M.B.; investigation, K.M.B., J.W.L., E.G., A.A, and A.X.; formal analysis, R.B.D.J. and K.M.B.; data curation, M.P., J.W.L., A.T.F., A.A., P.M.B., and U.T.; writing—original draft preparation, J.W.L., M.P., and J.T.B.; writing—review and editing, M.P., K.M.B., J.W.L., A.T.F., E.G., J.T.B., A.X., R.T.H., T.L.J., P.M.B., C.M.F., and U.T.; visualization, K.M.B., J.W.L., A.T.F., E.G., C.J., and A.H.S.; supervision, M.P., W.Z., R.B.D.J., R.T.H., T.L.J., C.M.F., and U.T. All authors have read and agreed to the published version of the manuscript.

Funding: Biostatistical and bioinformatics services were supported by the Comprehensive Cancer Center of Wake Forest University National Cancer Institute Cancer Center Support Grant P30CA012197. Cristina M. Furdui and Mercedes Porosnicu's effort was partly supported by NIH/NCI U01 CA215848.

Institutional Review Board Statement: The study was conducted according to the guidelines of the Declaration of Helsinki and approved by the Wake Forest School of Medicine Institutional Review Board (IRB00057787).

Informed Consent Statement: Patient consent was waived in this retrospective study, as the research involved no risk for participants, and waiving consent did not adversely affect the subjects. Furthermore, all data were completely deidentified from time of its collection from the electronic medical record.

Data Availability Statement: The datasets analyzed are available from the corresponding author upon request.

Conflicts of Interest: The authors declare no conflict of interest. No outsider funding source contributed to this research, and therefore, there was no conflict of interest from a funding source.

References

1. Ferris, R.L. Immunology and immunotherapy of head and neck cancer. *J. Clin. Oncol.* **2015**, *33*, 3293. [CrossRef]
2. Mandal, R.; Şenbabaoğlu, Y.; Desrichard, A.; Havel, J.J.; Dalin, M.G.; Riaz, N.; Lee, K.-W.; Ganly, I.; Hakimi, A.A.; Chan, T.A.; et al. The head and neck cancer immune landscape and its immunotherapeutic implications. *JCI Insight* **2016**, *1*, e89829. [CrossRef] [PubMed]
3. Perri, F.; Ionna, F.; Longo, F.; Scarpati, G.D.V.; De Angelis, C.; Ottaiano, A.; Botti, G.; Caponigro, F. Immune response against head and neck cancer: Biological mechanisms and implication on therapy. *Transl. Oncol.* **2020**, *13*, 262–274. [CrossRef]
4. Seiwert, T.Y.; Burtness, B.; Mehra, R.; Weiss, J.; Berger, R.; Eder, J.P.; Heath, K.; McClanahan, T.; Lunceford, J.; Gause, C. Safety and clinical activity of pembrolizumab for treatment of recurrent or metastatic squamous cell carcinoma of the head and neck (KEYNOTE-012): An open-label, multicentre, phase 1b trial. *Lancet Oncol.* **2016**, *17*, 956–965. [CrossRef]
5. Ferris, R.L.; Blumenschein Jr, G.; Fayette, J.; Guigay, J.; Colevas, A.D.; Licitra, L.; Harrington, K.; Kasper, S.; Vokes, E.E.; Even, C. Nivolumab for recurrent squamous-cell carcinoma of the head and neck. *N. Engl. J. Med.* **2016**, *375*, 1856–1867. [CrossRef]
6. Chow, L.Q.M.; Haddad, R.; Gupta, S.; Mahipal, A.; Mehra, R.; Tahara, M.; Berger, R.; Eder, J.P.; Burtness, B.; Lee, S.-H. Antitumor activity of pembrolizumab in biomarker-unselected patients with recurrent and/or metastatic head and neck squamous cell carcinoma: Results from the phase Ib KEYNOTE-012 expansion cohort. *J. Clin. Oncol.* **2016**, *34*, 3838. [CrossRef] [PubMed]
7. Soulieres, D.; Cohen, E.; Le Tourneau, C.; Dinis, J.; Licitra, L.; Ahn, M.-J.; Soria, A.; Machiels, J.-P.; Mach, N.; Mehra, R. Abstract CT115: Updated survival results of the KEYNOTE-040 study of pembrolizumab vs standard-of-care chemotherapy for recurrent or metastatic head and neck squamous cell carcinoma 2018. In Proceedings of the AACR Annual Meeting 2018, Chicago, IL, USA, 14–18 April 2018.
8. Larkins, E.; Blumenthal, G.M.; Yuan, W.; He, K.; Sridhara, R.; Subramaniam, S.; Zhao, H.; Liu, C.; Yu, J.; Goldberg, K.B. FDA approval summary: Pembrolizumab for the treatment of recurrent head and neck squamous cell carcinoma with disease progression on or after platinum-containing chemotherapy. *Oncologist* **2017**, *22*, 873. [CrossRef]
9. Oliva, M.; Spreafico, A.; Taberna, M.; Alemany, L.; Coburn, B.; Mesia, R.; Siu, L.L. Immune biomarkers of response to immune-checkpoint inhibitors in head and neck squamous cell carcinoma. *Ann. Oncol.* **2019**, *30*, 57–67. [CrossRef]
10. Bauml, J.; Seiwert, T.Y.; Pfister, D.G. Pembrolizumab for platinum- and cetuximab-refractory head and neck cancer: Results from a single-arm, phase II study. *J. Clin. Oncol.* **2017**, *35*, 1542–1549. [CrossRef]
11. Le, X.; Ferrarotto, R.; Wise-Draper, T.; Gillison, M. Evolving Role of Immunotherapy in Recurrent Metastatic Head and Neck Cancer. *J. Natl. Compr. Cancer Netw.* **2020**, *18*, 899–906. [CrossRef]
12. Ulrich, B.C.; Guibert, N. Non-invasive assessment of tumor PD-L1 status with circulating tumor cells. *Ann. Transl. Med.* **2018**, *6*, S48. [CrossRef] [PubMed]
13. Campesato, L.F.; Barroso-Sousa, R.; Jimenez, L.; Correa, B.R.; Sabbaga, J.; Hoff, P.M.; Reis, L.F.L.; Galante, P.A.F.; Camargo, A.A. Comprehensive cancer-gene panels can be used to estimate mutational load and predict clinical benefit to PD-1 blockade in clinical practice. *Oncotarget* **2015**, *6*, 34221. [CrossRef]
14. Johnson, D.B.; Frampton, G.M.; Rioth, M.J.; Yusko, E.; Xu, Y.; Guo, X.; Ennis, R.C.; Fabrizio, D.; Chalmers, Z.R.; Greenbowe, J. Targeted next generation sequencing identifies markers of response to PD-1 blockade. *Cancer Immunol. Res.* **2016**, *4*, 959–967. [CrossRef]
15. George, T.J.; Frampton, G.M.; Sun, J.; Gowen, K.; Kennedy, M.; Greenbowe, J.R.; Schrock, A.B.; Ali, S.M.; Klempner, S.J.; Hezel, A.F. Tumor mutational burden as a potential biomarker for PD1/PD-L1 therapy in colorectal cancer. *J. Clin. Oncol.* **2016**, *34*, 3587. [CrossRef]
16. Alexandrov, L.B.; Nik-Zainal, S.; Wedge, D.C.; Aparicio, S.A.J.R.; Behjati, S.; Biankin, A.V.; Bignell, G.R.; Bolli, N.; Borg, A.; Børresen-Dale, A.-L. Signatures of mutational processes in human cancer. *Nature* **2013**, *500*, 415–421. [CrossRef] [PubMed]
17. Kowanetz, M.; Zou, W.; Shames, D.S.; Cummings, C.; Rizvi, N.; Spira, A.I.; Frampton, G.M.; Leveque, V.; Flynn, S.; Mocci, S. Tumor mutation load assessed by FoundationOne (FM1) is associated with improved efficacy of atezolizumab (atezo) in patients with advanced NSCLC. *Ann. Oncol.* **2016**, *27*, vi23. [CrossRef]
18. Rosenberg, J.E.; Hoffman-Censits, J.; Powles, T.; Van Der Heijden, M.S.; Balar, A.V.; Necchi, A.; Dawson, N.; O'Donnell, P.H.; Balmanoukian, A.; Loriot, Y. Atezolizumab in patients with locally advanced and metastatic urothelial carcinoma who have progressed following treatment with platinum-based chemotherapy: A single-arm, multicentre, phase 2 trial. *Lancet* **2016**, *387*, 1909–1920. [CrossRef]

19. Rosenberg, J.E.; Petrylak, D.P.; Van Der Heijden, M.S.; Necchi, A.; O'Donnell, P.H.; Loriot, Y.; Retz, M.; Perez-Gracia, J.L.; Bellmunt, J.; Grivas, P. PD-L1 expression, Cancer Genome Atlas (TCGA) subtype, and mutational load as independent predictors of response to atezolizumab (atezo) in metastatic urothelial carcinoma (mUC; IMvigor210). *J. Clin. Oncol.* **2016**, *34*, 104. [CrossRef]
20. Hellmann, M.D.; Ciuleanu, T.-E.; Pluzanski, A.; Lee, J.S.; Otterson, G.A.; Audigier-Valette, C.; Minenza, E.; Linardou, H.; Burgers, S.; Salman, P. Nivolumab plus ipilimumab in lung cancer with a high tumor mutational burden. *N. Engl. J. Med.* **2018**, *378*, 2093–2104. [CrossRef]
21. Legrand, F.A.; Gandara, D.R.; Mariathasan, S.; Powles, T.; He, X.; Zhang, W.; Jhunjhunwala, S.; Nickles, D.; Bourgon, R.; Schleifman, E.; et al. Association of High Tissue TMB and Atezolizumab Efficacy across Multiple Tumor Types. *J. Clin. Oncol.* **2018**, *36*, 12000. [CrossRef]
22. Snyder, A.; Makarov, V.; Merghoub, T.; Yuan, J.; Zaretsky, J.M.; Desrichard, A.; Walsh, L.A.; Postow, M.A.; Wong, P.; Ho, T.S. Genetic basis for clinical response to CTLA-4 blockade in melanoma. *N. Engl. J. Med.* **2014**, *371*, 2189–2199. [CrossRef] [PubMed]
23. Rizvi, N.A.; Hellmann, M.D.; Snyder, A.; Kvistborg, P.; Makarov, V.; Havel, J.J.; Lee, W.; Yuan, J.; Wong, P.; Ho, T.S. Mutational landscape determines sensitivity to PD-1 blockade in non–small cell lung cancer. *Science* **2015**, *348*, 124–128. [CrossRef]
24. Cristescu, R.; Mogg, R.; Ayers, M.; Albright, A.; Murphy, E.; Yearley, J.; Sher, X.; Liu, X.Q.; Lu, H.; Nebozhyn, M.; et al. Pan-tumor genomic biomarkers for PD-1 checkpoint blockade–based immunotherapy. *Science* **2018**, *362*, eaar3593. [CrossRef] [PubMed]
25. McGrail, D.J.; Pilié, P.G.; Rashid, N.U.; Voorwerk, L.; Slagter, M.; Kok, M.; Jonasch, E.; Khasraw, M.; Heimberger, A.B.; Lim, B.; et al. High tumor mutation burden fails to predict immune checkpoint blockade response across all cancer types. *Ann. Oncol.* **2021**, *32*, 661–672. [CrossRef] [PubMed]
26. Goodman, A.M.; Kato, S.; Bazhenova, L.; Patel, S.P.; Frampton, G.M.; Miller, V.; Stephens, P.J.; Daniels, G.A.; Kurzrock, R. Tumor mutational burden as an independent predictor of response to immunotherapy in diverse cancers. *Mol. Cancer Ther.* **2017**, *16*, 2598–2608. [CrossRef] [PubMed]
27. Seiwert, T.Y.; Haddad, R.; Bauml, J.; Weiss, J.; Pfister, D.G.; Gupta, S.; Mehra, R.; Gluck, I.; Kang, H.; Worden, F.; et al. Abstract LB-339: Biomarkers predictive of response to pembrolizumab in head and neck cancer (HNSCC). *Cancer Res.* **2018**, *78*, LB-339. [CrossRef]
28. Hanna, G.J.; Lizotte, P.; Cavanaugh, M.; Kuo, F.C.; Shivdasani, P.; Frieden, A.; Chau, N.G.; Schoenfeld, J.D.; Lorch, J.H.; Uppaluri, R. Frameshift events predict anti–PD-1/L1 response in head and neck cancer. *JCI Insight* **2018**, *3*, e98811. [CrossRef]
29. Haddad, R.I.; Seiwert, T.Y.; Chow, L.Q.M.; Gupta, S.; Weiss, J.; Gluck, I.; Eder, J.P.; Burtness, B.; Tahara, M.; Keam, B.; et al. Genomic Determinants of Response to Pembrolizumab in Head and Neck Squamous Cell Carcinoma (HNSCC). *J. Clin. Oncol.* **2017**, *35*, 6009. [CrossRef]
30. Li, W.; Wildsmith, S.; Ye, J.; Si, H.; Morsli, N.; He, P.; Shetty, J.; Yovine, A.J.; Holoweckyj, N.; Raja, R. Plasma-based tumor mutational burden (bTMB) as predictor for survival in phase III EAGLE study: Durvalumab (D)± tremelimumab (T) versus chemotherapy (CT) in recurrent/metastatic head and neck squamous cell carcinoma (R/M HNSCC) after platinum failure. *J. Clin. Oncol.* **2020**, *38*, 6511. [CrossRef]
31. Wang, Z.; Duan, J.; Cai, S.; Han, M.; Dong, H.; Zhao, J.; Zhu, B.; Wang, S.; Zhuo, M.; Sun, J.; et al. Assessment of Blood Tumor Mutational Burden as a Potential Biomarker for Immunotherapy in Patients with Non–Small Cell Lung Cancer with Use of a Next-Generation Sequencing Cancer Gene Panel. *JAMA Oncol.* **2019**, *5*, 696–702. [CrossRef]
32. Burtness, B.; Harrington, K.J.; Greil, R.; Soulières, D.; Tahara, M.; de Castro, G., Jr.; Psyrri, A.; Basté, N.; Neupane, P.; Bratland, Å. Pembrolizumab alone or with chemotherapy versus cetuximab with chemotherapy for recurrent or metastatic squamous cell carcinoma of the head and neck (KEYNOTE-048): A randomised, open-label, phase 3 study. *Lancet* **2019**, *394*, 1915–1928. [CrossRef]
33. Chalmers, Z.R.; Connelly, C.F.; Fabrizio, D.; Gay, L.; Ali, S.M.; Ennis, R.; Schrock, A.; Campbell, B.; Shlien, A.; Chmielecki, J. Analysis of 100,000 human cancer genomes reveals the landscape of tumor mutational burden. *Genome Med.* **2017**, *9*, 34. [CrossRef]
34. Kumar, G.; South, A.P.; Curry, J.M.; Linnenbach, A.; Harshyne, L.A.; Ertel, A.; Fortina, P.; Luginbuhl, A. Multimodal genomic markers predict immunotherapy response in the head and neck squamous cell carcinoma. *bioRxiv* **2021**. [CrossRef]
35. Zhang, Y.; Lin, A.; Li, Y.; Ding, W.; Meng, H.; Luo, P.; Zhang, J. Age and mutations as predictors of the response to immunotherapy in head and neck squamous cell cancer. *Front. Cell Dev. Biol.* **2020**, *8*, 608969. [CrossRef]
36. Lenouvel, D.; González-Moles, M.Á.; Ruiz-Ávila, I.; Gonzalez-Ruiz, L.; Gonzalez-Ruiz, I.; Ramos-García, P. Prognostic and clinicopathological significance of PD-L1 overexpression in oral squamous cell carcinoma: A systematic review and comprehensive meta-analysis. *Oral. Oncol.* **2020**, *106*, 104722. [CrossRef] [PubMed]
37. Lin, Y.-M.; Sung, W.-W.; Hsieh, M.-J.; Tsai, S.-C.; Lai, H.-W.; Yang, S.-M.; Shen, K.-H.; Chen, M.-K.; Lee, H.; Yeh, K.-T. High PD-L1 expression correlates with metastasis and poor prognosis in oral squamous cell carcinoma. *PLoS ONE* **2015**, *10*, e0142656. [CrossRef]
38. Kim, H.S.; Lee, J.Y.; Lim, S.H.; Park, K.; Sun, J.-M.; Ko, Y.H.; Baek, C.-H.; Son, Y.; Jeong, H.S.; Ahn, Y.C.; et al. Association Between PD-L1 and HPV Status and the Prognostic Value of PD-L1 in Oropharyngeal Squamous Cell Carcinoma. *Cancer Res. Treat.* **2016**, *48*, 527–536. [CrossRef] [PubMed]
39. Lenouvel, D.; González-Moles, M.Á.; Ruiz-Ávila, I.; Chamorro-Santos, C.; González-Ruiz, L.; Gonzalez-Ruiz, I.; Ramos-García, P. Clinicopathological and prognostic significance of PD-L1 in oral cancer: A preliminary retrospective immunohistochemistry study. *Oral. Dis.* **2021**, *27*, 173–182. [CrossRef]

40. Balermpas, P.; Rödel, F.; Krause, M.; Linge, A.; Lohaus, F.; Baumann, M.; Tinhofer, I.; Budach, V.; Sak, A.; Stuschke, M. The PD-1/PD-L1 axis and human papilloma virus in patients with head and neck cancer after adjuvant chemoradiotherapy: A multicentre study of the German Cancer Consortium Radiation Oncology Group (DKTK-ROG). *Int. J. Cancer* **2017**, *141*, 594–603. [CrossRef] [PubMed]
41. Steuer, C.E.; Griffith, C.C.; Nannapaneni, S.; Patel, M.R.; Liu, Y.; Magliocca, K.R.; El-Deiry, M.W.; Cohen, C.; Owonikoko, T.K.; Shin, D.M. A correlative analysis of PD-L1, PD-1, PD-L2, EGFR, HER2, and HER3 expression in oropharyngeal squamous cell carcinoma. *Mol. Cancer Ther.* **2018**, *17*, 710–716. [CrossRef]
42. Zhang, L.; Li, B.; Peng, Y.; Wu, F.; Li, Q.; Lin, Z.; Xie, S.; Xiao, L.; Lin, X.; Ou, Z.; et al. The prognostic value of TMB and the relationship between TMB and immune infiltration in head and neck squamous cell carcinoma: A gene expression-based study. *Oral. Oncol.* **2020**, *110*, 104943. [CrossRef]
43. Cortellini, A.; Bersanelli, M.; Buti, S.; Cannita, K.; Santini, D.; Perrone, F.; Giusti, R.; Tiseo, M.; Michiara, M.; Di Marino, P.; et al. A multicenter study of body mass index in cancer patients treated with anti-PD-1/PD-L1 immune checkpoint inhibitors: When overweight becomes favorable. *J. Immunother. Cancer* **2019**, *7*, 57. [CrossRef]
44. Cui, J.; Wang, D.; Nie, D.; Liu, W.; Sun, M.; Pei, F.; Han, F. Difference in tumor mutation burden between squamous cell carcinoma in the oral cavity and larynx. *Oral. Oncol.* **2021**, *114*, 105142. [CrossRef]
45. Maruse, Y.; Kawano, S.; Jinno, T.; Matsubara, R.; Goto, Y.; Kaneko, N.; Sakamoto, T.; Hashiguchi, Y.; Moriyama, M.; Toyoshima, T. Significant association of increased PD-L1 and PD-1 expression with nodal metastasis and a poor prognosis in oral squamous cell carcinoma. *Int. J. Oral. Maxillofac. Surg.* **2018**, *47*, 836–845. [CrossRef] [PubMed]
46. Yang, W.; Wong, M.C.M.; Thomson, P.J.; Li, K.-Y.; Su, Y. The prognostic role of PD-L1 expression for survival in head and neck squamous cell carcinoma: A systematic review and meta-analysis. *Oral. Oncol.* **2018**, *86*, 81–90. [CrossRef] [PubMed]
47. Chen, S.-W.; Li, S.-H.; Shi, D.-B.; Jiang, W.-M.; Song, M.; Yang, A.-K.; Li, Y.-D.; Bei, J.-X.; Chen, W.-K.; Zhang, Q. Expression of PD-1/PD-L1 in head and neck squamous cell carcinoma and its clinical significance. *Int. J. Biol. Markers* **2019**, *34*, 398–405. [CrossRef] [PubMed]
48. Müller, T.; Braun, M.; Dietrich, D.; Aktekin, S.; Höft, S.; Kristiansen, G.; Göke, F.; Schröck, A.; Brägelmann, J.; Held, S.A.E. PD-L1: A novel prognostic biomarker in head and neck squamous cell carcinoma. *Oncotarget* **2017**, *8*, 52889. [CrossRef]
49. Hanna, G.J.; Woo, S.-B.; Li, Y.Y.; Barletta, J.A.; Hammerman, P.S.; Lorch, J.H. Tumor PD-L1 expression is associated with improved survival and lower recurrence risk in young women with oral cavity squamous cell carcinoma. *Int. J. Oral. Maxillofac. Surg.* **2018**, *47*, 568–577. [CrossRef]
50. Moreira, A.; Poulet, A.; Masliah-Planchon, J.; Lecerf, C.; Vacher, S.; Chérif, L.L.; Dupain, C.; Marret, G.; Girard, E.; Syx, L. Prognostic value of tumor mutational burden in patients with oral cavity squamous cell carcinoma treated with upfront surgery. *ESMO Open* **2021**, *6*, 100178. [CrossRef] [PubMed]
51. Eder, T.; Hess, A.K.; Konschak, R.; Stromberger, C.; Jöhrens, K.; Fleischer, V.; Hummel, M.; Balermpas, P.; Von Der Grün, J.; Linge, A. Interference of tumour mutational burden with outcome of patients with head and neck cancer treated with definitive chemoradiation: A multicentre retrospective study of the German Cancer Consortium Radiation Oncology Group. *Eur. J. Cancer* **2019**, *116*, 67–76. [CrossRef] [PubMed]
52. Mehra, R.; Seiwert, T.Y.; Gupta, S.; Weiss, J.; Gluck, I.; Eder, J.P.; Burtness, B.; Tahara, M.; Keam, B.; Kang, H.; et al. Efficacy and safety of pembrolizumab in recurrent/metastatic head and neck squamous cell carcinoma: Pooled analyses after long-term follow-up in KEYNOTE-012. *Br. J. Cancer* **2018**, *119*, 153–159. [CrossRef] [PubMed]
53. Cohen, E.E.W.; Soulières, D.; Le Tourneau, C.; Dinis, J.; Licitra, L.; Ahn, M.-J.; Soria, A.; Machiels, J.-P.; Mach, N.; Mehra, R. Pembrolizumab versus methotrexate, docetaxel, or cetuximab for recurrent or metastatic head-and-neck squamous cell carcinoma (KEYNOTE-040): A randomised, open-label, phase 3 study. *Lancet* **2019**, *393*, 156–167. [CrossRef]

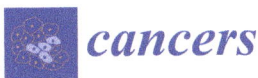

Article

Primary Driver Mutations in *GTF2I* Specific to the Development of Thymomas

Rumi Higuchi [1], Taichiro Goto [1,*], Yosuke Hirotsu [2], Yujiro Yokoyama [1], Takahiro Nakagomi [1], Sotaro Otake [1], Kenji Amemiya [2,3], Toshio Oyama [3], Hitoshi Mochizuki [2] and Masao Omata [2,4]

1. Lung Cancer and Respiratory Disease Center, Yamanashi Central Hospital, Yamanashi 400-8506, Japan; lumi.hgc.236@gmail.com (R.H.); dooogooodooo@me.com (Y.Y.); nakagomi.takahiro@gmail.com (T.N.); sotaro.otake@gmail.com (S.O.)
2. Genome Analysis Center, Yamanashi Central Hospital, Yamanashi 400-8506, Japan; hirotsu-bdyu@ych.pref.yamanashi.jp (Y.H.); amemiya-bdcd@ych.pref.yamanashi.jp (K.A.); h-mochiduki2a@ych.pref.yamanashi.jp (H.M.); m-omata0901@ych.pref.yamanashi.jp (M.O.)
3. Department of Pathology, Yamanashi Central Hospital, Yamanashi 400-8506, Japan; t-oyama@ych.pref.yamanashi.jp
4. Department of Gastroenterology, The University of Tokyo Hospital, Tokyo 113-8655, Japan
* Correspondence: taichiro@1997.jukuin.keio.ac.jp; Tel.: +81-55-253-7111

Received: 16 June 2020; Accepted: 22 July 2020; Published: 24 July 2020

Abstract: Thymomas are rare mediastinal tumors that are difficult to treat and pose a major public health concern. Identifying mutations in target genes is vital for the development of novel therapeutic strategies. Type A thymomas possess a missense mutation in *GTF2I* (chromosome 7 c.74146970T>A) with high frequency. However, the molecular pathways underlying the tumorigenesis of other thymomas remain to be elucidated. We aimed to detect this missense mutation in *GTF2I* in other thymoma subtypes (types B). This study involved 22 patients who underwent surgery for thymomas between January 2014 and August 2019. We isolated tumor cells from formalin-fixed paraffin-embedded tissues from the primary lesions using laser-capture microdissection. Subsequently, we performed targeted sequencing to detect mutant *GTF2I* coupled with molecular barcoding. We used PyClone analysis to determine the fraction of tumor cells harboring mutant *GTF2I*. We detected the missense mutation (chromosome 7 c.74146970T>A) in *GTF2I* in 14 thymomas among the 22 samples (64%). This mutation was harbored in many type B thymomas as well as type A and AB thymomas. The allele fraction for the tumors containing the mutations was variable, primarily owing to the coexistence of normal lymphocytes in the tumors, especially in type B thymomas. PyClone analysis revealed a high cellular prevalence of mutant *GTF2I* in tumor cells. Mutant *GTF2I* was not detected in other carcinomas (lung, gastric, colorectal, or hepatocellular carcinoma) or lymphomas. In conclusion, the majority of thymomas harbor mutations in *GTF2I* that can be potentially used as a novel therapeutic target in patients with thymomas.

Keywords: thymoma; driver mutation; sequencing; molecular barcoding

1. Introduction

Thymoma is a relatively rare mediastinal tumor that is difficult to treat [1,2]. Based on the histological classification by the World Health Organization, thymomas can be categorized into the types A, AB, B1, B2, and B3 depending on the tumor cell morphology and proportion of coexisting lymphocytes [3]. Thymomas of the A category are the least aggressive with the best prognosis; the extent of aggressiveness increases and the prognosis worsens according the order: type A, AB, B1, B2, and B3 [4,5]. Owing to the absence of effective treatment other than surgical resection, there is an urgent need to develop novel drug therapies for patients with inoperable advanced-stage thymomas and those with postoperative relapses of the tumor [6–9].

Analyzing the mutant genes present in thymomas is important in identifying novel treatment strategies. Recent studies showed a missense mutation (chromosome 7 c.74146970T>A) in *GTF2I* (GTF: general transcription factor) present with high frequency in type A thymomas [10,11]. Thymomas are encapsulated tumors. Type AB thymomas histologically comprise a complex mixture of type A and B thymomas. Thus, it seemed unreasonable to hypothesize that mutations in *GTF2I* account for the development of the type A component, with other mechanisms responsible for the development of the type B component. Thus, we focused on the importance of mutations in *GTF2I* in the development of type B thymomas using targeted sequencing coupled with techniques in molecular barcoding: more sensitive and specific assays than the whole-exome sequencing approach used in previous studies [10,11]. We expect that candidates that are commonly mutated in the majority of thymomas will help develop novel therapeutic targets in molecular targeting and gene therapies in the future.

2. Results

2.1. Patient Characteristics

We analyzed samples from 22 patients with thymomas who had undergone surgery ($n = 21$) or surgical biopsy ($n = 1$) at Yamanashi Central Hospital between January 2014 and August 2019. Table 1 shows the clinicopathologic characteristics of the patients, such as the age, sex, histology, tumor size, stage, smoking status, and diagnosis of myasthenia gravis. Among the 22 patients, 12 and 10 were males and females, respectively, and 14 and 8 were smokers and non-smokers, respectively. Using histological examination, there were five, three, seven, five, and two patients with type A, AB, B1, B2, and B3 tumors (Table 1). There were no cases of micronodular thymoma. The 22 patients recruited in this study were divided according to the Masaoka stages: stage I ($n = 7$), II ($n = 12$), III ($n = 2$), and IV ($n = 1$). The maximum tumor diameter ranged from 20 mm to 95 mm (mean tumor diameter, 43.6 ± 22.8 mm). The age of the patients ranged between 42 and 81 years (66.5 ± 12.6 years). One patient with type B2 thymoma exhibited comorbidity with myasthenia gravis (Case 16; Table 2).

Table 1. Patient Characteristics.

Parameter		Number of Patients	Overall Percentage
Total number		22	
Age (years), median (range)		66 (42–81)	
Sex			
	Male	12	54.5%
	Female	10	45.5%
Histology			
	Type A	5	22.7%
	Type AB	3	13.6%
	Type B1	7	31.8%
	Type B2	5	22.7%
	Type B3	2	9.1%
Tumor size (cm)			
	≤ 3	9	40.9%
	3 < size ≤ 5	9	40.9%
	5 <	4	18.2%

Table 1. Cont.

Parameter		Number of Patients	Overall Percentage
Masaoka Stage			
	I	7	31.8%
	II	12	54.5%
	III	2	9.1%
	IV	1	4.5%
Smoking Status (B.I.) [a]			
	0	8	36.4%
	1 < B.I. ≤ 600	10	45.5%
	600<	4	18.2%
Myasthenia gravis			
	+	1	4.5%
	−	21	95.5%

[a] B.I., Brinkman index.

Table 2. Characteristics of the Genomic Clusters.

Patient	Age	Sex	Masaoka Stage	Histology	GTF2I AF [b] (%)	Coverage (Nucleotides)	PD-L1 (%)
1	71	M [a]	I	A	40.6	1651	1<
2	65	M	I	A	45.7	1793	0
3	80	F [a]	III	A	66.7	1801	0
4	65	M	I	A	36.3	3401	30
5	68	F	II	A	42.8	3343	80
6	76	M	II	AB-A	34.3	2149	0
				AB-B	11.4	2780	3
7	62	M	I	AB-A	35.8	2675	0
				AB-B	9.4	2342	0
8	45	F	I	AB-A	38.8	7557	0
				AB-B	16.0	6065	10
9	42	F	II	B1	4.5	5639	0
10	76	F	II	B1	5.0	1623	1
11	48	F	II	B1	2.0	1867	0
12	73	M	II	B1	N.D [c]	−	−
13	46	M	II	B1	4.3	5158	7
14	76	F	II	B1	N.D	−	70
15	66	M	II	B1	N.D	−	55
16	76	M	I	B2	N.D	−	70
17	65	M	II	B2	14.1	1652	70
18	53	F	I	B2	N.D	−	50
19	67	M	IV	B2	N.D	−	70
20	44	F	II	B2	N.D	−	60
21	81	M	III	B3	N.D	−	90
22	81	F	II	B3	40.5	9140	80

[a] M, male; F, female. [b] AF, allele fraction. [c] N.D, not detected.

2.2. Targeted Sequencing

Table 2 shows the data obtained from the sequencing. The sequencing coverage ranged between 1623–9140 (mean ± SD: 3566 ± 2309). We detected point mutations in *GTF2I* in all the type A and

AB thymomas; several type B thymomas were also positive for these *GTF2I* mutations. The type A and B portions of the type AB thymomas harbored mutant *GTF2I*. The allele fraction with the mutant *GTF2I* was lower in type B thymomas compared to in type A thymomas; this could be attributed to the presence of normal cells in the tumor specimens. Mutations in *GTF2I* were detected in 14 out of 22 patients with thymomas (64%). Mutant *GTF2I* was detected in at least one sample from all the subtypes of thymomas (A, AB, B1, B2, and B3). Thus, the *GTF2I* mutation may well be called a prevalent mutation in thymomas in general.

2.3. PyClone Analysis

In our analysis of somatic mutations, there was a need to alleviate the allelic imbalances due to normal-cell contamination, especially in lymphocyte-rich type B thymomas. In this context, PyClone analysis was performed to estimate the cellular frequency patterns of mutations in a population of tumor cells. Mutant *GTF2I* was harbored in ~20%–90% of the tumor cells among all the thymomas (Figure 1), suggesting a high cellular prevalence of mutant *GTF2I*. This *GTF2I* mutation appeared to trigger clonal expansion and is retained ubiquitously within the tumors of the same clone.

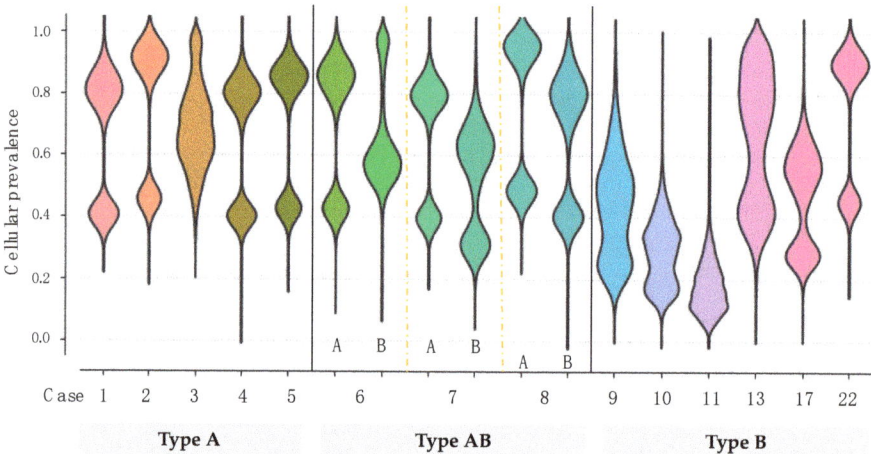

Figure 1. The cellular prevalence of *GTF2I* in the clonal population. The estimated cellular frequency for mutant *GTF2I* is represented by the distribution of the posterior probability using the PyClone model. The colored part represents the distribution of mutant *GTF2I* in each tumor.

2.4. PD-L1 Expression

PD-L1 expression was evaluated immunohistochemically in thymomas with the *GTF2I* mutation (*GTF2I*+) and without (*GTF2I*−; Figure 2A,B). Samples from the *GTF2I*+ group included 3 PD-L1-positive and 11 negative cases, whereas those in the *GTF2I*− group comprised 7 PD-L1-positive and 1 negative case. The distribution of positive and negative cases was significantly different between the two groups ($p < 0.05$; Chi-square test). The staining intensity of PD-L1 was significantly higher in the *GTF2I*+ group compared to in the *GTF2I*− group (Figure 2C), which suggests the mutually exclusive presence of PD-L1 expression and the *GTF2I* mutation in tumor cells.

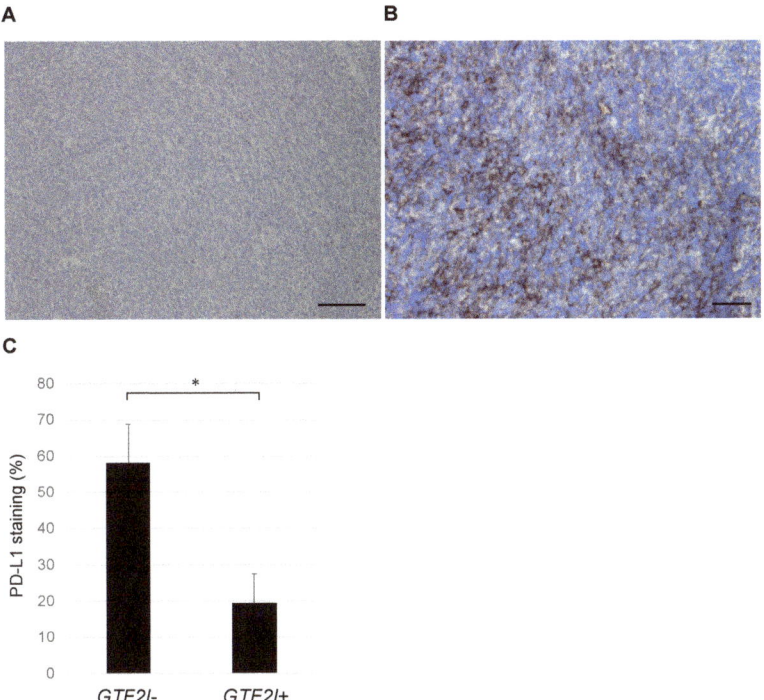

Figure 2. Immunostaining for PD-L1 in thymomas with and without mutant *GTF2I*. (**A**) A representative thymoma with mutant *GTF2I* (Case 1, type A) shows weak staining for PD-L1. (**B**) A representative thymoma without mutant *GTF2I* (Case 15, type B1) shows relatively strong PD-L1 expression. Each scale bar indicates 100 µm. (**C**) The PD-L1 levels were significantly higher in thymomas without mutant *GTF2I*. *, $p < 0.05$.

2.5. Correlation between the Clinical Factors and Genomic Profiles of Patients

The age, sex, smoking habits, tumor size, histological type, Masaoka stage, and PD-L1 expression were assessed using multivariate analysis to identify factors affecting the mutation status of *GTF2I*. Based on a Cox proportional hazards model, the histology and PD-L1 expression were factors that determined the presence of mutations in *GTF2I*; sex ($p = 0.41$), age ($p = 0.43$), smoking habit ($p = 0.68$), tumor size ($p = 0.97$), and tumor stage ($p = 0.46$) did not correlate with the mutation status of *GTF2I*. In essence, mutant *GTF2I* was detected at a higher extent in type A and AB thymomas compared to in types B1–B3. PD-L1-negative thymomas harbored mutant *GTF2I* significantly more frequently when compared to PD-L1-positive thymomas (HR: 12.60, 95% CI: 1.19–133.89).

2.6. Peripheral Blood Parameters

Peripheral blood markers were examined to better characterize the cases in reference to the clinical benefits in immunotherapy. An elevated lactate dehydrogenase (LDH) level was reported to be indicator of tumor burden that is typically associated with lower response rates to immunotherapy, while an elevated platelet-lymphocyte ratio (PLR) was also associated with lower response rates in patients treated with immunotherapy [12]. The pre-surgery blood exam data were analyzed, which revealed that serum LDH levels were significantly higher in thymomas with mutant *GTF2I* than those with wildtype *GTF2I* (thymomas with mutant *GTF2I*, 224.3 ± 13.3; thymomas with wildtype *GTF2I*, 183.7 ± 12.1; $p < 0.05$). In addition, the PLR was significantly higher in thymomas with mutant

GTF2I than those with wildtype *GTF2I* (thymomas with mutant *GTF2I*, 137.2 ± 13.1; thymomas with wildtype *GTF2I*, 97.0 ± 15.7; $p < 0.05$).

2.7. Specificity of GTF2I Mutations in Thymoma

In order to examine the specificity of the *GTF2I* mutation, patients with other malignant diseases were also enrolled in the study. The patients who underwent surgery or biopsy at our hospital between January 2014 and August 2019 were enrolled without bias, and they exhibited a wide range of histology and stages. Mutant *GTF2I* was not detected in other carcinomas, such as brain cancer, lung cancer, gastric cancer, colorectal cancer, hepatocellular carcinoma, and breast cancer, or in lymphomas ($n = 20$ for each, Table 3), indicating the specificity of mutant *GTF2I* in thymomas.

Table 3. The Presence of Mutant *GTF2I* in Other Cancers.

Type of Malignancy	Age (Mean ± SD)	Sex (Male/Female)	Frequency of Mutant *GTF2I*
Brain cancer	51.0 ± 15.5	12/8	0/20
Lung cancer	69.4 ± 8.6	13/7	0/20
Gastric cancer	71.2 ± 11.5	11/9	0/20
Colorectal cancer	65.8 ± 10.6	13/7	0/20
Hepatocellular carcinoma	68.2 ± 11.0	19/1	0/20
Breast cancer	52.7 ± 12.6	0/20	0/20
Lymphoma	58.9 ± 14.1	12/8	0/20

3. Discussion

In this study, we investigated the presence of point mutations in *GTF2I* in thymomas using targeted sequencing coupled with molecular barcoding to validate previous findings obtained by whole-exome sequencing [10,11]. We demonstrated a widespread distribution of mutant *GTF2I* in all types of thymomas, including type B. The SIFT and Polyphen 2 algorithms predicted that the *GTF2I* mutation (p.L424H) was somatic and altered protein structure and function [13,14]. Mutant *GTF2I* did not induce anchorage-independent growth but accelerated cell proliferation in vitro [10]. Type A thymomas were reported to harbor this point mutation [10,11]; however, our study also demonstrated the prevalence of this mutation in type B thymomas.

The presence of mutant *GTF2I* in type B thymomas, in addition to type A thymomas, in this study, unlike previous studies, can be attributed to three reasons. First, previous studies used macrodissection on formalin-fixed paraffin-embedded surgical specimens, whereas we performed laser-capture microdissection. Thymomas comprise tumor and normal cells. In particular, type B thymomas consist of a significant proportion of lymphocytes [15,16]. Contamination with normal cells reduces the probability of detecting mutations in tumor cells. We used laser-capture microdissection to select tumor cells to maximize the chances of detecting the point mutation.

Second, previous reports used whole-exome sequencing, whereas we performed deep-targeted sequencing with the molecular-barcoding technique. The sequence coverage was more extensive in our study compared to that in previous studies, and thus the sensitivity and specificity of detecting mutant *GTF2I* were theoretically much higher in our study. Third, we excluded the influence of pseudogenes and manually counted the DNA strands harboring the mutation in the real *GTF2I* gene. The pseudogenes could have potentially biased the measurement, thereby reducing the chance of detecting *GTF2I* since the heterozygous mutations were present in 1 out 6 (17%) of the amplicons. Thus, by eliminating such bias, we increased the chances of detecting mutations in *GTF2I* by approximately six-fold. Meanwhile, Feng et al. demonstrated that the *GTF2I* mutation was detected by quantitative real time PCR and the fraction of mutant *GTF2I* was the highest in type A and AB thymomas, followed by type B1, B2, and B3, consistent with our results [17].

The findings in this study will help in developing molecular *GTF2I*-targeted therapies. Over recent years, targeted drugs have been shown to exert dramatic effects on various carcinomas and have revolutionized cancer treatment [18,19]. For example, first-line therapy can be selected based on the gene mutation profiles of individual tumors, including epidermal growth factor receptor-tyrosine kinase inhibitors for lung cancer, mammalian target of rapamycin inhibitors for renal cell carcinoma, and human epidermal growth factor receptor-2 inhibitors for breast cancer [20–23]. However, there are no efficacious therapeutic agents for thymomas owing to the lack of knowledge regarding driver mutations. Empiric therapies constitute the currently available treatment strategies for advanced-stage thymoma; the outcomes of these therapies are mostly unsatisfactory. The common driver mutation in *GTF2I* was detected in ~64% of all thymomas; thus, molecular targeted therapy for *GTF2I* may be developed as the primary therapeutic strategy for patients with thymomas in the future.

Immunotherapy has been used in treating various carcinomas. Thus, the *GTF2I* point mutation may serve as a neoantigen for use as a therapeutic target. Treatment strategies using this cancer antigen, such as gene therapy, vaccine therapy, and chimeric antigen receptor T cell therapy coupled with the antibody against PD-1, may be promising for patients in the future [24,25]. In this study, PD-L1 expression and the presence of mutant *GTF2I* were inversely correlated; very few patients were positive for both PD-L1 and mutant *GTF2I*. In addition, blood marker data (serum LDH and PLR) in our study suggested that thymomas without the *GTF2I* mutation exhibited a higher response rate to immunotherapy. We hope that, with further studies, molecular targeted therapy and immunotherapy can be non-redundantly used in different subsets of patients [26].

However, this study is associated with some limitations. First, the patient cohort was relatively small owing to the rarity of the tumor. Second, patient survival could not be analyzed as no patients have shown recurrence in the cohort. Third, we sequenced the cell-free DNA in the serum of all patients, and mutant *GTF2I* could not be detected in these DNA samples. Liquid biopsies utilizing this mutation are deemed unavailable based on our data. In this context, a larger series will be needed to more comprehensively evaluate the genomic landscape of thymomas and more clearly elucidate associations with clinical parameters in a more comprehensive multivariate analysis. However, as the major aim of this preliminary analysis was to identify the driver mutation that should be prioritized for clinical development, the modestly sized sample can still provide useful insights.

4. Methods

4.1. Patient Cohort and Sample Preparation

In this study, we unbiasedly enrolled 22 patients who underwent surgical resection for thymoma at our hospital between January 2014 and August 2019. We obtained written informed consent for genetic research from all the patients in accordance with the protocols approved by the Institutional Review Board at our hospital (Institutional Review Board at Yamanashi Central Hospital). The specimens were categorized histologically based on the classification guidelines by the World Health Organization [16,27], and staged according to the Masaoka staging system [7,15,28]. Sections of formalin-fixed and paraffin-embedded tissues were stained with hematoxylin-eosin and microdissected using the ArcturusXT laser-capture microdissection system (Thermo Fisher Scientific, Waltham, MA, USA). For type AB thymomas, the type A and B portions were microdissected and examined separately. The GeneRead DNA FFPE Kit (Qiagen, Hilden, Germany) was used according to the manufacturer's instructions, and the DNA quality was checked using primers against ribonuclease P.

4.2. Targeted Deep Sequencing and Data Analysis

There were two pseudogenes with 99.4% sequence homology within approximately 500 base pairs upstream and downstream of the mutation site in *GTF2I* that limited the detection of *GTF2I* mutations. A single base difference (cytosine (C) in *GTF2I* and thymine (T) in the pseudogenes) upstream of the mutation site was used to identify *GTF2I* (Figure 3). Thus, we designed our primers for the polymerase chain reaction of the region inclusive of this single nucleotide variation. The primers were designed for use in targeted sequencing using Ion AmpliSeq Designer (Thermo Fisher Scientific) as described previously [29–38].

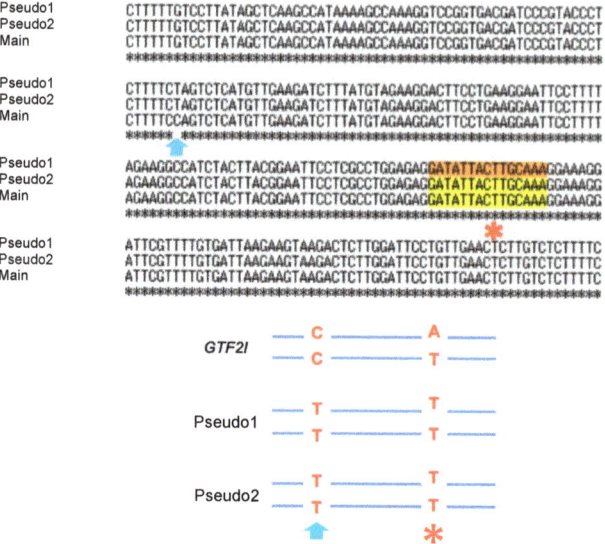

Figure 3. Sequence alignment of *GTF2I* (main) and its pseudogenes showing the single nucleotide variation (as indicated by the arrow) upstream of the point mutation (*). The substitution mutation (* mutation site, thymine (T)>adenine (A)) on the true *GTF2I* DNA strand with cytosine pointed by the arrow was categorized as the true mutation.

Multiplex PCR was performed with an Ion AmpliSeq HD primer and Ion AmpliSeq HD Library Kit (Thermo Fisher Scientific) in accordance with the manufacturer's instruction. Primer sets comprised two different primer pools. The reaction mixture comprised 3.7 µL of 4× Amplification Mix, 1.5 µL of 10× forward primer mix, 1.5 µL of 10× reverse primer mix, 1–20 ng of FFPE or plasma DNA, and nuclease-free water up to a 15 µL total volume. PCR was performed to amplify the target regions with the following cycling conditions: three cycles of 99 °C for 30 s, 64 °C for 2 min, 60 °C for 6 min, and 72 °C for 30 s; 72 °C for 2 min; and a final hold at 4 °C. After combining the PCR products, the amplicons were partially digested with 5 µL of SUPA reagent. The reactions were performed using the following conditions: 30 °C for 15 min, 50 °C for 15 min, 55 °C for 15 min, 25 °C for 10 min, 98 °C for 2 min, and a hold at 4 °C. The libraries were amplified with 4 µL of Ion AmpliSeq HD Dual Barcode Kit with the following conditions: 99 °C for 15 s; 5 cycles of 99 °C for 15 s, 62 °C for 20 s, and 72 °C for 20 s; 15–17 cycles of 99 °C for 15 sec and 70 °C for 40 s; 72 °C for 5 min; and a hold at 4 °C.

The sequencing libraries were prepared using the Ion AmpliSeq™ HD Library Kit (Thermo Fisher Scientific) as previously described [39]. After barcoding with Ion AmpliSeq HD Dual Barcode Kit (Thermo Fisher Scientific), the libraries were purified using Agencourt AMPure XP (Beckman Coulter, Brea, CA, USA) and quantified using the Ion Library Quantitation Kit (Thermo Fisher Scientific). Emulsion PCR and chip loading was performed on the Ion Chef with the Ion 540 Kit-Chef or Ion PI Hi-Q Chef kit; sequencing was performed using Ion 540 Kit-Chef on the Ion GeneStudio S5 Prime System or Ion PI Hi-Q Sequencing Kit on an Ion Proton Sequencer (Thermo Fisher Scientific).

4.3. Molecular Barcoding

The raw data were analyzed using Torrent Suite version 5.10.0 and processed using the standard Ion Torrent Suite Software running on the Torrent Server. The pipeline consisted of signal processing, base calling, quality score assignment, read alignment to the human genome 19, quality control of the mapping, and coverage analysis. Single nucleotide variants, insertions, and deletions were annotated using the Ion Reporter Server System (Thermo Fisher Scientific). The data were visualized with the Ion Reporter™ Genomic Viewer. We manually counted the *GTF2I* DNA strands with C at the site of the single nucleotide variation. In such DNA strands, the substitution of T>adenine (A) at the hotspot (c.74146970) was considered as a true mutation in *GTF2I* and used for analysis (Figure 3).

4.4. PyClone Analysis

PyClone is a Bayesian clustering tool to group sets of deep sequenced somatic mutations into putative clonal clusters while estimating their cellular prevalence. This method accounts for allelic imbalances introduced by changes in the segment copy number and sample contamination by normal cells [40]. In this study, PyClone analysis was performed to estimate the fraction of cancer cells harboring mutant *GTF2I* [40–42].

4.5. Immunohistochemistry for PD-L1

Specimens from 20 patients obtained between January 2000 and December 2013 were fixed with 10% buffered formalin. Formalin-fixed paraffin-embedded tissues were cut into 5 μm sections, deparaffinized, rehydrated, and stained in an automated system (Ventana Benchmark ULTRA system; Roche, Tucson, AZ, USA) using commercially available detection kits and antibodies against PD-L1 (28-8, ab205921; Abcam, Cambridge, MA, USA). PD-L1 was primarily localized to the cell membrane of tumor cells, and its expression was determined quantitatively by two pathologists based on the proportion of PD-L1-positive tumor cells. Cells were considered PD-L1-positive based on a ≥1% PD-L1 expression.

4.6. Presence or Absence of Gtf2i Mutation in Other Malignant Diseases

Other samples, such as brain cancer, lung cancer, gastric cancer, colorectal cancer, hepatocellular carcinoma, breast cancer, and lymphoma, were collected at our institution during regular clinical practice. After obtaining signed informed consent, their sample tissues were analyzed for the presence of the *GTF2I* mutation.

4.7. Statistical Analyses

Continuous variables were represented as the mean and standard deviation. Categorical variables were compared using the Chi-square test. Multivariate analyses and calculation of the hazard ratio (HR) and 95.0% confidence interval (CI) were performed using JMP (SAS Institute, Cary, NC, USA). Two-tailed $p < 0.05$ was considered statistically significant.

5. Conclusions

A missense mutation in *GTF2I* was detected with high prevalence in and specific to thymomas. This mutation may be a major driver mutation in the tumorigenesis of thymomas and serve as a promising therapeutic candidate to be used in "precision medicine" for patients with thymomas.

Author Contributions: T.G., Y.H. and R.H. wrote the manuscript. T.G., T.N., R.H., Y.Y. and S.O. performed the surgery. T.O., K.A. and R.H. carried out the pathological examination. Y.H., K.A., T.G., T.N., H.M., R.H., S.O. and M.O. participated in the genomic analyses. M.O. and T.G. edited the final manuscript. All authors have read and agreed to the published version of the manuscript.

Funding: This study was supported by a Grant-in-Aid for Genome Research Project from Yamanashi Prefecture (to Y.H. and M.O.).

Acknowledgments: The authors greatly appreciate Yumiko Kakizaki, Toshiharu Tsutsui, and Yoshihiro Miyashita for their helpful scientific discussion.

Conflicts of Interest: The authors declare no conflict of interest.

References

1. Engels, E.A. Epidemiology of thymoma and associated malignancies. *J. Thorac. Oncol.* **2010**, *5* (Suppl. S4), S260–S265. [CrossRef]
2. Venuta, F.; Anile, M.; Diso, D.; Vitolo, D.; Rendina, E.A.; De Giacomo, T.; Francioni, F.; Coloni, G.F. Thymoma and thymic carcinoma. *Eur. J. Cardiothorac. Surg.* **2010**, *37*, 13–25. [CrossRef] [PubMed]
3. Marx, A.; Chan, J.K.; Coindre, J.M.; Detterbeck, F.; Girard, N.; Harris, N.L.; Jaffe, E.S.; Kurrer, M.O.; Marom, E.M.; Moreira, A.L.; et al. The 2015 World Health Organization Classification of Tumors of the Thymus: Continuity and Changes. *J. Thorac. Oncol.* **2015**, *10*, 1383–1395. [CrossRef]
4. Marx, A.; Strobel, P.; Badve, S.S.; Chalabreysse, L.; Chan, J.K.; Chen, G.; de Leval, L.; Detterbeck, F.; Girard, N.; Huang, J.; et al. ITMIG consensus statement on the use of the WHO histological classification of thymoma and thymic carcinoma: Refined definitions, histological criteria, and reporting. *J. Thorac. Oncol.* **2014**, *9*, 596–611. [CrossRef]
5. Moon, J.W.; Lee, K.S.; Shin, M.H.; Kim, S.; Woo, S.Y.; Lee, G.; Han, J.; Shim, Y.M.; Choi, Y.S. Thymic epithelial tumors: Prognostic determinants among clinical, histopathologic, and computed tomography findings. *Ann. Thorac. Surg.* **2015**, *99*, 462–470. [CrossRef] [PubMed]
6. Girard, N.; Lal, R.; Wakelee, H.; Riely, G.J.; Loehrer, P.J. Chemotherapy definitions and policies for thymic malignancies. *J. Thorac. Oncol.* **2011**, *6* (Suppl. S3), S1749–S1755. [CrossRef]
7. Litvak, A.M.; Woo, K.; Hayes, S.; Huang, J.; Rimner, A.; Sima, C.S.; Moreira, A.L.; Tsukazan, M.; Riely, G.J. Clinical characteristics and outcomes for patients with thymic carcinoma: Evaluation of Masaoka staging. *J. Thorac. Oncol.* **2014**, *9*, 1810–1815. [CrossRef] [PubMed]
8. Schmitt, J.; Loehrer, P.J., Sr. The role of chemotherapy in advanced thymoma. *J. Thorac. Oncol* **2010**, *5* (Suppl. S4), S357–S360. [CrossRef]
9. Zhao, Y.; Shi, J.; Fan, L.; Hu, D.; Yang, J.; Zhao, H. Surgical treatment of thymoma: An 11-year experience with 761 patients. *Eur. J. Cardiothorac. Surg.* **2016**, *49*, 1144–1149. [CrossRef]
10. Petrini, I.; Meltzer, P.S.; Kim, I.K.; Lucchi, M.; Park, K.S.; Fontanini, G.; Gao, J.; Zucali, P.A.; Calabrese, F.; Favaretto, A.; et al. A specific missense mutation in *GTF2I* occurs at high frequency in thymic epithelial tumors. *Nat. Genet.* **2014**, *46*, 844–849. [CrossRef]
11. Radovich, M.; Pickering, C.R.; Felau, I.; Ha, G.; Zhang, H.; Jo, H.; Hoadley, K.A.; Anur, P.; Zhang, J.; McLellan, M.; et al. The Integrated Genomic Landscape of Thymic Epithelial Tumors. *Cancer Cell* **2018**, *33*, 244–258. [CrossRef]
12. Espinosa, E.; Marquez-Rodas, I.; Soria, A.; Berrocal, A.; Manzano, J.L.; Gonzalez-Cao, M.; Martin-Algarra, S.; Spanish Melanoma, G. Predictive factors of response to immunotherapy-a review from the Spanish Melanoma Group (GEM). *Ann. Transl. Med.* **2017**, *5*, 389. [CrossRef]
13. Adzhubei, I.A.; Schmidt, S.; Peshkin, L.; Ramensky, V.E.; Gerasimova, A.; Bork, P.; Kondrashov, A.S.; Sunyaev, S.R. A method and server for predicting damaging missense mutations. *Nat. Methods* **2010**, *7*, 248–249. [CrossRef]
14. Kumar, P.; Henikoff, S.; Ng, P.C. Predicting the effects of coding non-synonymous variants on protein function using the SIFT algorithm. *Nat. Protoc.* **2009**, *4*, 1073–1081. [CrossRef]
15. Ruffini, E.; Fang, W.; Guerrera, F.; Huang, J.; Okumura, M.; Kim, D.K.; Girard, N.; Bille, A.; Boubia, S.; Cangir, A.K.; et al. The International Association for the Study of Lung Cancer Thymic Tumors Staging Project: The Impact of the Eighth Edition of the Union for International Cancer Control and American Joint Committee on Cancer TNM Stage Classification of Thymic Tumors. *J. Thorac. Oncol.* **2020**, *15*, 436–447. [CrossRef]
16. Travis, W.D.; Brambilla, E.; Nicholson, A.G.; Yatabe, Y.; Austin, J.H.M.; Beasley, M.B.; Chirieac, L.R.; Dacic, S.; Duhig, E.; Flieder, D.B.; et al. The 2015 World Health Organization Classification of Lung Tumors: Impact of Genetic, Clinical and Radiologic Advances Since the 2004 Classification. *J. Thorac. Oncol.* **2015**, *10*, 1243–1260. [CrossRef]
17. Feng, Y.; Lei, Y.; Wu, X.; Huang, Y.; Rao, H.; Zhang, Y.; Wang, F. GTF2I mutation frequently occurs in more indolent thymic epithelial tumors and predicts better prognosis. *Lung Cancer* **2017**, *110*, 48–52. [CrossRef]
18. Ayati, A.; Moghimi, S.; Salarinejad, S.; Safavi, M.; Pouramiri, B.; Foroumadi, A. A review on progression of epidermal growth factor receptor (EGFR) inhibitors as an efficient approach in cancer targeted therapy. *Bioorg. Chem.* **2020**, *99*, 103811. [CrossRef]

19. Domagala-Kulawik, J. New Frontiers for Molecular Pathology. *Front. Med.* **2019**, *6*, 284. [CrossRef]
20. Huang, J.J.; Hsieh, J.J. The Therapeutic Landscape of Renal Cell Carcinoma: From the Dark Age to the Golden Age. *Semin. Nephrol.* **2020**, *40*, 28–41. [CrossRef]
21. Osawa, T.; Takeuchi, A.; Kojima, T.; Shinohara, N.; Eto, M.; Nishiyama, H. Overview of current and future systemic therapy for metastatic renal cell carcinoma. *Jpn. J. Clin. Oncol.* **2019**, *49*, 395–403. [CrossRef]
22. Roskoski, R., Jr. Properties of FDA-approved small molecule protein kinase inhibitors. *Pharmacol. Res.* **2019**, *144*, 19–50. [CrossRef]
23. Wang, J.; Xu, B. Targeted therapeutic options and future perspectives for HER2-positive breast cancer. *Signal Transduct. Target Ther.* **2019**, *4*, 34. [CrossRef]
24. Goto, T. Radiation as an In Situ Auto-Vaccination: Current Perspectives and Challenges. *Vaccines* **2019**, *7*, 100. [CrossRef]
25. Kunimasa, K.; Goto, T. Immunosurveillance and Immunoediting of Lung Cancer: Current Perspectives and Challenges. *Int. J. Mol. Sci.* **2020**, *21*, 597. [CrossRef]
26. Higuchi, R.; Goto, T.; Hirotsu, Y.; Nakagomi, T.; Yokoyama, Y.; Otake, S.; Amemiya, K.; Oyama, T.; Omata, M. PD-L1 Expression and Tumor-Infiltrating Lymphocytes in Thymic Epithelial Neoplasms. *J. Clin. Med.* **2019**, *8*, 1833. [CrossRef]
27. Gibbs, A.R.; Thunnissen, F.B. Histological typing of lung and pleural tumours: Third edition. *J. Clin. Pathol.* **2001**, *54*, 498–499. [CrossRef]
28. Chansky, K.; Detterbeck, F.C.; Nicholson, A.G.; Rusch, V.W.; Vallieres, E.; Groome, P.; Kennedy, C.; Krasnik, M.; Peake, M.; Shemanski, L.; et al. The IASLC Lung Cancer Staging Project: External Validation of the Revision of the TNM Stage Groupings in the Eighth Edition of the TNM Classification of Lung Cancer. *J. Thorac. Oncol.* **2017**, *12*, 1109–1121. [CrossRef]
29. Hirotsu, Y.; Nakagomi, H.; Sakamoto, I.; Amemiya, K.; Oyama, T.; Mochizuki, H.; Omata, M. Multigene panel analysis identified germline mutations of DNA repair genes in breast and ovarian cancer. *Mol. Genet. Genom. Med.* **2015**, *3*, 459–466. [CrossRef]
30. Hirotsu, Y.; Nakagomi, H.; Sakamoto, I.; Amemiya, K.; Mochizuki, H.; Omata, M. Detection of BRCA1 and BRCA2 germline mutations in Japanese population using next-generation sequencing. *Mol. Genet. Genom. Med.* **2015**, *3*, 121–129. [CrossRef]
31. Goto, T.; Hirotsu, Y.; Amemiya, K.; Nakagomi, T.; Shikata, D.; Yokoyama, Y.; Okimoto, K.; Oyama, T.; Mochizuki, H.; Omata, M. Distribution of circulating tumor DNA in lung cancer: Analysis of the primary lung and bone marrow along with the pulmonary venous and peripheral blood. *Oncotarget* **2017**, *8*, 59268–59281. [CrossRef] [PubMed]
32. Goto, T.; Hirotsu, Y.; Mochizuki, H.; Nakagomi, T.; Shikata, D.; Yokoyama, Y.; Oyama, T.; Amemiya, K.; Okimoto, K.; Omata, M. Mutational analysis of multiple lung cancers: Discrimination between primary and metastatic lung cancers by genomic profile. *Oncotarget* **2017**, *8*, 31133–31143. [CrossRef]
33. Goto, T.; Hirotsu, Y.; Oyama, T.; Amemiya, K.; Omata, M. Analysis of tumor-derived DNA in plasma and bone marrow fluid in lung cancer patients. *Med. Oncol.* **2016**, *33*, 29. [CrossRef] [PubMed]
34. Amemiya, K.; Hirotsu, Y.; Goto, T.; Nakagomi, H.; Mochizuki, H.; Oyama, T.; Omata, M. Touch imprint cytology with massively parallel sequencing (TIC-seq): A simple and rapid method to snapshot genetic alterations in tumors. *Cancer Med.* **2016**, *5*, 3426–3436. [CrossRef] [PubMed]
35. Goto, T.; Hirotsu, Y.; Mochizuki, H.; Nakagomi, T.; Oyama, T.; Amemiya, K.; Omata, M. Stepwise addition of genetic changes correlated with histological change from "well-differentiated" to "sarcomatoid" phenotypes: A case report. *BMC Cancer* **2017**, *17*, 65. [CrossRef]
36. Higuchi, R.; Nakagomi, T.; Goto, T.; Hirotsu, Y.; Shikata, D.; Yokoyama, Y.; Otake, S.; Amemiya, K.; Oyama, T.; Mochizuki, H.; et al. Identification of Clonality through Genomic Profile Analysis in Multiple Lung Cancers. *J. Clin. Med.* **2020**, *9*, 573. [CrossRef]
37. Nakagomi, T.; Goto, T.; Hirotsu, Y.; Shikata, D.; Yokoyama, Y.; Higuchi, R.; Otake, S.; Amemiya, K.; Oyama, T.; Mochizuki, H.; et al. Genomic Characteristics of Invasive Mucinous Adenocarcinomas of the Lung and Potential Therapeutic Targets of B7-H3. *Cancers* **2018**, *10*, 478. [CrossRef]
38. Nakagomi, T.; Hirotsu, Y.; Goto, T.; Shikata, D.; Yokoyama, Y.; Higuchi, R.; Otake, S.; Amemiya, K.; Oyama, T.; Mochizuki, H.; et al. Clinical Implications of Noncoding Indels in the Surfactant-Encoding Genes in Lung Cancer. *Cancers* **2019**, *11*, 552. [CrossRef]

39. Hirotsu, Y.; Otake, S.; Ohyama, H.; Amemiya, K.; Higuchi, R.; Oyama, T.; Mochizuki, H.; Goto, T.; Omata, M. Dual-molecular barcode sequencing detects rare variants in tumor and cell free DNA in plasma. *Sci. Rep.* **2020**, *10*, 3391. [CrossRef]
40. Roth, A.; Khattra, J.; Yap, D.; Wan, A.; Laks, E.; Biele, J.; Ha, G.; Aparicio, S.; Bouchard-Cote, A.; Shah, S.P. PyClone: Statistical inference of clonal population structure in cancer. *Nat. Methods* **2014**, *11*, 396–398. [CrossRef]
41. Nakagomi, T.; Goto, T.; Hirotsu, Y.; Shikata, D.; Amemiya, K.; Oyama, T.; Mochizuki, H.; Omata, M. Elucidation of radiation-resistant clones by a serial study of intratumor heterogeneity before and after stereotactic radiotherapy in lung cancer. *J. Thorac. Dis.* **2017**, *9*, E598–E604. [CrossRef]
42. Nakagomi, T.; Goto, T.; Hirotsu, Y.; Shikata, D.; Yokoyama, Y.; Higuchi, R.; Amemiya, K.; Okimoto, K.; Oyama, T.; Mochizuki, H.; et al. New therapeutic targets for pulmonary sarcomatoid carcinomas based on their genomic and phylogenetic profiles. *Oncotarget* **2018**, *9*, 10635–10649. [CrossRef]

© 2020 by the authors. Licensee MDPI, Basel, Switzerland. This article is an open access article distributed under the terms and conditions of the Creative Commons Attribution (CC BY) license (http://creativecommons.org/licenses/by/4.0/).

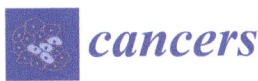

Article

A Novel Comprehensive Clinical Stratification Model to Refine Prognosis of Glioblastoma Patients Undergoing Surgical Resection

Tamara Ius [1,*], Fabrizio Pignotti [2], Giuseppe Maria Della Pepa [3], Giuseppe La Rocca [2,3], Teresa Somma [4], Miriam Isola [5], Claudio Battistella [5], Simona Gaudino [6], Maurizio Polano [7], Michele Dal Bo [7], Daniele Bagatto [8], Enrico Pegolo [9], Silvia Chiesa [10], Mauro Arcicasa [11], Alessandro Olivi [3], Miran Skrap [1] and Giovanni Sabatino [2,3]

1. Neurosurgery Unit, Department of Neuroscience, Santa Maria della Misericordia University Hospital, 33100 Udine, Italy; skrap@asuiud.sanita.fvg.it
2. Department of Neurosurgery, Mater Olbia Hospital, 07026 Olbia, Italy; fabrizio.pignotti@materolbia.com (F.P.); giovanni.sabatino@policlinicogemelli.it (G.S.); Giuseppe.larocca@policlinicogemelli.it (G.L.R.)
3. Institute of Neurosurgery, Catholic University, 00168 Rome, Italy; giuseppemaria.dellapepa@policlinicogemelli.it (G.M.D.P.); alessandro.olivi@policlinicogemelli.it (A.O.)
4. Division of Neurosurgery, Department of Neurosciences, Reproductive and Odontostomatological Sciences, Università degli Studi di Napoli Federico II, 80131 Naples, Italy; teresa.somma85@gmail.com
5. Department of Medicine, Santa Maria della Misericordia University Hospital, 33100 Udine, Italy; miriam.isola@uniud.it (M.I.); claudio.battistella@uniud.it (C.B.)
6. Institute of radiology, Fondazione Policlinico Universitario A. Gemelli IRCCS, 00168 Rome, Italy; simona.gaudino@policlinicogemelli.it
7. Experimental and Clinical Pharmacology Unit, Centro di Riferimento Oncologico di Aviano (CRO) IRCCS, 33081 Aviano, Italy; mpolano@cro.it (M.P.); mdalbo@cro.it (M.D.B.)
8. Neuroradiology Unit, Department of Diagnostic Imaging ASUIUD Udine, 33100 Udine, Italy; daniele.bagatto@asuiud.sanita.fvg.it
9. Institute of Pathology, Santa Maria della Misericordia University Hospital, 33100 Udine, Italy; enrico.pegolo@asuiud.sanita.fvg.it
10. Radiation Oncology Unit, Fondazione Policlinico Universitario A. Gemelli IRCCS, 00168 Rome, Italy; Silvia.chiesa@policlinicogemelli.it
11. Department of Oncology, Centro di Riferimento Oncologico di Aviano (CRO) IRCCS, 33081 Aviano, Italy; marcicasa@cro.it
* Correspondence: tamara.ius@gmail.com or tamara.ius@asuiud.sanita.fvg.it; Tel.: 0039-347-0178730/0039-0432

Received: 11 December 2019; Accepted: 5 February 2020; Published: 7 February 2020

Abstract: Despite recent discoveries in genetics and molecular fields, glioblastoma (GBM) prognosis still remains unfavorable with less than 10% of patients alive 5 years after diagnosis. Numerous studies have focused on the research of biological biomarkers to stratify GBM patients. We addressed this issue in our study by using clinical/molecular and image data, which is generally available to Neurosurgical Departments in order to create a prognostic score that can be useful to stratify GBM patients undergoing surgical resection. By using the random forest approach [CART analysis (classification and regression tree)] on Survival time data of 465 cases, we developed a new prediction score resulting in 10 groups based on extent of resection (EOR), age, tumor volumetric features, intraoperative protocols and tumor molecular classes. The resulting tree was trimmed according to similarities in the relative hazard ratios amongst groups, giving rise to a 5-group classification tree. These 5 groups were different in terms of overall survival (OS) ($p < 0.000$). The score performance in predicting death was defined by a Harrell's c-index of 0.79 (95% confidence interval [0.76–0.81]). The proposed score could be useful in a clinical setting to refine the prognosis of GBM patients after surgery and prior to postoperative treatment.

Keywords: glioblastoma prognosis; overall survival; extent of resection; random forest; Decision tree; personalized precision oncology

1. Introduction

Glioblastoma (GBM) is the most common primary malignant central nervous system (CNS) tumor in adults, representing about 25% of primary CNS tumors and 50%–55% of adult gliomas [1–3]. The current standard of care for GBM includes maximal safe surgical resection followed by concomitant chemoradiation therapy and adjunct chemotherapy [4–8]. Despite decades of advances in surgery and discovery in the molecular landscape, encouraging outcomes are not typically observed; patients diagnosed with these tumors generally have a dismal prognosis and poor quality of life as the disease progresses. The median survival time has been reported to be less than 15 months in cases. Survival longer than 3 years and 5 years have been reported for approximately 3%–5% and 0.5% of GBM patients, respectively. There is thus a pressing need to identify new systemic therapies [9–11]. The variety in overall survival and response to treatment in GBM is largely due to the high heterogeneity of GBM with a different distribution of aggressive biological traits across tumors, as well as within a single tumor [12–14]. To classify GBM cases according to this heterogeneity, different prognostic factors have been suggested for GBM, including age, performance status, specific molecular markers [e.g., MGMT methylation (O^6-methylguanine-DNA methyl-transferase), mutation of IDH1, IDH2(isocitrate dehydrogenase) or TERT (telomerase reverse transcriptase), 1p19q codeletion, overexpression of EGFR (epidermal growth factor receptor)], the size of necrosis and the extent of resection (EOR) [15–22]. The role of EOR in improving survival in patients with GBM has widely been demonstrated, with more extensive resections providing added advantages [8,9,16,18,19,23–33].

In this context, survival benefit based on extent of tumor resection has been reported to be as low as 78% and the greatest survival advantage has been seen in patients with EOR >95% [9]. Despite the infiltrative nature of this tumor, it still remains unclear if the resection beyond the contrast enhancement portion of the tumor translates into improved outcomes for patients with GBM [23].

In a clinical setting, the need for classification tools based on the prognostic stratification of GBM cases undergoing surgical protocols is of increasing importance. Numerous attempts have been developed to classify GBM patients, which include combination models of clinical, molecular and radiomic variables used in daily clinical practice [34–38].

Given the importance of each individual factor, it is often difficult to establish how these interact with each other and how they impact survival in the complexity of the clinical settings. In other words, classical survival models do not concomitantly evaluate multiple variables and establish the burden of different combinations of determinants on survival.

In the present investigation, we proposed a novel prognostic model comprehensively evaluating clinical, surgical volumetric and molecular factors to define prognosis of GBM-affected patients undergoing surgery.

2. Results

Demographic, clinical, neurophysiological and radiological features of the study population are summarized in Tables A1 and A2.

2.1. Survival Analysis and Risk Factors

The 1- and 2- year overall survival (OS) and progression-free survival (PFS) rates for the assessed patients were estimated to be 54.78% and 22.28%, and 33.05% and 13.82%, respectively (Figure 1).

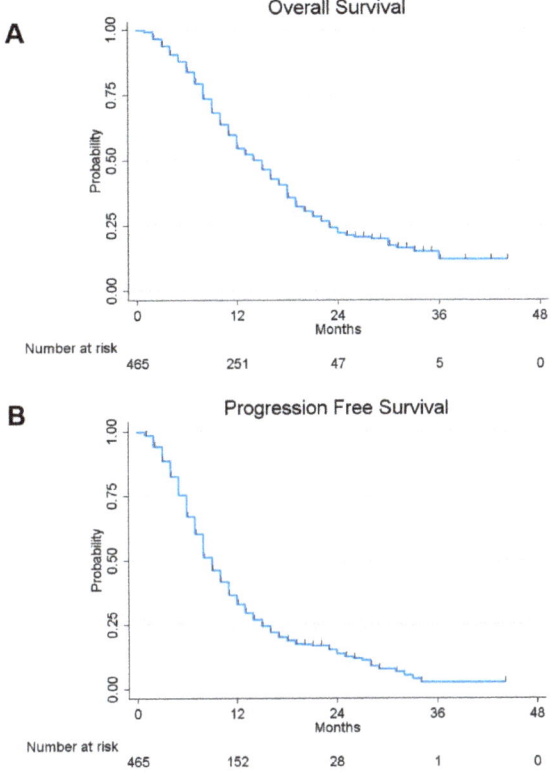

Figure 1. Kaplan–Meier curves displaying overall survival (OS) (**A**) and progression-free survival (PFS) (**B**) in the whole sample of 465 glioblastoma (GBM) included in the study.

Univariate analysis showed a significant better survival in patients with a younger age ($p = 0.000$), higher EOR ($p = 0.000$), methylated MGMT promoter ($p = 0.000$), mutation of IDH1/IDH2 genes ($p = 0.033$), presence of lower residual tumor ($p = 0.000$) and lower preoperative ΔT1/T2 MRI Index ($p = 0.000$) (Figure 2). Gender, tumoral side and tumoral site, however, did not statistically influence OS.

At multivariate Cox analysis, considering the variables with a significant p value in univariate analysis, EOR ($p = 0.000$), age ($p = 0.000$), MGMT methylation status ($p = 0.000$) and preoperative ΔT1/T2 MRI Index ($p = 0.000$) were confirmed as independent predictors for OS (Table 1).

Table 1. Univariate and multivariate analysis of OS in GBM patients.

Variable	Univariate Analysis			Multivariate Analysis		
	Hazard Ratio	95% CI	*p*-Value	Hazard Ratio	95% CI	*p*-Value
Age (yrs)	1.029	1.018–1.040	**0.000**	1.028	1.017–1.039	0.000
Sex						
Male	1					
Female	0.900	0.713–1.137	0.377			
Side						
Left	1					
Right	1.124	0.898–1.406	0.308			

Table 1. Cont.

Variable	Univariate Analysis			Multivariate Analysis		
	Hazard Ratio	95% CI	p-Value	Hazard Ratio	95% CI	p-Value
Tumor Site						
Precentral	1					
Retrocentral	1.092	0.825–1.446	0.539	0.954	0.718–1.267	0.745
Temporal + Insular	1.250	0.961–1.626	0.097	1.286	0.986–1.677	0.063
Radiological Features						
Ependymal involvement (yes vs no)	1.135	0.890–1.448	0.309			
Corpus Callosum involvement (yes vs no)	1.012	0.799–1.281	0.922			
Necrotic-cystic component (yes vs no)	0.923	0.725–1.176	0.517			
Midline shift (yes vs no)	0.970	0.775–1.214	0.789			
Preoperative Tumoral Volume computed on postcontrast T1-weighted images, cm^3	1.001	0.996–1.006	0.652			
Preoperative Tumoral Volume computed on T2-weighted images, cm^3	0.993	0.991–0.995	0.000	0.997	0.995–1.000	0.058
Preoperative ΔT1/T2 MRI Index	1.022	1.017–1.026	0.000	1.016	1.009–1.022	0.000
Residual tumor, cm^3	1.085	1.067–1.103	0.000	0.962	0.925–1.000	0.053
EOR (continuous variable)	0.946	0.938–0.954	0.000	0.937	0.923–0.950	0.000
EOR (categorical variable)						
EOR = 100%	1					
99% ≤ EOR ≤ 90%	1.755	1.314–2.343	0.000			
89% ≤ EOR ≤ 80%	2.477	1.757–3.492	0.000			
EOR ≤ 79%	6.300	4.537–8.748	0.000			
Biological Features						
MGMT promoter methylation (yes vs no)	0.605	0.482–0.760	0.000	0.606	0.480–0.765	0.000
IDH 1/2 mutation (yes vs no)	0.638	0.423–0.964	0.033	0.925	0.605–1.416	0.721
Ki67	1.001	0.995–1.007	0.725			

Table showing the influence of different factors on the OS rates as per univariate survival analysis and multivariate analysis on the entire GBM patients cohort. (p-value < 0.05 at Log-rank test). Boldfacing values represent statistical significant results ($p < 0.05$). CI = confidence interval; p-value = level of marginal significance; MRI = magnetic resonance image; preoperative ΔT1/T2 MRI Index = ratio between pre-operative tumoral volume on post-contrast T1-weighted and T2 weighted images; EOR = extent of resection; CWs = Carmustine Wafers; RT = radiotherapy; CT = chemotherapy; MGMT = O^6-methylguanine-DNA methyl-transferase; IDH = isocitrate dehydrogenase; OS = overall survival.

Similarly, when PFS was considered, univariate Cox regression analyses confirmed age ($p = 0.000$), EOR ($p = 0.000$), methylation status of MGMT promoter ($p = 0.000$) and preoperative ΔT1/T2 MRI Index ($p = 0.000$) as factors influencing the tumor progression. By performing multivariate Cox analysis considering the variables with a significant p value in univariate analysis, EOR ($p = 0.000$), age ($p = 0.002$), methylation status of MGMT promoter ($p = 0.000$) and preoperative ΔT1/T2 MRI Index ($p = 0.000$) were confirmed as independent predictors for PFS, however, no correlation was observed with other observed variables such as sex, tumor size and site, IDH-1 status and Ki67% (Figure 3, Table 2).

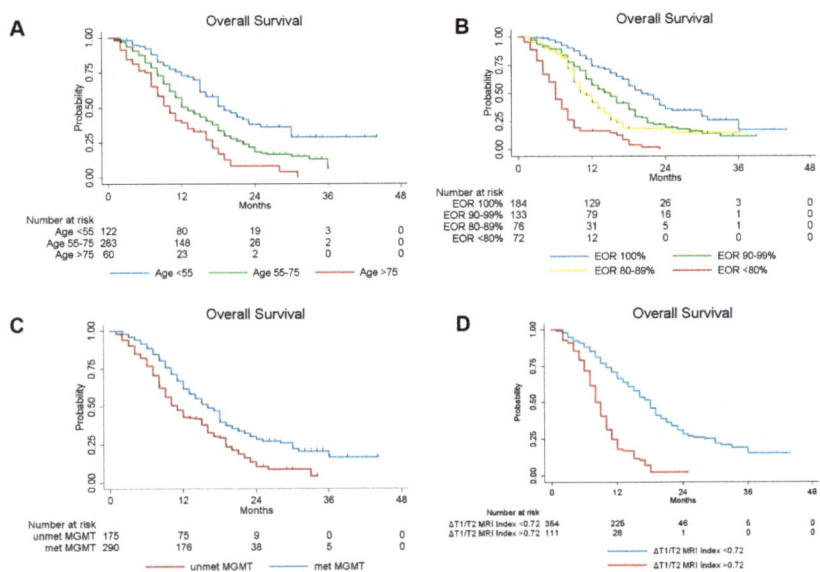

Figure 2. Kaplan-Meier curves displaying OS of GBM patients according to Age (**A**); EOR (**B**); MGMT promoter methylation status(**C**); and preoperative ΔT1/T2 MRI Index (**D**).

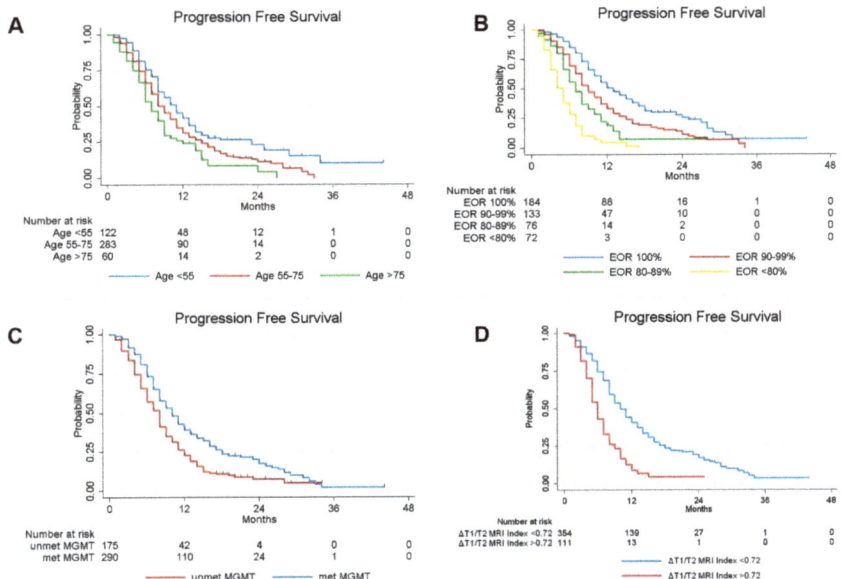

Figure 3. Kaplan-Meier curves displaying PFS of GBM patients according to Age (**A**); EOR (**B**): MGMT promoter methylation status (**C**); and preoperative ΔT1/T2 MRI Index (**D**).

Table 2. Univariate and Multivariate Analysis of PFS in GBM patients.

Variable	Univariate Analysis			Multivariate Analysis		
	Hazard Ratio	95% CI	p-Value	Hazard Ratio	95% CI	p-Value
Age (yrs)	1.017	1.008–1.027	0.000	1.015	1.006–1.024	0.002
Sex						
Male	1					
Female	0.851	0.687–1.054	0.140			
Side						
Left	1					
Right	1.091	0.889–1.339	0.404			
Tumor Site						
Precentral	1					
Retrocentral	1.045	0.811–1.347	0.733			
Temporal + Insular	1.031	0.810–1.312	0.806			
Radiological Features						
Ependymal involvement (yes vs no)	1.114	0.893–1.390	0.338			
Corpus Callosum involvement (yes vs no)	0.917	0.737–1.142	0.439			
Necrotic-cystic component (yes vs no)	0.974	0.781–1.215	0.816			
Midline shift (yes vs no)	0.979	0.797–1.202	0.838			
Preoperative Tumoral Volume computed on postcontrast T1-weighted images, cm^3	1.003	0.999–1.008	0.170			
Preoperative Tumoral Volume computed on T2-weighted images, cm^3	0.996	0.994–0.998	0.000	0.999	0.996–1.001	0.311
Preoperative ΔT1/T2 MRI Index	1.016	1.012–1.020	0.000	1.011	1.005–1.016	0.000
Residual tumor, cm^3	1.083	1.067–1.100	0.000	0.977	0.943–1.013	0.208
EOR (continuous variable)	0.949	0.942–0.957	0.000	0.948	0.935–0.961	0.000
EOR (categorical variable)						
EOR = 100%	1					
99% ≤ EOR ≤ 90%	1.622	1.254–2.098	0.000			
89% ≤ EOR ≤ 80%	2.425	1.783–3.298	0.000			
EOR ≤ 79%	5.245	3.854–7.138	0.000			
Biological Features						
MGMT promoter methylation (yes vs no)	0.639	0.518–0.787	0.000	0.673	0.544–0.833	0.000
IDH 1/2 mutation (yes vs no)	0.706	0.488–1.023	0.066	0.894	0.612–1.305	0.561
Ki67	1.000	0.995–1.006	0.873			

Table showing the influence of different factors on the PFS rates as per univariate survival analysis and multivariate analysis on the entire GBM patients cohort. (p-value < 0.05 at Log-rank test). Boldfacing values represent statistical significant results ($p < 0.05$). CI = confidence interval; p-value = level of marginal significance; MRI = magnetic resonance image; preoperative ΔT1/T2 MRI Index = ratio between pre-operative tumoral volume on postcontrast T1-weighted and T2 weighted images; EOR = extent of resection; CWs = Carmustine Wafers; RT = radiotherapy; CT = chemoterapy; MGMT = O^6-methylguanine-DNA methyl-transferase; IDH = isocitrate dehydrogenase; OS = overall survival.

2.2. Classification and Regression Tree (CART) Model

In order to create a prognostic model comprehensively evaluating clinical, molecular and treatment-associated factors to stratify GBM-affected patients undergoing surgery, we used a classification and regression tree (CART) approach. The algorithm relied on the clinical variables that showed a significant impact as independent predictor factors in multivariate analysis (age, EOR, MGMT methylation status, preoperative ΔT1/T2 MRI Index, preoperative volumetric tumor volume on T2-weighted images. (Figure 4). The application of the CART analysis led to the definition of 10 terminal nodes (Figure 4). According to the relative hazard ratio (RHR) obtained by performing the CART analysis, a clinical predictive score (GAPS = GBM-associated prognostic score) was elaborated. In detail, a score from 0 to 4 was then assigned to the 11 terminal nodes (score 0, assigned to the nodes with RHR ≤ 0.40; score 1 assigned to the nodes with RHR between 0.40 and 1.00; score 2 assigned to the nodes with RHR between 1.00 and 2.00; score 3 assigned to the nodes with RHR between 2.00–4.00; score 4 was assigned to the nodes with RHR > 4.00). Each score group was defined based on the following characteristics: Score 0: patients with EOR > 96%, preoperative ΔT1/T2 MRI Index < 0.72 and age < 53; Score 1: patients with EOR > 96%, T1/T2 < 0.72 and age > 53; patients with EOR between 81% and 95% if they have a preoperative ΔT1/T2 MRI Index < 0.72 and preoperative T2-weight volume > 147 cm3; Score 2: patients with EOR between 81% and 95%, preoperative ΔT1/T2 MRI Index < 0.72 and preoperative T2-weight volume < 147 cm3; patients with EOR > 80%, preoperative ΔT1/T2 MRI Index > 0.72, if they have EOR between 91% and 100%; patients with EOR between 56% and 80% if they are aged < 59; Score 3: patients with preoperative ΔT1/T2 MRI Index > 0.72 and EOR between 81% and 90%; patients with EOR between 56% and 80% if they have age > 60; Score 4: all patients with EOR < 55%. The obtained 5 groups of GBM cases were associated with different OS: score 0 group included 45 cases (accounting to the 9.68% of cases), score 1 included 157 cases (33.76%), score 2 included 165 cases (35.48%), score 3 included 79 cases (16.99%), and score 4 included 19 cases (4.09%).

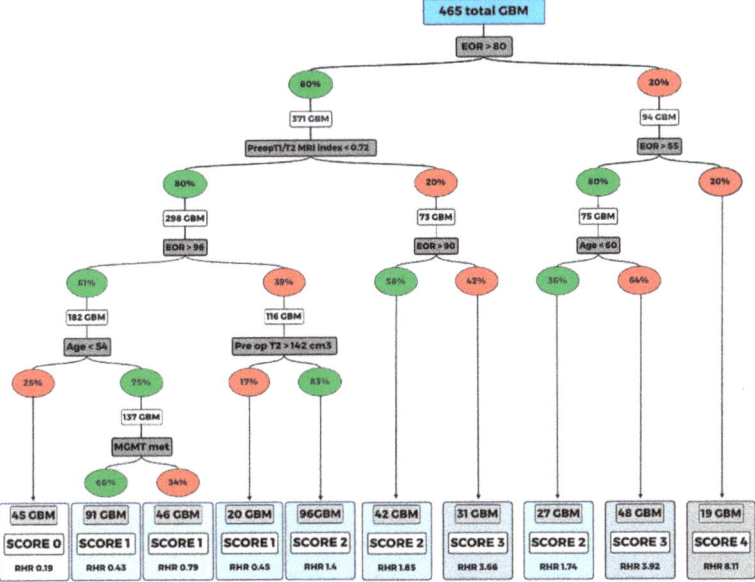

Figure 4. Random forest (classification and regression tree, CART).

Once the scores were obtained, a univariate Cox regression was performed to evaluate the predictive ability of the score.

Compared to score 0 (low risk), score 1 had hazard ratio (HR) = 2.6 (95% CI: [1.4–5.0], p = 0.003); score 2 had HR = 9.6 (95% CI: [5.1–18.3], p = 0.000); score 3 had HR = 28.1 (95% CI: [14.4–54.7], p = 0.000); score 4 had HR = 85.4 (95% CI: [38.5–189.3], p = 0.000).

The goodness of fit of the score model in predicting death was estimated with a Harrell's c-index of 0.78 (95% IC [0.76–0.81]). The 1-yr estimated OS was computed for each score category (Table 3).

Table 3. One-year estimated overall survival and hazard ratios for each score with relative 95% confidence intervals. A score (GBM-associated prognostic score, GAPS) from 0 to 4 was then assigned to the 10 terminal nodes thus defined based on the relative hazard ratio (RHR).

Score	Variables	OS% (95% CI)	HR (95%CI)	p-Value
0	Preoperative ΔT1/T2 MRI Index < 0.72; EOR > 96%; Age < 53	92.24 (77.82–97.43)	1	-
1	Preoperative ΔT1/T2 MRI Index < 0.72; EOR > 96%; Age > 53	84.36 (77.39–89.33)	2.6 (1.4–5.0)	0.003
	Preoperative ΔT1/T2 MRI Index < 0.72; EOR: 81%–95%; Preop T2-w vol > 147 cm^3			
2	Preoperative ΔT1/T2 MRI Index < 0.72; EOR: 81%–95%; Preop T2-w vol < 147cm^3	43.85 (35.94–51.48)	9.6 (5.1–18.3)	0.000
	Preoperative ΔT1/T2 MRI Index > 0.72; EOR >91%			
	EOR: 56%–80%; Age < 59			
3	Preoperative ΔT1/T2 MRI Index > 0.72; EOR 81%–90%	11.58 (5.69–19.76)	28.1 (14.4–54.7)	0.000
	EOR: 56%–80%; age > 60			
4	EOR < 55%	5.26 (0.36–21.43)	85.4 (38.5–189.3)	0.000

The algorithm relied on six clinical variables that shows the interaction between the significant variables at multivariate analysis (age, EOR, MGMT methylation status, preoperative ΔT1/T2 MRI index, pre-operative volumetric tumor volume on T2-weighted images and intraoperative protocol).

The score (GAPS) from 0 to 4 was then assigned to the 10 terminal nodes thus defined based on the relative hazard ratio (RHR). Percent values indicated in the in green ovals represent the presence of the variable considered; the red color indicates absence of that variable.

2.3. Treatment at Tumor Progression

In this study, a population of 369 cases experienced tumor progression; 298 were treated with salvage treatments, while the others with supportive care (SC).

Among patients treated with salvage treatments (298), the impact of treatment type (TMZ, second surgery, TMZ + RT, RT alone, photemustine-lomustine) on OS was analyzed.

At tumor progression, TMZ was administered in 215 patients, 43 patients underwent a second surgery. Twenty-four patients were treated with TMZ + RT, 8 patients with RT alone and 8 patients with photemustine-lomustine.

By applying the Kaplan–Meier survival estimates and the logrank test, there were no differences in survival on the basis of the treatment adopted at tumor progression ($p = 0.236$ considering all the subgroups taken separately; $p = 0.199$ combining TMZ + RT, RT and photemustine-lomustine). The Cox regression analysis also confirmed this evidence taking the TMZ treatment as a reference and combining the others salvage treatments. There was no association for intervention (HR = 0.760 [95% CI: 0.513–1.126], $p = 0.172$); TMZ+RT (HR = 0.670 [95% CI: 0.394–1.140], $p = 0.140$); RT (HR = 1.280 [95% CI: 0.628–2.608], $p = 0.496$); photemustine-lomustine (HR = 0.643 [95% CI: 0.263–1.571], $p = 0.332$).

One-year estimated PFS was computed in all generated GAPS class scores, resulting in being significantly different in each score class (Kruskall–Wallis test, $p = 0.001$) (Table 4).

Table 4. One-year estimated PFS according to GAPS score.

GAPS Score	1-Year Estimated PFS
Score 0	65.60%
Score 1	55.54%
Score 2	13.09%
Score 3–4	3.93%

3. Discussion

Despite decades of therapeutic, surgical and genetics refinements, GBM still remains the highest-grade malignant primary tumor of the central nervous system with an extremely poor prognosis [4,10,11,19,39].

Age, performance status, extent of surgical resection and MGMT methylation status are well known prognostic factors for GBM patients [4,21–34,39–44]. Nevertheless, the high degree of clinical/molecular heterogeneity found among GBM patients do not generally allow us to correctly classify GBM patients with the use of a single predictor or a few predictors. There is thus an increasing need of comprehensive predictive classification models, which concomitantly evaluate multiple clinical/molecular/radiomic biomarkers. Moreover, given the high degree of heterogeneity in survival rates among GBM patients, it becomes essential to use tools that are capable of considering the possible interaction between the significant independent survival variables as further possible source of differences in the survival outcome.

In the present study, we set up a prognostic model that comprehensively evaluated clinical, molecular and treatment-associated factors to stratify GBM-affected patients undergoing surgery using a random forest approach (CART). This model generated an integrative visualization of risk factors, giving rise to an easy and immediate interactive interpretation of results.

The analysis consisted of 3 main steps: first, the most informative variables were identified; then, a decision tree algorithm was applied to differentiate the survival and lastly the GAPS score was generated.

Five variables were selected as the most informative amongst the 20 variables considered. The highest classification accuracy included age, preoperative tumor volume computed on T2-wheighted MRI, preoperative ΔT1/T2 MRI Index, EOR, and MGMT methylation status. The interactions were analyzed using the CART model.

There has been an increasing number of volumetric investigations highlighting the association between the EOR and survival [8,9,16,18,19,23,25,33]. Nowadays an increasing variety of neurosurgical methods are available (e.g., frameless navigational systems, intraoperative imaging, ultrasonography, and functional mapping) to achieve the optimum balance between a maximal resection and a safe resection.

By performing the random forest approach, the EOR was placed on top of the decision tree. Specifically, the obtained results showed that cases with EOR >80% were associated with a longer survival rate. This finding is in keeping with previously published retrospective investigations suggesting that at least 70%–78% of the contrast-enhancing tumor volume represents the ideal resection target for survival benefit [9,25]. Sanai and colleagues were the first that have highlighted the importance of EOR threshold in GBM survival [9]. In line with their contribution, our study reported the best survival rate in patients with an EOR higher than 96% with estimated 1-yr OS of 92%.

Another important finding highlighted by the CART was the relevant impact on GBM prognosis for preoperative volumetric radiological features. The hallmarks of GBM on MRI are the contrast-enhancing tumor with its central necrosis and surrounding peritumoral edema. Each tumoral component could represent a potential imaging marker to predict the OS.

There is still open discussion among neuroncologists regarding which tumoral component has to be considered (e.g., contrast enhancement, peritumoral edema, central necrosis [13,23,45].

In this investigation, the preoperative MRI index based on the ΔT1/T2 MRI ratio was computed as previously described [45], resulting as being an independent predictor both for OS and PFS. Specifically, patients with a preoperative ΔT1/T2 MRI Index ratio close to 1 had a poor prognosis compared to those with preoperative T1/T2 MRI ratio close to 0, in other words lesions with ratio close to 1 should have more aggressive growth, as opposed to lesions with a ratio close to 0. However, we cannot ultimately identify which aspects of tumoral behavior determine the preoperative ΔT1/T2 MRI Index and given the wide heterogeneity of GBM, future investigations based on texture features from multiparametric MRI and next generation sequences analysis, may further clarify this issue.

Elderly age negatively affected the prognosis only in cases of limited resection, supporting the role of surgery in fit older patients when a safe and large resection can be planned [42–44].

Regarding the molecular features, the MGMT methylation status positively influenced the prognosis only in patients younger than 54 years with an EOR higher than 96%, thus suggesting the possibility of other genetic abnormalities potentially affecting survivals of GBM patients.

CART analysis provided 10 terminal nodes; the RHR of which were used to generate the score (GAPS) with the purpose of facilitating the survival stratification before patients were discharged postoperatively.

GAPS were elaborated to detect the impact of variables interaction on the overall survival giving rise to an easy and immediate interpretation score. Patients belonging to score 0 (preoperative ΔT1/T2 MRI Index < 0.72; EOR > 96%; Age < 53) had the better survival with a 3 years estimated OS of 25%, otherwise, the worse survival was for patients with score 3 and 4 (preoperative ΔT1/T2 MRI Index > 0.72; EOR 81%–90%, or EOR: 56%–80%; age > 60; or EOR < 55) with 1 year-estimated OS of 11.58% and 5.26% respectively after surgery being equal with regards to the post-operative treatments.

The novelty of this approach is that the focus is on the interaction of different factors rather than the single determinant. This allows the building of a model as close as possible to the real clinical setting.

The GAPS score could be useful in a day-to-day clinical environment and in a research setting to draw future prospective clinical trials. Moreover, GAPS score could be useful when deciding and discussing prognosis to better handle the entire GBM management.

We aware that our study has several limits, which include the retrospective nature of the investigation and the different treatments performed at tumor progression. Moreover, the retrospective study did not permit a standardized follow-up.

The GAPS score could be useful in a day-to-day clinical environment and in a research setting to draw future prospective clinical trials. Moreover, GAPS score could be adopted in discussing prognosis to better handle the entire GBM management.

We aware that our study has several limits, which include the retrospective nature of the investigation and the different treatments performed at tumor progression. Moreover, the retrospective study did not permit a standardized follow-up.

The statistical limitations of such a retrospective analysis are well known and cannot be completely controlled with any statistical model.

Treatments at GBM relapse represents a crucial issue. The recurrence of GBM is inevitable, in which management often tend to be unclear and case-dependent. Although re-radiation, re-resection, bevacizumab, and chemotherapy are still the most widely used therapies for treating recurrent GBM, the clinical benefit from these treatments is still not well established [46–50].

It is well known that to improve the prediction models, salvage treatments information should be updated in the analysis at the time of tumor progression.

Longer PFS resulted in late tumor recurrence and consequently in better OS [46].

In this investigation, patients with lower GAPS score had a longer PFS and consequent better OS. The predictive survival score computed in this investigation can, thus, be considered as an indirect measure of tumor progression. Patients with GAPS score of 0 had a better survival and prolonged PFS determined by the combination of radiological, surgical and molecular factors before tumor recurrence. The score was analyzed based on the characteristics of the patients included in the model. This tool provides information regarding a more or less rapid risk of progression before the administration of salvage treatments at tumor progression itself. For this reason, the salvage treatments cannot be considered. In addition, progression time is different in the different GAPS score classes and time dependent analysis should be applied to evaluate the effect of salvage treatments on OS.

Data regarding selection criteria adopted at tumor recurrence to plan the salvage treatment were not available. Each patient underwent an individualized management at tumor progression. We have not developed standardized protocols for treatments at tumor progression, which is another drawback of this study that requires future investigation.

Future prospective multicenter studies in a larger group of patients with a long follow-up are needed to overcome the inherent limitations of a retrospective study and to confirm the potential clinical usefulness of this tool in the management of GBM patients. Genetic studies could be integrated in this preliminary model in order to improve the accuracy of the score in the stratification of GBM patient prognosis.

4. Materials and Methods

A shared co-operative record databased 520 adult patients who underwent surgery for newly diagnosed GMB between January 2015 and December 2018; 465 GBM patients were enrolled in the case cohort according to the following inclusion criteria: age $\geq$ 18 years; no previous surgery; no preoperative chemo- or radiotherapy; objective evaluation of preoperative tumor volume on MRI images in DICOM format based on post-contrast T1-weighted MRI sequences and T2-weighted MRI sequences; objective estimation of EOR on post-contrast T1-weighted MRI sequences; revision of histopathological specimens by using the new 2016 World Health Organization (WHO) Classification of Tumors of the Central Nervous System [51]; MGMT promoter methylation and IDH1/IDH2 mutation status assessment. Cases were excluded from the case cohort if one or more of the following criteria were present: incomplete imaging data, follow-up interval, and multicentric tumors. Clinical, histopathological and molecular data were collected at the time of diagnosis from medical records. No central histopathological review and no additional molecular analyses were performed for the purpose of the study

Histological examination, immunohistochemistry for Ki67 and IDH1R132H, analysis of the genetic status of O6-methylguanine-DNA-methyltransferase (MGMT) promoter and isocitrate dehydrogenase (IDH1/2) genes were performed as previously described. Gliomas were defined as methylated when the average percentage of methylation of CpG islands was $\geq$8% [52].

Patients were clinically evaluated both prior to discharge, and at subsequent 4-monthly intervals. Patients that exhibited no clinical improvement by 6 months after surgery were considered to have a permanent deficit. In the follow-up period MRI images were obtained at regular (4-monthly) intervals.

The present study was approved by the local Ethics Committee (protocol N. 0036566 /P/ GEN/ EGAS, ID study 2538). Written informed consent was obtained for surgery. Considering that the study was retrospective, written consent to participate in the study was not applicable.

4.1. Volumetric Analysis

All pre and postoperative tumor segmentations were performed manually across all MRI slices using the OsiriX software tool [53].

The achieved EOR in each case was objectively evaluated using preoperative and postoperative MRI images (DICOM format), based on the contrast area of post-contrast T1 MRI sequences, using the below formula: (Pre-operative tumor volume – Post-operative tumor volume)/Pre-operative tumor volume) [54].

With the aim of evaluating the role of tumor growing pattern on OS, a novel predictive preoperative MRI index was defined as follows T1/T2 = preoperative volumetric tumor volume on post contrast T1-weighted images/ preoperative volumetric tumor volume on T2-weighted images.

4.2. Post-Operative Treatment

After surgery, all patients were treated with combinations of concomitant adjuvant radiotherapy and chemotherapy, followed by adjuvant chemotherapy, as recommended by Stupp [5].

External-beam (either conformal or stereotactic) radiotherapy was used to administer a total dose of 60 Gy (delivered in 30 fractions of 2 Gy over a 6-week period), followed by adjuvant oral chemotherapy with temozolomide (75 mg/m^2/day, 7 days/wk). Four weeks after the end of this treatment protocol, patients underwent at least six cycles of consolidation chemotherapy with oral temozolomide (150–200 mg/m^2/day, for 5 days/28 days).

4.3. Statistical Analysis

Categorical variables were reported as percentages, continuous variables were reported as mean ± standard deviation or median and range as appropriate, according with the data distribution. Normality of the continuous variables was tested using the Shapiro–Wilk test. The OS time was defined as extending from surgery until patient death; PFS time was defined as extending from surgery until the demonstration of gadolinium enhancement on follow-up imaging. OS and PFS were estimated using the Kaplan–Meier approach. The association between variables and survival distribution was tested using univariate and multivariate Cox proportional hazard models (after verification of proportional hazard assumptions). Patients with unknown survival were censored as of their last scan date. The variables we considered for univariate analysis were age, sex, KPS score, preoperative tumor volume computed on post contrast T1-wheighted images and on T2- weighted images MRI, tumor location, tumor side, EOR, postoperative adjuvant protocol used, IDH $\frac{1}{2}$ mutation, MGMT mutilation status and Ki-67. The EOR was modeled both as a continuous and an ordinal variable ($\leq$79%, 80%–89%, 90%–99%, 100%) in univariate analysis to ensure consistency with the previous 46 studies that focused on the impact of glioma resection in terms of volumes. The preoperative ΔT1/T2 MRI Index was calculated by the ratio between pre- operative tumor volume calculated on post-contrast T1-wheighted images MRI and the pre-operative tumor volume calculated on T2-weighted images MRI. In the univariate Cox regression, the preoperative ΔT1/T2 MRI Index was initially analyzed as a continuous variable. To better understand the variable's association pattern, the Cox regression was then applied to the quintiles splitted variable. Subsequently, the variable was dichotomized using a cut-off we identified at the quintile that showed a significant hazard ratio. The variables resulted in being significantly associated in the univariate model with $p < 0.05$. All statistical analyses were performed by Stata/IC 13.0 (StataCorp LP, College Station, TX, USA).

4.4. Classification and Regression Tree (CART) Method

To determine subgroups patients with different clinical prognosis, we used the decision tree model using the CART method [55,56].

This method is a machine learning model, composed of hierarchic decision rules involving optimal cutoff values that recursively split independent factors into different groups. The groups of individuals are called nodes, and form a branch node tree. Terminal nodes are groups of individuals that cannot be further subdivided on the basis of the established parameters (minimum size of subgroup, minimum number of events, maximum p-value required) to proceed in further subdivisions. The CART algorithm was performed on the entire sample (465 cases). In our study, nodes were required to have a minimum size of 15 patients, a minimum of 10 events and a maximum p-value of 0.05. Factors initially introduced into this CART analysis are the following: EOR, preoperative ΔT1/T2 MRI Index, age, MGMT methylation, pre-operative volumetric tumor volume on T2-weighted images and intraoperative protocol. Once the regression tree was generated, the nodes of the terminal branches were pruned (aggregated) on the basis of their relative hazard ratios (RHRs) in order to obtain final groups with homogeneous mortality risk. The final groups were converted in a score ordered according to their hazard ratios (HRs).

Differences in terms of overall survival probability among the score categories were investigated using univariate Cox regression analysis. The performance of the score in predicting time to death was estimated through Harrell's c-index [57]. All statistical analyses were performed by Stata/IC 13.0 (StataCorp LP, College Station, TX, USA).

5. Conclusions

Nowadays, the current standard of care for GBM still includes maximal safe surgical resection followed by concomitant chemoradiation therapy and adjunct of chemotherapy. The high degree of clinical heterogeneity found among GBM highlights a rising need for comprehensive predictive classification models concomitantly evaluating multiple clinical/molecular/radiomic biomarkers. The CART prediction model allowed to elaborate a novel comprehensive clinical score (GAPS) to stratify prognosis of glioblastoma patients undergoing surgical resection. Although GAPS needs to be validated in further multicenter studies, it could facilitate the survival-risk grading, guiding clinicians in the decision-making process.

Author Contributions: Data curation, T.I., F.P., G.M.D.P., S.G., G.L.R., T.S., C.B., M.P., M.D.B., D.B., E.P., S.C., M.A., G.S.; Formal analysis, M.I., C.B.; Investigation, T.I., S.G.; Methodology, T.I., F.P., G.M.D.P., S.G., G.L.R., T.S., M.I., G.S.; Software, M.I.; Supervision, T.I., A.O., M.S., G.S.; Validation, T.I., S.G.; Writing—original draft, TI; Writing—review and editing, T.I., F.P., G.M.D.P., S.G., G.L.R., T.S., C.B., M.P., M.D.B., M.I., D.B., E.P., S.C., A.O., M.S., M.A., G.S. All authors have read and agreed to the published version of the manuscript.

Funding: This work has been supported by: Progetto Ministero della Salute, Giovani Ricercatori 2016 GR-2016-02364678. Application of GLIADEL wafers (BCNU, carmustine) followed by temozolomide and radiotherapy in patients with high-grade glioma: a precision medicine based on molecular landscape. CUP: J26C16000000005

Acknowledgments: We acknowledge the support by the medical staff of the Departments of Pathology and Neuroradiology (Santa Maria della Misericordia University Hospital, Udine, Policlinico Gemelli, Rome).

Conflicts of Interest: The authors declare no conflict of interest. The funders had no role in the design of the study; in the collection, analyses, or interpretation of data; in the writing of the manuscript; or in the decision to publish the results.

Appendix A

Table A1. Baseline characteristics of the study population.

Parameters	Value (N and %, Mean ± Standard Deviation (SD) or Median and Range)
No. of patients	465
Age (years)	63 (20–85)
Sex	
Female	176 (37.85%)
Male	289 (62.15%)
Side	
Left	228 (49.03%)
Right	237 (50.97%)
Tumor Site	
Precentral	182 (39.14%)
Postcentral	128 (27.53%)
Temporal + Insular	155 (33.33%)
Intra-operative protocol	
CEUS + / 5-ALA +	43 (9.25%)
CEUS - / 5-ALA +	35 (7.53%)
CEUS + / 5-ALA -	34 (7.31%)
CEUS - / 5-ALA -	353 (75.91%)
Radiological Features	
Ependymal involvement (*yes vs. no*)	143 vs. 322 (30.75% vs 69.25%)
Corpus Callosum involvement (*yes vs. no*)	155 vs. 310 (33.33% vs 66.67%)
Necrotic-cystic component (*yes vs. no*)	319 vs. 146 (68.60% vs 31.40%)

Table A1. *Cont.*

Parameters	Value (N and %, Mean ± Standard Deviation (SD) or Median and Range)
Midline shift (*yes vs no*)	222 vs. 243 (47.74% vs 52.26%)
Preoperative Tumoral Volume computed on postcontrast T1-weighted images, cm^3	31 (0.682–136)
Preoperative Tumoral Volume computed on T2-weighted images, cm^3	65 (3–497)
Preoperative ΔT1/T2 MRI Index	48.55 (1.13–100)
Residual tumor, cm^3	0.959 (0–37.506)
EOR (continuous variable)	95 (38–100)
EOR (categorical variable)	
EOR = 100%	184 (39.57%)
99% ≤ EOR ≤ 90%	133 (28.6%)
89% ≤ EOR ≤ 80%	76 (16.34%)
EOR ≤ 79%	72 (15.48%)
Biological Features	
MGMT methylation (*yes vs no*)	290 vs. 175 (62.37% vs. 37.63%)
IDH 1/2 mutation (*yes vs no*)	38 vs. 427 (8.17% vs. 91.83%)
Ki-67	25 (2-95)
Two-gene model	
MGMT met and IDH 1/2 mut	27 (5.81%)
MGMT met and IDH 1/2 wt	263 (56.56%)
MGMT unmet and IDH 1/2 mut	10 (2.15%)
MGMT unmet and IDH 1/2 wt	165 (35.48%)
Postoperative Protocol	
Stupp protocol	345 (74.2%)
Stupp protocol + CWs	60 (12.9 %)
Stupp interrupted for side effects	60 (12.9 %)

Features of the study population are described using means ± standard deviation or median and range for continuous variables, number of cases with relative percentages reported in parentheses for categorical variables. EOR = extent of resection; MRI = magnetic resonance image; preoperative ΔT1/T2 MRI Index = ratio between pre-operative tumoral volume on postcontrast T1-weighted and T2 weighted images; CWs = Carmustine Wafers; MGMT =O^6-methylguanine-DNA methyl-transferase; IDH = isocitrate dehydrogenase.

Table A2. Clinical and follow-up characteristics of the study population.

	Value (N and %, Mean ± SD or Median and Range)
Clinical presentation	
No deficits	41 (8.82%)
Not-specific symptoms (headache, nausea, vomiting, disorientation etc.)	165 (35.48%)
Motor deficits	89 (19.14%)

Table A2. Cont.

	Value (N and %, Mean ± SD or Median and Range)
Sensory deficits	16 (3.44%)
Visual/speech deficits	66 (14.19%)
Seizures	88 (18.92%)
Post-operative course	
No deficits	263 (56.56%)
Not-specific symptoms (headache, nausea, vomiting, disorientation etc.)	64 (13.76%)
Motor deficits	80 (17.20%)
Sensory deficits	3 (0.65%)
Visual/speech deficits	52 (11.18%)
Seizures	3 (0.65%)
6-monts follow-up (in 394 pts alive)	
No deficits	245 (62.18%)
Not-specific symptoms (headache, nausea, vomiting, disorientation etc.)	94 (23.86%)
Motor deficits	35 (8.88%)
Sensory deficits	1 (0.25%)
Visual/speech deficits	17 (4.31%)
Seizures	2 (0.51%)
KPS	
Pre-operative	90 (50–100)
Immediate post-operative	90 (50–100)
6-monts follow-up (in 394 pts alive)	90 (50–100)
OS (alive vs dead)	158 vs. 307 (33.98% vs. 66.02%)
OS at 1-year follow-up	54.78%
OS at 2-year follow-up	22.28%
PFS (no recurrence vs recurrence)	96 vs. 369 (20.65% vs. 79.35%)
PFS at 1 year follow-up	33.05%
PFS at 2 year follow-up	13.82%

Characteristics of the study population are described using means ± s.d. (standard deviation) or median and range for continuous variables, number of cases with relative percentages reported in parentheses for categorical variables. KPS = Karnofsky Performance Status; OS = overall survival; PFS = progression-free survival.

References

1. Guden, M.; Ayata, H.B.; Ceylan, C.; Kilic, A.; Engin, K. Prognostic factors effective on survival of patients with glioblastoma: Anadolu Medical Center experience. *Indian J. Cancer* **2016**, *53*, 382–386.
2. Nam, J.Y.; De Groot, J.F. Treatment of Glioblastoma. *J. Oncol. Pr.* **2017**, *13*, 629–638. [CrossRef] [PubMed]
3. Ohgaki, H. Epidemiology of Brain Tumors. *Methods Mol. Biol.* **2009**, *472*, 323–342. [PubMed]
4. Weller, M.; Bent, M.V.D.; Hopkins, K.; Tonn, J.C.; Stupp, R.; Falini, A.; Cohen-Jonathan-Moyal, E.; Frappaz, D.; Henriksson, R.; Balaña, C.; et al. EANO guideline for the diagnosis and treatment of anaplastic gliomas and glioblastoma. *Lancet Oncol.* **2014**, *15*, 395–403. [CrossRef]

5. Stupp, R.; Mason, W.P.; van den Bent, M.J.; Weller, M.; Fisher, B.; Taphoorn, M.J.; Belanger, K.; Brandes, A.A.; Marosi, C.; Bogdahn, U.; et al. Radiotherapy plus concomitant and adjuvant temozolomide for glioblastoma. *N. Engl. J. Med.* **2005**, *352*, 987–996. [CrossRef] [PubMed]
6. Stupp, R.; Brada, M.; Bent, M.J.V.D.; Tonn, J.-C.; Pentheroudakis, G. High-grade glioma: ESMO Clinical Practice Guidelines for diagnosis, treatment and follow-up. *Ann. Oncol.* **2014**, *25*, 93–101. [CrossRef] [PubMed]
7. Stupp, R.; Hegi, M.E.; Gorlia, T.; Erridge, S.C.; Perry, J.; Hong, Y.-K.; Aldape, K.D.; Lhermitte, B.; Pietsch, T.; Grujicic, D.; et al. Cilengitide combined with standard treatment for patients with newly diagnosed glioblastoma with methylated MGMT promoter (CENTRIC EORTC 26071-22072 study): A multicentre, randomised, open-label, phase 3 trial. *Lancet Oncol.* **2014**, *15*, 1100–1108. [CrossRef]
8. Sanai, N.; Berger, M. Extent of resection influences outcomes for patients with gliomas. *Rev. Neurol.* **2011**, *167*, 648–654. [CrossRef]
9. Lacroix, M.; Abi-Said, D.; Fourney, D.R.; Gokaslan, Z.L.; Shi, W.; Demonte, F.; Lang, F.F.; McCutcheon, I.E.; Hassenbusch, S.J.; Holland, E.; et al. A multivariate analysis of 416 patients with glioblastoma multiforme: Prognosis, extent of resection, and survival. *J. Neurosurg.* **2001**, *95*, 190–198. [CrossRef]
10. McGirt, M.J.; Than, K.D.; Weingart, J.D.; Chaichana, K.L.; Attenello, F.J.; Olivi, A.; Laterra, J.; Kleinberg, L.R.; Grossman, S.A.; Brem, H.; et al. Gliadel (BCNU) wafer plus concomitant temozolomide therapy after primary resection of glioblastoma multiforme. *J. Neurosurg.* **2009**, *110*, 583–588. [CrossRef]
11. Chaudhry, N.S.; Shah, A.H.; Ferraro, N.; Snelling, B.M.; Bregy, A.; Madhavan, K.; Komotar, R.J. Predictors of long-term survival in patients with glioblastoma multiforme: Advancements from the last quarter century. *Cancer Invest.* **2013**, *31*, 287–308. [CrossRef]
12. Wijnenga, M.M.J.; French, P.J.; Dubbink, H.J.; Dinjens, W.N.M.; Atmodimedjo, P.N.; Kros, J.M.; Smits, M.; Gahrmann, R.; Rutten, G.J.; Verheul, J.B.; et al. The impact of surgery in molecularly defined low-grade glioma: An integrated clinical, radiological, and molecular analysis. *Neuro Oncol.* **2018**, *20*, 103–112. [CrossRef]
13. Gillies, R.J.; Kinahan, P.E.; Hricak, H. Radiomics: Images Are More than Pictures, They Are Data. *Radiology* **2016**, *278*, 563–577. [CrossRef]
14. O'Connor, J.P.; Aboagye, E.O.; Adams, J.E.; Aerts, H.J.; Barrington, S.F.; Beer, A.J.; Boellaard, R.; Bohndiek, S.E.; Brady, M.; Brown, G.; et al. Imaging biomarker roadmap for cancer studies. *Nat. Rev. Clin. Oncol.* **2017**, *14*, 169–186. [CrossRef] [PubMed]
15. Gittleman, H.; Lim, D.; Kattan, M.W.; Chakravarti, A.; Gilbert, M.R.; Lassman, A.B.; Lo, S.S.; Machtay, M.; Sloan, A.E.; Sulman, E.P.; et al. An independently validated nomogram for individualized estimation of survival among patients with newly diagnosed glioblastoma: NRG Oncology RTOG 0525 and 0825. *Neuro-Oncology* **2016**, *19*, 669–677.
16. Brown, T.J.; Brennan, M.C.; Li, M.; Church, E.W.; Brandmeir, N.J.; Rakszawski, K.L.; Patel, A.S.; Rizk, E.B.; Suki, D.; Sawaya, R.; et al. Association of the Extent of Resection With Survival in Glioblastoma: A Systematic Review and Meta-analysis. *JAMA Oncol.* **2016**, *2*, 1460–1469. [CrossRef] [PubMed]
17. Rahman, M.; Abbatematteo, J.; De Leo, E.K.; Kubilis, P.S.; Vaziri, S.; Bova, F.; Sayour, E.; Mitchell, D.; Quinones-Hinojosa, A. The effects of new or worsened postoperative neurological deficits on survival of patients with glioblastoma. *J. Neurosurg.* **2017**, *127*, 123–131. [CrossRef]
18. Chaichana, K.L.; Cabrera-Aldana, E.E.; Jusue-Torres, I.; Wijesekera, O.; Olivi, A.; Rahman, M.; Quiñones-Hinojosa, A. When Gross Total Resection of a Glioblastoma Is Possible, How Much Resection Should Be Achieved? *World Neurosurg.* **2014**, *82*, 257–265. [CrossRef]
19. Awad, A.-W.; Karsy, M.; Sanai, N.; Spetzler, R.; Zhang, Y.; Xu, Y.; Mahan, M.A. Impact of removed tumor volume and location on patient outcome in glioblastoma. *J. Neuro-Oncol.* **2017**, *135*, 161–171. [CrossRef]
20. Ng, K.; Kim, R.; Kesari, S.; Carter, B.; Chen, C.C. Genomic profiling of glioblastoma: Convergence of fundamental biologic tenets and novel insights. *J. Neurooncol.* **2012**, *107*, 1–12. [CrossRef]
21. Weller, M.; Felsberg, J.; Hartmann, C.; Berger, H.; Steinbach, J.P.; Schramm, J.; Westphal, M.; Schackert, G.; Simon, M.; Tonn, J.C.; et al. Molecular Predictors of Progression-Free and Overall Survival in Patients With Newly Diagnosed Glioblastoma: A Prospective Translational Study of the German Glioma Network. *J. Clin. Oncol.* **2009**, *27*, 5743–5750. [CrossRef] [PubMed]

22. Gessler, F.; Bernstock, J.D.; Braczynski, A.; Lescher, S.; Baumgarten, P.; Harter, P.N.; Mittelbronn, M.; Wu, T.; Seifert, V.; Senft, C. Surgery for Glioblastoma in Light of Molecular Markers: Impact of Resection and MGMT Promoter Methylation in Newly Diagnosed IDH-1 Wild-Type Glioblastomas. *Neurosurgery* **2019**, *84*, 190–197. [CrossRef] [PubMed]
23. Mampre, D.; Ehresman, J.; Pinilla-Monsalve, G.; Osorio, M.A.G.; Olivi, A.; Quinones-Hinojosa, A.; Chaichana, K.L. Extending the resection beyond the contrast-enhancement for glioblastoma: Feasibility, efficacy, and outcomes. *Br. J. Neurosurg.* **2018**, *32*, 528–535. [CrossRef] [PubMed]
24. Grabowski, M.M.; Recinos, P.F.; Nowacki, A.S.; Schroeder, J.L.; Angelov, L.; Barnett, G.H.; Vogelbaum, M.A. Residual tumor volume versus extent of resection: Predictors of survival after surgery for glioblastoma. *J. Neurosurg.* **2014**, *121*, 1115–1123. [CrossRef] [PubMed]
25. Chaichana, K.L.; Jusue-Torres, I.; Navarro-Ramirez, R.; Raza, S.M.; Pascual-Gallego, M.; Ibrahim, A.; Hernandez-Hermann, M.; Gomez, L.; Ye, X.; Weingart, J.D.; et al. Establishing percent resection and residual volume thresholds affecting survival and recurrence for patients with newly diagnosed intracranial glioblastoma. *Neuro-Oncology* **2014**, *16*, 113–122. [CrossRef] [PubMed]
26. Coburger, J.; Hagel, V.; Wirtz, C.R.; König, R. Surgery for Glioblastoma: Impact of the Combined Use of 5-Aminolevulinic Acid and Intraoperative MRI on Extent of Resection and Survival. *PLoS ONE* **2015**, *10*, e0131872. [CrossRef]
27. Cordova, J.S.; Gurbani, S.S.; Holder, C.A.; Olson, J.J.; Schreibmann, E.; Shi, R.; Guo, Y.; Shu, H.-K.G.; Shim, H.; Hadjipanayis, C.G. Semi-Automated Volumetric and Morphological Assessment of Glioblastoma Resection with Fluorescence-Guided Surgery. *Mol. Imaging Boil.* **2016**, *18*, 454–462. [CrossRef]
28. Suchorska, B.; Weller, M.; Tabatabai, G.; Senft, C.; Hau, P.; Sabel, M.C.; Herrlinger, U.; Ketter, R.; Schlegel, U.; Marosi, C.; et al. Complete resection of contrast-enhancing tumor volume is associated with improved survival in recurrent glioblastoma—Results from the DIRECTOR trial. *Neuro-Oncology* **2016**, *18*, 549–556. [CrossRef]
29. Grossman, R.; Shimony, N.; Shir, D.; Gonen, T.; Sitt, R.; Kimchi, T.J.; Harosh, C.B.; Ram, Z. Dynamics of FLAIR Volume Changes in Glioblastoma and Prediction of Survival. *Ann. Surg. Oncol.* **2017**, *24*, 794–800. [CrossRef]
30. Fukui, A.; Muragaki, Y.; Saito, T.; Maruyama, T.; Nitta, M.; Ikuta, S.; Kawamata, T. Volumetric Analysis Using Low-Field Intraoperative Magnetic Resonance Imaging for 168 Newly Diagnosed Supratentorial Glioblastomas: Effects of Extent of Resection and Residual Tumor Volume on Survival and Recurrence. *World Neurosurg.* **2017**, *98*, 73–80. [CrossRef]
31. Eseonu, C.I.; Refaey, K.; Garcia, O.; Raghuraman, G.; Quinones-Hinojosa, A. Volumetric Analysis of Extent of Resection, Survival, and Surgical Outcomes for Insular Gliomas. *World Neurosurg.* **2017**, *103*, 265–274. [CrossRef]
32. Henker, C.; Kriesen, T.; Glass, Ä.; Schneider, B.; Piek, J. Volumetric quantification of glioblastoma: Experiences with different measurement techniques and impact on survival. *J. Neuro-Oncol.* **2017**, *135*, 391–402. [CrossRef]
33. Coburger, J.; Segovia, J.; Ganslandt, O.; Ringel, F.; Wirtz, C.R.; Renovanz, M. Counseling Patients with a Glioblastoma Amenable Only for Subtotal Resection: Results of a Multicenter Retrospective Assessment of Survival and Neurologic Outcome. *World Neurosurg.* **2018**, *114*, 1180–1185. [CrossRef]
34. Zacharaki, E.; Morita, N.; Bhatt, P.; O'Rourke, D.; Melhem, E.R.; Davatzikos, C. Survival analysis of patients with high-grade gliomas based on data mining of imaging variables. *Am. J. Neuroradiol.* **2012**, *33*, 1065–1071. [CrossRef] [PubMed]
35. Ganggayah, M.D.; Taib, N.A.; Har, Y.C.; Lio, P.; Dhillon, S.K. Predicting factors for survival of breast cancer patients using machine learning techniques. *BMC Med. Inform. Decis. Mak.* **2019**, *19*, 48. [CrossRef] [PubMed]
36. Sudhamathy, G.; Thilagu, M.; Padmavathi, G. Comparative analysis of R package classifiers using breast cancer dataset. *Int. J. Eng. Technol.* **2016**, *8*, 2127–2136.
37. Chen, W.; Xie, X.; Wang, J.; Pradhan, B.; Hong, H.; Bui, D.T.; Duan, Z.; Ma, J. A comparative study of logistic model tree, random forest, and classification and regression tree models for spatial prediction of landslide susceptibility. *CATENA* **2017**, *151*, 147–160. [CrossRef]
38. Muchlinski, D.; Siroky, D.; He, J.; Kocher, M. Comparing Random Forest with Logistic Regression for Predicting Class-Imbalanced Civil War Onset Data. *Polit. Anal.* **2016**, *24*, 87–103. [CrossRef]

39. Ahmadipour, Y.; Jabbarli, R.; Gembruch, O.; Pierscianek, D.; Darkwah Oppong, M.; Dammann, P.; Wrede, K.; Özkan, N.; Müller, O.; Sure, U.; et al. Impact of Multifocality and Molecular Markers on Survival of Glioblastoma. *World Neurosurg.* **2019**, *122*, 461–466. [CrossRef]
40. Molenaar, R.J.; Verbaan, D.; Lamba, S.; Zanon, C.; Jeuken, J.W.; Boots-Sprenger, S.H.; Wesseling, P.; Hulsebos, T.J.; Troost, D.; Van Tilborg, A.A.; et al. The combination of IDH1 mutations and MGMT methylation status predicts survival in glioblastoma better than either IDH1 or MGMT alone. *Neuro-Oncology* **2014**, *16*, 1263–1273. [CrossRef]
41. Wee, C.W.; Kim, E.; Kim, I.H.; Kim, I.A.; Kim, N.; Suh, C.O. Novel Recursive Partitioning Analysis Classification for Newly Diagnosed Glioblastoma: A Multi-institutional Study Highlighting the MGMT Promoter Methylation and IDH1 Gene Mutation Status. *Radiother. Oncol.* **2017**, *123*, 106–111. [CrossRef] [PubMed]
42. Minniti, G.; Lombardi, G.; Paolini, S. Glioblastoma in Elderly Patients: Current Management and Future Perspectives. *Cancers* **2019**, *11*, 336. [CrossRef] [PubMed]
43. Cunha, M.L.V.D.; Esmeraldo, A.C.S.; Henriques, L.A.W.; Santos, M.A.M.D.J.; Medeiros, R.T.R.; Botelho, R.V. Elderly patients with glioblastoma: The impact of surgical resection extent on survival. *Rev. Assoc. Med. Bras.* **2019**, *65*, 937–945. [CrossRef] [PubMed]
44. Tanaka, S.; Meyer, F.B.; Buckner, J.C.; Uhm, J.H.; Yan, E.S.; Parney, I.F. Presentation, management, and outcome of newly diagnosed glioblastoma in elderly patients. *J. Neurosurg.* **2012**, *118*, 786–798. [CrossRef]
45. Ius, T.; Pignotti, F.; Della Pepa, G.M.; Bagatto, D.; Isola, M.; Battistella, C.; Gaudino, S.; Pegolo, E.; Chiesa, S.; Arcicasa, M.; et al. Glioblastoma: From volumetric analysis to molecular predictors. *J. Neurosurg. Sci.* **2020**, in press.
46. Gorlia, T.; Stupp, R.; Brandes, A.A.; Rampling, R.R.; Fumoleau, P.; Dittrich, C.; Campone, M.M.; Twelves, C.C.; Raymond, E.; Hegi, M.E.; et al. New prognostic factors and calculators for outcome prediction in patients with recurrent glioblastoma: A pooled analysis of EORTC Brain Tumour Group phase I and II clinical trials. *Eur. J. Cancer* **2012**, *48*, 1176–1184. [CrossRef]
47. Roy, S.; Lahiri, D.; Maji, T.; Biswas, J. Recurrent Glioblastoma: Where we stand. *South Asian J. Cancer* **2015**, *4*, 163–173. [CrossRef]
48. Zhao, Y.-H.; Wang, Z.-F.; Pan, Z.-Y.; Péus, D.; Delgado-Fernandez, J.; Pallud, J.; Li, Z.-Q. A Meta-Analysis of Survival Outcomes Following Reoperation in Recurrent Glioblastoma: Time to Consider the Timing of Reoperation. *Front. Neurol.* **2019**, *10*, 286. [CrossRef]
49. Chaul-Barbosa, C.; Marques, D.F. How We Treat Recurrent Glioblastoma Today and Current Evidence. *Curr. Oncol. Rep.* **2019**, *21*, 94. [CrossRef]
50. Azoulay, M.; Santos, F.; Shenouda, G.; Petrecca, K.; Oweida, A.; Guiot, M.C.; Owen, S.; Panet-Raymond, V.; Souhami, L.; Abdulkarim, B.S. Benefit of re-operation and salvage therapies for recurrent glioblastoma multiforme: Results from a single institution. *J. Neuro-Oncol.* **2017**, *97*, 377–426. [CrossRef]
51. Louis, D.N.; Perry, A.; Reifenberger, G.; Von Deimling, A.; Figarella-Branger, M.; Cavenee, W.K.; Ohgaki, H.; Wiestler, O.D.; Kleihues, P.; Ellison, D.W. The 2016 World Health Organization Classification of Tumors of the Central Nervous System: A summary. *Acta Neuropathol.* **2016**, *131*, 803–820. [CrossRef] [PubMed]
52. Preusser, M.; Berghoff, A.S.; Manzl, C.; Filipits, M.; Weinhäusel, A.; Pulverer, W.; Dieckmann, K.; Widhalm, G.; Wöhrer, A.; Knosp, E.; et al. Clinical Neuropathology practice news 1-2014: Pyrosequencing meets clinical and analytical performance criteria for routine testing of MGMT promoter methylation status in glioblastoma. *Clin. Neuropathol.* **2014**, *33*, 6–14. [CrossRef] [PubMed]
53. Ius, T.; Angelini, E.; De Schotten, M.T.; Mandonnet, E.; Duffau, H. Evidence for potentials and limitations of brain plasticity using an atlas of functional resectability of WHO grade II gliomas: Towards a "minimal common brain". *Neuroimage* **2011**, *56*, 992–1000. [CrossRef] [PubMed]
54. Smith, J.S.; Chang, E.F.; Lamborn, K.R.; Chang, S.M.; Prados, M.D.; Cha, S.; Tihan, T.; Vandenberg, S.; McDermott, M.W.; Berger, M.S. Role of Extent of Resection in the Long-Term Outcome of Low-Grade Hemispheric Gliomas. *J. Clin. Oncol.* **2008**, *26*, 1338–1345. [CrossRef] [PubMed]
55. Breiman, L.; Friedman, J.H.; Olshen, R.A.; Stone, C.J. *Classification Regression Trees*; Wadsworth International Group: Belmont, CA, USA, 1984.

56. Yohannes, Y.; Hoddinott, J. *Classification and Regression Tree: An Introduction*; International Food Policy Research Institute: Washington, DC, USA, 1999.
57. Schmid, M.; Wright, M.N.; Ziegler, A. On the use of Harrell's C for clinical risk prediction via random survival forests. *Expert Syst. Appl.* **2016**, *63*, 450–459. [CrossRef]

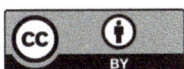

© 2020 by the authors. Licensee MDPI, Basel, Switzerland. This article is an open access article distributed under the terms and conditions of the Creative Commons Attribution (CC BY) license (http://creativecommons.org/licenses/by/4.0/).

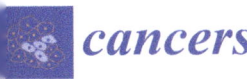

Review

Precision Medicine and Triple-Negative Breast Cancer: Current Landscape and Future Directions

Fokhrul Hossain [1,2,*], Samarpan Majumder [1,2], Justin David [3] and Lucio Miele [1,2,3]

1. Department of Genetics, Louisiana State University Health Sciences Center (LSUHSC), New Orleans, LA 70112, USA; smaju1@lsuhsc.edu (S.M.); lmiele@lsuhsc.edu (L.M.)
2. Stanley S. Scott Cancer Center, Louisiana State University Health Sciences Center (LSUHSC), New Orleans, LA 70112, USA
3. School of Medicine, Louisiana State University Health Sciences Center (LSUHSC), New Orleans, LA 70112, USA; jdav45@lsuhsc.edu
* Correspondence: fhossa@lsuhsc.edu

Simple Summary: The implementation of precision medicine will revolutionize cancer treatment paradigms. Notably, this goal is not far from reality: genetically similar cancers can be treated similarly. The heterogeneous nature of triple-negative breast cancer (TNBC) made it a suitable candidate to practice precision medicine. Using TNBC molecular subtyping and genomic profiling, a precision medicine-based clinical trial is ongoing. This review summarizes the current landscape and future directions of precision medicine and TNBC.

Abstract: Triple-negative breast cancer (TNBC) is an aggressive and heterogeneous subtype of breast cancer associated with a high recurrence and metastasis rate that affects African-American women disproportionately. The recent approval of targeted therapies for small subgroups of TNBC patients by the US 'Food and Drug Administration' is a promising development. The advancement of next-generation sequencing, particularly somatic exome panels, has raised hopes for more individualized treatment plans. However, the use of precision medicine for TNBC is a work in progress. This review will discuss the potential benefits and challenges of precision medicine for TNBC. A recent clinical trial designed to target TNBC patients based on their subtype-specific classification shows promise. Yet, tumor heterogeneity and sub-clonal evolution in primary and metastatic TNBC remain a challenge for oncologists to design adaptive precision medicine-based treatment plans.

Keywords: triple-negative breast cancer (TNBC); precision medicine; breast cancer; targeted therapy; TNBC subtypes; immunotherapy

Citation: Hossain, F.; Majumder, S.; David, J.; Miele, L. Precision Medicine and Triple-Negative Breast Cancer: Current Landscape and Future Directions. *Cancers* **2021**, *13*, 3739. https://doi.org/10.3390/cancers13153739

Academic Editors: Nandini Dey, Pradip De and Paola Marcato

Received: 15 April 2021
Accepted: 13 July 2021
Published: 26 July 2021

Publisher's Note: MDPI stays neutral with regard to jurisdictional claims in published maps and institutional affiliations.

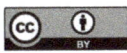

Copyright: © 2021 by the authors. Licensee MDPI, Basel, Switzerland. This article is an open access article distributed under the terms and conditions of the Creative Commons Attribution (CC BY) license (https://creativecommons.org/licenses/by/4.0/).

1. Precision Medicine: Perspective and Challenges

The human genome project opened a path to understanding human gene structure and function and identifying disease-associated mutations in our DNA. Since the human genome project, there have been dramatic advancements in genetic technology, with continuous progress towards more cost-efficient and powerful techniques [1]. The development of the chip-based microarray allowed early gene expression profiling studies as well as genome-wide association studies for millions of single nucleotide polymorphisms (SNPs). Still, it was eventually replaced for most non-SNP applications by the high-throughput next-generation sequencing (NGS) of genomic DNA and RNA-derived cDNA [2]. These advancements have paved the way for genomic medicine. Genomic medicine is an integral part of precision medicine, defined by the NIH as an emerging approach of tailoring treatment and prevention based on individual variability in genes, environments, and lifestyle to classify individuals into specific subgroups susceptible to one particular treatment plan [3]. Although some think of precision medicine and personalized medicine interchangeably, the two concepts are not identical. "Precision" medicine uses data and genomics to tailor treatments to specific groups sharing genetic and/or clinical, environmental and lifestyle features. "Personalized" medicine would imply treatments designed specifically for individual patients. Except in unique circumstances, such as tumor vaccines or tumor-infiltrating lymphocytes (TIL) produced from individual tumors, truly personalized medicine remains an aspirational goal. In 2015, US President Barack Obama announced an NIH-funded precision medicine initiative to assemble the most significant medical research cohort in history, collecting health and behavioral data as well as DNA and other biospecimens from one million or more Americans reflecting the diversity of our population. The centerpiece of the precision medicine initiative is the "All of US" research program [3]. This program is expected to collect and share data from genome sequencing, electronic medical records, personal reported information, and digital health technologies [3]. Using these integrated datasets, researchers will assess the effectiveness of treatments and identify genetic variations associated with a higher or lower risk of disease or adverse medication events of any particular group of people. This information can form the basis for the design of novel biomarker studies and therapeutic trials. In effect, the goal is to stimulate a progressive transition away from generalized, broad-spectrum therapies to more precise treatments in well-defined patient populations [4].

Knowing the genetics of diseases will allow physicians to make health care decisions that are more effective for the patient to improve the quality of care and decrease unnecessary screenings or procedures [3]. For example, genetic analysis revealed that there are subgroups of type I and II diabetes that differ in medication responsiveness due to genetic differences. Thiazolidinedione use has declined, but genetic analysis could identify patients who are more likely to respond to this group of drugs [5]. Genome-wide association studies (GWAS) analyze human DNA variation to identify risk factors and improve treatment strategies [2]. One of the first GWAS studies identified polymorphisms in the cytochrome P450 2C9 (CYP2C9) complex and the vitamin K epoxide reductase complex 1 (VKORC1), which are both correlated with Warfarin pharmacokinetics [6]. Pharmacogenomics studies have revealed several other genetic variants associated with differential drug metabolism [7–9]. Despite advancements in precision medicine, there are many obstacles to its routine clinical deployment. One significant barrier to the clinical use of genomic data is the high number of variants of unknown significance in the human genome and the difficulty in attaining sufficiently large sample sizes to analyze their possible roles [10]. Additionally, identifying risk factors is not always straightforward, as the relationship between risk factors and their biology is often more complex than previously anticipated. Two patients with the same risk factors do not necessarily share the same disease [11]. There is also difficulty in identifying the standard features of polymorphisms between ancestral groups. For instance, African genomes are more polymorphic and have less linkage disequilibrium in single nucleotide polymorphisms than Europeans [2]. Another barrier to the advancement of precision medicine is the lack of infrastructure and education in clinical-based settings. Routine precision medicine practice will require highly integrated patient datasets, including clinical, lifestyle, and genetic data [3], and there is a lack of genetics professionals in hospitals [12]. Finally, cost and reimbursement issues must be solved before fully integrating genetic data into the clinical setting [12,13]. Solutions to these barriers include developing technology infrastructure, outcome-based reimbursement policies, education and promotion to personnel in clinical-based settings [14], and patient willingness to participate in precision medicine [3]. There is a promising future for precision medicine, but it must overcome a number of obstacles before it is fully integrated into the healthcare system.

One field that is currently benefiting from the development of clinical genomics is oncology. Many new cancer therapies [4] use precision medicine and genomic tests based on NGS as a strategy to identify cancers that are more likely to respond, as opposed to anatomical sites. Whole-exome sequencing (WES) helped discover and understand driver mutations and copy number variants in cancers, and WGS is slowly improving our limited knowledge of mutations in non-coding regions [15]. One of the earliest therapeutics developed based on genetic alterations was trastuzumab for cancers carrying genomic amplification of a region of chromosome 17 containing the ERBB2/HER2 gene, which led to better outcomes than first-line chemotherapy [16]. Subsequently, genetic analysis revealed that cetuximab effectively treated colorectal cancers in patients without KRAS mutations [17]. Targetable prostate cancer mutations have been lacking, but PARP-1 inhibition has been effective in certain patients [18]. The discovery of specific mutations can advance the development of therapeutics for the treatment of other cancers with the same mutation, though context can make a difference. For example, trastuzumab also benefits gastric cancers with HER2 amplification [19]. In contrast, BRAF inhibitors were effective in hairy cell leukemia with BRAF mutations but not in colorectal cancer, highlighting the limitations of single gene-based approaches and the importance of clinical trials for targeted therapy [20]. Prevention strategies have also been proposed for patients with a genetic predisposition to some cancers, such as sulindac and celecoxib causing polyp regression in patients with Familial Adenomatous Polyposis [21]. Despite the development of potentially effective therapies based on mutational profiles, tumor heterogeneity adds another barrier to precision medicine in oncology. The clonal heterogeneity of tumors and the evolution of clones carrying additional mutations compared to the original drivers is a significant obstacle to the effectiveness of targeted cancer therapies, particularly as monotherapy. Frequently, after targeted treatment based on a driver mutation produced clinical responses, the tumor will circumvent the targeted pathway blockade through genetic evolution or epigenetic plasticity and will find a way to resume progression [22]. Clonal heterogeneity is often based on mutational heterogeneity, with some cells showing specific mutations, while other cancer cells display different mutational profiles [23]. Evolutionary "trees" of tumor clones under the form of "tropical fish plots" effectively show this phenomenon [24]. Usually, the development of new mutations under therapy-imposed selection results in treatment resistance [25]. One group of cancers that would greatly benefit from precision oncology is triple-negative breast cancer (TNBC).

2. Triple-Negative Breast Cancer (TNBC)

Triple-negative breast cancer (TNBC) is an aggressive and heterogeneous subtype of breast cancer. TNBC was found to be negative for the estrogen receptor α (ER−), the progesterone receptor (PR−), and the human epidermal growth factor receptor two loci (HER2−) by immunohistological analysis [26–30]. TNBC constitutes 11–20% of all breast cancers and typically affects premenopausal women, especially African American women [26,30,31]. TNBC has a higher rate of mortality and recurrence than other types of breast cancer, especially in the first five years [26]. There are currently a few targeted therapies available for TNBC, but chemotherapy remains the mainstay of treatment, while immunotherapy is a recent and increasingly important addition [27,31–33]. Optimizing the treatment of TNBC based on genomic and possibly immunological features would be a significant advancement.

Comorbidities have significant effects on the risk and outcomes of TNBC, in part by affecting tumor biology. Obesity is linked with increased incidence and a worse prognosis of triple-negative breast cancer [34]. One theory of obesity's relation to TNBC biology is that obesity increases the development of a pro-inflammatory and metabolically activated phenotype of macrophages (MMe). MMe macrophages are dominant in obese human and mouse mammary adipose tissue. They are tumorigenic due to the increased secretion of IL-6 in a NADPH oxidase-2 (NOX2)-dependent fashion. IL-6 signals through glycoprotein-130 induce stem-like properties in TNBC cells [34]. Another study concluded that the increased inflammation and reactive oxygen species from obesity drive the increased expression of a splicing variant of methyl-CpG-binding domain 2 (MBD2_v2), increasing the stem cell-like properties of TNBC cells [35]. Increased adipose tissue caused by obesity also increases the secretion of the hormone leptin, which enhances the expression of genes linked to stem cell-like properties and epithelial–mesenchymal transition [36]. Another theory is that hyperinsulinemia secondary to insulin resistance increases the activation of the

AKT/mTOR pathway, promoting proliferation and survival in TNBC cells. Additionally, the AKT/mTOR pathway increases glucose uptake and promotes the Warburg effect, a shift from aerobic oxidation in the mitochondria to anaerobic glycolysis, which allows for rapid growth and resistance to apoptosis [37–39]. The development of targeted therapies for TNBC must consider these factors, including the cross-talk between the adipose tissue, metabolism, and tumor biology.

The progression of a primary tumor to a metastatic tumor is based on its ability to leave the original site and spread into the blood and/or the lymphatic system, potentially forming new tumors in other locations in the body. Breast tumors start in the mammary ducts or lobules but can spread into the surrounding adipose tissue and migrate to other parts of the body, escaping immune surveillance mechanisms [40]. Metastatic TNBC is more aggressive compared to other breast cancers, and the average rate of patient survival is lower than other subtypes [41]. Understanding the biological differences between a primary TNBC tumor and a metastatic TNBC tumor could benefit therapy. Primary TNBC is associated with relatively few somatic single-nucleotide variants, but numerous somatic copy number variations (CNV) [42]. The cell cycle's loss of function mutations and the apoptosis regulator p53 [42–45] as well as the gain-of-function PIK3CA mutations are common in primary TNBC [43,44]. However, the possible mutational landscape for TNBC is very broad and contains numerous other genes associated with the control of cell shape, motility, and extracellular signaling [43]. Metastatic TNBC is associated with p53, LRP1B, HERC1, CDH5, RB1, and NF1 mutations in general [45]. The biology of the progression from a primary tumor to metastasis is not completely understood. Comprehensive gene expression profiles in primary and metastatic breast cancer revealed many differentially expressed genes in metastatic versus primary disease [46]. Metastatic breast cancer, including metastatic TNBC (mTNBC), is a major concern in the inpatient treatment regimen. Recent advancements in immunotherapy and targeted therapies in breast cancer improve the longevity of cancer patients. In addition to the advancement of targeted therapies, locoregional resection also plays an important role in preventing metastasis [47,48]. Further understanding of the genetic landscape associated with primary and secondary TNBC is an urgent need.

3. TNBC Subtypes and Current Treatment Options

TNBC molecular subtypes are a useful starting point on the road to TNBC precision treatment [26–31,49–51]. Based on the gene expression profiles of TNBC samples, Lehmann et al. classified TNBC patients into six subtypes: basal-like 1 (BL1), basal-like 2 (BL2), mesenchymal (M), mesenchymal stem-like (MSL), immunomodulatory (IM), and luminal androgen receptor (LAR) [52]. These authors also developed a web-based subtyping tool (TNBCtype) to predict subtype assignment for new TNBC samples to guide biomarker or treatment studies [53]. Subsequently, Burstein et al. classified TNBC into four subtypes: LAR, M, BLIS (basal-like immunosuppressed), and BLIA (basal-like immune-activated) [54]. They reported that the prognosis was the worst for BLIS tumors and the best for BLIA tumors in terms of disease-free survival (DFS) and disease-specific survival (DSS). The order from best to worst prognosis was BLIA > M > LAR > BLIS for both DFS and DSS [54]. Liu et al. classified TNBC tumors based on the expression profiles of both mRNAs and lncRNAs and proposed the Fudan University Shanghai Cancer Center (FUSCC) classification as well as the analysis of its interaction with the Lehman/Pietenpol subtypes [55]. They divided TNBC tumors into four subtypes including the immunomodulatory subtype (IM), the mesenchymal-like subtype (MES), the luminal androgen receptor subtype (LAR), and the basal-like and immune-suppressed (BLIS) subtype [55]. In 2016, Lehmann et al. re-classified the TNBC molecular subtypes from six (TNBCtype: (BL1, BL2, IM, M, MSL and LAR)) to four (TNBCtype-4) tumor-specific subtypes (BL1, BL2, M, and LAR) based upon the complexity and overlapping of the varying histological landscapes of tumor samples [56]. The IM and MSL subtypes were dependent upon transcripts from immune infiltrates and other tumor stromal cells. While these transcripts may affect tumor biology, their reproducibility was linked to levels of tumor infiltration. These authors demonstrated that TNBC subtypes had a significantly different response to neo-adjuvant chemotherapy and suggested that the classification will benefit future clinical trial design [56]. Different TNBC subtype classifications are presented in Figure 1.

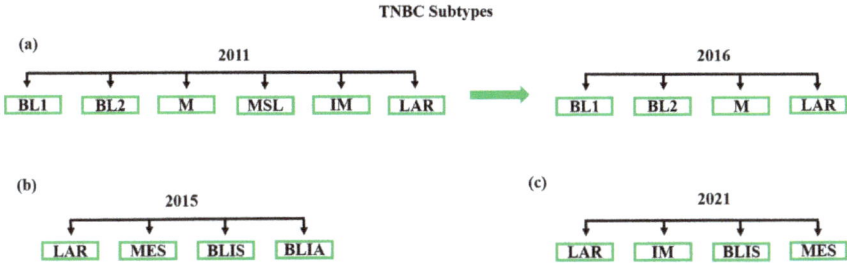

Figure 1. Major TNBC subtypes based on gene expression profiles. (**a**) Lehmann et al. classified TNBC patients into six subtypes (TNBCtype) in 2011: basal-like 1 (BL1), basal-like 2 (BL2), mesenchymal (M), mesenchymal stem-like (MSL), immunomodulatory (IM), and luminal androgen receptor (LAR) [52]. In 2016, Lehman et al. re-classified the TNBC molecular subtypes from six (TNBCtype) to four (TNBCtype-4) tumor-specific subtypes: BL1, BL2, M, and LAR [56]. (**b**) Burstein el al. suggested four subtypes: luminal androgen receptor (LAR), mesenchymal (MES), basal-like immunosuppressed (BLIS), and basal-like immune-activated (BLIA) [54]. (**c**) FUTURE trial schema: LAR, immunomodulatory (IM), mesenchymal-like (MES), and basal-like immune-suppressed (BLIS) [57].

TNBC has higher rates of early recurrence and mortality than other types of breast cancer. The reason for the poor outcomes of TNBC is the lack of effective targeted therapies. Endocrine agents such as aromatase inhibitors or HER2 targeted monoclonal antibodies or small molecules are not effective for TNBC patients [58–61]. Therefore, standard cytotoxic chemotherapy (doxorubicin, docetaxel, 5-fluorouracil, platinum drugs, and/or cyclophosphamide and other agents in different combinations) remains the standard of care for TNBC patients [62–65]. It is essential to consider the risks and benefits of treating early-stage TNBC patients. Over-treatment increases toxicity and undesirable adverse effects, compromising the patient's quality of life. Early-stage TNBC patients without lymph node involvement generally have a good prognosis in terms of five-year relapse-free survival (RFS) and five-year distant recurrence-free survival (DRFS) [66,67]. Chemotherapy is the choice of care for TNBC patients with a tumor size > 5 mm with or without lymph node (LN) metastases. Combinations of anthracyclines, alkylators, and taxanes with carboplatin are common chemotherapy regimens for TNBC [68]. The ABC trial suggested that the addition of an anthracycline to docetaxel and cyclophosphamide therapy significantly improves invasive disease-free survival (IDFS) for early stage TNBC patients [69].

In the adjuvant (post-surgical) setting, the treatment of eight weeks of paclitaxel followed by the standard regimen of adjuvant fluorouracil, epirubicin, and cyclophosphamide (FEC) decreased tumor relapse and improved DFS in LN-positive breast cancer [70]. Neoadjuvant chemotherapy (NACT) is now used as the standard of care to treat high-risk TNBC to reduce tumor volume before surgery [71–79]. Patients treated with standard NACT have approximately 30–40% pathologic complete response rates (pCR) [49,80–82]. Tumors that do not achieve pCR have significantly higher recurrence rates than tumors that do. The ability to predict which patients achieve pCR and/or to increase pCR rates without increasing toxicity would be major advances in the treatment of TNBC. Tumor-infiltrating lymphocytes (TIL) within residual tumors post-NACT are considered as a semi-quantitative assessment of immune response [83–90]. In a landmark study, Denkert et al. [91], analyzed the results of the GEPAR-Sixto clinical trial and, determined that increased levels of stromal TILs predicted pCR. Gene expression profiling revealed three immune subtypes with different pCR rates. The most predictive transcripts were PD-L1 and CCL5. Subsequent studies confirmed the predictive value of immunophenotyping and TILs, suggesting a role of the immune system in clearing tumor cells during chemotherapy [92]. Another gene signature consisting of HLF, CXCL13, SULT1E1, and GBP1 in pre-treatment samples predicted the extent of lymphocytic infiltration after NACT [93]. Tumor mutational burden, possibly resulting in higher numbers of tumor-associated antigens, was identified as an independent predictor of pCR in addition to TIL [94]. Conversely, the presence of a PIK3CA H1047R mutation was associated with lower rates of pCR [95].

Following NACT, the most commonly used prognostic factor in TNBC is pCR. However, pCR is not an absolute predictor, as some TNBC patients who achieve pCR develop relapses [96–99]. Studies from the MD Anderson Cancer Center have reported a more quantitative evaluation scale called the Residual Cancer Burden (RCB), which is based on tumor size, invasive cancer cellularity, and node status post-NACT [100,101]. RCB is classified on a 0-III range, with the higher values indicating the probability of subsequent recurrence, metastatic spread, and increased mortality.

4. Recently FDA-Approved Therapies for TNBC

Chemotherapy and surgery remain the standard of care for most TNBC patients. However, a few classes of agents, such as Immune Checkpoint Blockers (ICBs), PARP inhibitors (PARPi), and Antibody Drug Conjugates (ADC), have demonstrated clear benefits in TNBC patients, and in some cases, have received FDA approval. Nonetheless, response rates with the new agents are variable, and predicting the response to these new classes of agents will be the focus of a major precision oncology effort.

4.1. Approved Checkpoint Inhibitors

Many TNBC tumors are immunologically "cold", meaning they lack sizeable TIL infiltrates (see above for biomarkers of tumor immunity). Converting "cold" TNBC to "hot" tumors and making them amenable to treatment with ICBs would be a potentially valuable treatment strategy. Approximately 40% of TNBC expresses PD-L1 in TILs, and PD-L1 positive tumors (PD-L1 positivity is defined by PD-L1 expression on tumor-infiltrating immune cells covering ≥1% of the tumor area) tend to respond favorably to treatment with anti-PD-L1 therapy [102–104]. In an analysis of a PD-L1-positive TNBC cohort, the addition of atezolizumab, a humanized monoclonal antibody to PD-L1, in combination with nab-paclitaxel compared to chemotherapy (nab-paclitaxel)-alone significantly improved median progression-free survival (PFS) to 7.5 months versus 5.0 months, respectively (HR 0.62; 95% CI, 0.49–0.78), and improved OS to 25 months from 15.5 months, respectively (HR, 0.62; 95% CI, 0.45–0.86) [105]. Based on this compelling data, on 8 March 2019, the FDA granted the accelerated approval of atezolizumab (Tecentriq) in combination with nab-paclitaxel (Abraxane) for the treatment of PD-L1-positive unresectable locally advanced and metastatic TNBC tumors [106]. The FDA also granted accelerated approval to Merck's anti-PD-1 monoclonal antibody, pembrolizumab (Keytruda), in combination with chemotherapy for locally recurrent or metastatic TNBC in November, 2020 [107]. A first-line treatment regimen of pembrolizumab with chemotherapy extended PFS by 35% compared to a placebo. However, the FDA declined to grant accelerated approval to Keytruda in either neoadjuvant or adjuvant settings for high-risk, early-stage TNBC. The FDA panel reasoned that a 15% increase in pCR would not necessarily be indicative of an increase in overall survival (OS).

Other Immune Checkpoint Inhibitors in Clinical Trials

A recent paper described details about clinical trials involving PD-1/PD-L1 blockade either as monotherapy, in combination with chemotherapy, or with other targeted therapies [108]. Gagliato et al. also described the success and challenges of PD-1/PD-L1 immunotherapy for TNBC patients [109]. In addition to PD-1 and its ligand (PD-L1), other immune checkpoint inhibitors are also being investigated in TNBC clinical trials, including cytotoxic T lymphocyte-associated protein 4 (CTLA-4), Lymphocyte-activation gene 3 (LAG-3), and T cell immunoglobulin and mucin-domain containing-3 (TIM-3) [110]. Ipilimumab, a CTLA4 blocking antibody, is in a phase 2 TNBC clinical trial with nivolumab, a PD-1 blocking antibody with taxane-based neoadjuvant chemotherapy (Clinicaltrials.gov: NCT03546686). Another phase 2 clinical trial is ongoing with nivolumab in combination with ipilimumab for advanced or metastatic solid tumors, including TNBC (Clinicaltrials.gov: NCT01928394). Tremelimumab, another anti-CTLA-4 monoclonal antibody, is in a phase I clinical trial with durvalumab (anti-PD-L1 monoclonal antibody) in combination with chemotherapy in advanced solid tumors, including TNBC (Clinicaltrials.gov: NCT02658214). Tremelimumab is also being tested in phase 2 clinical trials as a monotherapy or with MEDI4736 for advanced solid tumors, including in TNBC (Clinicaltrials.gov: NCT02527434).

Bottai et al. suggested that LAG-3 and PD1 were co-expressed in approximately 15% of TNBC patients, and their co-expression positively correlated with the presence of tumor-infiltrating lymphocytes (TILs) [111]. LAG525 (IMP701), an anti-LAG-3 antibody in combination with spartalizumab (an anti-PD-1 checkpoint inhibitor) is under a phase I clinical investigation in patients with advanced or metastatic TNBC (Clinicaltrials.gov: NCT03742349). TSR-033, an anti-LAG-3 monoclonal antibody, is in a phase 1 clinical trial alone and in combination with the anti-PD-1 antibody dostarlimab in patients with advanced solid tumors (Clinicaltrials.gov: NCT03250832). Another anti-LAG-3 antibody (INCAGN02385) is under a phase I clinical investigation in patients with advanced malignancies, including TNBC (Clinicaltrials.gov: NCT03538028). TIM-3, another immune checkpoint, plays an important role in tumor immunity [112]. An anti-TIM-3 antibody, INCAGN02390, is in phase I clinical trials in select advanced malignancies, including TNBC (Clinicaltrials.gov: NCT03652077).

4.2. Poly-ADP-Ribose Polymerase (PARP) Inhibitors

The loss of function mutations in the BRCA1 and BRCA2 genes have long been known to confer a high risk of TNBC. The loss of BRCA1/BRCA2 function mutations impairs DNA double-stranded break (DSB) repair in normal cells, leading to the accumulation of genetic damage and chromosomal aberrations. About 19.5% of TNBC cases are associated with germline BRCA1/BRCA2 gene mutations [113]. Cancer cells that are defective in DSB repair are susceptible to other mechanisms of DNA damage. Poly-ADP-Ribose Polymerase (PARP) is an enzyme involved in single strand break (SSB) DNA repair. Cells with DSB repair defects are vulnerable to SSBs, which trigger apoptosis. PARP inhibitors (PARPi) exploit this vulnerability. PARPi are well-tolerated and improve both progression free survival (PFS) and OS in TNBC patients with germline BRCA1/BRCA2 mutations, which is reviewed in [114,115]. The FDA approved two PARP inhibitors to treat TNBC patients with BRCA-mutant tumors. In January 2018, olaparib (Lynparza) was approved for the treatment of patients with BRCA-positive, HER2-negative metastatic breast cancer [116]. Talazoparib (Talzenna) was also approved in the same year for the treatment of patients with BRCA-mutated and HER2-negative locally advanced or metastatic breast cancer [117].

4.3. Antibody-Drug Conjugates (ADC)

Antibody-Drug Conjugates (ADC) are chemically modified monoclonal antibodies (mAb) usually linked to high-potency cytotoxic payloads. In such cases, the mAb is used to selectively target the toxic payload of cancer cells. ADCs are one of the fastest-growing classes of cancer therapeutics in the past few decades [118]. In 2020, the FDA granted accelerated approval to sacituzumab govitecan, an ADC sold under the brand name Trodelvy [119]. Accelerated approval was granted for the treatment of adults with TNBC that has metastasized and has received at least two prior therapies. Sacituzumab govitecan (Trodelvy) received regular approval from the FDA on 7 April 2021 for unresectable locally advanced or metastatic TNBC (mTNBC) [120]. Trodelvy is a Trop-2-directed antibody conjugated to govitecan, a topoisomerase inhibitor. However, despite mAb-mediated selective delivery, this agent has significant toxicity that has prompted a boxed warning: severe neutropenia and severe diarrhea are common. Patients experiencing neutropenia are advised to receive treatment with G-CSF to stimulate bone marrow hematopoiesis. A recent review paper highlighted the use of the ADCs, including sacituzumab govitecan (SG), ladiratuzumab vedotin (LV), and trastuzumab deruxtecan (T-DXd) in mTNBC [121]. Although T-Dxd has proven efficacy in HER2-overexpressing metastatic breast cancer, it has also shown better clinical responses in patients with low HER2-expressing metastatic breast cancers, including TNBC [121]. A phase Ib clinical trial (Clinicaltrials.gov: NCT04556773) is currently recruiting patients with metastatic HER2-low advanced or metastatic breast cancer to evaluate the efficacy of T-DXd in combination with other therapies.

5. Precision Medicine in TNBC: Emerging Therapies and Ongoing Studies

5.1. Receptor Tyrosine Kinases (RTKs) and Downstream Signaling Pathways

RTKs in TNBC signaling operates through two main downstream signaling cascades: the RAS/MAPK and the PI3K/AKT/mTOR signaling axis. RTKs in TNBC cells transduce signals downstream of EGFR, PDEGFR, VEGFR, IGFR, TGF-β, and FGFR. Almost 60–80% of TNBC tumors have dysregulated EGFR expression [122]. EGFR expression is associated with aggressive TNBC. Post NACT, EGFR expression frequently persisted in TNBC, suggesting that anti-EGFR therapy may offer an additional window of opportunity for patients with therapy-refractory EGFR-positive TNBC tumors [123]. The KRAS/SIAH/EGFR pathway is frequently upregulated in TNBC. The seven in absentia homolog (SIAH), an E3 ligase and the most downstream "gatekeeper" of the EGFR/KRAS signaling cascade, is often upregulated in TNBC along with EGFR [58,123]. Paired gene expression of SIAH and EGFR has been proposed as a prognostic biomarker in TNBC [123]. A decrease in SIAH and EGFR expression in a patient-derived specimen post-NACT compared to pre-NACT levels predicts treatment benefits.

Targeting EGFR would thus appear to be a potentially attractive strategy for TNBC. However, EGFR inhibitors have significant off-target toxicities [124], and multi-center clinical trials have not shown cetuximab, an anti-EGFR, to be an effective therapy for TNBC, probably due to the activation of compensatory signaling mechanisms such as PI3K-AKT (see below) [58].

Lapatinib, a dual EGFR/HER2 RTK inhibitor effective in HER2- positive breast cancer, was not effective in TNBC [125]. The MEK inhibitor selumetinib blocked the motility and invasiveness of the MDA-MB-231 and SUM149 TNBC cell lines in vitro [122]. Furthermore, selumetinib appeared to decrease lung metastasis in a TNBC-bearing mouse xenograft model [126], supporting the study of MEK inhibitors in TNBC. Compared to monotherapy, combining MEK inhibition with PD-L1/PD-1 inhibition increased therapeutic efficacy in a murine syngeneic TNBC model [127].

5.2. PI3K/AKT/mTOR Targeted Therapy

The PI3K/AKT/mTOR pathway is one of the most active cell survival pathways in cancer, often leading to chemoresistance [128]. This pathway, which is initiated by PI3K family kinases and receives input from EGFR family receptors, insulin, and insulin-like growth factor receptors, is a significant player in regulating apoptosis and metabolism. It also perpetuates the effect of BRCA mutations by stabilizing DNA double-stranded breaks [68]. PI3K/AKT/mTOR pathway dysregulation frequently occurs in TNBC. The PI3KCA-gain of function mutations is observed in 23.7% of TNBC patients [129]. Notably, the loss of function mutations or epigenetic silencing of the gene encoding PI3K negative regulator phosphatase PTEN, including promoter silencing and functional suppression, are detected in 25–30% of TNBC cases [122]. AKT and mTOR hyperactivation portend a poor prognosis in TNBC patients. The dual inhibition of AKT and mTOR (necessary to avoid feedback activation of AKT by mTORC2 after inhibition of mTORC1) may offer a promising therapeutic option for TNBC treatment [122,130] based on preclinical results. Investigational AKT inhibitors like ipatasertib and capivasertib have demonstrated incremental benefits in improving outcomes for patients with high-risk TNBC [131,132]. The FDA-approved mTORC1 inhibitor everolimus increases progression-free survival when combined with the non-steroidal aromatase inhibitor exemestane for patients with HR(+)

and HER2(−) advanced breast cancer [133]. Everolimus combined with carboplatin has been proposed as an effective therapy for metastatic TNBC patients [134,135] because of the link between mTOR activation and platinum resistance [136]. PI3K inhibition can also decrease the expression of BRCA1 and 2 and can sensitize BRCA1/2 wild-type TNBC tumors for PARP inhibition [137]. Based on this observation, a clinical trial with BKM120 (buparlisib) and olaparib was initiated [122]. Interestingly, resistance to mTOR inhibitors in TNBC was accompanied by the appearance of Notch-dependent cancer stem-like cells (CSCs) [138], suggesting that Notch inhibitors may be combined with mTOR/AKT inhibitors.

5.3. Notch Signaling and TNBC

Notch signaling activation is correlated with TNBC tumor growth, CSCs maintenance, expansion, tumor invasiveness, and metastasis [139–142]. Notably, ~10% of TNBC carry driver Notch1/Notch2 chromosomal rearrangements that produce constitutively active, oncogenic forms of Notch1 or Notch2 [143]. Efforts to target Notch signaling in cancers, including in TNBC, have been ongoing for the past 15 years. However, an FDA-approved Notch inhibitor/drug is still elusive, though at least one of them is currently in phase 3. For an extensive review of the field, readers are directed to [142]. An abundance of preclinical data provided a compelling case for the use of gamma-secretase inhibitors (GSIs) to inhibit Notch signaling and reverse tumor progression in TNBC. However, GSI demonstrated mechanism-based dose-dependent gastrointestinal (GI) toxicities that limited their clinical applications [142,143]. Intermittent dosing of GSIs to circumvent their GI toxicities has been adopted in numerous clinical trials. Still, we do not know whether intermittent dosing is sufficient to eliminate TNBC CSCs [142,143]. Non-GSI, new generation Notch inhibitors are in clinical development. Among them, CB-103 appears particularly promising.

CB-103 (Cellestia biotech, Basel, Switzerland; https://www.cellestia.com/, accessed on 16 July 2021) is a first-in class, oral pan-Notch small molecule inhibitor with a unique mode of action. CB-103 inhibits the Notch transcriptional complex assembly and blocks Notch signaling in receiving cells [142,143]. Importantly, CB-103 does not induce mechanism-based dose-dependent GI toxicity, unlike GSIs. Furthermore, its action mechanism implies that CB-103 would be effective against the truncated forms of Notch1 or Notch2 produced by genetic rearrangements associated with ~10% of TNBC. The safety and efficacy of CB-103 in Notch-dependent advanced or metastatic solid tumors or hematological malignancies are being investigated in a phase I/II clinical trial (Clinicaltrials.gov: NCT03422679).

5.4. Cyclin-Dependent Kinases (CDKs)

Cyclin-dependent kinases (CDKs) play an essential role in modulating cell division by regulating cell cycle and transcriptional activities. Similar to many tumors, the aberrant expression of CDKs (e.g., CDK4 and CDK6) are also common in TNBC. CDK inhibitors have been used successfully to inhibit TNBC growth in preclinical settings. Dinaciclib, a pan-CDK inhibitor, is in phase I clinical trial in combination with pembrolizumab (Clinicaltrials.gov: NCT01676753) for TNBC and advanced or metastatic breast cancer. Trilaciclib, a CDK 4/6 Inhibitor, is in phase 1 clinical trial in combination with gemcitabine and carboplatin for metastatic TNBC (mTNBC) (Clinicaltrials.gov: NCT02978716). Ribociclib, another CDK 4/6 Inhibitor, is in phase I/II clinical trial in combination with bicalutamide, an androgen receptor (AR) inhibitor for advanced AR+ TNBC (Clinicaltrials.gov: NCT03090165). A phase II study of PF-06873600 (CDK inhibitor) in combination with endocrine therapy is ongoing for metastatic breast cancer, ovarian cancer, and TNBC (NCT03519178). Another phase II study of abemaciclib (selective ATP-competitive inhibitor of CDK4 and CDK6 kinase activity) for TNBC is also ongoing (Clinicaltrials.gov: NCT03130439). CDK inhibitors (mainly CDK4/6) augment anti-tumor immunity through T-cell activation, supporting the rationale for combination with immunotherapy [108,144,145]. A phase Ib clinical breast cancer study of pembrolizumab with abemaciclib demonstrated tolerability with clinical benefits [108].

5.5. Androgen Receptor (AR) Expression and TNBC

There is a lack of consensus among breast cancer researchers on whether AR expression is a favorable prognostic indicator in TNBC [146]. AR expression is upregulated in 10–43% of the TNBCs andfalls into the LAR molecular subtype. Therapy with AR antagonists showed clinical benefits in some TNBC patients [58,147–150]. A phase II randomized clinical trial is currently investigating the efficacy of a new AR antagonist, darolutamide, for unresectable or metastatic TNBC patients (Clinicaltrials.gov: NCT03383679) [58].

5.6. Angiogenesis and TNBC

Angiogenesis is one of the necessary adaptations that cancer cells must adopt to form macroscopic tumors. VEGF-A is the most critical pro-angiogenic secretory factor produced by solid tumors (see [58,151] for recent reviews). Elevated VEGF expression in TNGC is linked to poor prognosis independent of tumor size, histological grade, or nodal status [152]. The use of an anti-VEGF antibody, bevacizumab, in combination with chemotherapy was shown to improve PFS but failed to provide statistically meaningful improvements in OS in TNBC compared to chemotherapy alone [58,153]. The combined inhibition of VEGF and Notch ligand DLL4, which is also required for angiogenesis, through bispecific monoclonal antibodies is currently being investigated [142].

5.7. Investigational Antibody-Drug Conjugates (ADC)

Following the FDA approval of Trodelvy in 2020, several pharmaceutical companies are interested in ADC for TNBC treatment. In addition, the phase I study demonstrated favorable efficacy and tolerability using ladiratuzumab vedotin [118]. Recent review papers described other ADCs under clinical investigations [118,154].

6. Other Targeted Therapies

Recent progress in preclinical studies with small-molecule agents for the targeted therapy of TNBC has been summarized in recent publications [28,110,155]. Islam et al. described targeting the Bcl-2 family, proteasome, STAT3, histone deacetylase (HDACs), Src in TNBC in detail [155]. P53 mutations are prevalent in TNBC, which lead the cells to rely on checkpoint kinase 1 (ChK1) and ataxia telangiectasia related to Rad3 (ATR) for DNA repair management [110]. LY2606368, a ChK1/2 inhibitor, is under a phase 2 clinical trial for various tumors (ovarian, breast, and prostate), including TNBC (Clinicaltrials.gov: NCT02203513). Another phase 2 clinical trial is ongoing with olaparib in combination with an ATR inhibitor (ceralasertib) and adavosertib for metastatic TNBC patients (Clinicaltrials.gov: NCT03330847).

6.1. Cancer Vaccines

Apart from ICBs, an immunotherapeutic strategy that has been in development for decades but has yet to achieve its full clinical potential is cancer vaccines. Despite preclinical successes and the safety and immunogenicity in humans that have been documented in many clinical trials [156], cancer vaccines have yet to produce meaningful and reproducible clinical responses in TNBC [157]. This may be due to immune editing, a phenotypic and genetic adaptation process whereby cancers evade the immune system [157] and/or insufficiently robust T cell responses [156]. Perhaps the rapid evolution in vaccine technology sparked by the COVID19 pandemic, which borrowed from the field of cancer immunology, will eventually produce clinically effective cancer vaccines. Table 1 lists the active clinical trials from Clinicaltrials.gov as of 18 June 2021.

Table 1. Active TNBC clinical trials using targeted therapy and Immunotherapy (Clinicaltrials.gov, accessed on 18 June 2021).

Title	Phase	Status	Age	ID
Evaluation of IPI-549 combined with front-line treatments in patients with TNBCr or Renal Cell Carcinoma (MARIO-3)	Phase II	Active	18 and over	NCT03961698
Testing the addition of Copanlisib to Eribulin for the Treatment of Advanced-Stage Triple Negative Breast Cancer	Phase I/II	Active	18 and over	NCT04345913
Study of Pembrolizumab (MK-3475) plus chemotherapy vs. placebo plus chemotherapy for previously untreated locally recurrent inoperable or metastatic TNBC	Phase III	Active, not recruiting	18 and over	NCT02819518
Atorvastatin in treating patients with stage IIb-III TNBC who did not achieve a PCR after receiving neoadjuvant chemotherapy	Phase II	Active	18 and over	NCT03872388
A Study of Atezolizumab in combination with Nab-Paclitaxel compared with placebo with Nab-paclitaxel for participants with previously untreated metastatic TNBC	Phase III	Active, not recruiting	18 and over	NCT02425891
Avelumab With Binimetinib, Sacituzumab Govitecan, or Liposomal Doxorubicin in treating patients with stage IV or unresectable recurrent TNBC (InCITe)	Phase II	Active	18 and over	NCT03971409
A Study of Atezolizumab and Paclitaxel versus placebo and paclitaxel in participants with previously untreated locally advanced or metastatic TNBC (Impassion131)	Phase III	Active, not recruiting	18 and over	NCT03125902
A Study evaluating the efficacy and safety of multiple immunotherapy-based treatment combinations in patients with metastatic or inoperable locally advanced TNBC (Morpheus-TNBC)	Phase I/II	Active	18 and over	NCT03424005
A Study of Cobimetinib plus paclitaxel, Cobimetinib plus Atezolizumab plus Paclitaxel, or Cobimetinib plus Atezolizumab plus Nab-Paclitaxel as initial treatment for participants with TNBC that has spread	Phase II	Active, not recruiting	18 and over	NCT02322814
Women's MoonShot: Neoadjuvant treatment with PaCT for patients with locally advanced TNBC	Phase II	Active	18 and over	NCT02593175
A phase II study of Nivolumab in combination with Cabozantinib for metastatic TNBC	Phase II	Active, not recruiting	18 and over	NCT03316586
FUSCC Refractory TNBC Umbrella (FUTURE)	Phase I/II	Active	18 to 75 years	NCT03805399
Peri-Operative Ipilimumab + Nivolumab and Cryoablation in women with TNBC	Phase II	Active	18 and over	NCT03546686
Trilaciclib (G1T28), a CDK 4/6 Inhibitor, in Combination with Gemcitabine and Carboplatin in metastatic TNBC	Phase II	Active, not recruiting	18 and over	NCT02978716

6.2. Combination Regimens

The molecular heterogeneity and frequent multi-clonality of TNBC strongly suggest that precision combination therapies are more likely to be successful than monotherapeutic strategies. The use of targeted agents plus standard chemotherapy or other targeted agents has shown promising results. One study found that olaparib, a PARP inhibitor, combined with the PI3K inhibitor buparlisib and carboplatin caused cytotoxic effects by promoting of non-homologous DNA end joining in TNBC cells [158]. A phase I study is assessing an olaparib–buparlisib combination regimen in TNBC and ovarian cancer (Clinicaltrials.gov: NCT01623349). PARP inhibitors have also shown activity with ADCs and chemotherapy, such as olaparib with sacitzumab govetican in TNBC cells with and without BRCA mutations [159] and iniparib in combination with gemcitabine and carboplatin [160]. PARPi have also been explored in combination with immunotherapy. PARPi have been shown to upregulate PD-L1, and PD-L1 inhibitors were documented to restore breast cancer sensitivity to PARP inhibitors [156]. In contrast, Higuchi et al. found no improvement of the efficacy of PARPi in BRCA-negative ovarian cancer with PD-1/PD-L1 inhibition, but they [161] did find improvement if PARPi were used in combination with CTLA-4 inhibitors [161]. Buparlisib in combination with DSF/Cu (Disulfiram/copper) and paclitaxel caused decreased tumor burden and recurrence rates in TNBC compared to paclitaxel alone [162]. In addition, a clinical trial involving the AKT inhibitor ipatasertib combined with paclitaxel has shown promising results (Clinicaltrials.gov: NCT02162719).

Combination therapy involving Notch targeting may be an attractive strategy. A late clinical development stage GSI, PF-03084014 combined with the AKT inhibitor MK-2206 or the NF-kB inhibitor Bay11-7082 effectively treated TNBC cells with a Notch mutation and wild-type PTEN [163]. Another study found a correlation between Notch3 inhibition and the increased effectiveness of the tyrosine kinase inhibitor gefitinib targeting EGFR in TNBC cells [164].

Combinations of immunotherapeutics with chemotherapy or with targeted agents are potentially promising. The I-SPY trial found success in combining the PD-1 inhibitor pembrolizumab with paclitaxel (Clinicaltrials.gov: NCT01042379), and the KEYNOTE 173 trial is seeing antitumor activity with pembrolizumab and neoadjuvant chemotherapy (Clinicaltrials.gov: NCT02622074). Another clinical trial is investigating PD-1 (nivolumab) and CTLA-4 inhibitors (ipilimumab) together along with cryoablation (Clinicaltrials.gov: NCT02833233). Many potential immunogenic tumors do not respond to immune checkpoint blockers. Kim et al. found significant improvement in outcomes when ICBs were used in combination with epigenetic-modulating drugs targeting myeloid-derived suppressor cells (MDSCs) or a PI3K inhibitor that reduced MDSCs [165].

7. Design of Precision Medicine-Based Clinical Trials in TNBC: The Path Forward

The future of TNBC developmental therapeutics depends on increasingly precise, biomarker-based, adaptive clinical trials. A perfect example is the ongoing FUTURE trial (Clinicaltrials.gov: NCT03805399) [57]. This is a phase I/II subtyping-based and genomic biomarker-guided umbrella trial where the investigators have classified metastatic TNBC patients based on molecular subtyping and genomic profiling. Patient classification for this trial relies on an integrative analysis that combines somatic mutations, copy number aberrations (CNAs), and gene expression profiles as well as validated immunohistochemistry surrogates. Based on these criteria, TNBC patients are stratified into four subtypes: (1) luminal androgen receptor (LAR), (2) immunomodulatory (IM), (3) basal-like immune-suppressed (BLIS), and (4) mesenchymal-like (MES) [57]. Within the LAR group, patients with HER2 mutations are treated with pyrotinib and capecitabine, while patients without HER2 mutations are treated with an androgen receptor antagonist and a CDK4/6 inhibitor. For the IM group, patients are treated with anti-PD-1 immunotherapy plus nab-paclitaxel. If the patients have BRCA1/2 germline mutation within the BLIS group, they are treated with a PARP inhibitor. If no BRCA1/2 germline mutations are detected, the patients are treated with anti-VEGFR therapy. Within the MES group, if patients have PI3K/AKT pathway mutations, they are treated with an mTOR inhibitor (Everolimus) with nab-paclitaxel. In contrast, patients without PI3K/AKT pathway mutations are treated with anti-VEGFR therapy. New arms can be added or existing arms can be terminated based on the ongoing examination of the study results. This type of study design is likely to become standard in TNBC and beyond.

8. Conclusions

The rapid evolution of targeted therapy and immunotherapy guided by somatic and in some cases germline genomics gives us realistic hopes for the more effective, more precise, and less toxic treatment of TNBC in the near future. However, further research is necessary to realize the full potential of precision medicine in TNBC. Somatic NGS alone has limitations, and we must move beyond simplistic one-gene-one therapy paradigms. Mutational landscapes change with time, and a single NGS test performed before treatment may not be representative of the tumor after chemotherapy or radiation. Longitudinal testing, if accessible tumor or perhaps circulating tumor cells are available, is likely to provide more accurate information. Many genotyped tumors reveal no targetable mutations, or, even when such mutations are identified, the patient may not respond to treatment [166]. This may be due to compensatory mutations, epigenetic changes, phenotypic plasticity, or clonal heterogeneity. Despite these limitations, genomic-driven therapy is already improving outcomes. An MD Anderson study found a higher response rate and more prolonged survival when treating single-mutation cancers with matched therapy [167].

Phenotypic screening using 3D tumor organotypic spheroids [168] may offer a promising alternative or complementary strategy, provided that results can be obtained rapidly, and treatment can potentially be adapted to tumor evolution using more than one round of screening. Pauli et al. were able to improve drug sensitivity screening using 3-D cultures and PDX models, showing that integration of exome sequencing with these methods could help better identify the best therapy [166]. An important limitation of these methods is that they require accessible tumor tissue. "Liquid biopsy," a group of evolving methods to obtain circulating tumor cells or circulating tumor DNA from patient blood, could be an avenue for therapeutic screening and the longitudinal monitoring of molecular tumor profiles [169]. Single-cell RNA sequencing to identify resistant clones is now a reality [170]. Proteogenomics combining proteomic and genomic results is an attractive strategy if costs can be brought down [171]. The study of tumor metabolism and metabolomics is another highly promising precision medicine field that can be combined with genomics. A recent manuscript described a targetable retinoblastoma tumor suppressor, (RB1)-glucose transporter 1 (GLUT1) metabolic axis, in TNBC and suggested targeting GLUT1 in TNBC patients based on their RB1 protein expression levels [172]. The promise of precision medicine in the treatment of TNBC and other solid tumors is undeniable, and combinations of increasingly sensitive "omics" and phenotypic screening may significantly accelerate the development of novel therapeutics.

Author Contributions: F.H. developed the idea and concept. He also wrote and reviewed the manuscript. S.M. wrote and reviewed the manuscript. J.D. wrote one chapter under the supervision of F.H., and L.M. wrote and reviewed the manuscript. All authors contributed to the editing, proofreading, and revising the manuscript. All authors have read and agreed to the published version of the manuscript.

Funding: This work was supported by US National Institutes of Health (NIH) (P20CA233374 to L.M.) and Louisiana Clinical and Translational Science (LA CaTs) Roadmap Scholar grant to F.H. (NIH U54 GM104940).

Conflicts of Interest: The authors declare no conflict of interests.

References

1. Goodwin, S.; McPherson, J.D.; McCombie, W.R. Coming of age: Ten years of next-generation sequencing technologies. *Nat. Rev. Genet.* **2016**, *17*, 333–351. [CrossRef]
2. Bush, W.S.; Moore, J.H. Chapter 11: Genome-wide association studies. *PLoS Comput. Biol.* **2012**, *8*, e1002822. [CrossRef]
3. Ginsburg, G.S.; Phillips, K.A. Precision Medicine: From Science To Value. *Health Aff. (Millwood)* **2018**, *37*, 694–701. [CrossRef]
4. Dugger, S.A.; Platt, A.; Goldstein, D.B. Drug development in the era of precision medicine. *Nat. Rev. Drug Discov.* **2018**, *17*, 183–196. [CrossRef]
5. Xie, F.; Chan, J.C.; Ma, R.C. Precision medicine in diabetes prevention, classification and management. *J. Diabetes Investig.* **2018**, *9*, 998–1015. [CrossRef] [PubMed]

6. Cooper, G.M.; Johnson, J.A.; Langaee, T.Y.; Feng, H.; Stanaway, I.B.; Schwarz, U.I.; Ritchie, M.D.; Stein, C.M.; Roden, D.M.; Smith, J.D.; et al. A genome-wide scan for common genetic variants with a large influence on warfarin maintenance dose. *Blood* **2008**, *112*, 1022–1027. [CrossRef] [PubMed]
7. Motsinger-Reif, A.A.; Jorgenson, E.; Relling, M.V.; Kroetz, D.L.; Weinshilboum, R.; Cox, N.J.; Roden, D.M. Genome-wide association studies in pharmacogenomics: Successes and lessons. *Pharm. Genom.* **2013**, *23*, 383–394. [CrossRef] [PubMed]
8. Scharfe, C.P.I.; Tremmel, R.; Schwab, M.; Kohlbacher, O.; Marks, D.S. Genetic variation in human drug-related genes. *Genome Med.* **2017**, *9*, 117. [CrossRef]
9. Sim, S.C.; Kacevska, M.; Ingelman-Sundberg, M. Pharmacogenomics of drug-metabolizing enzymes: A recent update on clinical implications and endogenous effects. *Pharm. J.* **2013**, *13*, 1–11. [CrossRef]
10. Liu, X.; Luo, X.; Jiang, C.; Zhao, H. Difficulties and challenges in the development of precision medicine. *Clin. Genet.* **2019**, *95*, 569–574. [CrossRef]
11. Singh, R.S.; Gupta, B.P. Genes and genomes and unnecessary complexity in precision medicine. *NPJ Genom. Med.* **2020**, *5*, 21. [CrossRef]
12. Chanfreau-Coffinier, C.; Peredo, J.; Russell, M.M.; Yano, E.M.; Hamilton, A.B.; Lerner, B.; Provenzale, D.; Knight, S.J.; Voils, C.I.; Scheuner, M.T. A logic model for precision medicine implementation informed by stakeholder views and implementation science. *Genet. Med.* **2019**, *21*, 1139–1154. [CrossRef]
13. Reuter, C.M.; Kohler, J.N.; Bonner, D.; Zastrow, D.; Fernandez, L.; Dries, A.; Marwaha, S.; Davidson, J.; Brokamp, E.; Herzog, M.; et al. Yield of whole exome sequencing in undiagnosed patients facing insurance coverage barriers to genetic testing. *J. Genet. Couns.* **2019**, *28*, 1107–1118. [CrossRef]
14. Klein, M.E.; Parvez, M.M.; Shin, J.G. Clinical Implementation of Pharmacogenomics for Personalized Precision Medicine: Barriers and Solutions. *J. Pharm. Sci.* **2017**, *106*, 2368–2379. [CrossRef]
15. Nakagawa, H.; Fujita, M. Whole genome sequencing analysis for cancer genomics and precision medicine. *Cancer Sci.* **2018**, *109*, 513–522. [CrossRef]
16. Slamon, D.J.; Leyland-Jones, B.; Shak, S.; Fuchs, H.; Paton, V.; Bajamonde, A.; Fleming, T.; Eiermann, W.; Wolter, J.; Pegram, M.; et al. Use of chemotherapy plus a monoclonal antibody against HER2 for metastatic breast cancer that overexpresses HER2. *N. Engl. J. Med.* **2001**, *344*, 783–792. [CrossRef] [PubMed]
17. Karapetis, C.S.; Khambata-Ford, S.; Jonker, D.J.; O'Callaghan, C.J.; Tu, D.; Tebbutt, N.C.; Simes, R.J.; Chalchal, H.; Shapiro, J.D.; Robitaille, S.; et al. K-ras mutations and benefit from cetuximab in advanced colorectal cancer. *N. Engl. J. Med.* **2008**, *359*, 1757–1765. [CrossRef] [PubMed]
18. Mullane, S.A.; Van Allen, E.M. Precision medicine for advanced prostate cancer. *Curr. Opin. Urol.* **2016**, *26*, 231–239. [CrossRef]
19. Zhao, D.; Klempner, S.J.; Chao, J. Progress and challenges in HER2-positive gastroesophageal adenocarcinoma. *J. Hematol. Oncol.* **2019**, *12*, 50. [CrossRef]
20. Hall, R.D.; Kudchadkar, R.R. BRAF mutations: Signaling, epidemiology, and clinical experience in multiple malignancies. *Cancer Control.* **2014**, *21*, 221–230. [CrossRef] [PubMed]
21. Arber, N.; Levin, B. Chemoprevention of colorectal neoplasia: The potential for personalized medicine. *Gastroenterology* **2008**, *134*, 1224–1237. [CrossRef]
22. Mennel, R.G. Precision medicine: Hype or hoax? *Proc. (Bayl. Univ. Med. Cent.)* **2015**, *28*, 397–400. [CrossRef]
23. Dagogo-Jack, I.; Shaw, A.T. Tumour heterogeneity and resistance to cancer therapies. *Nat. Rev. Clin. Oncol.* **2018**, *15*, 81–94. [CrossRef] [PubMed]
24. Miller, C.A.; McMichael, J.; Dang, H.X.; Maher, C.A.; Ding, L.; Ley, T.J.; Mardis, E.R.; Wilson, R.K. Visualizing tumor evolution with the fishplot package for R. *BMC Genom.* **2016**, *17*, 880. [CrossRef] [PubMed]
25. Jackson, S.E.; Chester, J.D. Personalised cancer medicine. *Int. J. Cancer* **2015**, *137*, 262–266. [CrossRef] [PubMed]
26. Dent, R.; Trudeau, M.; Pritchard, K.I.; Hanna, W.M.; Kahn, H.K.; Sawka, C.A.; Lickley, L.A.; Rawlinson, E.; Sun, P.; Narod, S.A. Triple-negative breast cancer: Clinical features and patterns of recurrence. *Clin. Cancer Res.* **2007**, *13*, 4429–4434. [CrossRef] [PubMed]
27. Aysola, K.; Desai, A.; Welch, C.; Xu, J.; Qin, Y.; Reddy, V.; Matthews, R.; Owens, C.; Okoli, J.; Beech, D.J.; et al. Triple Negative Breast Cancer—An Overview. *Hered. Genet.* **2013**, *2013*. [CrossRef]
28. Yin, L.; Duan, J.J.; Bian, X.W.; Yu, S.C. Triple-negative breast cancer molecular subtyping and treatment progress. *Breast Cancer Res.* **2020**, *22*, 61. [CrossRef]
29. Garrido-Castro, A.C.; Lin, N.U.; Polyak, K. Insights into Molecular Classifications of Triple-Negative Breast Cancer: Improving Patient Selection for Treatment. *Cancer Discov.* **2019**, *9*, 176–198. [CrossRef]
30. Sporikova, Z.; Koudelakova, V.; Trojanec, R.; Hajduch, M. Genetic Markers in Triple-Negative Breast Cancer. *Clin. Breast Cancer* **2018**, *18*, e841–e850. [CrossRef]
31. Bianchini, G.; Balko, J.M.; Mayer, I.A.; Sanders, M.E.; Gianni, L. Triple-negative breast cancer: Challenges and opportunities of a heterogeneous disease. *Nat. Rev. Clin. Oncol.* **2016**, *13*, 674–690. [CrossRef] [PubMed]
32. Salas-Benito, D.; Perez-Gracia, J.L.; Ponz-Sarvise, M.; Rodriguez-Ruiz, M.E.; Martinez-Forero, I.; Castanon, E.; Lopez-Picazo, J.M.; Sanmamed, M.F.; Melero, I. Paradigms on Immunotherapy Combinations with Chemotherapy. *Cancer Discov.* **2021**. [CrossRef]
33. Singh, S.; Numan, A.; Maddiboyina, B.; Arora, S.; Riadi, Y.; Md, S.; Alhakamy, N.A.; Kesharwani, P. The emerging role of immune checkpoint inhibitors in the treatment of triple-negative breast cancer. *Drug Discov. Today* **2021**. [CrossRef]

34. Tiwari, P.; Blank, A.; Cui, C.; Schoenfelt, K.Q.; Zhou, G.; Xu, Y.; Khramtsova, G.; Olopade, F.; Shah, A.M.; Khan, S.A.; et al. Metabolically activated adipose tissue macrophages link obesity to triple-negative breast cancer. *J. Exp. Med.* **2019**, *216*, 1345–1358. [CrossRef] [PubMed]
35. Teslow, E.A.; Mitrea, C.; Bao, B.; Mohammad, R.M.; Polin, L.A.; Dyson, G.; Purrington, K.S.; Bollig-Fischer, A. Obesity-induced MBD2_v2 expression promotes tumor-initiating triple-negative breast cancer stem cells. *Mol. Oncol.* **2019**, *13*, 894–908. [CrossRef]
36. Bowers, L.W.; Rossi, E.L.; McDonell, S.B.; Doerstling, S.S.; Khatib, S.A.; Lineberger, C.G.; Albright, J.E.; Tang, X.; deGraffenried, L.A.; Hursting, S.D. Leptin Signaling Mediates Obesity-Associated CSC Enrichment and EMT in Preclinical TNBC Models. *Mol. Cancer Res.* **2018**, *16*, 869–879. [CrossRef]
37. Dietze, E.C.; Chavez, T.A.; Seewaldt, V.L. Obesity and Triple-Negative Breast Cancer: Disparities, Controversies, and Biology. *Am. J. Pathol.* **2018**, *188*, 280–290. [CrossRef] [PubMed]
38. Elstrom, R.L.; Bauer, D.E.; Buzzai, M.; Karnauskas, R.; Harris, M.H.; Plas, D.R.; Zhuang, H.; Cinalli, R.M.; Alavi, A.; Rudin, C.M.; et al. Akt stimulates aerobic glycolysis in cancer cells. *Cancer Res.* **2004**, *64*, 3892–3899. [CrossRef] [PubMed]
39. Robey, R.B.; Hay, N. Is Akt the "Warburg kinase"?-Akt-energy metabolism interactions and oncogenesis. *Semin. Cancer Biol.* **2009**, *19*, 25–31. [CrossRef] [PubMed]
40. Steenbrugge, J.; Vander Elst, N.; Demeyere, K.; De Wever, O.; Sanders, N.N.; Van Den Broeck, W.; Dirix, L.; Van Laere, S.; Meyer, E. Comparative Profiling of Metastatic 4T1- vs. Non-metastatic Py230-Based Mammary Tumors in an Intraductal Model for Triple-Negative Breast Cancer. *Front. Immunol.* **2019**, *10*, 2928. [CrossRef]
41. Khosravi-Shahi, P.; Cabezon-Gutierrez, L.; Custodio-Cabello, S. Metastatic triple negative breast cancer: Optimizing treatment options, new and emerging targeted therapies. *Asia Pac. J. Clin. Oncol.* **2018**, *14*, 32–39. [CrossRef] [PubMed]
42. Stover, D.G.; Parsons, H.A.; Ha, G.; Freeman, S.S.; Barry, W.T.; Guo, H.; Choudhury, A.D.; Gydush, G.; Reed, S.C.; Rhoades, J.; et al. Association of Cell-Free DNA Tumor Fraction and Somatic Copy Number Alterations With Survival in Metastatic Triple-Negative Breast Cancer. *J. Clin. Oncol.* **2018**, *36*, 543–553. [CrossRef] [PubMed]
43. Shah, S.P.; Roth, A.; Goya, R.; Oloumi, A.; Ha, G.; Zhao, Y.; Turashvili, G.; Ding, J.; Tse, K.; Haffari, G.; et al. The clonal and mutational evolution spectrum of primary triple-negative breast cancers. *Nature* **2012**, *486*, 395–399. [CrossRef]
44. Cancer Genome Atlas, N. Comprehensive molecular portraits of human breast tumours. *Nature* **2012**, *490*, 61–70. [CrossRef] [PubMed]
45. Brewster, A.M.; Chavez-MacGregor, M.; Brown, P. Epidemiology, biology, and treatment of triple-negative breast cancer in women of African ancestry. *Lancet Oncol.* **2014**, *15*, e625–e634. [CrossRef]
46. Cejalvo, J.M.; Martinez de Duenas, E.; Galvan, P.; Garcia-Recio, S.; Burgues Gasion, O.; Pare, L.; Antolin, S.; Martinello, R.; Blancas, I.; Adamo, B.; et al. Intrinsic Subtypes and Gene Expression Profiles in Primary and Metastatic Breast Cancer. *Cancer Res.* **2017**, *77*, 2213–2221. [CrossRef]
47. Amabile, M.I.; Frusone, F.; De Luca, A.; Tripodi, D.; Imbimbo, G.; Lai, S.; D'Andrea, V.; Sorrenti, S.; Molfino, A. Locoregional Surgery in Metastatic Breast Cancer: Do Concomitant Metabolic Aspects Have a Role on the Management and Prognosis in this Setting? *J. Pers. Med.* **2020**, *10*, 227. [CrossRef]
48. Ma, L.; Mi, Y.; Cui, S.; Wang, H.; Fu, P.; Yin, Y.; Jin, F.; Li, J.; Liu, Y.; Fan, Z.; et al. Role of locoregional surgery in patients with de novo stage IV breast cancer: Analysis of real-world data from China. *Sci. Rep.* **2020**, *10*, 18132. [CrossRef]
49. Carey, L.; Winer, E.; Viale, G.; Cameron, D.; Gianni, L. Triple-negative breast cancer: Disease entity or title of convenience? *Nat. Rev. Clin. Oncol.* **2010**, *7*, 683–692. [CrossRef]
50. Marra, A.; Trapani, D.; Viale, G.; Criscitiello, C.; Curigliano, G. Practical classification of triple-negative breast cancer: Intratumoral heterogeneity, mechanisms of drug resistance, and novel therapies. *NPJ Breast Cancer* **2020**, *6*, 54. [CrossRef]
51. Rakha, E.A.; El-Sayed, M.E.; Green, A.R.; Lee, A.H.; Robertson, J.F.; Ellis, I.O. Prognostic markers in triple-negative breast cancer. *Cancer* **2007**, *109*, 25–32. [CrossRef] [PubMed]
52. Lehmann, B.D.; Bauer, J.A.; Chen, X.; Sanders, M.E.; Chakravarthy, A.B.; Shyr, Y.; Pietenpol, J.A. Identification of human triple-negative breast cancer subtypes and preclinical models for selection of targeted therapies. *J. Clin. Investig.* **2011**, *121*, 2750–2767. [CrossRef] [PubMed]
53. Chen, X.; Li, J.; Gray, W.H.; Lehmann, B.D.; Bauer, J.A.; Shyr, Y.; Pietenpol, J.A. TNBCtype: A Subtyping Tool for Triple-Negative Breast Cancer. *Cancer Inform.* **2012**, *11*, 147–156. [CrossRef] [PubMed]
54. Burstein, M.D.; Tsimelzon, A.; Poage, G.M.; Covington, K.R.; Contreras, A.; Fuqua, S.A.; Savage, M.I.; Osborne, C.K.; Hilsenbeck, S.G.; Chang, J.C.; et al. Comprehensive genomic analysis identifies novel subtypes and targets of triple-negative breast cancer. *Clin. Cancer Res.* **2015**, *21*, 1688–1698. [CrossRef] [PubMed]
55. Liu, Y.R.; Jiang, Y.Z.; Xu, X.E.; Yu, K.D.; Jin, X.; Hu, X.; Zuo, W.J.; Hao, S.; Wu, J.; Liu, G.Y.; et al. Comprehensive transcriptome analysis identifies novel molecular subtypes and subtype-specific RNAs of triple-negative breast cancer. *Breast Cancer Res.* **2016**, *18*, 33. [CrossRef] [PubMed]
56. Lehmann, B.D.; Jovanovic, B.; Chen, X.; Estrada, M.V.; Johnson, K.N.; Shyr, Y.; Moses, H.L.; Sanders, M.E.; Pietenpol, J.A. Refinement of Triple-Negative Breast Cancer Molecular Subtypes: Implications for Neoadjuvant Chemotherapy Selection. *PLoS ONE* **2016**, *11*, e0157368. [CrossRef]
57. Jiang, Y.Z.; Liu, Y.; Xiao, Y.; Hu, X.; Jiang, L.; Zuo, W.J.; Ma, D.; Ding, J.; Zhu, X.; Zou, J.; et al. Molecular subtyping and genomic profiling expand precision medicine in refractory metastatic triple-negative breast cancer: The FUTURE trial. *Cell Res.* **2021**, *31*, 178–186. [CrossRef]

58. Gupta, G.K.; Collier, A.L.; Lee, D.; Hoefer, R.A.; Zheleva, V.; Siewertsz van Reesema, L.L.; Tang-Tan, A.M.; Guye, M.L.; Chang, D.Z.; Winston, J.S.; et al. Perspectives on Triple-Negative Breast Cancer: Current Treatment Strategies, Unmet Needs, and Potential Targets for Future Therapies. *Cancers* **2020**, *12*, 2392. [CrossRef]
59. Hutchinson, L. Breast cancer: TNBC: Can we treat the untargetable? *Nat. Rev. Clin. Oncol.* **2014**, *11*, 379. [CrossRef]
60. Pal, S.K.; Childs, B.H.; Pegram, M. Triple negative breast cancer: Unmet medical needs. *Breast Cancer Res. Treat.* **2011**, *125*, 627–636. [CrossRef] [PubMed]
61. Sharma, P. Biology and Management of Patients With Triple-Negative Breast Cancer. *Oncologist* **2016**, *21*, 1050–1062. [CrossRef] [PubMed]
62. Andreopoulou, E.; Schweber, S.J.; Sparano, J.A.; McDaid, H.M. Therapies for triple negative breast cancer. *Expert Opin. Pharmacother.* **2015**, *16*, 983–998. [CrossRef] [PubMed]
63. Ciriello, G.; Gatza, M.L.; Beck, A.H.; Wilkerson, M.D.; Rhie, S.K.; Pastore, A.; Zhang, H.; McLellan, M.; Yau, C.; Kandoth, C.; et al. Comprehensive Molecular Portraits of Invasive Lobular Breast Cancer. *Cell* **2015**, *163*, 506–519. [CrossRef]
64. Gradishar, W.J.; Anderson, B.O.; Balassanian, R.; Blair, S.L.; Burstein, H.J.; Cyr, A.; Elias, A.D.; Farrar, W.B.; Forero, A.; Giordano, S.H.; et al. NCCN Guidelines Insights: Breast Cancer, Version 1.2017. *J. Natl. Compr. Canc. Netw.* **2017**, *15*, 433–451. [CrossRef]
65. Isakoff, S.J.; Mayer, E.L.; He, L.; Traina, T.A.; Carey, L.A.; Krag, K.J.; Rugo, H.S.; Liu, M.C.; Stearns, V.; Come, S.E.; et al. TBCRC009: A Multicenter Phase II Clinical Trial of Platinum Monotherapy With Biomarker Assessment in Metastatic Triple-Negative Breast Cancer. *J. Clin. Oncol.* **2015**, *33*, 1902–1909. [CrossRef]
66. Theriault, R.L.; Litton, J.K.; Mittendorf, E.A.; Chen, H.; Meric-Bernstam, F.; Chavez-Macgregor, M.; Morrow, P.K.; Woodward, W.A.; Sahin, A.; Hortobagyi, G.N.; et al. Age and survival estimates in patients who have node-negative T1ab breast cancer by breast cancer subtype. *Clin. Breast Cancer* **2011**, *11*, 325–331. [CrossRef]
67. Vaz-Luis, I.; Ottesen, R.A.; Hughes, M.E.; Mamet, R.; Burstein, H.J.; Edge, S.B.; Gonzalez-Angulo, A.M.; Moy, B.; Rugo, H.S.; Theriault, R.L.; et al. Outcomes by tumor subtype and treatment pattern in women with small, node-negative breast cancer: A multi-institutional study. *J. Clin. Oncol.* **2014**, *32*, 2142–2150. [CrossRef]
68. Park, J.H.; Ahn, J.H.; Kim, S.B. How shall we treat early triple-negative breast cancer (TNBC): From the current standard to upcoming immuno-molecular strategies. *ESMO Open* **2018**, *3*, e000357. [CrossRef]
69. Blum, J.L.; Flynn, P.J.; Yothers, G.; Asmar, L.; Geyer, C.E., Jr.; Jacobs, S.A.; Robert, N.J.; Hopkins, J.O.; O'Shaughnessy, J.A.; Dang, C.T.; et al. Anthracyclines in Early Breast Cancer: The ABC Trials-USOR 06-090, NSABP B-46-I/USOR 07132, and NSABP B-49 (NRG Oncology). *J. Clin. Oncol.* **2017**, *35*, 2647–2655. [CrossRef] [PubMed]
70. Martin, M.; Rodriguez-Lescure, A.; Ruiz, A.; Alba, E.; Calvo, L.; Ruiz-Borrego, M.; Santaballa, A.; Rodriguez, C.A.; Crespo, C.; Abad, M.; et al. Molecular predictors of efficacy of adjuvant weekly paclitaxel in early breast cancer. *Breast Cancer Res. Treat.* **2010**, *123*, 149–157. [CrossRef]
71. Arteaga, C.L.; Sliwkowski, M.X.; Osborne, C.K.; Perez, E.A.; Puglisi, F.; Gianni, L. Treatment of HER2-positive breast cancer: Current status and future perspectives. *Nat. Rev. Clin. Oncol.* **2011**, *9*, 16–32. [CrossRef]
72. DeMichele, A.; Yee, D.; Berry, D.A.; Albain, K.S.; Benz, C.C.; Boughey, J.; Buxton, M.; Chia, S.K.; Chien, A.J.; Chui, S.Y.; et al. The Neoadjuvant Model Is Still the Future for Drug Development in Breast Cancer. *Clin. Cancer Res.* **2015**, *21*, 2911–2915. [CrossRef] [PubMed]
73. Haddad, T.C.; Goetz, M.P. Landscape of neoadjuvant therapy for breast cancer. *Ann. Surg. Oncol.* **2015**, *22*, 1408–1415. [CrossRef]
74. King, T.A.; Morrow, M. Surgical issues in patients with breast cancer receiving neoadjuvant chemotherapy. *Nat. Rev. Clin. Oncol.* **2015**, *12*, 335–343. [CrossRef] [PubMed]
75. Nagayama, A.; Hayashida, T.; Jinno, H.; Takahashi, M.; Seki, T.; Matsumoto, A.; Murata, T.; Ashrafian, H.; Athanasiou, T.; Okabayashi, K.; et al. Comparative effectiveness of neoadjuvant therapy for HER2-positive breast cancer: A network meta-analysis. *J. Natl. Cancer Inst.* **2014**, *106*. [CrossRef] [PubMed]
76. Prat, A.; Fan, C.; Fernandez, A.; Hoadley, K.A.; Martinello, R.; Vidal, M.; Viladot, M.; Pineda, E.; Arance, A.; Munoz, M.; et al. Response and survival of breast cancer intrinsic subtypes following multi-agent neoadjuvant chemotherapy. *BMC Med.* **2015**, *13*, 303. [CrossRef] [PubMed]
77. Tevaarwerk, A.J.; Gray, R.J.; Schneider, B.P.; Smith, M.L.; Wagner, L.I.; Fetting, J.H.; Davidson, N.; Goldstein, L.J.; Miller, K.D.; Sparano, J.A. Survival in patients with metastatic recurrent breast cancer after adjuvant chemotherapy: Little evidence of improvement over the past 30 years. *Cancer* **2013**, *119*, 1140–1148. [CrossRef] [PubMed]
78. Thompson, A.M.; Moulder-Thompson, S.L. Neoadjuvant treatment of breast cancer. *Ann. Oncol.* **2012**, *23* (Suppl. 10), x231–x236. [CrossRef]
79. Zardavas, D.; Baselga, J.; Piccart, M. Emerging targeted agents in metastatic breast cancer. *Nat. Rev. Clin. Oncol.* **2013**, *10*, 191–210. [CrossRef]
80. Foulkes, W.D.; Smith, I.E.; Reis-Filho, J.S. Triple-negative breast cancer. *N. Engl. J. Med.* **2010**, *363*, 1938–1948. [CrossRef]
81. Isakoff, S.J. Triple-negative breast cancer: Role of specific chemotherapy agents. *Cancer J.* **2010**, *16*, 53–61. [CrossRef]
82. Santonja, A.; Sanchez-Munoz, A.; Lluch, A.; Chica-Parrado, M.R.; Albanell, J.; Chacon, J.I.; Antolin, S.; Jerez, J.M.; de la Haba, J.; de Luque, V.; et al. Triple negative breast cancer subtypes and pathologic complete response rate to neoadjuvant chemotherapy. *Oncotarget* **2018**, *9*, 26406–26416. [CrossRef]

33. Asano, Y.; Kashiwagi, S.; Goto, W.; Takada, K.; Takahashi, K.; Hatano, T.; Noda, S.; Takashima, T.; Onoda, N.; Tomita, S.; et al. Prediction of survival after neoadjuvant chemotherapy for breast cancer by evaluation of tumor-infiltrating lymphocytes and residual cancer burden. *BMC Cancer* **2017**, *17*, 888. [CrossRef]
34. Asano, Y.; Kashiwagi, S.; Goto, W.; Takada, K.; Takahashi, K.; Morisaki, T.; Fujita, H.; Takashima, T.; Tomita, S.; Ohsawa, M.; et al. Prediction of treatment responses to neoadjuvant chemotherapy in triple-negative breast cancer by analysis of immune checkpoint protein expression. *J. Transl. Med.* **2018**, *16*, 87. [CrossRef] [PubMed]
35. Byrne, A.; Savas, P.; Sant, S.; Li, R.; Virassamy, B.; Luen, S.J.; Beavis, P.A.; Mackay, L.K.; Neeson, P.J.; Loi, S. Tissue-resident memory T cells in breast cancer control and immunotherapy responses. *Nat. Rev. Clin. Oncol.* **2020**, *17*, 341–348. [CrossRef] [PubMed]
36. Dieci, M.V.; Criscitiello, C.; Goubar, A.; Viale, G.; Conte, P.; Guarneri, V.; Ficarra, G.; Mathieu, M.C.; Delaloge, S.; Curigliano, G.; et al. Prognostic value of tumor-infiltrating lymphocytes on residual disease after primary chemotherapy for triple-negative breast cancer: A retrospective multicenter study. *Ann. Oncol.* **2015**, *26*, 1518. [CrossRef] [PubMed]
37. Dieci, M.V.; Radosevic-Robin, N.; Fineberg, S.; van den Eynden, G.; Ternes, N.; Penault-Llorca, F.; Pruneri, G.; D'Alfonso, T.M.; Demaria, S.; Castaneda, C.; et al. Update on tumor-infiltrating lymphocytes (TILs) in breast cancer, including recommendations to assess TILs in residual disease after neoadjuvant therapy and in carcinoma in situ: A report of the International Immuno-Oncology Biomarker Working Group on Breast Cancer. *Semin. Cancer Biol.* **2018**, *52*, 16–25. [CrossRef] [PubMed]
38. Garcia-Martinez, E.; Gil, G.L.; Benito, A.C.; Gonzalez-Billalabeitia, E.; Conesa, M.A.; Garcia Garcia, T.; Garcia-Garre, E.; Vicente, V.; Ayala de la Pena, F. Tumor-infiltrating immune cell profiles and their change after neoadjuvant chemotherapy predict response and prognosis of breast cancer. *Breast Cancer Res.* **2014**, *16*, 488. [CrossRef] [PubMed]
39. Ladoire, S.; Mignot, G.; Dabakuyo, S.; Arnould, L.; Apetoh, L.; Rebe, C.; Coudert, B.; Martin, F.; Bizollon, M.H.; Vanoli, A.; et al. In situ immune response after neoadjuvant chemotherapy for breast cancer predicts survival. *J. Pathol.* **2011**, *224*, 389–400. [CrossRef]
40. Pinard, C.; Debled, M.; Ben Rejeb, H.; Velasco, V.; Tunon de Lara, C.; Hoppe, S.; Richard, E.; Brouste, V.; Bonnefoi, H.; MacGrogan, G. Residual cancer burden index and tumor-infiltrating lymphocyte subtypes in triple-negative breast cancer after neoadjuvant chemotherapy. *Breast Cancer Res. Treat.* **2020**, *179*, 11–23. [CrossRef]
41. Denkert, C.; von Minckwitz, G.; Brase, J.C.; Sinn, B.V.; Gade, S.; Kronenwett, R.; Pfitzner, B.M.; Salat, C.; Loi, S.; Schmitt, W.D.; et al. Tumor-infiltrating lymphocytes and response to neoadjuvant chemotherapy with or without carboplatin in human epidermal growth factor receptor 2-positive and triple-negative primary breast cancers. *J Clin Oncol* **2015**, *33*, 983–991. [CrossRef] [PubMed]
42. Filho, O.M.; Stover, D.G.; Asad, S.; Ansell, P.J.; Watson, M.; Loibl, S.; Geyer, C.E., Jr.; Bae, J.; Collier, K.; Cherian, M.; et al. Association of Immunophenotype With Pathologic Complete Response to Neoadjuvant Chemotherapy for Triple-Negative Breast Cancer: A Secondary Analysis of the BrighTNess Phase 3 Randomized Clinical Trial. *JAMA Oncol.* **2021**. [CrossRef] [PubMed]
43. Criscitiello, C.; Bayar, M.A.; Curigliano, G.; Symmans, F.W.; Desmedt, C.; Bonnefoi, H.; Sinn, B.; Pruneri, G.; Vicier, C.; Pierga, J.Y.; et al. A gene signature to predict high tumor-infiltrating lymphocytes after neoadjuvant chemotherapy and outcome in patients with triple-negative breast cancer. *Ann. Oncol.* **2018**, *29*, 162–169. [CrossRef]
44. Karn, T.; Denkert, C.; Weber, K.E.; Holtrich, U.; Hanusch, C.; Sinn, B.V.; Higgs, B.W.; Jank, P.; Sinn, H.P.; Huober, J.; et al. Tumor mutational burden and immune infiltration as independent predictors of response to neoadjuvant immune checkpoint inhibition in early TNBC in GeparNuevo. *Ann. Oncol.* **2020**, *31*, 1216–1222. [CrossRef] [PubMed]
45. Guo, S.; Loibl, S.; von Minckwitz, G.; Darb-Esfahani, S.; Lederer, B.; Denkert, C. PIK3CA H1047R Mutation Associated with a Lower Pathological Complete Response Rate in Triple-Negative Breast Cancer Patients Treated with Anthracycline-Taxane-Based Neoadjuvant Chemotherapy. *Cancer Res. Treat.* **2020**, *52*, 689–696. [CrossRef] [PubMed]
46. Cain, H.; Macpherson, I.R.; Beresford, M.; Pinder, S.E.; Pong, J.; Dixon, J.M. Neoadjuvant Therapy in Early Breast Cancer: Treatment Considerations and Common Debates in Practice. *Clin. Oncol. (R Coll Radiol)* **2017**, *29*, 642–652. [CrossRef]
47. Gass, P.; Lux, M.P.; Rauh, C.; Hein, A.; Bani, M.R.; Fiessler, C.; Hartmann, A.; Haberle, L.; Pretscher, J.; Erber, R.; et al. Prediction of pathological complete response and prognosis in patients with neoadjuvant treatment for triple-negative breast cancer. *BMC Cancer* **2018**, *18*, 1051. [CrossRef]
48. Lee, J.S.; Yost, S.E.; Yuan, Y. Neoadjuvant Treatment for Triple Negative Breast Cancer: Recent Progresses and Challenges. *Cancers* **2020**, *12*, 1404. [CrossRef]
49. Pelizzari, G.; Gerratana, L.; Basile, D.; Fanotto, V.; Bartoletti, M.; Liguori, A.; Fontanella, C.; Spazzapan, S.; Puglisi, F. Post-neoadjuvant strategies in breast cancer: From risk assessment to treatment escalation. *Cancer Treat. Rev.* **2019**, *72*, 7–14. [CrossRef]
100. Symmans, W.F.; Peintinger, F.; Hatzis, C.; Rajan, R.; Kuerer, H.; Valero, V.; Assad, L.; Poniecka, A.; Hennessy, B.; Green, M.; et al. Measurement of residual breast cancer burden to predict survival after neoadjuvant chemotherapy. *J. Clin. Oncol.* **2007**, *25*, 4414–4422. [CrossRef]
101. Symmans, W.F.; Wei, C.; Gould, R.; Yu, X.; Zhang, Y.; Liu, M.; Walls, A.; Bousamra, A.; Ramineni, M.; Sinn, B.; et al. Long-Term Prognostic Risk After Neoadjuvant Chemotherapy Associated With Residual Cancer Burden and Breast Cancer Subtype. *J. Clin. Oncol.* **2017**, *35*, 1049–1060. [CrossRef] [PubMed]
102. Leon-Ferre, R.A.; Polley, M.Y.; Liu, H.; Gilbert, J.A.; Cafourek, V.; Hillman, D.W.; Elkhanany, A.; Akinhanmi, M.; Lilyquist, J.; Thomas, A.; et al. Impact of histopathology, tumor-infiltrating lymphocytes, and adjuvant chemotherapy on prognosis of triple-negative breast cancer. *Breast Cancer Res. Treat.* **2018**, *167*, 89–99. [CrossRef] [PubMed]

103. Marra, A.; Viale, G.; Curigliano, G. Recent advances in triple negative breast cancer: The immunotherapy era. *BMC Med.* **2019**, *17*, 90. [CrossRef]
104. Planes-Laine, G.; Rochigneux, P.; Bertucci, F.; Chretien, A.S.; Viens, P.; Sabatier, R.; Goncalves, A. PD-1/PD-L1 Targeting in Breast Cancer: The First Clinical Evidences Are Emerging. A Literature Review. *Cancers* **2019**, *11*, 1033. [CrossRef] [PubMed]
105. Schmid, P.; Adams, S.; Rugo, H.S.; Schneeweiss, A.; Barrios, C.H.; Iwata, H.; Dieras, V.; Hegg, R.; Im, S.A.; Shaw Wright, G.; et al. Atezolizumab and Nab-Paclitaxel in Advanced Triple-Negative Breast Cancer. *N. Engl. J. Med.* **2018**, *379*, 2108–2121. [CrossRef]
106. Schmid, P.; Rugo, H.S.; Adams, S.; Schneeweiss, A.; Barrios, C.H.; Iwata, H.; Dieras, V.; Henschel, V.; Molinero, L.; Chui, S.Y.; et al. Atezolizumab plus nab-paclitaxel as first-line treatment for unresectable, locally advanced or metastatic triple-negative breast cancer (IMpassion130): Updated efficacy results from a randomised, double-blind, placebo-controlled, phase 3 trial. *Lancet Oncol.* **2020**, *21*, 44–59. [CrossRef]
107. FDA, K. FDA Grants Accelerated Approval to Pembrolizumab. Available online: https://www.fda.gov/drugs/resources-information-approved-drugs/fda-grants-accelerated-approval-pembrolizumab-locally-recurrent-unresectable-or-metastatic-triple (accessed on 18 June 2021).
108. Heeke, A.L.; Tan, A.R. Checkpoint inhibitor therapy for metastatic triple-negative breast cancer. *Cancer Metastasis Rev.* **2021**. [CrossRef] [PubMed]
109. De Melo Gagliato, D.; Buzaid, A.C.; Perez-Garcia, J.; Cortes, J. Immunotherapy in Breast Cancer: Current Practice and Clinical Challenges. *BioDrugs* **2020**, *34*, 611–623. [CrossRef]
110. Nakhjavani, M.; Hardingham, J.E.; Palethorpe, H.M.; Price, T.J.; Townsend, A.R. Druggable Molecular Targets for the Treatment of Triple Negative Breast Cancer. *J. Breast Cancer* **2019**, *22*, 341–361. [CrossRef] [PubMed]
111. Bottai, G.; Raschioni, C.; Losurdo, A.; Di Tommaso, L.; Tinterri, C.; Torrisi, R.; Reis-Filho, J.S.; Roncalli, M.; Sotiriou, C.; Santoro, A.; et al. An immune stratification reveals a subset of PD-1/LAG-3 double-positive triple-negative breast cancers. *Breast Cancer Res.* **2016**, *18*, 121. [CrossRef]
112. Du, W.; Yang, M.; Turner, A.; Xu, C.; Ferris, R.L.; Huang, J.; Kane, L.P.; Lu, B. TIM-3 as a Target for Cancer Immunotherapy and Mechanisms of Action. *Int. J. Mol. Sci.* **2017**, *18*, 645. [CrossRef]
113. Gonzalez-Angulo, A.M.; Timms, K.M.; Liu, S.; Chen, H.; Litton, J.K.; Potter, J.; Lanchbury, J.S.; Stemke-Hale, K.; Hennessy, B.T.; Arun, B.K.; et al. Incidence and outcome of BRCA mutations in unselected patients with triple receptor-negative breast cancer. *Clin. Cancer Res.* **2011**, *17*, 1082–1089. [CrossRef] [PubMed]
114. Cortesi, L.; Rugo, H.S.; Jackisch, C. An Overview of PARP Inhibitors for the Treatment of Breast Cancer. *Target. Oncol.* **2021**. [CrossRef] [PubMed]
115. Pop, L.; Suciu, I.; Ionescu, O.; Bacalbasa, N.; Ionescu, P. The role of novel poly (ADP-ribose) inhibitors in the treatment of locally advanced and metastatic Her-2/neu negative breast cancer with inherited germline BRCA1/2 mutations. A review of the literature. *J. Med. Life* **2021**, *14*, 17–20. [CrossRef] [PubMed]
116. FDA, L. FDA Granted Regular Approval to Olaparib Tablets Lynparza. Available online: https://www.fda.gov/drugs/resources-information-approved-drugs/fda-approves-olaparib-germline-brca-mutated-metastatic-breast-cancer (accessed on 17 June 2021).
117. FDA, T. FDA Approves Talazoparib. Available online: https://www.fda.gov/drugs/drug-approvals-and-databases/fda-approves-talazoparib-gbrcam-her2-negative-locally-advanced-or-metastatic-breast-cancer (accessed on 17 June 2021).
118. Nagayama, A.; Vidula, N.; Ellisen, L.; Bardia, A. Novel antibody-drug conjugates for triple negative breast cancer. *Ther. Adv. Med. Oncol.* **2020**, *12*. [CrossRef] [PubMed]
119. FDA, T. FDA Granted Accelerated Approval to Trodelvy. Available online: https://www.fda.gov/news-events/press-announcements/fda-approves-new-therapy-triple-negative-breast-cancer-has-spread-not-responded-other-treatments (accessed on 17 June 2021).
120. FDA, S.G. FDA Grants Regular Approval to Sacituzumab Govitecan. Available online: https://www.fda.gov/drugs/resources-information-approved-drugs/fda-grants-regular-approval-sacituzumab-govitecan-triple-negative-breast-cancer (accessed on 17 June 2021).
121. McGuinness, J.E.; Kalinsky, K. Antibody-drug conjugates in metastatic triple negative breast cancer: A spotlight on sacituzumab govitecan, ladiratuzumab vedotin, and trastuzumab deruxtecan. *Expert Opin. Biol. Ther.* **2021**, *21*, 903–913. [CrossRef]
122. Wu, N.; Zhang, J.; Zhao, J.; Mu, K.; Zhang, J.; Jin, Z.; Yu, J.; Liu, J. Precision medicine based on tumorigenic signaling pathways for triple-negative breast cancer. *Oncol. Lett.* **2018**, *16*, 4984–4996. [CrossRef]
123. Van Reesema, L.L.S.; Zheleva, V.; Winston, J.S.; Jansen, R.J.; O'Connor, C.F.; Isbell, A.J.; Bian, M.; Qin, R.; Bassett, P.T.; Hinson, V.J.; et al. SIAH and EGFR, Two RAS Pathway Biomarkers, are Highly Prognostic in Locally Advanced and Metastatic Breast Cancer. *EBioMedicine* **2016**, *11*, 183–198. [CrossRef]
124. Bayraktar, S.; Gluck, S. Molecularly targeted therapies for metastatic triple-negative breast cancer. *Breast Cancer Res. Treat.* **2013**, *138*, 21–35. [CrossRef]
125. Hsiao, Y.C.; Yeh, M.H.; Chen, Y.J.; Liu, J.F.; Tang, C.H.; Huang, W.C. Lapatinib increases motility of triple-negative breast cancer cells by decreasing miRNA-7 and inducing Raf-1/MAPK-dependent interleukin-6. *Oncotarget* **2015**, *6*, 37965–37978. [CrossRef] [PubMed]

26. Bartholomeusz, C.; Xie, X.; Pitner, M.K.; Kondo, K.; Dadbin, A.; Lee, J.; Saso, H.; Smith, P.D.; Dalby, K.N.; Ueno, N.T. MEK Inhibitor Selumetinib (AZD6244; ARRY-142886) Prevents Lung Metastasis in a Triple-Negative Breast Cancer Xenograft Model. *Mol. Cancer Ther.* **2015**, *14*, 2773–2781. [CrossRef] [PubMed]
27. Loi, S.; Dushyanthen, S.; Beavis, P.A.; Salgado, R.; Denkert, C.; Savas, P.; Combs, S.; Rimm, D.L.; Giltnane, J.M.; Estrada, M.V.; et al. Correction: RAS/MAPK Activation Is Associated with Reduced Tumor-Infiltrating Lymphocytes in Triple-Negative Breast Cancer: Therapeutic Cooperation Between MEK and PD-1/PD-L1 Immune Checkpoint Inhibitors. *Clin. Cancer Res.* **2019**, *25*, 1437. [CrossRef] [PubMed]
28. Khan, M.A.; Jain, V.K.; Rizwanullah, M.; Ahmad, J.; Jain, K. PI3K/AKT/mTOR pathway inhibitors in triple-negative breast cancer: A review on drug discovery and future challenges. *Drug Discov. Today* **2019**, *24*, 2181–2191. [CrossRef]
29. Cossu-Rocca, P.; Orru, S.; Muroni, M.R.; Sanges, F.; Sotgiu, G.; Ena, S.; Pira, G.; Murgia, L.; Manca, A.; Uras, M.G.; et al. Analysis of PIK3CA Mutations and Activation Pathways in Triple Negative Breast Cancer. *PLoS ONE* **2015**, *10*, e0141763. [CrossRef]
30. Shrivastava, S.; Kulkarni, P.; Thummuri, D.; Jeengar, M.K.; Naidu, V.G.; Alvala, M.; Redddy, G.B.; Ramakrishna, S. Piperlongumine, an alkaloid causes inhibition of PI3 K/Akt/mTOR signaling axis to induce caspase-dependent apoptosis in human triple-negative breast cancer cells. *Apoptosis* **2014**, *19*, 1148–1164. [CrossRef]
31. Killock, D. AKT inhibition improves OS in TNBC. *Nat. Rev. Clin. Oncol.* **2020**, *17*, 135. [CrossRef]
32. Lin, J.; Sampath, D.; Nannini, M.A.; Lee, B.B.; Degtyarev, M.; Oeh, J.; Savage, H.; Guan, Z.; Hong, R.; Kassees, R.; et al. Targeting activated Akt with GDC-0068, a novel selective Akt inhibitor that is efficacious in multiple tumor models. *Clin. Cancer Res.* **2013**, *19*, 1760–1772. [CrossRef]
33. Baselga, J.; Campone, M.; Piccart, M.; Burris, H.A., 3rd; Rugo, H.S.; Sahmoud, T.; Noguchi, S.; Gnant, M.; Pritchard, K.I.; Lebrun, F.; et al. Everolimus in postmenopausal hormone-receptor-positive advanced breast cancer. *N. Engl. J. Med.* **2012**, *366*, 520–529. [CrossRef]
34. Ganesan, P.; Moulder, S.; Lee, J.J.; Janku, F.; Valero, V.; Zinner, R.G.; Naing, A.; Fu, S.; Tsimberidou, A.M.; Hong, D.; et al. Triple-negative breast cancer patients treated at MD Anderson Cancer Center in phase I trials: Improved outcomes with combination chemotherapy and targeted agents. *Mol. Cancer Ther.* **2014**, *13*, 3175–3184. [CrossRef]
35. Singh, J.; Novik, Y.; Stein, S.; Volm, M.; Meyers, M.; Smith, J.; Omene, C.; Speyer, J.; Schneider, R.; Jhaveri, K.; et al. Phase 2 trial of everolimus and carboplatin combination in patients with triple negative metastatic breast cancer. *Breast Cancer Res.* **2014**, *16*, R32. [CrossRef]
36. Beuvink, I.; Boulay, A.; Fumagalli, S.; Zilbermann, F.; Ruetz, S.; O'Reilly, T.; Natt, F.; Hall, J.; Lane, H.A.; Thomas, G. The mTOR inhibitor RAD001 sensitizes tumor cells to DNA-damaged induced apoptosis through inhibition of p21 translation. *Cell* **2005**, *120*, 747–759. [CrossRef] [PubMed]
37. Ibrahim, Y.H.; Garcia-Garcia, C.; Serra, V.; He, L.; Torres-Lockhart, K.; Prat, A.; Anton, P.; Cozar, P.; Guzman, M.; Grueso, J.; et al. PI3K inhibition impairs BRCA1/2 expression and sensitizes BRCA-proficient triple-negative breast cancer to PARP inhibition. *Cancer Discov.* **2012**, *2*, 1036–1047. [CrossRef]
38. Bhola, N.E.; Jansen, V.M.; Koch, J.P.; Li, H.; Formisano, L.; Williams, J.A.; Grandis, J.R.; Arteaga, C.L. Treatment of Triple-Negative Breast Cancer with TORC1/2 Inhibitors Sustains a Drug-Resistant and Notch-Dependent Cancer Stem Cell Population. *Cancer Res.* **2016**, *76*, 440–452. [CrossRef] [PubMed]
39. Giuli, M.V.; Giuliani, E.; Screpanti, I.; Bellavia, D.; Checquolo, S. Notch Signaling Activation as a Hallmark for Triple-Negative Breast Cancer Subtype. *J. Oncol.* **2019**, *2019*, 8707053. [CrossRef] [PubMed]
40. Qiu, M.; Peng, Q.; Jiang, I.; Carroll, C.; Han, G.; Rymer, I.; Lippincott, J.; Zachwieja, J.; Gajiwala, K.; Kraynov, E.; et al. Specific inhibition of Notch1 signaling enhances the antitumor efficacy of chemotherapy in triple negative breast cancer through reduction of cancer stem cells. *Cancer Lett.* **2013**, *328*, 261–270. [CrossRef]
41. Zhu, H.; Bhaijee, F.; Ishaq, N.; Pepper, D.J.; Backus, K.; Brown, A.S.; Zhou, X.; Miele, L. Correlation of Notch1, pAKT and nuclear NF-kappaB expression in triple negative breast cancer. *Am. J. Cancer Res.* **2013**, *3*, 230–239. [PubMed]
42. Majumder, S.; Crabtree, J.S.; Golde, T.E.; Minter, L.M.; Osborne, B.A.; Miele, L. Targeting Notch in oncology: The path forward. *Nat. Rev. Drug Discov.* **2021**, *20*, 125–144. [CrossRef] [PubMed]
43. Lehal, R.; Zaric, J.; Vigolo, M.; Urech, C.; Frismantas, V.; Zangger, N.; Cao, L.; Berger, A.; Chicote, I.; Loubery, S.; et al. Pharmacological disruption of the Notch transcription factor complex. *Proc. Natl. Acad. Sci. USA* **2020**, *117*, 16292–16301. [CrossRef] [PubMed]
44. Deng, J.; Wang, E.S.; Jenkins, R.W.; Li, S.; Dries, R.; Yates, K.; Chhabra, S.; Huang, W.; Liu, H.; Aref, A.R.; et al. CDK4/6 Inhibition Augments Antitumor Immunity by Enhancing T-cell Activation. *Cancer Discov.* **2018**, *8*, 216–233. [CrossRef]
45. Goel, S.; DeCristo, M.J.; Watt, A.C.; BrinJones, H.; Sceneay, J.; Li, B.B.; Khan, N.; Ubellacker, J.M.; Xie, S.; Metzger-Filho, O.; et al. CDK4/6 inhibition triggers anti-tumour immunity. *Nature* **2017**, *548*, 471–475. [CrossRef]
46. Bhattarai, S.; Klimov, S.; Mittal, K.; Krishnamurti, U.; Li, X.B.; Oprea-Ilies, G.; Wetherilt, C.S.; Riaz, A.; Aleskandarany, M.A.; Green, A.R.; et al. Prognostic Role of Androgen Receptor in Triple Negative Breast Cancer: A Multi-Institutional Study. *Cancers* **2019**, *11*, 995. [CrossRef] [PubMed]
47. Chan, J.J.; Tan, T.J.Y.; Dent, R.A. Novel therapeutic avenues in triple-negative breast cancer: PI3K/AKT inhibition, androgen receptor blockade, and beyond. *Ther. Adv. Med. Oncol.* **2019**, *11*. [CrossRef] [PubMed]

148. Ricciardi, G.R.; Adamo, B.; Ieni, A.; Licata, L.; Cardia, R.; Ferraro, G.; Franchina, T.; Tuccari, G.; Adamo, V. Androgen Receptor (AR), E-Cadherin, and Ki-67 as Emerging Targets and Novel Prognostic Markers in Triple-Negative Breast Cancer (TNBC) Patients. *PLoS ONE* **2015**, *10*, e0128368. [CrossRef]
149. Bonnefoi, H.; Grellety, T.; Tredan, O.; Saghatchian, M.; Dalenc, F.; Mailliez, A.; L'Haridon, T.; Cottu, P.; Abadie-Lacourtoisie, S.; You, B.; et al. A phase II trial of abiraterone acetate plus prednisone in patients with triple-negative androgen receptor positive locally advanced or metastatic breast cancer (UCBG 12-1). *Ann. Oncol.* **2016**, *27*, 812–818. [CrossRef]
150. Gucalp, A.; Tolaney, S.; Isakoff, S.J.; Ingle, J.N.; Liu, M.C.; Carey, L.A.; Blackwell, K.; Rugo, H.; Nabell, L.; Forero, A.; et al. Phase II trial of bicalutamide in patients with androgen receptor-positive, estrogen receptor-negative metastatic Breast Cancer. *Clin. Cancer Res.* **2013**, *19*, 5505–5512. [CrossRef] [PubMed]
151. Madu, C.O.; Wang, S.; Madu, C.O.; Lu, Y. Angiogenesis in Breast Cancer Progression, Diagnosis, and Treatment. *J. Cancer* **2020**, *11*, 4474–4494. [CrossRef] [PubMed]
152. Ribatti, D.; Nico, B.; Ruggieri, S.; Tamma, R.; Simone, G.; Mangia, A. Angiogenesis and Antiangiogenesis in Triple-Negative Breast cancer. *Transl. Oncol.* **2016**, *9*, 453–457. [CrossRef]
153. Hutchinson, L. Breast cancer: BEATRICE bevacizumab trial—Every cloud has a silver lining. *Nat. Rev. Clin. Oncol.* **2013**, *10*, 548. [CrossRef]
154. Barroso-Sousa, R.; Tolaney, S.M. Clinical Development of New Antibody-Drug Conjugates in Breast Cancer: To Infinity and Beyond. *BioDrugs* **2021**, *35*, 159–174. [CrossRef]
155. Islam, R.; Lam, K.W. Recent progress in small molecule agents for the targeted therapy of triple-negative breast cancer. *Eur. J. Med. Chem.* **2020**, *207*, 112812. [CrossRef]
156. Emens, L.A. Breast Cancer Immunotherapy: Facts and Hopes. *Clin. Cancer Res.* **2018**, *24*, 511–520. [CrossRef] [PubMed]
157. Vikas, P.; Borcherding, N.; Zhang, W. The clinical promise of immunotherapy in triple-negative breast cancer. *Cancer Manag. Res.* **2018**, *10*, 6823–6833. [CrossRef]
158. Zhao, H.; Yang, Q.; Hu, Y.; Zhang, J. Antitumor effects and mechanisms of olaparib in combination with carboplatin and BKM120 on human triplenegative breast cancer cells. *Oncol. Rep.* **2018**, *40*, 3223–3234. [CrossRef] [PubMed]
159. Cardillo, T.M.; Sharkey, R.M.; Rossi, D.L.; Arrojo, R.; Mostafa, A.A.; Goldenberg, D.M. Synthetic Lethality Exploitation by an Anti-Trop-2-SN-38 Antibody-Drug Conjugate, IMMU-132, Plus PARP Inhibitors in BRCA1/2-wild-type Triple-Negative Breast Cancer. *Clin. Cancer Res.* **2017**, *23*, 3405–3415. [CrossRef] [PubMed]
160. Bergin, A.R.T.; Loi, S. Triple-negative breast cancer: Recent treatment advances. *F1000Res* **2019**, *8*. [CrossRef]
161. Higuchi, T.; Flies, D.B.; Marjon, N.A.; Mantia-Smaldone, G.; Ronner, L.; Gimotty, P.A.; Adams, S.F. CTLA-4 Blockade Synergizes Therapeutically with PARP Inhibition in BRCA1-Deficient Ovarian Cancer. *Cancer Immunol. Res.* **2015**, *3*, 1257–1268. [CrossRef] [PubMed]
162. Wu, L.; Meng, F.; Dong, L.; Block, C.J.; Mitchell, A.V.; Wu, J.; Jang, H.; Chen, W.; Polin, L.; Yang, Q.; et al. Disulfiram and BKM120 in Combination with Chemotherapy Impede Tumor Progression and Delay Tumor Recurrence in Tumor Initiating Cell-Rich TNBC. *Sci. Rep.* **2019**, *9*, 236. [CrossRef]
163. Hossain, F.; Sorrentino, C.; Ucar, D.A.; Peng, Y.; Matossian, M.; Wyczechowska, D.; Crabtree, J.; Zabaleta, J.; Morello, S.; Del Valle, L.; et al. Notch Signaling Regulates Mitochondrial Metabolism and NF-kappaB Activity in Triple-Negative Breast Cancer Cells via IKKalpha-Dependent Non-canonical Pathways. *Front. Oncol.* **2018**, *8*, 575. [CrossRef]
164. Diluvio, G.; Del Gaudio, F.; Giuli, M.V.; Franciosa, G.; Giuliani, E.; Palermo, R.; Besharat, Z.M.; Pignataro, M.G.; Vacca, A.; d'Amati, G.; et al. NOTCH3 inactivation increases triple negative breast cancer sensitivity to gefitinib by promoting EGFR tyrosine dephosphorylation and its intracellular arrest. *Oncogenesis* **2018**, *7*, 42. [CrossRef]
165. Kim, K.; Skora, A.D.; Li, Z.; Liu, Q.; Tam, A.J.; Blosser, R.L.; Diaz, L.A., Jr.; Papadopoulos, N.; Kinzler, K.W.; Vogelstein, B.; et al. Eradication of metastatic mouse cancers resistant to immune checkpoint blockade by suppression of myeloid-derived cells. *Proc. Natl. Acad. Sci. USA* **2014**, *111*, 11774–11779. [CrossRef] [PubMed]
166. Pauli, C.; Hopkins, B.D.; Prandi, D.; Shaw, R.; Fedrizzi, T.; Sboner, A.; Sailer, V.; Augello, M.; Puca, L.; Rosati, R.; et al. Personalized In Vitro and In Vivo Cancer Models to Guide Precision Medicine. *Cancer Discov.* **2017**, *7*, 462–477. [CrossRef]
167. Tsimberidou, A.M.; Wen, S.; Hong, D.S.; Wheler, J.J.; Falchook, G.S.; Fu, S.; Piha-Paul, S.; Naing, A.; Janku, F.; Aldape, K.; et al. Personalized medicine for patients with advanced cancer in the phase I program at MD Anderson: Validation and landmark analyses. *Clin. Cancer Res.* **2014**, *20*, 4827–4836. [CrossRef] [PubMed]
168. Aref, A.R.; Campisi, M.; Ivanova, E.; Portell, A.; Larios, D.; Piel, B.P.; Mathur, N.; Zhou, C.; Coakley, R.V.; Bartels, A.; et al. 3D microfluidic ex vivo culture of organotypic tumor spheroids to model immune checkpoint blockade. *Lab Chip* **2018**, *18*, 3129–3143. [CrossRef] [PubMed]
169. Low, S.K.; Zembutsu, H.; Nakamura, Y. Breast cancer: The translation of big genomic data to cancer precision medicine. *Cancer Sci.* **2018**, *109*, 497–506. [CrossRef]
170. Sehgal, K.; Portell, A.; Ivanova, E.V.; Lizotte, P.H.; Mahadevan, N.R.; Greene, J.R.; Vajdi, A.; Gurjao, C.; Teceno, T.; Taus, L.J.; et al. Dynamic single-cell RNA sequencing identifies immunotherapy persister cells following PD-1 blockade. *J. Clin. Investig.* **2021**, *131*. [CrossRef] [PubMed]

71. Mertins, P.; Mani, D.R.; Ruggles, K.V.; Gillette, M.A.; Clauser, K.R.; Wang, P.; Wang, X.; Qiao, J.W.; Cao, S.; Petralia, F.; et al. Proteogenomics connects somatic mutations to signalling in breast cancer. *Nature* **2016**, *534*, 55–62. [CrossRef]
72. Wu, Q.; Ba-Alawi, W.; Deblois, G.; Cruickshank, J.; Duan, S.; Lima-Fernandes, E.; Haight, J.; Tonekaboni, S.A.M.; Fortier, A.M.; Kuasne, H.; et al. GLUT1 inhibition blocks growth of RB1-positive triple negative breast cancer. *Nat. Commun.* **2020**, *11*, 4205. [CrossRef] [PubMed]

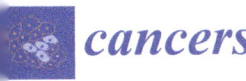

Article

Regulations, Open Data and Healthcare Innovation: A Case of MSK-IMPACT and Its Implications for Better Cancer Care

Takaharu Jibiki [1], Hayato Nishimura [1,2], Shintaro Sengoku [1,3,*] and Kota Kodama [4]

1. Department of Innovation Science, School of Environment and Society, Tokyo Institute of Technology, Tokyo 108-0023, Japan; jibiki.t.aa@m.titech.ac.jp (T.J.); nishih@riken.jp (H.N.)
2. Policy Planning Division, RIKEN, Saitama 351-0198, Japan
3. Life Style by Design Research Unit, Institute for Future Initiatives, University of Tokyo, Tokyo 113-0033, Japan
4. Graduate School of Technology Management, Ritsumeikan University, Osaka 567-8570, Japan; kkodama@fc.ritsumei.ac.jp
* Correspondence: sengoku.s.aa@m.titech.ac.jp; Tel.: +81-3-3454-8907

Simple Summary: The advancement in both science and technology has contributed to the development of novel diagnostic technologies; such technologies enable medical practitioners to diagnose diseases that could not be previously detected. However, in order to translate new technologies into practical applications, various types of challenges need to be overcome. To address these challenges, including those in clinical management and regulatory science, healthcare policies have been constantly implemented to promote the practical application of outcomes generated by healthcare innovation. This study conducted comparative analyses of three tumor profiling tests approved by the U.S. Food and Drug Administration (FDA) in 2017, hypothesizing that the FDA's regulatory reforms, early application of new technologies to both research and clinical settings, and open data accumulated as a result of large-scale research programs have promoted new drug development in oncology. The study then discussed the implications potentially suggested by the outcomes and challenges of the three tests.

Abstract: This study investigated a case of Memorial Sloan Kettering-Integrated Mutation Profiling of Actionable Cancer Targets (MSK-IMPACT), a tumor profiling test approved by the U.S. Food and Drug Administration (FDA) in 2017, to examine what factors would contribute to healthcare innovation. First, we set the following three parameters to observe cases: (i) the FDA regulatory reforms, (ii) early application of new technologies, such as next-generation sequencing (NGS), to both research and clinical settings, and (iii) accumulation of open data. Then, we performed a comparative analysis of MSK-IMPACT with FoundationOne CDx and Oncomine Dx Target Test, both of which were FDA-approved tumor profiling tests launched in 2017. As a result, we found that MSK-IMPACT secures neutrality as a non-profit organization, achieves the active incorporation of basic research results, and performs superiorly in clinical operations, such as patient enrollment. On the contrary, we confirmed that FoundationOne CDx was the most prominent case in terms of the number of new drugs and expanded indications approved in which the FDA's expedited approval programs were considerably utilized. Consequently, to uncover the full potential of MSK-IMPACT, it is suggested that more intersectoral collaborative activities between various healthcare stakeholders, in particular, pharmaceutical companies, for driving clinical development must be carried out based on an organizational framework that facilitates collaboration.

Keywords: new drug development; next-generation sequencing (NGS); open data; regulatory reform; tumor profiling test

Citation: Jibiki, T.; Nishimura, H.; Sengoku, S.; Kodama, K. Regulations, Open Data and Healthcare Innovation: A Case of MSK-IMPACT and Its Implications for Better Cancer Care. *Cancers* 2021, *13*, 3448. https://doi.org/10.3390/cancers13143448

Academic Editors: Nandini Dey and Pradip De

Received: 27 April 2021
Accepted: 7 July 2021
Published: 9 July 2021

Publisher's Note: MDPI stays neutral with regard to jurisdictional claims in published maps and institutional affiliations.

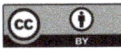

Copyright: © 2021 by the authors. Licensee MDPI, Basel, Switzerland. This article is an open access article distributed under the terms and conditions of the Creative Commons Attribution (CC BY) license (https://creativecommons.org/licenses/by/4.0/).

1. Introduction

1.1. Next-Generation Sequencing (NGS) for Advanced Medicine

As genome science advances, personalized medicine, which would enable tailor-made medical solutions based on personal biological information, is expected to become a reality. The 2015 State of the Union Address announced that the United States would make nationwide efforts to realize the Precision Medicine Initiative, which sought to establish healthcare, considering differences among individuals that could be caused by genes, environment, lifestyle, and so forth [1]. The initiative covered a variety of issues, such as the development and delivery of cancer care, establishment of a nationwide research cohort leveraging over 1 million volunteers, development of new validation methods for Next Generation Sequencing (NGS) instruments and data sharing platforms, and regulatory reforms [1].

NGS is known to have dramatically reduced sequencing costs [2] and has contributed to the practice of large collaborative research projects worldwide. Since this technology has enabled researchers to efficiently analyze the genetic information of target samples at a reasonable cost, the application of NGS now ranges from analysis of genetic mutations of cancer patients to that of information on microbial samples, such as the human microbiome. NGS can surely extend the frontier of healthcare by practically helping researchers realize the application of personalized medicine in a clinical setting.

Although new technologies, such as NGS, allow scientists to explore new research areas, they do not necessarily ensure safety due to the lack of data and precedents. Therefore, the development and further application of new therapeutic options to a clinical setting based on bioinformatics requires, to a certain extent, regulatory efforts by relevant authorities that can simultaneously ensure both the safety and efficacy. In addition, it is recommended that biological data necessary for the development of new therapeutic options be open to the public. It is reasonable to assume that the researchers can be encouraged to access a database of biological information if they can use it at any given time. It is also recommended that such data be regularly updated, with a certain degree of standardization and compatibility between different datasets. In general, no researcher wants to use either obsolete or unstandardized data without their compatibility with other datasets, as these are factors that can affect the quality of the scientific research.

1.2. Regulatory Reforms for the Pharmaceutical Industry

Healthcare innovation can be induced by implementing efficient regulations [3]. This can apply not only to pharmaceuticals, but also to new technological fields, such as mobile health (mHealth). Onodera et al. 2018 revealed that the regulatory reforms implemented by the FDA indirectly contributed to the increase in the number of FDA-cleared mobile medical apps during the mid-2010s [4]. This implies that regulations can even stimulate innovation in such an emerging field with uncertainly if they are appropriately implemented to support innovators. The question here is to what extent pharmaceutical regulations in the United States have facilitated innovation in terms of conventional pharmaceutical development and commercialization.

The U.S. Food and Drug Administration (FDA) has started making regulatory reforms in drug approvals with a certain degree of organizational efforts since the early 1980s. Such reforms are supposed to have partly contributed to promoting innovation. For example, the distribution of orphan drugs among all FDA-approved drugs increased from 17 percent (1984–1988) to 31 percent (2004–2008) after the Orphan Drug Act of 1983, which was enacted at the earliest stage of the regulatory reforms by the FDA [5]. Moreover, the proportion of approved drugs that qualified for the FDA's expedited approval programs (i.e., Orphan Drug Act (1983) [6], Fast Track Designation (1988) [7], Accelerated Approval Program (1992) [8], and Breakthrough Therapy Designation (2012) [9]) has increased from 1984 to 2018 [10]. For example, 22 out of the 39 FDA-approved drugs in 2012 were reported to have utilized such programs [11].

On the other hand, Golodner et al. 1998 raised a concern that expedited approval programs, which were intended to shortcut a drug review process toward approval, would deliver "dangerous or unnecessary drugs" to the users [12]. Since data obtained through the use of such programs rely on early-stage clinical trials, the quantity of clinical evidence tends to be limited and unstable [11]. The trade-off between the speed of the approval process and the efficacy of a drug candidate has remained a critical issue for the FDA to overcome.

Meanwhile, the FDA has succeeded in shortening the drug review time from more than 3 years in 1983 to less than 1 year in 2017 [10]; the major strategies were (1) to collect user fees from pharmaceutical companies to raise funds needed to review the increasing number of new drug applications under the Prescription Drug User Fee Act (PDUFA) of 1992 [10,13], and (2) to encourage the use of surrogate measures for clinical trials [10,14]. Nonetheless, the total time needed for clinical trials, which ranges from the application for Investigational New Drug (IND) to the FDA approval, has not been reduced from 1986 to 2017 [10]; it averaged at approximately 8 years during this period [10]. As expedited programs were utilized for the development of drugs for rare diseases, recruitment challenges for clinical trials and therapeutic challenges, both of which were found to be the typical difficulties specific to the drug development for such diseases, have arisen; these may have prolonged the overall clinical development time [10].

In addition, a series of regulatory reforms have not necessarily led to a dramatic increase in the number of new drugs approved between 1982 and 2018 [10]. The mean number of new drug approvals per annum, including those for biologics, between 1990 and 1999, was 34 [10]. However, the number remained at 41 between 2010 and 2018 [10]. To summarize, the FDA has taken certain actions to implement the regulatory reforms for the past three decades while undergoing some occasional setbacks.

1.3. Open Data and Healthcare Innovation

Previous research on the association between healthcare innovation and open data has been scarce. Goodsell et al. 2019 clarified in their study that the Protein Data Bank (PDB) archive, which was the "first open-access digital data resource" that provided researchers with data on three-dimensional (3D) protein structures, has contributed to new drug development since its establishment in 1971 [15]. The PDB database, which allowed open access to approximately 6000 protein structures, contributed to the FDA's new drug approval of "88% of 210 new molecular entities" from 2010 to 2016 [15]. The PDB archive has grown dramatically over time through the accumulation of data on protein structures and other relevant topics. PDB users and data depositors, including a global expert community in structural biology, deposit data regarding protein structures into the archive [15]. Moreover, PDB data are updated on a weekly basis by integrating them with multiple external databases [15].

NGS technologies, in turn, generate biological data on target samples that a researcher intends to analyze. However, the contribution of such technologies to innovation is yet to be adequately discussed. Kahn et al. 2014 reported that the discussions were held on how NGS should be utilized for scientific research at the NGS for Cancer Drug Development conference held in Boston, USA, in September 2013 [16]. Participants from both the industry and academia discussed how they utilized data generated by NGS, such as the utilization of biomarker data for cancer drug development [16]. The use of "publicly available NGS data for target discovery," along with the importance of "data integration" and "quality control," were also discussed at this conference [16]. However, whether such data have contributed to facilitating innovation is yet to be thoroughly discussed.

1.4. Purpose of the Study

This study aimed to identify the institutional and organizational factors that can facilitate (or hinder) the development and dissemination of novel bioinformatics-based therapies. Considering the uniqueness of the product and its early practical utilization as a catalyst for an entry into cancer care services with NGS technologies, this study specifically focused on the case of Memorial Sloan Kettering-Integrated Mutation Profiling of Actionable Cancer Targets (MSK-IMPACT) to discuss how clinical sequencing and genomic cancer medicine could be promoted.

MSK-IMPACT, one of the first three FDA-approved tumor profiling tests launched in the market [17], is unique in that it was developed by the Memorial Sloan Kettering Cancer Center (MSKCC), a private cancer center located in Manhattan, New York City, USA; this was unlike FoundationOne CDx (Foundation Medicine, Inc., Cambridge, MA, USA) and Oncomine Dx Target Test (Life Technologies Corporation, Carlsbad, CA, USA), both of which were developed by companies and approved in the same year. MSK-IMPACT was a product developed by a hospital and had indeed been applied to a clinical setting before it was approved by the FDA as an in vitro diagnostic (IVD) test.

This study was centered around the following two questions: (i) How have the FDA's regulatory reforms facilitated the development of new drug candidates identified by MSK-IMPACT? and (ii) how has MSK-IMPACT helped identify new drug candidates in oncology, leveraging open data accumulated through global research projects. To better answer these questions, this study particularly investigated the following regulatory and technological aspects: (i) FDA's regulatory reforms and their outcomes, (ii) the contribution of publicly accessible open databases, specifically those based on the genetic mutations provided by cancer patients and established through large-scale research projects, and (iii) early application of new technologies (i.e., MSK-IMPACT) to both research and clinical settings. To ensure both fairness and objectiveness and to better clarify the outcomes of each panel test, we carried out a comparison between MSK-IMPACT and the other two panel tests, all of which were the first marketed products [17].

Based on the analysis of such comparisons, we then attempted to understand the characteristics and challenges associated with MSK-IMPACT by comparing them with those associated with FoundationOne CDx. Furthermore, we have also discussed how clinical sequencing in oncology should be further promoted to deliver and maximize the benefits of the technology in an efficient manner.

2. Materials and Methods

2.1. The Case

Following a review of the existing literature, this study sought to consider whether the FDA's regulatory reforms have led to an early application of new technologies in both research and clinical settings, with a specific focus on the case of MSK-IMPACT. It also aimed to examine whether bioinformatics-driven innovation had been promoted in clinical sequencing in oncology as a result of the accumulation and utilization of publicly accessible open data on genetic information. Overall, research was conducted by referring to the public information released by the relevant organizations and employing a semi-structured interview with a key individual in the clinical oncology sequencing community. To offer a better understanding of the results of the research, Table 1 summarizes various types of relevant stakeholders and catalysts for cancer care innovation identified by the investigation of this study.

Table 1. Major stakeholders and catalysts.

Category	Stakeholders/Catalysts	Major Roles in Cancer Care Innovation
Regulatory authority	U.S. Food and Drug Administration (FDA)	Take responsibilities to set out and periodically reform pharmaceutical and medical devices regulations
Assay developer	Foundation Medicine, Inc., Life Technologies Corporation, Memorial Sloan Kettering Cancer Center (MSKCC)	Develop and commercialize tumor profiling tests
Developer of public data sharing platform	National Center for Biotechnology Information (NCBI), National Human Genome Research Institute	Establish and provide access to publicly accessible open data through international research programs/projects
International research program/project	Cancer Genome Atlas, Genome Reference Consortium, International HapMap Project, Personal Genome Project, 1000 Genome Project	Help researchers obtain genetic information from cancer patients
Drug manufacturer	Pharmaceutical companies (i.e., Roche Holding AG, Basel, Switzerland)	Develop new drugs and/or add new indications to the existing drugs on the basis of the use of tumor profiling tests
Healthcare institution	Hospitals providing healthcare services (i.e., MSKCC)	Provide cancer patients with opportunities for cancer care and clinical trials
Direct beneficiary of healthcare innovation	Cancer patients	Provide genetic data and use newly developed cancer therapies through clinical trials

2.2. Document-Based Analysis

Considering the nature of the study, we mostly referred to qualitative information released by the FDA and MSKCC as well as to other relevant articles as the major sources of information.

For the first step of a literature search, this study employed the Patient, Intervention, Comparison, Outcome (PICO) framework for a preliminary search to gain a better understanding about the case, and to develop literature search strategies. Some of the typical search terms used were as follows: "cancer patients," "MSK-IMPACT," "FoundationOne CDx," "Oncomine Dx Target Test," and "new drug development." Second, we hypothesized that (i) regulations, (ii) publicly accessible open data, and (iii) early application of new technologies induced by the regulations as key drivers of bioinformatics-driven innovation. After that, we performed database searches to obtain relevant articles that cover issues of the above 3 hypotheses; we performed each database search on Web of Science (https://www.webofscience.com/wos/woscc/basic-search, accessed on 7 March 2020) by using up to any of the 3 search terms at a time from the following: "bioinformatics," "innovation," "facilitate," "facilitation," "new drug development," "NGS," and "regulation." As a result, we found 148 articles in total. Of these, we selected and examined 13 articles that were considered most relevant to the topics and hypotheses for this study. Furthermore, we conducted an issue-specific literature search on Scopus (https://www.scopus.com/search/form.uri?display=basic#basic, accessed on 21 June 2020) and Google Scholar (https://scholar.google.com/, accessed on 21 June 2020), focusing on a single issue relating to any of the above 3 hypotheses (i.e., a combination of issue-specific search terms "FDA Modernization Act" and "drug development").

We also conducted a database search using PubMed (https://pubmed.ncbi.nlm.nih.gov/, accessed on 3 January 2019) and ClinicalTrials.gov (https://clinicaltrials.gov/, accessed on 3 January 2019) to gain quantitative implications and sought to confirm the number of scientific publications relating to data on genetic information and the number of clinical trials relating to cancer genomic medicine from the early 2000s to the late 2010s. In order to confirm the former, we used the search terms "GWAS" (genome-wide association study) and "SNP" (single nucleotide polymorphism) to separately investigate the numbers of publications regarding these technological issues on PubMed. Regarding the latter, we applied a combination of the search terms "cancer/NGS or WES (whole exome sequencing) or WGS (whole genome sequencing)" to confirm the number of clinical trials relating to cancer genomic medicine on ClinicalTrials.gov.

2.3. Comparative Analysis

Based on the information collected from the above research and analyses, this study sought to confirm whether MSK-IMPACT had made a certain contribution to promoting innovation in clinical sequencing in oncology. To ensure the fairness of the research, a comparative analysis between MSK-IMPACT, FoundationOne CDx, and Oncomine Dx Target Test was performed to gain objective insights.

First, this study investigated the characteristics of MSK-IMPACT and other tests to better understand if they have particular foundations to promote scientific research for innovation, which would help pharmaceutical companies conduct clinical trials and develop new cancer therapies.

Second, it also investigated whether these tests helped in the facilitation of healthcare innovation, particularly analyzing whether new drugs were successfully developed based on the use of such tests. For better clarification, this study defined the outcomes of the tests as "drugs identified using three panel tests as a result of either patient screening or confirmatory testing of gene expressions upon the onset of clinical trials." Overall, it appeared to be difficult to fully cover such outcomes in this study. As of 30 November 2020, ClinicalTrials.gov suggested only 2 observational studies through a keyword search using a single search term "MSK-IMPACT" [18]. Since observational studies were not considered as clinical trials, the search result did not indicate that the test had led to the development of new drugs for cancer treatment. Following this result, and due in part to the difficulties in accessing certain information on the outcomes of the tests, this study took different approaches to investigate the outcomes of MSK-IMPACT and those of the other tests, as illustrated in Figure 1. It then examined whether the new drugs among these outcomes identified by this investigation method utilized any of the FDA's expedited approval programs using a drug development database Cortellis.com (https://www.cortellis.com/intelligence/home.do, accessed on 24 April 2021). This was intended to confirm the impact of the FDA's regulatory reforms on the outcomes of each test.

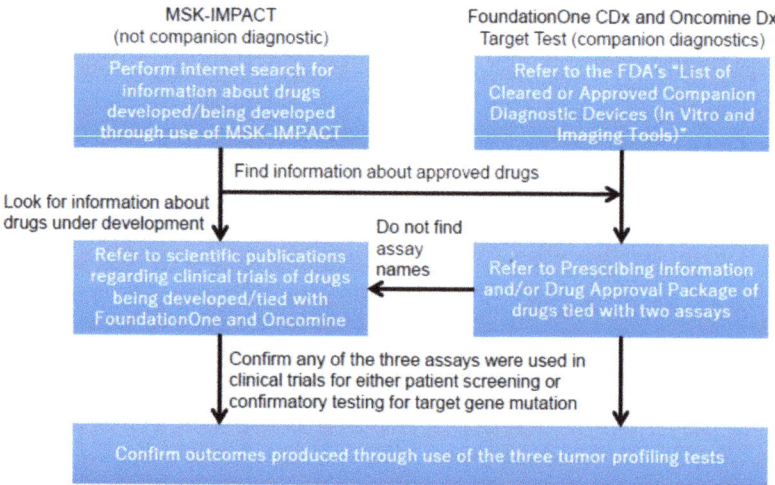

Figure 1. Investigation methods to define contribution to new drug development by the three tumor profiling tests.

2.4. Interview-Based Analysis

A semi-structured interview was conducted with an anonymous expert, the president of a company that provided its customers with clinical sequencing services, such as analytical services using NGS and tumor profiling tests, including MSK-IMPACT. The interview was focused on 3 key topics: (1) FDA's regulatory reforms that have promoted the utilization and early application of new technologies in a clinical setting, (2) accumulation of publicly accessible open data on genetic information and its contribution to the development of new therapies in oncology, and (3) benefits and challenges of MSK-IMPACT in comparison with those associated with other tumor profiling tests from an innovation point of view. The interview was conducted for 1 h on 8 May 2020.

3. Results

3.1. FDA's Regulatory Reforms and Their Outcomes

Figure 2 illustrates the historical overview of the regulatory reforms implemented by the FDA over the last three decades. As explained earlier, the series of regulatory reforms implemented by the FDA began after the enactment of the Orphan Drug Act of 1983, followed by that of expedited programs as well as other relevant acts to promote comprehensive healthcare innovation. The FDA Modernization Act (FDAMA), which was enacted in 1997 to reduce the review time for new drug candidates by extending the PDUFA of 1992, also sought to cover the medical devices. Meanwhile, the FDA intended to balance the risks between the early approval of new drugs and lack of scientific data. Under the FDA Amendments Act of 2007, the Risk Evaluation and Mitigation Strategy (2007) and Sentinel Initiative (2008) were implemented [10]. These programs were implemented to promote the safe use of medications [10,19] and mitigate risks by monitoring data regarding the adverse effects of drugs in certain patient populations [20]. Equally important was that the 21st Century Cures Act [21] of 2016 had sought to promote the utilization of medical data for new drug development, which triggered the facilitation of data utilization and accumulation of data on genetic mutations obtained through clinical sequencing in oncology.

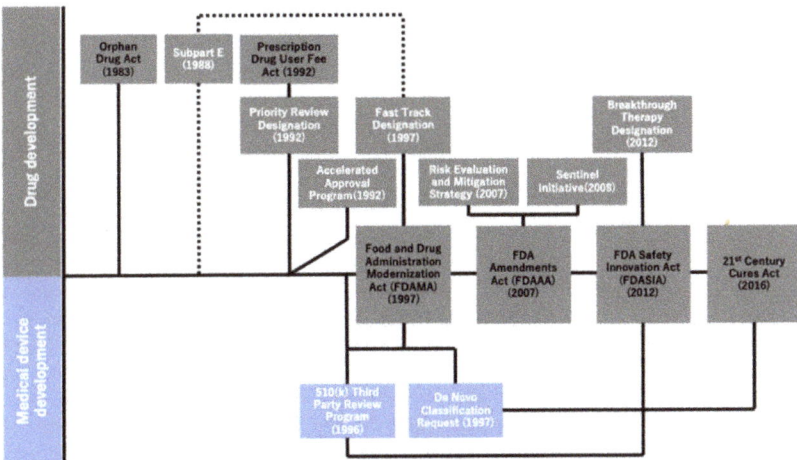

Figure 2. Historical overview of regulatory reforms by the U.S. Food and Drug Administration (FDA). This figure illustrates the association between the four major acts and relevant regulatory programs, actions, etc. in chronological order. The four major acts are lined up on the center line and are tied up with essential regulatory programs and actions implemented under any of such acts (i.e., the FDASIA and the Breakthrough Therapy Designation). The association between the subpart E regulations and the Fast Track Designation is expressed using the dotted lines because the former is the predecessor of the latter.

Not only did the FDA work on reforming the pharmaceutical regulations, but it also performed practical actions to modernize the regulations for medical devices. This study was only focused on the regulations that can be considered to have facilitated the approval process of MSK-IMPACT. By employing the combination of the De Novo pathway and 510(k) 3 PR Program, both of which were implemented under the FDAMA, the FDA approved MSK-IMPACT, taking lesser time than originally envisioned. The FDA saved time by approving the test as an IVD in 51 days, which was shorter than the 150 days duration [22] originally set by the organization as the performance goal for the review of De Novo applications (through an email query to the FDA on 24 November 2020, we have additionally confirmed that "150 days" was the performance goal for the FDA De Novo reviews). It was also remarkable to note that these regulations allowed the test, which was originally considered as a Laboratory Developed Test (LDT), to be approved as an IVD. Prior to the implementation of these programs, there was no formal IVD approval process for LDTs; these were merely not-for-sale products developed in laboratories certified by the Clinical Laboratory Improvement Amendments and were not allowed to be distributed for commercial purposes.

Furthermore, to realize precision medicine, the FDA held public workshops twice in 2015 to take practical measures to establish regulations for clinical testing based on the utilization of NGS, gathering various stakeholders, including the College of American Pathologists, National Institutes of Health (NIH), National Institute of Standards and Technology, and Centers for Disease Control (CDC), as well as those from academia and manufacturers of diagnostic tools and instruments [23,24]. Based on a series of discussions, the FDA released the guidance draft to establish a regulatory pathway for cancer genomic medicine in 2016 [25]. Further, referring to the public comments, the FDA released certain guidelines in 2018, which summarized issues of how the FDA would interpret the clinical validity and significance of a product upon consideration of its regulatory approval [26].

3.2. The Contribution of Open Databases

Datasets of genetic information have been accumulated over time and were disclosed to the public in parallel due to the large-scale collaborative research programs triggered by the political will, combined with the advancement in DNA sequencing and analytical technologies. In 1999, the National Center for Biotechnology Information (NCBI) collaborated with the National Human Genome Research Institute to establish dbSNP, a data-sharing platform that provides genetic data on single nucleotide polymorphisms (SNPs) [27]. The International HapMap Project, which began in 2003, allowed researchers to analyze the reference dataset using the Genome-Wide Association Study (GWAS), a method that enabled the analysis of the association between diseases and relevant SNPs along with quantitative traits. The utilization of the reference dataset, encouraged by the establishment of the analytical tool, has contributed to the radical increase in the number of scientific publications [28]. In fact, according to the search results yielded using the search term "genome wide association study" on PubMed, the number of scientific publications relating to GWAS increased from 1 to 1808 between 2002 and 2018 [29]. Similarly, as a result of a keyword search using the search term "SNP" on PubMed, the number of SNP-related publications was also shown an increase from 721 in 2002 to 3826 in 2018 [29]. Such an accumulation in scientific knowledge of the association between diseases and SNPs eventually fueled the practical application of relevant technologies to a clinical setting; typical examples included tumor profiling tests and direct-to-consumer genetic testing services [28].

The barrage of scientific outcomes was reinforced by the practical application of NGS technologies after the launch of the world's first NGS instrument in 2005. Some international collaborative research programs started using NGS, and the data obtained from these research programs were publicly released; the Genome Reference Consortium, the Personal Genome Project, and the 1000 Genome Project are some of the examples of such programs [30,31]. Data on genetic information obtained and accumulated from, both, basic research and clinical applications were further utilized. The NCBI has developed a data sharing platform by integrating different datasets with each other; it has become a foundation for further scientific research on and clinical applications of genetic testing [32]. Researchers are obliged to register data obtained from research programs supported by the NIH. Nevertheless, the platform has become popular among the global scientific community due to its user-friendliness. In the meantime, the rising tide of data disclosure further spilled over into the field of oncology. The Cancer Genome Atlas, which started in 2007, released a dataset of 4,938,362 genetic mutations from 7042 cases in 2013, accounting for 30 types of cancers [33].

As these genetic-information-based datasets continuously accumulated, activities to secure and improve the analytical validity of such data were also conducted through these large-scale, multicenter research programs by standardizing NGS instruments, tools, analytical protocols, and overall infrastructure required for scientific research. The CDC also organized the Next-Generation Sequencing: Standardization of Clinical Testing (NexStoCT), and published recommendations for the utilization of NGS in a clinical laboratory setting in 2012, specifically focusing on (1) validation, (2) quality control, (3) proficiency testing, and (4) reference materials [34].

Considering all these facts, it is worth paying attention to the recent trends in the field of cancer genomic medicine; a search result obtained using multiple search terms on ClinicalTrials.gov showed that the number of clinical trials in this field has gradually increased from 1 in 2008 to 30 in 2018 [18].

3.3. An Early Application of the New Technologies

The application of cancer genetic testing to both research and clinical settings was accelerated by the FDA's approvals for Oncomine Dx Target Test, MSK-IMPACT, and FoundationOne CDx as IVDs in 2017 [35–37]. The FDA then simplified the review process for additional biomarkers, which would be brought after the approval of these tests, by allowing the test developers to report claims "without an FDA submission [38]." The decision was made based on the FDA's approach that genetic mutations would fall into one of the three different evidence levels in accordance with the clinical significance, and that these evidence levels would be continuously updated as the science advances [38]. Companion diagnostics (CDx) were categorized as "Level 1" [38]. This level requires a genetic mutation to provide the highest clinical significance to be considered as a biomarker on the basis of clinical trials incorporating either "patient outcomes" or "clinical concordance to a previously approved CDx", along with "analytical validity" of the test for that mutation [38]. "Level 2" requires "analytical validity" and "clinical validity" of the test, which is typically "publicly available clinical evidence" [38]. "Level 3" merely requires "analytical validation" in combination with the minimal level of clinical significance, such as "peer-reviewed publications" and "in-vitro preclinical models [38]." Genetic mutations that are neither Level 1 or 2 are considered Level 3, and these are not considered as biomarkers [38].

Based on the concept of three-tiered clinical significance, the FDA has allowed the test developers to move a genetic mutation from Level 3 to 2 without an additional FDA submission, if it can be recognized within the clinical community based on the accumulation of clinical evidence [38]. In addition, not only has the FDA allowed for a genetic mutation that accounts for a specific cancer type to be considered as a biomarker, but it has also paved the way for its approval as a biomarker for other cancers that can result from the same mutation.

Aside from the FDA's regulatory efforts to simplify the review process for biomarkers, MSK-IMPACT was used as an LDT at MSKCC even before it was granted the FDA approval as an IVD in 2017 as stated earlier. It should also be emphasized again that MSK-IMPACT was approved in an accelerated manner as a result of the FDA's regulatory efforts to establish the regulatory pathways for LDTs as mentioned earlier.

3.4. The Utilization Structure of MSK-IMPACT

Figure 3 illustrates the overall structure of how MSK-IMPACT was utilized at MSKCC, which offers cancer care, diagnostic services, and opportunities for cancer patients to participate in the clinical trials in New York and New Jersey [39]. The utilization structure was gradually established as it was being used as an LDT. Genetic mutations data with clinical implications, collected from cancer patients, were accumulated and anonymously released to the public on "cBioPortal for Cancer Genomics" [40]. The hospital also developed an open source software that visualized data obtained through MSK-IMPACT; such data were released on GitHub to the public, and researchers are allowed to access them for free to facilitate further research for the development of novel therapeutic options in combination with the data released on cBioPortal [41,42]. Further, the spillover effect stemmed from the utilization of open data generated by MSK-IMPACT was found in a case of The Hyve B.V. (Utrecht, The Netherlands), a company that has developed free public software for cBioPortal [43]. Their software allows researchers to use data released on the data sharing platform [43]. Moreover, MSKCC has also established "OncoKB," a knowledge base that helps healthcare professionals determine therapies based on the diagnostic outcomes provided by MSK-IMPACT [44]; this knowledge base, in accordance with the evidence levels regularly updated by the FDA, constantly updates information and data that are beneficial for decision-making for cancer therapies, such as those on cancer genetic mutations, cancer types, and molecular target drugs that can be potentially used for cancer treatment.

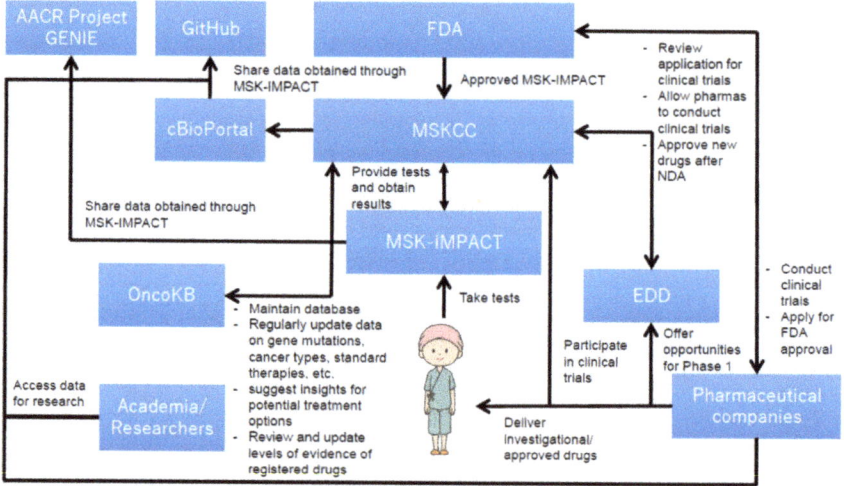

Figure 3. Key technological assets and their relationship in MSK-IMPACT [36,45,46]. Overall, this figure shows that the utilization structure of MSK-IMPACT contributes to both research and clinical settings. The structure helps genetic data obtained from cancer patients to be accumulated over time and be released to the public for further research. It also helps cancer patients participate in clinical trials. The structure has been established and reinforced based on interactions among various types of stakeholders (i.e., the FDA, MSKCC, cancer patients, pharmaceutical companies, etc.), and has provided research and clinical contributions, both of which are imperative for new drug development in oncology.

MSKCC has also established multiple processes to facilitate clinical trials by efficiently recruiting eligible patients in a timely manner, utilizing data collected through the applications of MSK-IMPACT. The hospital promotes phase 1 clinical trials by encouraging the treating physicians to introduce the Early Drug Development (EDD) Service to the eligible patients [45], which were identified by the DARWIN Cohort Management System, an original informatics platform used for the screening and management of patient cohorts for "genotype-matched clinical trials" [47]. In fact, the test suggested approximately 30% of patients would be eligible for clinical trials among more than 10,000 cancer patients in a study in which the clinical utility of MSK-IMPACT was evaluated using sequencing data obtained from such patients [48]. Furthermore, the hospital has recently initiated the Program for Drug Development in Leukemia (PDD-L) to promote the development of leukemia treatments by inducing leukemia patients to enroll in phase 1 clinical trials [49].

MSKCC has also functioned to conduct "basket trials," which cover various cancer types by focusing on a specific genetic mutation that is considered to cause tumors [50]. Rather than focusing on a specific cancer type, basket trials enable researchers and drug developers to simultaneously cover the patients with different types of cancers [50]. In such a setting, rare cancers, for which the patient populations were generally small, can also be covered [50]. Vemurafenib (ZELBORAF®) was developed through a basket trial. The drug was first approved in August 2011 for the treatment of unresectable or metastatic melanoma associated with the *BRAF* V600 mutation [51]. MSKCC further provided an additional opportunity to conduct a basket trial to test the drug for *BRAF* V600 mutation-positive nonmelanoma patients [52]. As a result, the FDA approved the drug for the treatment of Erdheim–Chester disease (ECD), an extremely rare cancer, in November 2017 [53,54].

3.5. Comparison between MSK-IMPACT and Other Panel Tests

The results of the comparative analyses are shown in Tables 2–4. Table 2 summarizes the basic information regarding MSK-IMPACT, FoundationOne CDx and Oncomine Dx Target Test. The remarkable difference between these three assays is that MSK-IMPACT was not approved as a companion diagnostic assay, while its competing IVDs were listed as FDA-approved companion diagnostic devices [55]. The other difference was found in their data management systems; FoundationOne CDx and MSK-IMPACT appeared to have their own data sharing platforms, while OncomineCDx Target Test was merely found to possess its data management system, which would not be intended for data sharing with others. Second, Table 3 reveals the contribution of these three assays to new drug development. FoundationOne CDx appeared to be the most prominent, while Oncomine Dx Target Test, the other companion diagnostic device, seemed to have struggled to produce certain outcomes. In addition, there were 24 FDA-approved drugs associated with FoundationOne CDx for cancer care, while the number of such drugs for Oncomine Dx Target Test remained at 5 [55]. Although there were no CDx-tied drugs with MSK-IMPACT, it helped in the production of two FDA-approved drugs and two other drug candidates, which are currently under development. The other finding was that three of these drugs were identified through basket trials. Third, Table 4 shows the expedited approval programs that were helpful in obtaining FDA approvals for the new drugs produced based on the use of each panel test; considering the significance as well as difficulties of innovation, this study only focused on the new drugs, and thus excluded the existing drugs with history of expanding additional indications. It should be noted that these new drugs were found to have utilized multiple programs to accelerate the drug development process. Moreover, the average time frame between IND and FDA approval for these drugs was found to be approximately 3.5 years, which was significantly shorter than approximately 8 years that averaged from 1986 to 2017 as explained earlier [10].

Table 2. Comparison of basic information.

Item	FoundationOne CDx [37,55–57]	MSK-IMPACT [36,45,46,58]	Oncomine Dx Target Test [35,55,59,60]
Developer	Foundation Medicine, Inc.	Memorial Sloan Kettering Cancer Center (MSKCC)	Life Technologies Corporation
Date of FDA approval as IVD	30 November 2017	15 November 2017	22 June 2017
Specimen type	FFPE tumor tissue	FFPE tumor tissue and patient-matched blood/normal tissue as a normal control	FFPE tumor tissue
Number of genes covered	324	468	23
Biomarker	SNVs, Indels, CNVs, gene rearrangements, TMB, MSI and HRD	SNVs, Indels, CNVs, Promoter mutation (TERT), Gene rearrangements, TMB and MSI	SNVs, Deletions and Fusion gene (ROS1)
FDA approval for CDx	Granted for diagnosis of breast cancer, cholangiocarcinoma, colon/rectum cancer, non-small cell lung cancer (NSCLC), malignant melanoma, ovary cancer, prostate cancer, and solid cancer	None	Granted for diagnosis of non-small cell lung cancer (NSCLC)
Availability and functions of data management and/or sharing platform for new drug development	Allows access to open data on cancer patients through FoundationInsights, a cloud-based data platform. Provides access to FoundationCore through FoundationInsights, a knowledgebase with data obtained from cancer patients	Facilitates research for the development of new therapies through cBioPortal for Cancer Genomics (open database) Provides and updates clinical data obtained from cancer patients through OncoKB (knowledgebase) Allows patients to access Phase 1 clinical trials for solid tumors identified by the DARWIN Cohort Management System Manages study cohorts for clinical trials on a timely basis	Analyzes and reports sequencing data through the Torrent Suit Dx Software, which works on Google Chrome browser Allows sequencing results and reports to be automatically archived to an external server

The abbreviations for the terminology in genome science indicated in this table originally stand for the following: formalin fixed paraffin embedded (FFPE), single nucleotide variant (SNV), insertion/detection (Indel), copy number variation (CNV), tumor mutational burden (TMB), microsatelite instability (MSI), homologous recombination deficiency (HRD).

Table 3. Comparison of outcomes.

Product Name	New Drugs					Expanded Additional Indications to Existing Drugs			
	Drug Name	Biomarker	Indication/Therapy Type	Status		Drug Name	Biomarker	Indication/Therapy Type	Status
FoundationOne CDx	PEMAZYRE® (pemigatinib) [61,62]	FGFR2	Cholangiocarcinoma/ Monotherapy	Approved (April 2020)		GILOTRIF® (afatinib) [63,64]	EGFR	Squamous cell carcinoma (lung)/Monotherapy	Approved (April 2016)
	ROZLYTREK® (entrectinib) [65,66]	NTRK	Solid tumors/Monotherapy	Approved (August 2019)		KEYTRUDA® (pembrolizumab) [67,68]	TMB	TMB-H solid tumors/Monotherapy	Approved (June 2020)
		ROS1	Non-small cell lung cancer (NSCLC)/Monotherapy			LYNPARZA® (olaparib)	BRCA1/2	Ovarian cancer/Monotherapy [69,70]	Approved (December 2018)
	TABRECTA™ (capmatinib) [71,72]	Mutation relating to MET exon 14 skipping	Non-small cell lung cancer (NSCLC)/Monotherapy	Approved (May 2020)			HRR genes	mCRPC/Monotherapy [73,74]	Approved (May 2020)
	VITRAKVI® (larotrectinib) [75,76]	NTRK	Solid tumors/Monotherapy	Approved (November 2018)		ZELBORAF® (vemulafenib) [52,54]	BRAF V600	Erdheim-Chester disease (ECD)/Monotherapy	Approved (November 2017)
MSK-IMPACT	AZD5363 (capivasertib) [18,77]	AKT1/2/3	Multiple indications (breast cancer, prostate cancer, solid tumors, etc.)/Either monotherapy or combination	Phase 1~ (as of April 2021)		NERLYNX® (neratinib) with XELODA® (capecitabine) [77,78]	HER2	Breast cancer/Combination	Approved (February 2020)
	LOXO-195 (selitrectinib) [18,79]	NTRK	Solid tumors (with resistance to Larotrectinib)/Monotherapy	Phase 1/2 (as of April 2021)		-	-	-	-
	VITRAKVI® (larotrectinib) [75,76]	NTRK	Solid tumors/Monotherapy	Approved (November 2018)		-	-	-	-
Oncomine Dx Target Test	GAVRETO™ (pralsetinib) [80,81]	RET	Non-small cell lung cancer (NSCLC)/Monotherapy	Approved (September 2020)		TAFINLAR® (dabrafenib) with MEKINIST® (trametinib) [82]	BRAF V600 E	Non-small cell lung cancer (NSCLC)/Combination	Approved (June 2017)

Table 4. Association between the FDA's expedited approval programs and the new drugs identified by the three tumor profiling tests. To a greater or lesser extent, all the new drugs identified by the tests were found to have succeeded in speeding up the review process by utilizing a combination of the expedited approval programs.

Drug Information					Expedited Approval Programs [83]				
Drug Name (Generic Name)	Assay Used for Clinical Trials	Indication	IND Submission Date	Approval Date	Orphan Drug	Fast Track	Breakthrough Therapy	Priority Review	Accelerated Approval
GAVRETO™ (pralsetinib)	Oncomine Dx Target Test	Non-small cell lung cancer (NSCLC)	August 2019 [84]	September 2020 [81]	Yes	No	Yes	Yes	Yes
PEMAZYRE® (pemigatinib)	FoundationOne CDx	Cholangio-carcinoma	January 2018 [85]	April. 2020 [62]	Yes	No	Yes	Yes	Yes
ROZLYTREK® (entrectinib)	FoundationOne CDx	Solid tumors	February 2014 [83]	August 2019 [66]	Yes	No	Yes	Yes	Yes
ROZLYTREK® (entrectinib)	FoundationOne CDx	Non-small cell lung cancer (NSCLC)	May 2017 [65]	August 2019 [66]	Yes	No	No	Yes	Yes
TABRECTA™ (capmatinib)	FoundationOne CDx	Non-small cell lung cancer (NSCLC)	January 2015 [86]	May 2020 [72]	Yes	No	Yes	No	Yes
VITRAKVI® (larotrectinib)	FoundationOne CDx, MSK-IMPACT™	Solid tumors	February 2014 [87]	November 2018 [76]	Yes	No	Yes	Yes	Yes

4. Discussion

4.1. Implications of Regulatory Reforms to Corporate Activities

The number of outcomes produced by each panel test implies that FoundationOne CDx has benefited from the FDA's regulatory reforms, early application of new technologies, and accumulation of publicly accessible open data. It would be reasonable to assume that the FDA has encouraged drug developers to facilitate drug development activities through the implementation of a series of regulatory reforms, including expedited approval programs. In the meantime, pharmaceutical regulations have become stringent in monitoring the safety of drug candidates under the FDA Amendments Act. The FDA's strategies to balance the flexibility and stringency in drug development should be considered to be a reasonable action because the efficacy and safety of new therapies need to be secured and appropriately balanced, especially when such therapies are developed based on the utilization of the new technologies. It would also be reasonable to assume that data accumulation and disclosure to the public, along with the efforts for standardization and compatibility development between different datasets, has facilitated drug development activities in which FoundationOne CDx was incorporated. On the contrary, MSK-IMPACT does not seem to have fully benefitted from these regulatory efforts, although it succeeded in shortening the FDA's review process for its IVD approval.

This may be because of the differences in the organizational interests and incentives between the developers. Foundation Medicine falls under the umbrella of the pharmaceutical giant Roche Holding AG (Basel, Switzerland), while MSKCC is a hospital. There is no doubt that the former has an interest in expanding collaborations with other players, such as pharmaceutical companies, to facilitate drug development activities using its products, considering the relationship with its parent company. On the other hand, the primary interest of MSKCC, as a healthcare provider, is to serve its patients.

In addition, the number of outcomes by Oncomine Dx Target Test was found to be inadequate despite its CDx approval. At this point, the fact that Life Technologies is a manufacturer of laboratory tools and is not directly involved in the drug development activities may account for this result. Therefore, it is reasonable to assume that, unlike the relationship between Foundation Medicine and Roche, the capital relationship of Life Technologies with its parent company, Thermo Fisher Scientific Inc. (Waltham, MA, USA), which is not a pharmaceutical company, has not functioned enough to motivate the company to be involved in new drug development.

4.2. Characteristics of MSK-IMPACT

Our study has identified tangible and intangible values of MSK-IMPACT. First, the test has been embedded into the patient recruitment activities of MSKCC for efficient enrollment in clinical trials. Second, there is an established utilization structure of data for genetic mutations in cancer patients collected using the test, which can be used for further research. Third, although the extent of the contribution of the test to basic cancer research has yet to be clear, the case of The Hyve, a free software developer, implies that MSK-IMPACT is believed to have contributed to basic research through its data sharing platform cBioPortal in combination with The Hyve's free software. It is likely that researchers have gained some benefits from these tools as they can access the open data for free. This case represents the differentiation of MSK-IMPACT from FoundationOne CDx, which provides similar benefits at the researchers' expense, such as the provision of data on a closed basis. Fourth, MSKCC and MSK-IMPACT have functioned as a catalyst to promote the practice of basket trials, which are an advanced form of clinical trials. Lastly, the test has thus far contributed to the development of both monotherapies and combination therapies for cancer. In contrast to FoundationOne CDx, the advantages associated with MSK-IMPACT were mostly identified in its integrated utilization structure within the MSKCC community.

Key challenges of MSK-IMPACT were pointed out from a marketing and business development point of view, considering the potential differences between this test and FoundationOne CDx. First, the test was basically used within the MSKCC community. This seems to have caused limitations for the test in gaining utilization opportunities outside the hospital group. Since the hospital has a well-established utilization structure of the test within its own community with a specific priority of saving patients, it has struggled to expand opportunities for the test to be used at other hospitals. The hospital may have also missed alliance and collaboration opportunities with other counterparts, such as pharmaceutical companies, for drug development activities. Second, cancer patients at MSKCC do not have to pay test fees because they are covered by donations [88]. This casts a concern about the sustainability of the testing practice. Since MSK-IMPACT has limitations in expanding marketing opportunities outside the MSKCC community, the hospital may have to consider alternative measures to ensure the sustainability of the testing practice for its patients.

4.3. Recommendations for a Better Clinical Sequencing in Oncology

Based on these considerations, we emphasize the importance of collaborations with external organizations, including other hospitals and pharmaceutical companies, for a non-profit model such as MSKCC to better promote drug development. Mirnezami et al. 2012 have pointed out that collaboration between various healthcare stakeholders, such as the governments, researchers, and pharmaceutical industries, would be required to promote precision medicine [89]. Looking at the comparison between MSK-IMPACT and FoundationOne CDx, the number of outcomes produced by the latter seems to be overwhelming, due in part to its CDx approval. The potential interest in drug development activities between Roche and Foundation Medicine should have been the major driving force. The difference in organizational interests can affect one's motivation to facilitate innovation and even its consequences. As a case of collaborative development of cancer drugs, Makino et al. 2018 argued in their quantitative research that there was a positive correlation between the number of alliances (i.e., R&D licensing, marketing licensing, etc.) and a number of patents relating to CDx [90]. This implies that a challenge for MSK-IMPACT is to promote collaborative opportunities with external counterparts for drug development activities.

Despite these issues, MSKCC has established the utilization structure of MSK-IMPACT over time. Patients with cancer at MSKCC can easily be notified regarding their eligibility for clinical trials. Data on genetic mutations in patients at the hospital can also be utilized for further research. These processes can both, directly and indirectly, contribute to saving patients. Based on these findings, this study insists that even more patients would be saved if the characteristics of these two tests were to be mixed. It is recommended that MSKCC considers reinforcing collaborations with other hospitals, pharmaceutical companies, and the like and providing relevant resources to them to promote drug development activities.

Equally importantly, regulatory authorities need to consider establishing a certain institutional framework that integrates different healthcare stakeholders to facilitate drug development activities. For example, in the field of cell and gene therapy in Japan, a double-track regulation of providing values through medical services based on translational research and products based on clinical trials has been implemented, guaranteeing a variety of opportunities for companies and non-profit institutions [91]. Such an innovative approach in regulatory science will provide more opportunities for cancer drug development, which will eventually contribute to providing more treatment options for cancer patients.

4.4. Study Limitations

This study had some potential limitations. First, ClinicalTrials.gov did not function to accurately find clinical trials that employed MSK-IMPACT for either screening or confirmatory purposes, as pointed out earlier. Second, the investigation method to find outcomes by FoundationOne CDx and Oncomine Dx Target Test was not intended to cover ongoing clinical trials for their pre-approval drugs, while it detected some for MSK-IMPACT. Third, the method was not intended to cover the outcomes of basket trials by FoundationOne CDx and Oncomine Dx Target Test, while it found that the majority of the outcomes of MSK-IMPACT were developed through this form of clinical trials. Since the study focused on investigating the CDx-tied drugs with these two tests, the results did not convey the extent to which they were being used in the basket trials. Overall, the fact that numerous clinical trials involving cancer clinical sequencing have already been conducted accounts for the difficulties in fully covering the outcomes of these three tests. At this point, there is still room for further research to investigate the contribution of these three tests to cancer care innovation.

5. Conclusions

The present study explored factors that contribute to facilitating innovation in cancer clinical sequencing with a particular focus on the case of MSK-IMPACT with two comparative cases, FoundationOne CDx and Oncomine Dx Target Test. Through comparative analyses between these three tests, FoundationOne CDx appeared to have outweighed the MSK-IMPACT and Oncomine Dx Target Test in terms of the number of generated outcomes, whereas MSK-IMPACT was functioning as a hub to efficiently enroll cancer patients in clinical trials with its in-house data management platform. These results suggest two key challenges that MSK-IMPACT needs to overcome. First, more collaborations with external organizations for drug development activities, including but not limited to other hospitals and pharmaceutical companies, need to be pursued. Another challenge lies in the sustainability of the testing practice: since the use of the test is limited within the MSKCC community, it is ideal for the hospital to secure alternative financial sources to ensure continued testing practice. To address these challenges, MSK-IMPACT should expand the use of the test for collaborations with external organizations to develop novel cancer therapies. It should also be noted from a regulatory perspective that pharmaceutical regulations need to be supportive of drug developers, while balancing the efficacy and safety of new therapies under development in an appropriate manner. All these efforts will eventually contribute to the development of novel therapies for cancer patients.

Author Contributions: Conceptualization, T.J. and H.N.; methodology, T.J. and H.N.; validation, T.J., H.N., S.S.; formal analysis, T.J. and H.N.; investigation, T.J.; writing—original draft preparation, T.J.; writing—review and editing, S.S.; visualization, T.J.; supervision, S.S. and K.K.; funding acquisition, K.K. and S.S. T.J. and H.N. equally contributed to this work as the co-first authors. All authors have read and agreed to the published version of the manuscript.

Funding: This research was financially and partially supported by MEXT/JSPS KAKENHI (the Grant-in-Aid for Scientific Research, 20 K20769 and 21 H00739), Japan.

Institutional Review Board Statement: Not applicable.

Informed Consent Statement: Not applicable.

Data Availability Statement: Our study did not generate any numerical data.

Acknowledgments: We would like to thank Naoto Kondo of RIKEN GENESIS CO., LTD. for his valuable comments and cooperation.

Conflicts of Interest: The authors hereby declare any personal circumstances or interests that may be perceived as inappropriately influencing the representation or interpretation of the reported research results. T.J. is an employee of ASKA Pharmaceutical Co., Ltd. (Tokyo, Japan). The funding bodies had no role in the design of the study, the collection, analyses, or interpretation of the data, or in the writing of the manuscript, or in the decision to publish the results.

References

1. The Precision Medicine Initiative. Available online: https://obamawhitehouse.archives.gov/precision-medicine (accessed on 18 September 2020).
2. Wetterstrand, K.A. DNA Sequencing Costs: Data from the NHGRI Genome Sequencing Program (GSP). Available online: https://www.genome.gov/about-genomics/fact-sheets/DNA-Sequencing-Costs-Data (accessed on 19 April 2021).
3. The OECD Innovation Strategy: Getting a Head Start on Tomorrow. Available online: https://read.oecd-ilibrary.org/science-and-technology/the-oecd-innovation-strategy_9789264083479-en#page1 (accessed on 20 April 2021).
4. Onodera, R.; Sengoku, S. Innovation process of mHealth: An overview of FDA-approved mobile medical applications. *Int. J. Med Inform.* **2018**, *118*, 65–71. [CrossRef]
5. Coté, T.; Kelkar, A.; Xu, K.; Braun, M.M.; Phillips, M.I. Orphan products: An emerging trend in drug approvals. *Nat. Rev. Drug Discov.* **2010**, *9*, 84. [CrossRef]
6. PUBLIC LAW 97-414. Available online: https://www.govinfo.gov/content/pkg/STATUTE-96/pdf/STATUTE-96-Pg2049.pdf (accessed on 8 July 2021).
7. Food and Drug Administration Modernization Act of 1997. Available online: https://www.govinfo.gov/content/pkg/PLAW-105publ115/pdf/PLAW-105publ115.pdf (accessed on 8 July 2021).
8. Accelerated Approval. Available online: https://www.fda.gov/patients/fast-track-breakthrough-therapy-accelerated-approval-priority-review/accelerated-approval (accessed on 8 July 2021).
9. PUBLIC LAW 112-144. Available online: https://www.govinfo.gov/content/pkg/PLAW-112publ144/pdf/PLAW-112publ144.pdf (accessed on 8 July 2021).
10. Darrow, J.J.; Avorn, J.; Kesselheim, A.S. FDA Approval and Regulation of Pharmaceuticals, 1983–2018. *Am. Med Assoc.* **2020**, *323*, 164–176. [CrossRef]
11. Darrow, J.J.; Avorn, J.; Kesselheim, A.S. New FDA Breakthrough-Drug Category—Implications for Patients. *N. Engl. J. Med.* **2014**, *370*, 1252–1258. [CrossRef]
12. Golodner, L.F. The US Food and Drug Administration Modernization Act of 1997: Impact on consumers. *Clin. Ther.* **1998**, *20*, C20–C25. [CrossRef]
13. Merrill, R.A. Modernizing the FDA: An Incremental Revolution. *Health Aff.* **1999**, *18*, 96–111. [CrossRef]
14. Goble, J.A. The Potential Effect of the 21st Century Cures Act on Drug Development. *J. Manag. Care Spec. Pharm.* **2018**, *24*, 677–681. [CrossRef]
15. Goodsell, D.S.; Zardecki, C.; Costanzo, L.D.; Duarte, J.M.; Hudson, B.P.; Persikova, I.; Segura, J.; Shao, C.; Voigt, M.; Westbrook, J.D.; et al. RCSB Protein Data Bank: Enabling biomedical research. *Protein Soc.* **2020**, *29*, 52–65. [CrossRef] [PubMed]
16. Kahn, S.M. Next-generation sequencing for cancer drug development: The present and visions for the future. *Pers. Med.* **2014**, *11*, 139–142. [CrossRef] [PubMed]
17. Patriquin, C.M. A Case Study of Next-Generation Sequencing Operationalization in an Oncology Companion Diagnostic Environment. Master's Thesis, Harvard Extension School, Cambridge, MA, USA, May 2020.
18. ClinicalTrials. Available online: https://clinicaltrials.gov/ (accessed on 19 January 2019).
19. Risk Evaluation and Mitigation Strategies | REMS. Available online: https://www.fda.gov/drugs/drug-safety-and-availability/risk-evaluation-and-mitigation-strategies-rems (accessed on 14 July 2020).
20. Platt, R.; Brown, J.S.; Robb, M.; McClellan, M.; Ball, R.; Nguyen, M.D.; Sherman, R.E. The FDA Sentinel Initiative—An Evolving National Resource. *N. Engl. J. Med.* **2018**, *379*, 2091–2093. [CrossRef] [PubMed]
21. 21st Century Cures Act. Available online: https://www.fda.gov/regulatory-information/selected-amendments-fdc-act/21st-century-cures-act (accessed on 8 July 2021).
22. Hillebrenner, E. Third Party Review: FDA Perspective. Available online: https://www.amdm.org/uploads/8/3/9/2/8392851/hillebrenner_3p_case_study.pdf (accessed on 25 June 2020).

23. Public Workshop—Optimizing FDA's Regulatory Oversight of Next Generation Sequencing Diagnostic Tests Public Workshop. Available online: https://wayback.archive-it.org/7993/20170406155937/https://www.fda.gov/MedicalDevices/NewsEvents/WorkshopsConferences/ucm427296.htm (accessed on 23 September 2020).
24. Public Workshop—Standards Based Approach to Analytical Performance Evaluation of Next Generation Sequencing In Vitro Diagnostic Tests. Available online: https://wayback.archive-it.org/7993/20170111165845/http://www.fda.gov/MedicalDevices/NewsEvents/WorkshopsConferences/ucm459449.htm (accessed on 23 September 2020).
25. Webinar—Next Generation Sequencing (NGS) Draft Guidances: Implications for Patients and Providers—27 July 2016. Available online: https://www.fda.gov/medical-devices/workshops-conferences-medical-devices/webinar-next-generation-sequencing-ngs-draft-guidances-implications-patients-and-providers-july-27 (accessed on 23 September 2020).
26. Use of Public Human Genetic Variant Databases to Support Clinical Validity for Genetic and Genomic-Based In Vitro Diagnostics. Available online: https://www.fda.gov/media/99200/download (accessed on 23 September 2020).
27. dbSNP Celebrates 20 Years! Available online: https://ncbiinsights.ncbi.nlm.nih.gov/2019/10/07/dbsnp-celebrates-20-years/ (accessed on 14 September 2020).
28. Empowering GWAS for a New Era of Discovery. Available online: https://jp.illumina.com/content/dam/illumina-marketing/documents/products/technotes/technote_empower_gwas.pdf (accessed on 14 September 2020).
29. PubMed. Available online: https://pubmed.ncbi.nlm.nih.gov/ (accessed on 7 October 2019).
30. Participating in the Harvard PGP. Available online: https://pgp.med.harvard.edu/participate (accessed on 16 September 2020).
31. McVean, G.A. An integrated map of genetic variation from 1092 human genomes. *Nature* **2012**, *491*, 56–65.
32. Mitsubishi Research Institute, Inc. Heisei Niju-Nana Nendo Kokunaigai ni Okeru Idenshi Shinryo no Jittai Chosa Houkokusyo—Kenkyu Iryomen ni Oite Yuyoh na Data Sharing Kiban no Kento. Available online: https://www.amed.go.jp/content/000004863.pdf (accessed on 17 September 2020). (In Japanese).
33. Alexandrov, L.B.; Nik-Zainal, S.; Stratton, M.R.; Wedge, D.C.; Aparicio, S.A.J.R.; Behjati, S.; Biankin, A.V.; Bignell, G.R.; Bolli, N.; Borg, A.; et al. Signatures of mutational processes in human cancer. *Nature* **2013**, *500*, 415–421. [CrossRef]
34. Gargis, A.S.; Kalman, L.; Berry, M.W.; Bick, D.P.; Dimmock, D.P.; Hambuch, T.; Lu, F.; Lyon, E.; Voelkerding, K.V.; Zehnbauer, B.A.; et al. Assuring the quality of next-generation sequencing in clinical laboratory practice. *Nat. Biotechnol.* **2012**, *30*, 1033–1036. [CrossRef] [PubMed]
35. FDA Approves First Companion Diagnostic Test to Simultaneously Screen for Multiple Non-Small Cell Lung Cancer Therapies. Available online: https://thermofisher.mediaroom.com/2017-06-22-FDA-Approves-First-Companion-Diagnostic-Test-to-Simultaneously-Screen-for-Multiple-Non-Small-Cell-Lung-Cancer-Therapies (accessed on 24 September 2020).
36. FDA Unveils a Streamlined Path for the Authorization of Tumor Profiling Tests Alongside Its Latest Product Action. Available online: https://www.fda.gov/news-events/press-announcements/fda-unveils-streamlined-path-authorization-tumor-profiling-tests-alongside-its-latest-product-action (accessed on 24 September 2020).
37. FDA Approves Foundation Medicine's FoundationOne CDx™, the First and Only Comprehensive Genomic Profiling Test for All Solid Tumors Incorporating Multiple Companion Diagnostics. Available online: https://www.foundationmedicine.com/press-releases/f2b20698-10bd-4ac9-a5e5-c80c398a57b5 (accessed on 24 September 2020).
38. Fda Fact Sheet Cdrh's Approach to Tumor Profiling Next Generation Sequencing Tests. Available online: https://www.fda.gov/media/109050/download (accessed on 24 September 2020).
39. Memorial Sloan Kettering Cancer Center. Available online: https://health.usnews.com/best-hospitals/area/ny/memorial-sloan-kettering-cancer-center-6213060 (accessed on 7 October 2020).
40. cBioPortal for Cancer Genomics. Available online: https://www.cbioportal.org/ (accessed on 8 October 2020).
41. cBioPortal. Available online: https://github.com/cBioPortal/ (accessed on 8 October 2020).
42. Hyman, D.M.; Solit, D.B.; Arcila, M.E.; Cheng, D.; Sabbatini, P.; Baselga, J.; Berger, M.F.; Ladanyi, M. Precision medicine at Memorial Sloan Kettering Cancer Center: Clinical next-generation sequencing enabling next-generation targeted therapy trials. *Drug Discov. Today* **2015**, *20*, 1422–1428. [CrossRef] [PubMed]
43. Cancer Genomics. Available online: https://www.thehyve.nl/focus-areas/cancer-genomics (accessed on 3 June 2021).
44. Chakravarty, D.; Gao, J.; Phillips, S.; Kundra, R.; Zhang, H.; Wang, J.; Rudolph, J.E.; Yaeger, R.; Soumerai, T.; Nissan, M.H.; et al. OncoKB: A Precision Oncology Knowledge Base. *JCO Precis. Oncol.* **2017**. [CrossRef] [PubMed]
45. Early Drug Development Service: Phase I Clinical Trials Program. Available online: https://www.mskcc.org/departments/division-solid-tumor-oncology/early-drug-development-service-phase-clinical-trials (accessed on 16 October 2020).
46. MSK-IMPACT: A Targeted Test for Mutations in Both Rare and Common Cancers. Available online: https://www.mskcc.org/msk-impact (accessed on 20 November 2020).
47. Eubank, M.H.; Hyman, D.M.; Kanakamedala, A.D.; Gardos, S.M.; Wills, J.M.; Stetson, P.D. Automated eligibility screening and monitoring for genotype-driven precision oncology trials. *J. Am. Med. Inform. Assoc.* **2016**, *23*, 777–781. [CrossRef]
48. Zehir, A.; Benayed, R.; Shah, R.H.; Syed, A.; Middha, S.; Kim, H.R.; Srinivasan, P.; Gao, J.; Chakravarty, D.; Delvin, S.M.; et al. Mutational landscape of metastatic cancer revealed from prospective clinical sequencing of 10,000 patients. *Nat. Med.* **2017**, *23*, 703–713. [CrossRef]
49. MSK Program Focuses on Speeding Up Development of New Leukemia Treatments. Available online: https://www.mskcc.org/news/msk-program-focuses-speeding-up-new-leukemia-treatments (accessed on 20 November 2020).

50. Clinical Trial Shows Promise of "Basket Studies" for Cancer Drugs. Available online: https://www.mskcc.org/news/clinical-trial-shows-promise-basket-studies-drugs (accessed on 10 December 2020).
51. Kim, G.; McKee, A.E.; Ning, Y.M.; Hazarika, M.; Theoret, M.; Johnson, J.R.; Xu, Q.C.; Tang, S.; Sridhara, R.; Jiang, X.; et al. FDA Approval Summary: Vemurafenib for Treatment of Unresectable or Metastatic Melanoma with the BRAFV600E Mutation. *Clin. Cancer Res.* **2014**, *20*, 4994–5000. [CrossRef]
52. Hyman, D.M.; Puzanov, I.; Subbiah, V.; Faris, J.E.; Chau, I.; Blay, J.Y.; Wolf, J.; Raje, N.S.; Diamond, E.L.; Hollebecque, A.; et al. Vemurafenib in Multiple Nonmelanoma Cancers with BRAF V600 Mutations. *N. Engl. J. Med.* **2015**, *373*, 726–736. [CrossRef]
53. Patricia, O.A.; Kwitkowski, V.; Luo, L.; Shen, Y.L.; Subramaniam, S.; Shord, S.; Goldberg, K.B.; McKee, A.E.; Kaminskas, E.; Farrell, A.; et al. FDA Approval Summary: Vemurafenib for the Treatment of Patients with Erdheim-Chester Disease with the BRAFV600 Mutation. *Oncologist* **2018**, *23*, 1520–1524.
54. FDA Approves First Treatment for Certain Patients with Erdheim-Chester Disease, a Rare Blood Cancer. Available online: https://www.fda.gov/news-events/press-announcements/fda-approves-first-treatment-certain-patients-erdheim-chester-disease-rare-blood-cancer#:~{}:text=The%20U.S.%20Food%20and%20Drug%20Administration%20today%20expanded,a%20specific%20genetic%20mutation%20known%20as%20BRAF%20V600 (accessed on 10 December 2020).
55. List of Cleared or Approved Companion Diagnostic Devices (In Vitro and Imaging Tools). Available online: https://www.fda.gov/medical-devices/vitro-diagnostics/list-cleared-or-approved-companion-diagnostic-devices-vitro-and-imaging-tools (accessed on 18 December 2020).
56. Genomic Data Solutions. Available online: https://www.foundationmedicine.com/service/genomic-data-solutions (accessed on 25 November 2020).
57. FoundationOne®CDx Technical Information. Available online: https://info.foundationmedicine.com/hubfs/FMI%20Labels/FoundationOne_CDx_Label_Technical_Info.pdf (accessed on 3 June 2021).
58. Evaluation of Automatic Class III Designation for Msk-Impact (Integrated Mutation Profiling of Actionable Cancer Targets) Decision Summary. Available online: https://www.accessdata.fda.gov/cdrh_docs/reviews/den170058.pdf (accessed on 3 June 2021).
59. Oncomine™ Dx Target Test Part I: Sample Preparation and Quantification User Guide. Available online: https://www.accessdata.fda.gov/cdrh_docs/pdf16/p160045c.pdf (accessed on 25 April 2021).
60. Summary of Safety and Effectiveness Data (SSED). Available online: https://www.accessdata.fda.gov/cdrh_docs/pdf16/p160045b.pdf (accessed on 3 June 2021).
61. Abou-Alfa, G.K.; Sahai, V.; Hollebecque, A.; Vaccaro, G.; Melisi, D.; Al-Rajabi, R.; Paulson, A.S.; Borad, M.J.; Gallinson, D.; Murphy, A.G.; et al. Pemigatinib for previously treated, locally advanced or metastatic cholangiocarcinoma: A multicentre, open-label, phase 2 study. *Lancet Oncol.* **2020**, *21*, 671–684. [CrossRef]
62. FDA Approves First Targeted Treatment for Patients with Cholangiocarcinoma, a Cancer of Bile Ducts. Available online: https://www.fda.gov/news-events/press-announcements/fda-approves-first-targeted-treatment-patients-cholangiocarcinoma-cancer-bile-ducts (accessed on 8 February 2021).
63. FDA Approves Gilotrif® (Afatinib) as New Oral Treatment Option for Patients with Squamous Cell Carcinoma of the Lung. Available online: https://www.boehringer-ingelheim.us/press-release/fda-approves-gilotrifr-afatinib-new-oral-treatment-option-patients-squamous-cell (accessed on 14 February 2021).
64. Soria, J.C.; Felip, E.; Cobo, M.; Lu, S.; Syrigos, K.; Lee, K.H.; Goker, E.; Georgoulias, V.; Li, W.; Isla, D.; et al. Afatinib versus erlotinib as second-line treatment of patients with advanced squamous cell carcinoma of the lung (LUX-Lung 8): An open-label randomised controlled phase 3 trial. *Lancet Oncol.* **2015**, *16*, 897–907. [CrossRef]
65. NDA/BLA Multi-Disciplinary Review and Evaluation NDA 212725 Rozlytrek (Entrectinib). Available online: https://www.accessdata.fda.gov/drugsatfda_docs/nda/2019/212725Orig1s000,%20212726Orig1s000MultidisciplineR.pdf (accessed on 1 February 2021).
66. FDA Approves Entrectinib for NTRK Solid Tumors and ROS-1 NSCLC. Available online: https://www.fda.gov/drugs/resources-information-approved-drugs/fda-approves-entrectinib-ntrk-solid-tumors-and-ros-1-nsclc#:~{}:text=On%20August%2015%2C%202019%2C%20the%20Food%20and%20Drug,following%20treatment%20or%20have%20no%20satisfactory%20standard%20th (accessed on 15 August 2019).
67. Prescribing Information of KEYTRUDA. Available online: https://www.accessdata.fda.gov/drugsatfda_docs/label/2020/125514s071s090lbl.pdf (accessed on 1 February 2021).
68. FDA Approves Pembrolizumab for Adults and Children with TMB-H Solid Tumors. Available online: https://www.fda.gov/drugs/drug-approvals-and-databases/fda-approves-pembrolizumab-adults-and-children-tmb-h-solid-tumors (accessed on 8 February 2021).
69. Arora, S.; Balasubramaniam, S.; Zhang, H.; Berman, T.; Narayan, P.; Suzman, D.; Bloomquist, E.; Tang, S.; Gong, Y.; Sridhara, R.; et al. FDA Approval Summary: Olaparib Monotherapy or in Combination with Bevacizumab for the Maintenance Treatment of Patients with Advanced Ovarian Cancer. *Oncologist* **2021**, *26*, e164–e172. [CrossRef]
70. FDA Approved Olaparib (LYNPARZA, AstraZeneca Pharmaceuticals LP). Available online: https://www.fda.gov/drugs/fda-approved-olaparib-lynparza-astrazeneca-pharmaceuticals-lp-maintenance-treatment-adult-patients (accessed on 18 February 2021).

71. Prescribing Information of TABRECTA. Available online: https://www.accessdata.fda.gov/drugsatfda_docs/label/2020/213591s000lbl.pdf (accessed on 8 February 2021).
72. FDA Approves First Targeted Therapy to Treat Aggressive Form of Lung Cancer. Available online: https://www.fda.gov/news-events/press-announcements/fda-approves-first-targeted-therapy-treat-aggressive-form-lung-cancer (accessed on 8 February 2021).
73. De Bono, J.; Mateo, J.; Fizazi, K.; Saad, F.; Shore, N.; Sandhu, S.; Chi, K.N.; Sartor, O.; Agarwal, N.; Olmos, D.; et al. Olaparib for Metastatic Castration-Resistant Prostate Cancer. *N. Engl. J. Med.* **2020**, *382*, 2091–2102. [CrossRef]
74. FDA Approves Olaparib for HRR Gene-Mutated Metastatic Castration-Resistant Prostate Cancer. Available online: https://www.fda.gov/drugs/drug-approvals-and-databases/fda-approves-olaparib-hrr-gene-mutated-metastatic-castration-resistant-prostate-cancer#:~{}:text=On%20May%2019%2C%202020%2C%20the,(mCRPC)%2C%20who%20have%20progressed (accessed on 18 February 2021).
75. Drilon, A.; Laetsch, T.W.; Kummar, S.; DuBois, S.G.; Lassen, U.N.; Demetri, G.D.; Nathenson, M.; Doebele, R.C.; Farago, A.F.; Pappo, A.S.; et al. Efficacy of Larotrectinib in TRK Fusion–Positive Cancers in Adults and Children. *N. Engl. J. Med.* **2018**, *378*, 731–739. [CrossRef] [PubMed]
76. FDA Approves Larotrectinib for Solid Tumors with NTRK Gene Fusions. Available online: https://www.fda.gov/drugs/fda-approves-larotrectinib-solid-tumors-ntrk-gene-fusions (accessed on 8 February 2021).
77. Cheng, M.L.; Berger, M.F.; Hyman, D.M.; Solit, D.B. Clinical tumour sequencing for precision oncology: Time for a universal strategy. *Nat. Rev. Cancer* **2018**, *18*, 527–528. [CrossRef] [PubMed]
78. FDA Approves Neratinib for Metastatic HER2-Positive Breast Cancer. Available online: https://www.fda.gov/drugs/resources-information-approved-drugs/fda-approves-neratinib-metastatic-her2-positive-breast-cancer (accessed on 18 February 2021).
79. O'Reilly, E.M.; Hechtman, J.H. Tumour response to TRK inhibition in a patient with pancreatic adenocarcinoma harbouring an *NTRK* gene fusion. *Ann. Oncol.* **2019**, *30*, viii36–viii40. [CrossRef]
80. Prescribing Information of GAVRETO. Available online: https://www.accessdata.fda.gov/drugsatfda_docs/label/2020/213721s000lbl.pdf (accessed on 8 February 2021).
81. FDA Approves Pralsetinib for Lung Cancer with RET Gene Fusions. Available online: https://www.fda.gov/drugs/resources-information-approved-drugs/fda-approves-pralsetinib-lung-cancer-ret-gene-fusions (accessed on 8 February 2021).
82. Odogwu, L.; Mathieu, L.; Blumenthal, G.; Larkins, E.; Goldberg, K.B.; Griffin, N.; Bijwaard, K.; Lee, E.Y.; Philip, R.; Jian, X.; et al. FDA Approval Summary: Dabrafenib and Trametinib for the Treatment of Metastatic Non-Small Cell Lung Cancers Harboring BRAF V600E Mutations. *Oncologist* **2018**, *23*, 740–745. [CrossRef] [PubMed]
83. Cortellis. Available online: https://www.cortellis.com/intelligence/home.do (accessed on 24 April 2021).
84. Application Number: 213721Orig1s000 Administrative and Correspondence Documents. Available online: https://www.accessdata.fda.gov/drugsatfda_docs/nda/2020/213721Orig1s000AdminCorres.pdf (accessed on 25 April 2021).
85. Application Number: 213736Orig1s000 Multi-Discipline Review. Available online: https://www.accessdata.fda.gov/drugsatfda_docs/nda/2020/213736Orig1s000MultidisciplineR.pdf (accessed on 25 April 2021).
86. Application Number: 213591Orig1s000 Administrative and Correspondence Documents. Available online: https://www.accessdata.fda.gov/drugsatfda_docs/nda/2020/213591Orig1s000AdminCorres.pdf (accessed on 25 April 2021).
87. Application Number: 210861Orig1s000 211710Orig1s000 MULTI-Discipline Review. Available online: https://www.accessdata.fda.gov/drugsatfda_docs/nda/2018/210861Orig1s000_211710Orig1s000MultidisciplineR.pdf (accessed on 25 April 2021).
88. Mirnezami, R.; Nicholson, J.; Darzi, A. Preparing for Precision Medicine. *N. Engl. J. Med.* **2012**, *366*, 489–491. [CrossRef] [PubMed]
89. Chakradhar, S. Tumor sequencing takes off, but insurance reimbursement lags. *Nat. Med.* **2014**, *20*, 1220–1221. [CrossRef]
90. Makino, T.; Lim, Y.; Kodama, K. Strategic R&D transactions in personalized drug development. *Drug Discov. Today* **2018**, *23*, 1334–1339. [PubMed]
91. Sengoku, S.; Sakurai, M.; Yashiro, Y. Japan's regulatory framework: Seeking to provide impetus to the commercialization of regenerative medicine products. *Cell Gene Ther. Insights* **2015**, *1*, 83–92. [CrossRef]

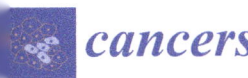

Opinion

Using Electronic Medical Records to Identify Potentially Eligible Study Subjects for Lung Cancer Screening with Biomarkers

Lamorna Brown *, Utkarsh Agrawal and Frank Sullivan

School of Medicine, University of St Andrews, St Andrews KY16 9AJ, UK; ua1@st-andrews.ac.uk (U.A.); fms20@st-andrews.ac.uk (F.S.)
* Correspondence: lb300@st-andrews.ac.uk; Tel.: +44-7824793243

Simple Summary: Recent cancer screening trials have found that using low-dose computed tomography (LDCT), compared to chest radiography, resulted in a significant reduction in lung cancer mortality. To effectively carry out this intervention, individuals at a high risk of developing lung cancer are targeted. However, accurately identifying and retaining these groups can be challenging. As electronic medical records (EMRs) contain important demographic and clinical information, they could be used to accurately identify subjects for screening. To determine whether EMRs can be used for this purpose, this paper examines the evidence around the use of EMRs in screening trials and the information contained in them that could be used to aid researchers in identifying eligible subjects.

Abstract: Lung cancer screening trials using low-dose computed tomography (LDCT) show reduced late-stage diagnosis and mortality rates. These trials have identified high-risk groups that would benefit from screening. However, these sub-populations can be difficult to access and retain in trials. Implementation of national screening programmes further suggests that there is poor uptake in eligible populations. A new approach to participant selection may be more effective. Electronic medical records (EMRs) are a viable alternative to population-based or health registries, as they contain detailed clinical and demographic information. Trials have identified that e-screening using EMRs has improved trial retention and eligible subject identification. As such, this paper argues for greater use of EMRs in trial recruitment and screening programmes. Moreover, this opinion paper explores the current issues in and approaches to lung cancer screening, whether records can be used to identify eligible subjects for screening and the challenges that researchers face when using EMR data.

Keywords: cancer; screening; smoking; electronic records

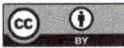

1. Introduction

Lung cancer remains one of the most aggressive and frequently diagnosed cancers in the UK [1]. Mortality rates for the disease remain high, at 21% for both males and females, making it the most common cause of cancer-related death [2]. As late-stage lung cancer (i.e., stage III/IV) is less susceptible to curative medical interventions, such as surgical resection, there is a low survival rate for individuals diagnosed at these stages (2–3%) [2]. The majority of lung cancer cases are diagnosed with late-stage cancer, leading to overall low survival rates at 1 (40%) and 5 years (16%) post-diagnosis [1,3,4].

To reduce late-stage diagnosis, lung cancer screening using low-dose computed tomography (LDCT) has been recommended [5]. Screening trials using LDCT, compared to usual care (i.e., chest X-rays), have provided evidence of a significant mortality benefit. Trials such as the NLST, NELSON and UK Lung Cancer Screening Trial found those undergoing LDCT scans had a reduced probability of dying from lung cancer [6–8]. The Early Detection of Cancer of the Lung Scotland (ECLS) trial also indicated that blood-based biomarkers are effective when used in conjunction with LDCT, significantly reducing late-stage diagnosis and lung cancer mortality [9].

While these trials support the use of LDCT in screening programmes to identify lung cancer, there are practical barriers that can reduce participant engagement, limiting the effectiveness of interventions [10]. These practical barriers include difficulties accessing target groups and identifying patients that fit screening inclusion criteria [10–12]. However, electronic medical records (EMRs) contain important clinical and demographic information that can reduce and resolve these issues [13].

This paper covers the current issues in and approaches to lung cancer screening and appraises the methods used and evidence for the effectiveness and appropriateness of using electronic medical records as a way of identifying those at high risk of developing cancer.

Defining high-risk groups for lung cancer screening is an ongoing challenge. Age, occupation, family history, some respiratory conditions (particularly emphysema) and environmental factors such as air pollution and radon exposure are important risk factors for lung cancer [14,15]. The strongest determinant of lung cancer, however, is smoking, with over 70% of cases in the UK linked to smoking [16,17]. As a result, smoking status has been used to identify eligible participants for lung cancer trials. In this article, we consider an important characteristic of high-risk groups to be whether they are current smokers, and thus papers which report on the recording of smoking in EMRs in order to identify eligible subjects are included in this article. Other health, sociodemographic and environmental risk factors for lung cancer that appear in EMRs are also examined.

2. Issues and Approaches to Current Lung Cancer Screening Programmes

Lung cancer screening programmes use a targeted approach, whereby those most at risk, and thus most likely to benefit from screening, are eligible for inclusion. Trials such as the NELSON and NLST use patient self-declared age and the number of pack years as bases for inclusion using a questionnaire [6,18]. Trials utilising risk models to identify high-risk groups have provided further risk factors to consider for screening criteria, such as family history of lung cancer and respiratory diseases [19]. The use of these models for participant selection has led to lower numbers of individuals eligible for selection but enabled greater prevention of lung cancer death in trials [15,20].

Despite progress in the identification of high-risk individuals, low participation and retention rates can hinder the effectiveness of interventions. Table 1 presents the approach response rates, methods of recruitment and percentage of respondents randomised for some of the major European lung cancer screening trials. Previous lung cancer trials have had approach response rates (i.e., the proportion of individuals who responded when approached) between 23 and 52% [21]. To improve these rates, the barriers and issues around lung cancer screening implementation must be explored.

There are both participant- and provider-related barriers to lung cancer screening engagement. The UK Lung Cancer Screening Pilot Trial identified participant demographic factors associated with a reduced likelihood of participation. It was found that those who were female, older, current smokers and from a lower socioeconomic group were less likely to participate [27]. Further, there are both emotional and practical barriers to participation. Practical barriers such as a participant's state of health and emotional barriers such as fear of screening and information avoidance are cited as reasons for non-participation by eligible subjects [27–29]. The stigma associated with lung cancer may also act as a barrier for both participants and providers [30,31]. Patients with lung cancer report feeling more stigmatised by themselves and others compared to individuals with cancers such as breast, cervical and skin cancer, as there is a perception that they have brought the illness upon themselves by smoking [32]. This can delay individuals seeking help and receiving timely investigation and treatment, which can have a detrimental effect on patient outcomes [33]. Stigma is also associated with reduced levels of screening uptake [34].

Table 1. The recruitment strategies, numbers of subjects approached, numbers of respondents and the percentage of respondents randomised in major European lung cancer screening trials.

Lung Cancer Screening Trial	Recruitment Period	Number of Subjects Approached	Number of Subjects That Responded	Approach Response Rate	Number of Eligible Subjects That Consented	% of Respondents Randomised	Method of Recruitment
NELSON [6]	2003–2006	606,409	150,920	24.9%	15,822	10.5%	Direct mail
ITALUNG [22]	2004–2006	71,232	17,055	23.9%	3206	18.8%	Direct mail
LUSI [23]	2007–2011	292,440	95,797	32.8%	4052	4.2%	Direct mail and mass media
NLST [18]	2002–2004	n/a	53,454	n/a	52,486	n/a	Direct mail, mass media and outreach
UKLS [8]	2011–2014	247,354	98,746	39.9%	4061	4.1%	Direct mail
LSUT [24]	2015–2017	2012	1058	52.6%	770	72.8%	Direct mail
LHC Manchester [25]	2016–2018	16,402	2827	17.2%	1384	49.0%	Searched GP records to send direct mail invitations
LHC Liverpool [26]	2016–2018	11,526	4566	39.6%	1318	28.9%	Searched GP records to send direct mail invitations
ECLS [9]	2013–2016	77,077	18,657	24.2%	12,209	65.4%	Searched GP records to send direct mail invitations, mass media and outreach

The significant barriers that providers face relate to identifying and recruiting eligible subjects. Previous lung cancer screening trials identified subjects through population-based registries [21]. Information that could aid in the identification of high-risk groups may not be present in these registries. Additionally, the information that is present may not be accurate and, as a result, researchers risk contacting individuals who do not meet trial eligibility criteria. Trials that use electronic medical records (EMRs) for identifying subjects have shown that both identification and uptake can match those of trials that have utilised population registries. The LHC Liverpool study utilised EMRs to search for eligible subjects before contacting them; this targeted approach resulted in the trial obtaining one of the highest approach response proportions out of recent lung cancer screening trials (40%) [21,26]. The ECLS trial similarly searched for eligible participants through primary care EMRs. This trial recruited 12,208 participants and is, consequently, the largest trial for the detection of lung cancer using blood-based biomarkers [9,35]. Additionally, the ECLS and both LHC trials had a lower percentage of respondents drop out between response to invitation and randomisation (see Table 1). This indicates that EMRs can potentially aid researchers in identifying and retaining eligible study subjects.

3. Can Records Be Used to Aid in Identifying Eligible Subjects for Screening?

EMRs have been used to aid in identifying patients eligible for screening. A large-scale study in Minhang District in China, conducted between 2008 and 2016, used EMRs of 5 million patients to identify those eligible for screening multiple cancers including colorectal, gastric, liver, lung, cervical and breast cancer [36]. As a result, more cases of cancer were detected at an early stage, including a number of individuals who were identified as being at high risk of cancer. Similarly, trials for Lung Health Check programmes, implemented in Liverpool and Manchester, were able to recruit and retain a significant proportion of respondents approached [9,26]. These studies indicate that EMRs could be used to conduct more focused interventions. In addition, previous studies have also used machine learning algorithms on smoking history information, identified from EMRs, to create a registry of patients eligible for cancer control efforts, such as smoking cessation and lung cancer screening, which could additionally aid in targeting eligible patients for screening [37,38].

3.1. What Codes Are Associated with LC and Appear in EMRs?

Codes are frequently used to identify patients with various health conditions. Published comorbidity indices and phenotype code lists, such as CALIBER, the Charlson Comorbidity Index, the Elixhauser Comorbidity Index and the Quality and Outcomes Framework (QOF), have compiled a list of codes for lung cancer [39–43]. Moreover, different coding formats are used within different data sources in the EMRs, for example, primary care settings use read codes and secondary care settings use ICD codes [44,45]. A sample code list is presented in Appendix A, Table A1.

Various smoking codes are present within EMRs. These can be used to identify high-risk smokers for screening. Wiley et al. (2013) and Atkinson et al. (2018) examined whether smoking read codes present in EMRs could be used to determine the smoking status of participants [46,47]. Wiley et al. used ICD-9 smoking codes and found that they could accurately detect true smokers in a general population [46]. The combination of codes and free text improved sensitivity to ever smokers, however. Atkinson et al. used smoking read codes found in primary care general practice records to assess participants' smoking history [47]. They found that read codes compared well with a population health survey (Kappa–0.64), indicating that read codes are moderately accurate and, thus, can be used in the identification of smokers.

Codes for health conditions and environmental factors present in EMRs could also be used to identify high-risk groups. A study utilising EMRs from general practices across the UK found that asbestos exposure, COPD and symptoms such as coughing and chest pain were frequently recorded in EMR documentation and prevalent among those diagnosed with lung cancer [48]. Further to this, COPD recording has been explored in

EMRs. Algorithms have been developed to determine the presence of COPD in patients. Quint et al. (2014) and Chu et al. (2021) developed two such algorithms that performed well, with positive predictive values (PPVs) of 86.5% and 93.5% [49,50].

Other risk factors such as alcohol consumption and asthma have also been examined. Read codes for alcohol consumption have been validated by comparing EMR data to a health survey. The study by Mansfield et al. (2019) found similar prevalence rates between both a health survey and an EMR dataset, indicating EMRs can be accurately used to identify both current and non-drinkers [51]. Asthma has been validated in EMRs, with the PPVs of studies comparing asthma codes to a reference ranging from 46 to 100% [52].

While there are other social and environmental determinants of lung cancer, such as air pollution and radon exposure, this detailed information is not routinely collected in EMRs. To examine environmental factors, recent studies have linked geospatial and environmental data to EMRs in order to examine related health outcomes [53–55]. Greater consensus on measures to be captured in EMRs, as well as improvements in the linking of external sources of environmental data, could address this issue.

3.2. Use of Free Text to Identify Eligible Participants?

Most studies have used structured variables such as smoking status (non-smoker; ex-smoker; light smoker; moderate smoker; heavy smoker), asthma diagnosed ever (yes/no), pneumonia diagnosed ever (yes/no) and family history of lung cancer (yes/no) to estimate the risk of having lung cancer and to identify participants eligible for lung cancer screening studies [19,56,57]. However, recent studies have begun to explore free text in EMRs to identify eligible patients [58–60].

Natural language processing provides a feasible way to extract various types of information from EMRs. This technique has been successfully used to extract and quantify smoking information in EMRs. De Silva et al. and Palmer et al. used text analysis to quantify pack years from EMR free text [61,62]. This was successfully performed for the majority of cases, but due to the heterogeneity of clinical notes, mis-categorisation and missing cases remained an issue. Smoking status can also be identified accurately from EMRs. Groenhof et al. extracted information on smoking behaviours from free text to categorise participants into current, past and never smokers. Smoking information was accurately retrieved for the majority of cases [63].

This method of smoker identification may be more accurate and less costly and time consuming compared to asking potential participants to fill out questionnaires or to assess their own eligibility for screening. Indeed, free text in EMRs has provided more accurate and comprehensive information on smoking than structured sources of data from EMRs [64]. As these papers indicate that smoking information is present in EMRs and that smokers and non-smokers can be accurately identified from the information contained in them, this method of identification may be feasible for participant identification.

4. What Are the Challenges in Using EMR Data to Detect and Identify High-Risk Populations?

While, when utilising EMR data, screening programmes may achieve better targeting of eligible subjects, there are significant challenges to using EMR data. Data completeness for certain coded data elements can vary, with diagnostic and lifestyle data being less populated than prescription data [62]. Indeed, two prevalent issues affecting data completeness are missing data elements and errors in the recording of health conditions/lifestyle factors. Martin found 43% of the electronic records examined contained errors. Indeed, multiple errors were found in participant records which resulted in a total of 229 errors in 169 participant records [65]. Marston et al.'s study found that 20% of their sample had missing smoking data [66]. While overall trends show that the recording of risk factors such as smoking status has improved, missing data are still a concern, with recorded information on health care indicators only present in 10–40% of sampled EMRs [67–70].

The accuracy and quality of EMR data are a further issue. This is usually examined by comparing coded or extracted EMR data against a "gold standard" reference. Studies examining data quality show mixed results. Booth et al. examined CPRD data compared to population survey data [71]. They found little difference between the prevalence of smoking in CPRD data compared to the population survey. Estimates for current smokers and non-smokers were similar to survey data estimates, but there was underreporting of former smokers in EMRs. Similarly, asthma recording in EMRs was found to compare moderately well with manual chart reviews, with NLP and diagnosis code-based algorithms generating PPVs of 88.0% and 57.1% [72]. Conversely, Modin et al. found significant discordance between pack years recorded in EMRs and pack years determined from a shared decision-making conversation [73]. This research highlights the difficulties in truly determining data accuracy as references may not contain accurate information.

Obtaining ethical approval to access EMRs is equally challenging. EMRs contain sensitive information which means it is imperative that the data are stored and accessed in a secure way. As a result, it can be both costly and time consuming to access and obtain EMR data. Given that the use of EMR data in clinical research has grown, the development and usage of Data Safe Havens to store EMR data have mitigated some of the ethical concerns around the accessibility and storage of the data.

5. Future Research

There has been significant research on the extraction and classification of smoking status in EMRs. However, further research on the use of EMR information to identify and flag patients for follow-ups or screening is required. Safety netting is viewed as a best practice for those at risk of cancer, although there is little evidence for its effectiveness for cancer detection [74]. The use of EMRs to detect and flag patients for follow-ups has been successfully implemented to detect risk of adverse events, delays in follow-ups to abnormal lung imaging findings and delays in cancer diagnosis [75–77]. Algorithms that detect delays in follow-ups have identified a lack of appropriate follow-up action based on four diagnostic cues. The same could be performed to investigate their use for flagging patients that either partially or fully meet screening criteria.

While there is a significant amount of research examining the validity of smoking behaviours in EMRs, further research could be conducted to examine quality for other data elements. There are few papers examining environmental factors such as asbestos and radon exposure. Examining the completeness, accuracy and frequency of recordings for these exposures could aid in identifying high-risk populations.

Further research on lung cancer risk modelling using EMR data is also required [6]. Many risk models have been developed which include clinical and demographic factors. These models utilise trial or registry data and, as a result, there is a lack of research examining the use of real-world EMR information and the use of linked datasets in risk modelling [78]. Wang et al. used EMR data to model the incidence of lung cancer, and they were able to extract a large number of features to include, demonstrating the usefulness of EMR data in modelling [79]. Additionally, further examination of risk models using EMR data would be useful to identify whether models apply well to other datasets.

6. Conclusions

Lung cancer screening using LDCT and biomarkers has the potential to reduce late diagnosis, thereby lowering mortality rates and improving survival of the disease. However, there are significant issues with the detection of subjects eligible for lung cancer screening. Screening trials and programmes have low approach response rates, despite targeting those at a higher risk of developing cancer.

EMRs have provided useful information for clinicians and researchers which has resulted in greater engagement. For example, both the LSUT study and ECLS trial recruited a large number of participants by identifying eligible patients through EMRs. Further, the research presented in this article has shown there are data features contained in EMRs that have the ability to aid screening, such as smoking information contained in codes and free clinical text. This information can ensure that eligible populations are easier to access for researchers/clinicians and that, as a result, these individuals can be better targeted.

There are significant challenges to using EMR data such as a lack of data completeness and data accuracy. With the advances in text analysis and improvements in EMR structure and codes, they may be a viable option that both health systems and researchers can use to identify populations for lung cancer screening.

Author Contributions: Conceptualisation, F.S. and L.B.; introduction, L.B.; Section 1, L.B.; Section 2, U.A.; Section 3, L.B.; future research, L.B.; conclusions, L.B. All authors have read and agreed to the published version of the manuscript.

Funding: This research was funded by Oncimmune Ltd. (grant number SMD0-ZGO002) nand The Melville Trust for the Care and Cure of Cancer (grant number M00109.0001/TZH/MHR).

Institutional Review Board Statement: Not applicable.

Informed Consent Statement: Not applicable.

Data Availability Statement: Not applicable.

Acknowledgments: Not applicable.

Conflicts of Interest: The authors declare no conflict of interest. The funders had no role in the design of the study; in the collection, analyses or interpretation of data; in the writing of the manuscript, or in the decision to publish the results.

Appendix A

Table A1. Read codes and their associated read terms and conditions.

Read Code	Read Term	Condition
B220100	Malignant neoplasm of mucosa of trachea	Primary Malignancy-Lung
B220.00	Malignant neoplasm of trachea	Primary Malignancy-Lung
B220z00	Malignant neoplasm of trachea NOS	Primary Malignancy-Lung
B221000	Malignant neoplasm of carina of bronchus	Primary Malignancy-Lung
B221100	Malignant neoplasm of hilus of lung	Primary Malignancy-Lung
B221.00	Malignant neoplasm of main bronchus	Primary Malignancy-Lung
B221z00	Malignant neoplasm of main bronchus NOS	Primary Malignancy-Lung
B222000	Malignant neoplasm of upper lobe bronchus	Primary Malignancy-Lung
B222100	Malignant neoplasm of upper lobe of lung	Primary Malignancy-Lung
B222.00	Malignant neoplasm of upper lobe, bronchus or lung	Primary Malignancy-Lung
B222.11	Pancoast's syndrome	Primary Malignancy-Lung
B222z00	Malignant neoplasm of upper lobe, bronchus or lung NOS	Primary Malignancy-Lung
B223000	Malignant neoplasm of middle lobe bronchus	Primary Malignancy-Lung
B223100	Malignant neoplasm of middle lobe of lung	Primary Malignancy-Lung
B223.00	Malignant neoplasm of middle lobe, bronchus or lung	Primary Malignancy-Lung
B223z00	Malignant neoplasm of middle lobe, bronchus or lung NOS	Primary Malignancy-Lung
B224000	Malignant neoplasm of lower lobe bronchus	Primary Malignancy-Lung
B224100	Malignant neoplasm of lower lobe of lung	Primary Malignancy-Lung
B224.00	Malignant neoplasm of lower lobe, bronchus or lung	Primary Malignancy-Lung
B224z00	Malignant neoplasm of lower lobe, bronchus or lung NOS	Primary Malignancy-Lung
B225.00	Malignant neoplasm of overlapping lesion of bronchus and lung	Primary Malignancy-Lung
B22..00	Malignant neoplasm of trachea, bronchus and lung	Primary Malignancy-Lung
B22y.00	Malignant neoplasm of other sites of bronchus or lung	Primary Malignancy-Lung
B22z.00	Malignant neoplasm of bronchus or lung NOS	Primary Malignancy-Lung
B22z.11	Lung cancer	Primary Malignancy-Lung
BB5S200	[M]Bronchiolo-alveolar adenocarcinoma	Primary Malignancy-Lung
BB5S211	[M]Alveolar cell carcinoma	Primary Malignancy-Lung
BB5S212	[M]Bronchiolar carcinoma	Primary Malignancy-Lung
BB5S400	[M]Alveolar adenocarcinoma	Primary Malignancy-Lung
Byu2000	[X]Malignant neoplasm of bronchus or lung, unspecified	Primary Malignancy-Lung
ZV10100	[V]Personal history of malig neop of trachea/bronchus/lung	Primary Malignancy-Lung
ZV10111	[V]Personal history of malignant neoplasm of bronchus	Primary Malignancy-Lung
ZV10112	[V]Personal history of malignant neoplasm of lung	Primary Malignancy-Lung
ICD10 code	ICD10 term	Condition
C33	Malignant neoplasm of trachea	Primary Malignancy-Lung
C34	Malignant neoplasm of bronchus and lung	Primary Malignancy-Lung

References

1. Cancer Research, U.K. Lung Cancer Statistics. 2021. Available online: https://www.cancerresearchuk.org/health-professional/cancer-statistics/statistics-by-cancer-type/lung-cancer#heading-Zero (accessed on 12 May 2021).
2. Cancer Research, U.K. Lung Cancer Mortality. 2021. Available online: https://www.cancerresearchuk.org/health-professional/cancer-statistics/statistics-by-cancer-type/lung-cancer/mortality#heading-Zero (accessed on 12 May 2021).
3. Birring, S.S.; Peake, M.D. Symptoms and the early diagnosis of lung cancer. *Thorax* **2005**, *60*, 268–269. [CrossRef] [PubMed]
4. Cancer Research, U.K. Advanced Stage Lung Cancer. 2021. Available online: https://www.cancerresearchuk.org/about-cancer/lung-cancer/advanced/about (accessed on 12 May 2021).
5. Oudkerk, M.; Devaraj, A.; Vliegenthart, R.; Henzler, T.; Prosch, H.; Heussel, C.P.; Bastarrika, G.; Sverzellati, N.; Mascalchi, M.; Delorme, S.; et al. European position statement on lung cancer screening. *Lancet Oncol.* **2017**, *18*, 754–766. [CrossRef]
6. De Koning, H.J.; van der Aalst, C.M.; de Jong, P.A.; Scholten, E.T.; Nackaerts, K.; Heuvelmans, M.A.; Lammers, J.W.; Weenink, C.; Yousaf-Khan, U.; Horeweg, N.; et al. Reduced lung-cancer mortality with volume CT screening in a randomized trial. *N. Engl. J. Med.* **2020**, *382*, 503–513. [CrossRef] [PubMed]
7. Xu, D.M.; Gietema, H.; de Koning, H.; Vernhout, R.; Nackaerts, K.; Prokop, M.; Weenink, C.; Lammers, J.W.; Groen, H.; Oudkerk, M.; et al. Nodule management protocol of the NELSON randomised lung cancer screening trial. *Lung Cancer* **2006**, *54*, 177–184. [CrossRef]
8. Field, J.K.; Duffy, S.W.; Baldwin, D.R.; Brain, K.E.; Devaraj, A.; Eisen, T.; Green, B.A.; Holemans, J.A.; Kavanagh, T.; Kerr, K.M.; et al. The, U.K. Lung Cancer Screening Trial: A pilot randomised controlled trial of low-dose computed tomography screening for the early detection of lung cancer. *Health Technol. Assess.* **2016**, *20*, 1–146. [CrossRef]
9. Sullivan, F.M.; Mair, F.S.; Anderson, W.; Armory, P.; Briggs, A.; Chew, C.; Dorward, A.; Haughney, J.; Hogarth, F.; Kendrick, D.; et al. Earlier diagnosis of lung cancer in a randomised trial of an autoantibody blood test followed by imaging. *Eur. Respir. J.* **2021**, *57*, 1–11. [CrossRef] [PubMed]
10. Wang, G.X.; Baggett, T.P.; Pandharipande, P.V.; Park, E.R.; Percac-Lima, S.; Shepard, J.A.; Fintelmann, F.J.; Flores, E.J. Barriers to lung cancer screening engagement from the patient and provider perspective. *Radiology* **2019**, *290*, 278–287. [CrossRef]
11. Lam, S.; Tammemagi, M. Contemporary issues in the implementation of lung cancer screening. *Eur. Respir. Rev.* **2021**, *30*, 1–17. [CrossRef]
12. Carter-Harris, L.; Gould, M.K. Multilevel barriers to the successful implementation of lung cancer screening: Why does it have to be so hard? *Ann. Am. Thorac. Soc.* **2017**, *14*, 1261–1265. [CrossRef]
13. Thadani, S.R.; Weng, C.; Bigger, J.T.; Ennever, J.F.; Wajngurt, D. Electronic screening improves efficiency in clinical trial recruitment. *J. Am. Med. Inform. Assoc.* **2009**, *16*, 869–873. [CrossRef]
14. Malhotra, J.; Malvezzi, M.; Negri, E.; La Vecchia, C.; Boffetta, P. Risk factors for lung cancer worldwide. *Eur. Respir. J.* **2016**, *48*, 889–902. [CrossRef]
15. Toumazis, I.; Bastani, M.; Han, S.S.; Plevritis, S.K. Risk-Based lung cancer screening: A systematic review. *Lung Cancer* **2020**, *147*, 154–186. [CrossRef]
16. Gandini, S.; Botteri, E.; Iodice, S.; Boniol, M.; Lowenfels, A.B.; Maisonneuve, P.; Boyle, P. Tobacco smoking and cancer: A meta-analysis. *Int. J. Cancer* **2008**, *122*, 155–164. [CrossRef]
17. Boyle, P.; Maisonneuve, P. Lung cancer and tobacco smoking. *Lung Cancer* **1995**, *12*, 167–181. [CrossRef]
18. Aberle, D.R.; Adams, A.M.; Berg, C.D.; Black, W.C.; Clapp, J.D.; Fagerstrom, R.M.; Gareen, I.F.; Gatsonis, C.; Marcus, P.M.; Sicks, J.D. Reduced lung-cancer mortality with low-dose computed tomographic screening. *N. Engl. J. Med.* **2011**, *365*, 395–409. [PubMed]
19. Katki, H.A.; Kovalchik, S.A.; Berg, C.D.; Cheung, L.C.; Chaturvedi, A.K. Development and validation of risk models to select ever-smokers for CT lung cancer screening. *JAMA* **2016**, *315*, 2300–2311. [CrossRef]
20. Ten Haaf, K.; Bastani, M.; Cao, P.; Jeon, J.; Toumazis, I.; Han, S.S.; Plevritis, S.K.; Blom, E.F.; Kong, C.Y.; Tammemägi, M.C.; et al. A comparative modeling analysis of risk-based lung cancer screening strategies. *JNCI J. Natl. Cancer Inst.* **2020**, *112*, 466–479. [CrossRef]
21. Rankin, N.M.; McWilliams, A.; Marshall, H.M. Lung cancer screening implementation: Complexities and priorities. *Respirology* **2020**, *25*, 5–23. [CrossRef] [PubMed]
22. Paci, E.; Puliti, D.; Pegna, A.L.; Carrozzi, L.; Picozzi, G.; Falaschi, F.; Pistelli, F.; Aquilini, F.; Ocello, C.; Zappa, M.; et al. Mortality, survival and incidence rates in the ITALUNG randomised lung cancer screening trial. *Thorax* **2017**, *72*, 825–831. [CrossRef]
23. Becker, N.; Motsch, E.; Trotter, A.; Heussel, C.P.; Dienemann, H.; Schnabel, P.A.; Kauczor, H.U.; Maldonado, S.G.; Miller, A.B.; Kaaks, R.; et al. Lung cancer mortality reduction by LDCT screening—Results from the randomized German, LUSI trial. *Int. J. Cancer* **2020**, *146*, 1503–1513. [CrossRef] [PubMed]
24. Quaife, S.L.; Ruparel, M.; Dickson, J.L.; Beeken, R.J.; McEwen, A.; Baldwin, D.R.; Bhowmik, A.; Navani, N.; Sennett, K.; Duffy, S.W.; et al. Lung Screen Uptake Trial (LSUT): Randomized Controlled Clinical Trial Testing Targeted Invitation Materials. *Am. J. Respir. Crit. Care Med.* **2020**, *201*, 965–975. [CrossRef]
25. Crosbie, P.A.; Balata, H.; Evison, M.; Atack, M.; Bayliss-Brideaux, V.; Colligan, D.; Duerden, R.; Eaglesfield, J.; Edwards, T.; Elton, P.; et al. Implementing lung cancer screening: Baseline results from a community-based 'Lung Health Check'pilot in deprived areas of Manchester. *Thorax* **2019**, *74*, 405–409. [CrossRef] [PubMed]

26. Ghimire, B.; Maroni, R.; Vulkan, D.; Shah, Z.; Gaynor, E.; Timoney, M.; Jones, L.; Arvanitis, R.; Ledson, M.; Lukehirst, L.; et al. Evaluation of a health service adopting proactive approach to reduce high risk of lung cancer: The Liverpool Healthy Lung Programme. *Lung Cancer* **2019**, *134*, 66–71. [CrossRef]
27. Ali, N.; Lifford, K.J.; Carter, B.; McRonald, F.; Yadegarfar, G.; Baldwin, D.R.; Weller, D.; Hansell, D.M.; Duffy, S.W.; Field, J.K.; et al. Barriers to uptake among high-risk individuals declining participation in lung cancer screening: A mixed methods analysis of the UK Lung Cancer Screening (UKLS) trial. *BMJ Open* **2015**, *5*, e008254. [CrossRef] [PubMed]
28. Patel, D.; Akporobaro, A.; Chinyanganya, N.; Hackshaw, A.; Seale, C.; Spiro, S.G.; Griffiths, C. Attitudes to participation in a lung cancer screening trial: A qualitative study. *Thorax* **2012**, *67*, 418–425. [CrossRef] [PubMed]
29. Quaife, S.L.; Marlow, L.A.; McEwen, A.; Janes, S.M.; Wardle, J. Attitudes towards lung cancer screening in socioeconomically deprived and heavy smoking communities: Informing screening communication. *Health Expect.* **2017**, *20*, 563–573. [CrossRef]
30. Chapple, A.; Ziebland, S.; McPherson, A. Stigma, shame, and blame experienced by patients with lung cancer: Qualitative study. *BMJ* **2004**, *328*, 1470. [CrossRef]
31. Van Hal, G.; Garcia, P.D. Lung cancer screening: Targeting the hard to reach—A review. *Transl. Lung Cancer Res.* **2021**, *10*, 2309–2322. [CrossRef]
32. Williamson, T.J.; Rawl, S.M.; Kale, M.S.; Carter-Harris, L. Lung cancer screening and stigma: Do smoking-related differences in perceived lung cancer stigma emerge prior to diagnosis? *Stigma Health* **2021**, *63*. [CrossRef]
33. Carter-Harris, L. Lung cancer stigma as a barrier to medical help-seeking behavior: Practice implications. *J. Am. Assoc. Nurse Pract.* **2015**, *27*, 240–245. [CrossRef]
34. Vrinten, C.; Gallagher, A.; Waller, J.; Marlow, L.A. Cancer stigma and cancer screening attendance: A population based survey in England. *BMC Cancer* **2019**, *19*, 566. [CrossRef] [PubMed]
35. Sullivan, F.M.; Farmer, E.; Mair, F.S.; Treweek, S.; Kendrick, D.; Jackson, C.; Robertson, C.; Briggs, A.; McCowan, C.; Bedford, L.; et al. Detection in blood of autoantibodies to tumour antigens as a case-finding method in lung cancer using the EarlyCDT®-Lung Test (ECLS): Study protocol for a randomized controlled trial. *BMC Cancer* **2017**, *17*, 1. [CrossRef] [PubMed]
36. He, D.; Xu, W.; Su, H.; Li, W.; Zhou, J.; Yao, B.; Xu, D.; He, N. Electronic health Record-Based screening for major cancers: A 9-year experience in Minhang district of Shanghai, China. *Front. Oncol.* **2019**, *9*, 375. [CrossRef]
37. Onega, T.; Nutter, E.L.; Sargent, J.; Doherty, J.A.; Hassanpour, S. Identifying patient smoking history for cessation and lung cancer screening through mining electronic health records. *Cancer Epidemiol. Prev. Biomark.* **2017**, *26*, 437. [CrossRef]
38. Hippisley-Cox, J.; Coupland, C. Identifying patients with suspected lung cancer in primary care: Derivation and validation of an algorithm. *Br. J. Gen. Pract.* **2011**, *61*, 715–723. [CrossRef]
39. Kuan, V.; Denaxas, S.; Gonzalez-Izquierdo, A.; Direk, K.; Bhatti, O.; Husain, S.; Sutaria, S.; Hingorani, M.; Nitsch, D.; Parisinos, C.A.; et al. A chronological map of 308 physical and mental health conditions from 4 million individuals in the English National Health Service. *Lancet Digit. Health* **2019**, *1*, 63–77. [CrossRef]
40. Charlson, M.E.; Pompei, P.; Ales, K.L.; MacKenzie, C.R. A new method of classifying prognostic comorbidity in longitudinal studies: Development and validation. *J. Chronic Dis.* **1987**, *40*, 373–383. [CrossRef]
41. Elixhauser, A.; Steiner, C.; Harris, D.R.; Coffey, R.M. Comorbidity measures for use with administrative data. *Med. Care* **1998**, *36*, 8–27. [CrossRef]
42. Metcalfe, D.; Masters, J.; Delmestri, A.; Judge, A.; Perry, D.; Zogg, C.; Gabbe, B.; Costa, M. Coding algorithms for defining Charlson and Elixhauser co-morbidities in Read-coded databases. *BMC Med. Res. Methodol.* **2019**, *19*, 115. [CrossRef]
43. NHS Digital, Quality and Outcomes Framework. 2020. Available online: https://digital.nhs.uk/data-and-information/publications/statistical/quality-and-outcomes-framework-achievement-prevalence-and-exceptions-data (accessed on 21 May 2021).
44. NHS Digital, Read Codes. 2020. Available online: https://digital.nhs.uk/services/terminology-and-classifications/read-codes (accessed on 21 May 2021).
45. NHS Digital, NHS Classification Service. *NHS Digit. Trud.* **2021**. Available online: https://isd.digital.nhs.uk/trud3/user/guest/group/0/home (accessed on 20 May 2021).
46. Wiley, L.K.; Shah, A.; Xu, H.; Bush, W.S. ICD-9 tobacco use codes are effective identifiers of smoking status. *J. Am. Med. Inform. Assoc.* **2013**, *20*, 652–658. [CrossRef]
47. Atkinson, M.D.; Kennedy, J.I.; John, A.; Lewis, K.E.; Lyons, R.A.; Brophy, S.T. Development of an algorithm for determining smoking status and behaviour over the life course from UK electronic primary care records. *BMC Med. Inform. Decis. Mak.* **2017**, *17*, 2. [CrossRef] [PubMed]
48. Soriano, L.C.; Zong, J.; Rodríguez, L.A. Feasibility and validity of The Health Improvement Network database of primary care electronic health records to identify and characterise patients with small cell lung cancer in the United Kingdom. *BMC Cancer* **2019**, *19*, 91. [CrossRef]
49. Quint, J.K.; Müllerova, H.; DiSantostefano, R.L.; Forbes, H.; Eaton, S.; Hurst, J.R.; Davis, K.; Smeeth, L. Validation of chronic obstructive pulmonary disease recording in the Clinical Practice Research Datalink (CPRD-GOLD). *BMJ Open* **2014**, *4*, e005540. [CrossRef] [PubMed]
50. Chu, S.H.; Wan, E.S.; Cho, M.H.; Goryachev, S.; Gainer, V.; Linneman, J.; Scotty, E.J.; Hebbring, S.J.; Murphy, S.; Lasky-Su, J.; et al. An independently validated, portable algorithm for the rapid identification of COPD patients using electronic health records. *Sci. Rep.* **2021**, *11*, 19959. [CrossRef]

51. Mansfield, K.; Crellin, E.; Denholm, R.; Quint, J.K.; Smeeth, L.; Cook, S.; Herrett, E. Completeness and validity of alcohol recording in general practice within the UK: A cross-sectional study. *BMJ Open* **2019**, *9*, e031537. [CrossRef] [PubMed]
52. Nissen, F.; Quint, J.K.; Wilkinson, S.; Mullerova, H.; Smeeth, L.; Douglas, I.J. Validation of asthma recording in electronic health records: A systematic review. *Clin. Epidemiol.* **2017**, *9*, 643. [CrossRef]
53. Schinasi, L.H.; Auchincloss, A.H.; Forrest, C.B.; Roux, A.V. Using electronic health record data for environmental and place based population health research: A systematic review. *Ann. Epidemiol.* **2018**, *28*, 493–502. [CrossRef]
54. Torres-Durán, M.; Casal-Mouriño, A.; Ruano-Ravina, A.; Provencio, M.; Parente-Lamelas, I.; Hernández-Hernández, J.; Vidal-García, I.; Varela-Lema, L.; Valdés Cuadrado, L.; Fernández-Villar, A.; et al. Residential radon and lung cancer characteristics at diagnosis. *Int. J. Radiat. Biol.* **2021**, 1–6. [CrossRef]
55. Boulos, M.N. Towards evidence-based, GIS-driven national spatial health information infrastructure and surveillance services in the United Kingdom. *Int. J. Health Geogr.* **2004**, *3*, 1–50. [CrossRef]
56. Okoli, G.N.; Kostopoulou, O.; Delaney, B.C. Is symptom-based diagnosis of lung cancer possible? A systematic review and meta-analysis of symptomatic lung cancer prior to diagnosis for comparison with real-time data from routine general practice. *PLoS ONE* **2018**, *13*, e0207686. [CrossRef]
57. Klingman, K.J.; Sprey, J. Insomnia disorder diagnosis and treatment patterns in primary care: A cross-sectional analysis of electronic medical records data. *J. Am. Assoc. Nurse Pract.* **2020**, *32*, 145–151. [CrossRef]
58. Solarte-Pabon, O.; Torrente, M.; Rodriguez-González, A.; Provencio, M.; Menasalvas, E.; Tuñas, J.M. Lung cancer diagnosis extraction from clinical notes written in spanish. In Proceedings of the 2020 IEEE 33rd International Symposium on Computer-Based Medical Systems (CBMS), Rochester, MN, USA, 28–30 July 2020; pp. 492–497.
59. Ruiz, E.M.; Tuñas, J.M.; Bermejo, G.; Martín, C.G.; Rodríguez-González, A.; Zanin, M.; de Pedro, C.G.; Méndez, M.; Zaretskaia, O.; Rey, J.; et al. Profiling lung cancer patients using electronic health records. *J. Med. Syst.* **2018**, *42*, 1–10.
60. Jensen, K.; Soguero-Ruiz, C.; Mikalsen, K.O.; Lindsetmo, R.O.; Kouskoumvekaki, I.; Girolami, M.; Skrovseth, S.O.; Augestad, K.M. Analysis of free text in electronic health records for identification of cancer patient trajectories. *Sci. Rep.* **2017**, *7*, 46226. [CrossRef] [PubMed]
61. Palmer, E.L.; Hassanpour, S.; Higgins, J.; Doherty, J.A.; Onega, T. Building a tobacco user registry by extracting multiple smoking behaviors from clinical notes. *BMC Med. Inform. Decis. Mak.* **2019**, *19*, 141. [CrossRef] [PubMed]
62. De Silva, L.; Ginter, T.; Forbush, T.; Nokes, N.; Fay, B.; Mikuls, T.; Cannon, G.; DuVall, S. Extraction and quantification of pack-years and classification of smoker information in semi-structured Medical Records. In Proceedings of the 28th International Conference on Machine Learning, Bellevue, WA, USA, 28 June 2011; pp. 1–8.
63. Groenhof, T.K.; Koers, L.R.; Blasse, E.; de Groot, M.; Grobbee, D.E.; Bots, M.L.; Asselbergs, F.W.; Lely, A.T.; Haitjema, S.; van Solinge, W.; et al. Data mining information from electronic health records produced high yield and accuracy for current smoking status. *J. Clin. Epidemiol.* **2020**, *118*, 100–106. [CrossRef]
64. Wang, L.; Ruan, X.; Yang, P.; Liu, H. Comparison of three information sources for smoking information in electronic health records. *Cancer Inform.* **2016**, *15*, 237–242. [CrossRef]
65. Martin, P.M. Can we trust electronic health records? The smoking test for commission errors. *BMJ Health Care Inform.* **2018**, *25*. [CrossRef]
66. Marston, L.; Carpenter, J.R.; Walters, K.R.; Morris, R.W.; Nazareth, I.; White, I.R.; Petersen, I. Smoker, ex-smoker or non-smoker? The validity of routinely recorded smoking status in UK primary care: A cross-sectional study. *BMJ Open* **2014**, *4*, e004958. [CrossRef]
67. Simpson, C.R.; Hippisley-Cox, J.; Sheikh, A. Trends in the epidemiology of smoking recorded in UK general practice. *Br. J. Gen. Pract.* **2010**, *60*, 121–127. [CrossRef]
68. Szatkowski, L.; Lewis, S.; McNeill, A.; Coleman, T. Is smoking status routinely recorded when patients register with a new GP? *Fam. Pract.* **2010**, *27*, 673–675. [CrossRef] [PubMed]
69. Thiru, K.; Hassey, A.; Sullivan, F. Systematic review of scope and quality of electronic patient record data in primary care. *BMJ* **2003**, *326*, 1070. [CrossRef]
70. Petersen, I.; Welch, C.A.; Nazareth, I.; Walters, K.; Marston, L.; Morris, R.W.; Carpenter, J.R.; Morris, T.P.; Pham, T.M. Health indicator recording in UK primary care electronic health records: Key implications for handling missing data. *Clin. Epidemiol.* **2019**, *11*, 157–167. [CrossRef] [PubMed]
71. Booth, H.P.; Prevost, A.T.; Gulliford, M.C. Validity of smoking prevalence estimates from primary care electronic health records compared with national population survey data for England, 2007 to 2011. *Pharmacoepidemiol. Drug Saf.* **2013**, *22*, 1357–1361. [CrossRef] [PubMed]
72. Wu, S.T.; Sohn, S.; Ravikumar, K.E.; Wagholikar, K.; Jonnalagadda, S.R.; Liu, H.; Juhn, Y.J. Automated chart review for asthma cohort identification using natural language processing: An exploratory study. *Ann. Allergy Asthma Immunol.* **2013**, *111*, 364–369. [CrossRef] [PubMed]
73. Modin, H.E.; Fathi, J.T.; Gilbert, C.R.; Wilshire, C.L.; Wilson, A.K.; Aye, R.W.; Farivar, A.S.; Louie, B.E.; Vallières, E.; Gorden, J.A. Pack-year cigarette smoking history for determination of lung cancer screening eligibility. Comparison of the electronic medical record versus a shared decision-making conversation. *Ann. Am. Thorac. Soc.* **2017**, *14*, 1320–1325. [CrossRef]
74. Nicholson, B.D.; Mant, D.; Bankhead, C. Can safety-netting improve cancer detection in patients with vague symptoms? *BMJ* **2016**, *355*, i5515. [CrossRef]

75. Murphy, D.R.; Laxmisan, A.; Reis, B.A.; Thomas, E.J.; Esquivel, A.; Forjuoh, S.N.; Parikh, R.; Khan, M.M.; Singh, H. Electronic health record-based triggers to detect potential delays in cancer diagnosis. *BMJ Qual. Saf.* **2014**, *23*, 8–16. [CrossRef]
76. Murphy, D.R.; Thomas, E.J.; Meyer, A.N.; Singh, H. Development and validation of electronic health record–based triggers to detect delays in follow-up of abnormal lung imaging findings. *Radiology* **2015**, *277*, 81–87. [CrossRef]
77. Hinrichsen, V.L.; Kruskal, B.; O'Brien, M.A.; Lieu, T.A.; Platt, R. Using electronic medical records to enhance detection and reporting of vaccine adverse events. *J. Am. Med. Inform. Assoc.* **2007**, *14*, 731–735. [CrossRef]
78. Department of Health and Social Care, Data Saves Lives: Reshaping Health an Social Care with Data (Draft). 2021. Available online: https://www.gov.uk/government/publications/data-saves-lives-reshaping-health-and-social-care-with-data-draft/data-saves-lives-reshaping-health-and-social-care-with-data-draft (accessed on 10 August 2021).
79. Wang, X.; Zhang, Y.; Hao, S.; Zheng, L.; Liao, J.; Ye, C.; Xia, M.; Wang, O.; Liu, M.; Weng, C.H.; et al. Prediction of the 1-year risk of incident lung cancer: Prospective study using electronic health records from the state of maine. *J. Med. Internet Res.* **2019**, *21*, 1–17. [CrossRef]

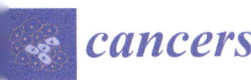

Article

Clinical Guideline-Guided Outcome Consistency for Surgically Resected Stage III Non-Small Cell Lung Cancer: A Retrospective Study

Hiroaki Kuroda [1,*], Yusuke Sugita [2], Katsuhiro Masago [3], Yusuke Takahashi [1], Takeo Nakada [1], Eiichi Sasaki [3], Noriaki Sakakura [1], Rui Yamaguchi [4], Hirokazu Matsushita [2] and Toyoaki Hida [5]

1. Department of Thoracic Surgery, Aichi Cancer Center Hospital, Nagoay 464-8681, Japan; y.takahashi@aichi-cc.jp (Y.T.); t.nakada@aichi-cc.jp (T.N.); nsakakura@aichi-cc.jp (N.S.)
2. Division of Oncoimmunology, Aichi Cancer Center Research Institute, Nagoya 464-8681, Japan; y.sugita07@gmail.com (Y.S.); h.matsushita@aichi-cc.jp (H.M.)
3. Department of Pathology and Molecular Diagnostics, Aichi Cancer Center, Nagoya 464-8681, Japan; masago@aichi-cc.jp (K.M.); esasaki@aichi-cc.jp (E.S.)
4. Division of Cancer Systems Biology, Aichi Cancer Center Research Institute, Nagoya 464-8681, Japan; r.yamaguchi@aichi-cc.jp
5. Department of Thoracic Oncology, Aichi Cancer Center, Nagoya 464-8681, Japan; 107974@aichi-cc.jp
* Correspondence: h-kuroda@aichi-cc.jp; Tel.: +81-52-762-6111; Fax: +81-52-763-5233

Simple Summary: Evidence-based guidelines provide valuable management recommendations that can significantly improve patient treatment and outcome, thereby reducing clinical variability. Recent clinical trials demonstrated that personalised treatments based on genomic and immune profiles can contribute to the prognosis of non-small cell lung cancer (NSCLC). This retrospective study investigated whether guideline-consistency, including adjuvant treatments after surgical resection (ATSR) and guideline-matched first-line treatment for recurrence (GMT-R), could influence overall survival (OS). From 2006 to 2017, 308 patients with pathological stage III NSCLC were eligible, among whom 207 (67.2%) recurrence cases were identified. ATSR and GMT-R were allowed in 164 (53.2%) and 129 (62.3%) cases, respectively. The 5-year OS in guideline-consistent cases receiving ATSR and GMT-R was significantly better than that in guideline-inconsistent cases ($p < 0.01$). Subgroup analyses further revealed that the 5-year OS after propensity adjustment was significantly better in guideline-consistent than in guideline-inconsistent cases ($p < 0.01$). Hence, guideline-consistent treatment alternatives effectively contribute to better outcomes.

Abstract: Clinical guidelines can help reduce the use of inappropriate therapeutics due to localism and individual clinician perspectives. Nevertheless, despite the intention of clinical guidelines to achieve survival benefit or desirable outcomes, they cannot ensure a robust outcome. This retrospective study aimed to investigate whether guideline-consistency, including adjuvant treatments after surgical resection (ATSR) and guideline-matched first-line treatment for recurrence (GMT-R), according to the genomic profiles and immune status, could influence overall survival (OS). From 2006 to 2017, the clinical data of 308 patients with stage III non-small cell lung cancer (NSCLC) after surgical resection were evaluated. ATSR and GMT-R were allowed in 164 (53.2%) and 129 (62.3%) patients cases after surgical pulmonary resection, among which 207 (67.2%) recurrences were identified. The 5-year OS in guideline-consistent cases was significantly better than that in guideline-inconsistent cases ($p < 0.01$). Subgroup analyses further showed that the 5-year OS after propensity adjustment was significantly better in guideline-consistent than in guideline-inconsistent cases ($p < 0.01$), but not in either ATSR or GMT-R ($p = 0.24$). These data suggest that the guideline-consistent alternatives, which comprise ATSR or GMT-R, can contribute to survival benefits in pathological stage III NSCLC. However, only either ATSR or GMT-R has a potential survival benefit in these patients.

Keywords: clinical guideline; non-small cell lung cancer; outcome; overall survival; adjuvant chemotherapy; epidermal growth factor receptor; anaplastic lymphoma receptor tyrosine kinase

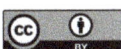

1. Introduction

The landscape of anticancer agents available in the clinical setting has significantly evolved over the past 50 years. In particular, the combination of chemotherapy with cisplatin to target non-small cell lung cancer (NSCLC) that has progressed has allowed the support of a mean length of life of 8–12 months. However, the outcome of these patients still remains poor and further therapeutic options are limited [1]. In the 21st century, due to the bright results of molecular targeted techniques, genome medicine, and immunobiology, the diagnostic and therapeutic efficacy for NSCLC has greatly progressed. These advances have paved the way for physicians and surgeons to be realistically able to see results from translational research. Therefore, a strategy to unify fragmented treatment and, thereby, improve treatment efficacy in clinical practice is indispensable.

The clinical evidence-based quality of treatment indicators for NSCLC is clinically required to ensure adequate management and better treatment strategies. The treatment of NSCLC at various stages is established by correct clinical staging, and treatment strategies are delineated by multidisciplinary teams. Therefore, evidence-based clinical guidelines can provide physicians and surgeons with the same basic principles for conducting lung cancer treatment. Various clinical practice guidelines have been developed to reduce inappropriate treatments, eliminate local and geographic deviations, and authorise the effective use of cancer treatment resources. If resistance to guideline-based first- or second-line treatments is quickly developed, physicians may suggest additional therapies or best supportive care to patients harbouring a more advanced stage.

Our previous report on 2756 NSCLC patients whose tumours were surgically resected between 1990 and 2012 revealed that the 5-year overall survival (OS) rates were 47.6% and 24.1% for patients with stage IIIA ($n = 536$, 19%) and IIIB (+IIIC) ($n = 146$, 5%) cancer, which mainly had lymph node metastasis or involvement of neighbouring structures, respectively [2]. Staged-III NSCLC has locally advanced non-metastatic assets as well as a heterogeneous profile. Accurate staging of patients being investigated by multidisciplinary teams can pave the way for most effective treatments, such as neoadjuvant or adjuvant chemotherapy, with or without surgery, chemotherapy, or additional radiotherapy. Alternatively, for patients with resectable tumours, multimodality treatment, including surgery, can be offered in an attempt to improve survival. Adjuvant chemotherapy has been approved for the treatment of surgically resected stage IB–IIIA NSCLC and is recommended as a standard treatment strategy according to various guidelines [3].

Clinical guidelines have the intention to promote survival benefit or desirable outcomes based on selected randomised studies; however, they cannot ensure a robust outcome. This study focused on two main key words in perioperative clinical guidelines: 'adjuvant treatments after surgically resection' (ATSR) and 'guideline-matched first-line treatment for recurrence' (GMT-R). The aim of this study was to explore whether guideline-consistency could provide specific outcomes according to these two therapeutic alternatives.

2. Materials and Methods

In this prospective cohort, we examined 308 patients with staged-III primary NSCLC who underwent pulmonary resection at the Aichi Cancer Hospital between January 2006 and December 2017. This study was conducted in accordance with the Declaration of Helsinki. The institutional review board of the Aichi Cancer Centre approved this study (2020-1-614). Informed consent obtained by individuals was waived because of the retrospective nature of this cohort. The following exclusion criteria were applied: (1) salvage surgery; (2) patients having final diagnosis as small cell lung cancer or carcinoid; (3) induction chemotherapy with or without radiotherapy; and (4) sublobar resection. All patients with NSCLC underwent lobectomy or more with mediastinal lymph node dissection or sampling. Data postoperatively collected from patient records included age, gender, era, clinical N stage determined by positron emission tomography and computed tomography, prognostic nutrition index or PNI (calculated using the following formula = serum albumin levels (g/dL) $\times$ 10 + total lymphocyte count (per mm^3) $\times$ 0.005)] [4], and smoking status (pack-years). Computed tomography is routinely used as the standard for preoperative lymph node staging, and the commonly used criterion for a clinical diagnosis of N evaluation is a short axis diameter > 10 mm. Resectable indication of cN2 is only single station. If multiple station metastases is clinically suspected, we performed endobronchial ultrasound-guided transbronchial needle aspiration. Pathological stages were defined according to the 8th edition of Union for the International Cancer Control (UICC)/American Joint Committee on Cancer (AJCC) TNM staging criteria [5].

The NCCN guideline [6] indicated these following recommendation: (a) The overall plan of treatment as well as needed imaging studies should be determined before any non-emergency treatment is initiated; (b) Anatomic pulmonary resection is preferred for the majority of patients with NSCLC. (c) N1 or N2 node resection and mapping should be a routine component of lung cancer resections—a minimum of three N2 stations sampled or complete lymph node dissection; (d) Patients with pathologic stage II or greater should be referred to medical oncology for evaluation; (e) The presence of N2-positive lymph nodes substantially increases the likelihood of positive N3 lymph nodes. Pathologic evaluation of the mediastinum must include evaluation of subcarinal station and contralateral lymph nodes; (f) Neoadjuvant chemotherapy would be considered, followed by surgery, when a patient is likely, based on initial evaluation, to require a pnumonectomy. According to guidelines, neoadjuvant treatment is recommended for cN2 disease, but we excluded the patients who had received neoadjuvant chemotherapy or chemoradiotherapy. Our institutional criteria for neoadjuvant therapy is mostly to escape the pnumonectomy. Therefore, we did not consider that enough evaluation of mediastinal lymph node was obtained, preoperatively.

Statistical Analyses

All computations relied on standard software (SPSS version25.0; SPSS Inc, Chicago, IL, USA). Comparisons between the two groups were performed by Mann–Whitney U-tests. Propensity adjustment is defined as the conditional probability calculated by preoperative covariates. Propensity adjustment was estimated using a logistic model including limited variables, which showed a significant difference ($p < 0.05$) by univariate analyses. The Kaplan–Meier method was used to analyse survival rates in the patient subsets; between-group differences in survival were assessed with the log-rank test. Potential correlates of survival were subjected to univariate and multivariate analyses using the Cox proportional hazards regression model.

3. Results

3.1. Patient Flow Algorism

Between January 2006 and December 2017, 308 patients with surgically resected NSCLC were diagnosed with pN2 (cancer spread to 1–4 lymph nodes). Patients who received neoadjuvant chemotherapy were excluded from the analysis because precise information on lymph node mapping could not be obtained. *EGFR* mutations (exons 18–21) have been assessed using the cycleave PCR method since 2006. *ALK* rearrangement and *ROS1* were first screened by immunochemistry, and the final definition was performed by fluorescence in situ hybridisation. Information on these fusion genes has been clinically used since 2007 and 2016. *BRAF* assessment (exons 11 to 15) was based on reverse transcription PCR, coupled with direct sequencing, as previously reported [7]. The expression status of the programmed death-ligand 1 (PD-L1) was determined by immunostaining using two antibodies, either 28-8 or 22C3 pharmDx kits (Dako North America, Carpinteria, CA, USA), and the total proportion score was calculated. Patient flow diagram of this study is shown in Figure 1. The cases were classified as guideline inconsistent or consistent based on the National Comprehensive Cancer Network (NCCN) guideline for NSCLC. Overall, 179 guideline-inconsistent and 129 guideline-inconsistent cases were identified.

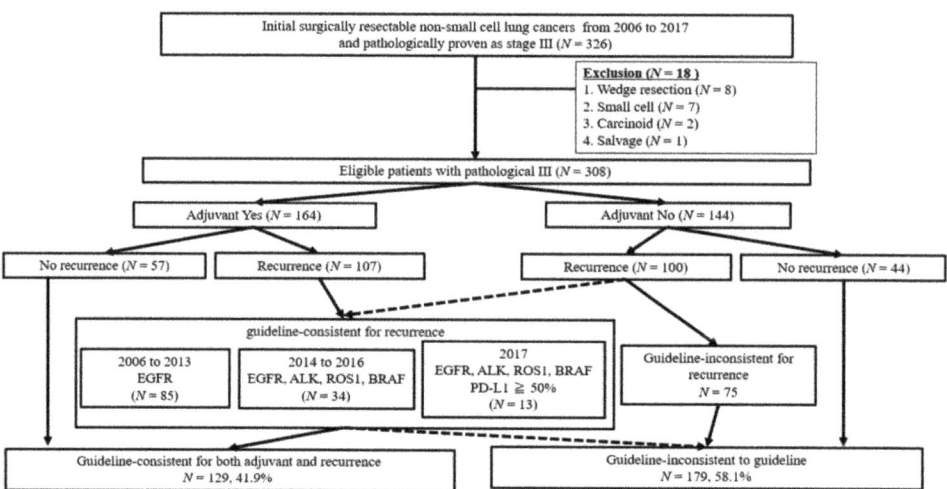

Figure 1. Patient flow diagram.

3.2. Patient Characteristics

Table 1 shows the relevant patient characteristics. According to clinical guidelines for recurrence, ATSR was established as follows: the molecular target drug for EGFR from 2006, for ALK from 2007, for BRAF from 2014, for ROS1 from 2016, for an immune checkpoint inhibitor from 2017, for tumour proportion score (TMS) $\geq$ 50% of program cell death protein 1 (PD-1). Guideline inconsistency was defined as patients with ATSR and GMT-R.

Table 1. Clinicopathological characteristics before propensity adjustment.

Characteristics	Inconsistent n = 179	Consistent n = 129	p-Value
Age (years old), median	67	63	<0.01
IQR	(61–73)	(58–67)	
Gender, male (%)	104 (58.1%)	73 (56.6%)	0.79
Era			0.82
2006–2013	116 (64.8%)	82 (63.6%)	
2014–2017	63 (35.2%)	47 (36.4%)	
Smoking history (pack-year), median	34.0	16.0	0.08
IQR	(0–52.0)	(0–46.5)	
Prognostic nutritional index, median	49.8	52.4	<0.01
IQR	(46.3–53.3)	(49.3–54.7)	
Clinical stage N (number, %)			0.31
cN0	98 (54.7%)	63 (48.8%)	
cN1–2	81 (45.3%)	66 (51.2%)	
Clinical stage			0.80
cI	68 (38.0%)	51 (39.5%)	
cII	46 (25.7%)	32 (24.8%)	
cIII	65 (36.3%)	46 (35.7%)	

Table 1. Cont.

Characteristics	Inconsistent n = 179	Consistent n = 129	p-Value
Histology (number, %)			0.05
Adenocarcinoma	117 (65.4%)	98 (76.0%)	
Others	62 (34.6%)	31 (24.0%)	
Type of procedures (number, %)			0.02
Lobectomy	149 (83.2%)	119 (92.2%)	
Pneumonectomy/Bilobectomy	30 (16.8%)	10 (7.8%)	
ATCR (yes, %)	35 (19.6%)	129 (100%)	<0.01
Pathological-Stage			<0.01
IIIA	167 (93.2%)	123 (95.3%)	
IIIB	12 (6.7%)	6 (4.7%)	
Single lymph node involvement (yes, %)	29 (16.2%)	16 (12.4%)	0.35
Mutation status (yes/no/uninformative)			
EGFR	68/111/0	55/74/0	0.41
ALK	5/140/34	6/95/28	0.35
BRAF	0/62/117	0/40/89	NA
ROS1	0/24/155	1/16/107	NA
Treatment after recurrence (yes, %)	136 (76.0%)	74 (57.4%)	0.04
Local control	26 (19.1%)	7 (9.0%)	
Chemotherapy ± Radiotherapy	55 (40.4%)	21 (28.4%)	
Molecular target drug	37 (27.2%)	44 (59.5%)	
Immune checkpoint inhibitor	4 (3.0%)	2 (2.7%)	
Others	14 (10.3%)	0 (0%)	

ALK, anaplastic lymphoma kinase; ATSR, adjuvant treatments after surgical resection; BRAF, v-raf murine sarcoma viral oncogene homolog B1; EGFR, epidermal growth factor receptor; IQR, interquartile range; NA, not available; ROS1, c-ros oncogene 1.

The methods for the analysis of each mutations, EGFR, ALK, BRAF, and ROS1 have been previously described [8]. EGFR (exons 18–21) mutations were identified using the cycleave polymerase chain reaction method. BRAF (exons 11–15) mutation was assessed using fragment analysis, and the results were validated by direct sequencing. ALK and ROS1 mutations were first screened using immunohistochemistry, and the final confirmation was performed using fluorescence in situ hybridization.

The guideline-inconsistent group ($n = 179$) comprised older patients ($p < 0.01$) and patients with lower prognostic nutritional index ($p < 0.01$) compared with guideline-consistent cases ($n = 128$). Patients within the guideline-consistent group were less likely to undergo lobectomy ($p = 0.02$) and were more like to have non-adenocarcinoma ($p = 0.05$). ATSR was performed in 35 (19.6%) guideline-inconsistent cases.

3.3. Surgical Outcomes and Therapeutic Efficacy in Recurred Patients

The median follow-up duration was 54.4 months (interquartile range (IQR): 30.1–92.5). The 5-year and median OS were significantly better in stage III cases who received ATSR ($n = 164$; 68.0% and 111.3 months, respectively) than in those who did not ($n = 144$; 47.6% and 56.0 months, respectively) ($p < 0.01$) (Figure 2a). Moreover, the 5-year and median disease-free survival (DFS) were significantly better in stage III patients who received ATSR (34.6% and 25 months, respectively) than in those who did not ($n = 23.8$% and 12.8%, respectively; $p = 0.02$) (Figure 2b).

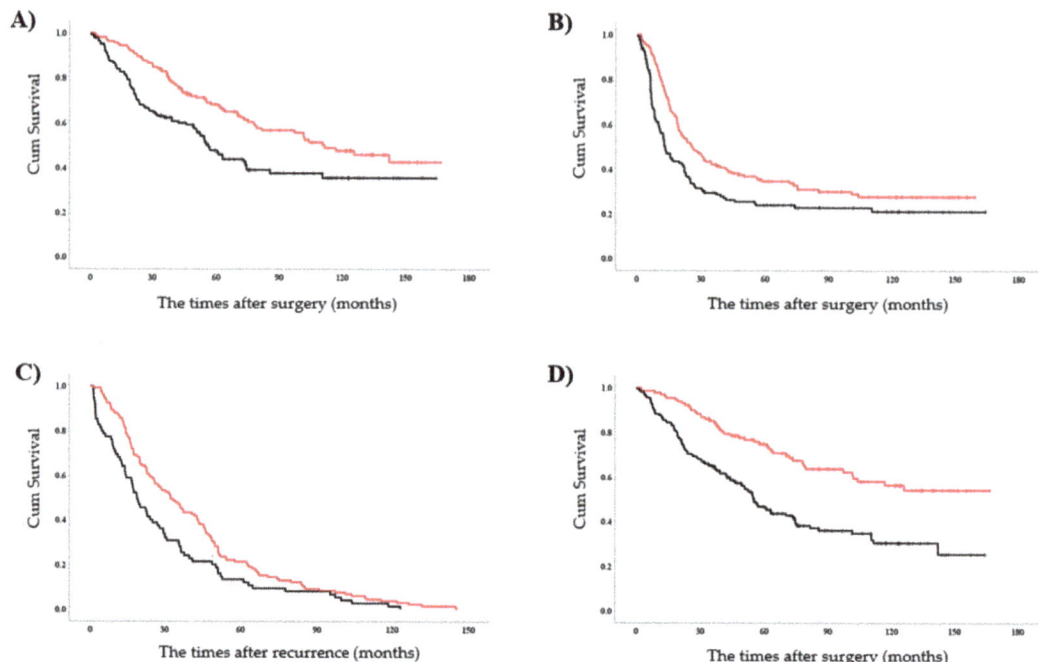

Figure 2. Kaplan–Meier curves. (**A**) Overall survival curve and (**B**) disease-free survival curve after surgical tumour resection stratified according to the adjuvant treatments. Red and black lines represent with and without adjuvant treatments, respectively. (**C**) Overall survival curve after recurrence stratified according to the guideline matched first-line treatment for recurrence. Red and black lines represent yes and no, respectively. (**D**) Overall survival after surgical tumour resection. Red and black lines represent guideline-consistent and guideline-inconsistent cases, respectively.

Overall, 207 patients (67.2%) experienced tumour recurrence during the study period. As shown in Appendix A, the frequent mutation was EGFR (n = 96, 46.4%), followed by ALK (n = 8, 3.8%) and ROS1 (n = 1, 0.5%), while total proportion score ≥ 50% were seen in 5 (2.4%). Among them, target therapy was performed in 69 (71.8%) of EGFR, in 5 (62.5%) of ALK, and in 1 (100%) of ROS1, while 3 patients (60.0%) received immunecheck point inhibitor as first-line treatment. Seventy-two patients from ATSR (67.2%) were subjected to GMT-R, including local therapy in 6 (8.3%), chemotherapy only in 16 (22.2%), chemoradiotherapy in 5 (7.0%), and targeted therapy in 45 (62.5%). The 5-year and median OS were significantly better in recurred patients who received GMT-R (n = 132; 21.2% and 32.1 months, respectively) than in those who did not (n = 75; 13.3% and 18.8 months, respectively; $p < 0.01$) (Figure 2c). Furthermore, the 5-year and median OS were significantly better in the guideline-consistent group (n = 129; 74.8% and not reached, respectively) than in the guideline-inconsistent group (n = 179; 46.5% and 54.9%, respectively; $p < 0.01$) (Figure 2d).

3.4. To Investigate the Prognostic Factor for OS

Multivariate Cox regression analysis of OS after surgical tumour resection was performed according to the results of the univariate analysis. Univariate analyses revealed that age, male sex, prognostic nutritional index (<50), era (2006–2013), guideline-inconsistency, and any genetic mutations were independent OS predictors (Table 2). Multivariate analyses further confirmed that age, era (2006–2013), and guideline inconsistency were independent predictors (Table 2).

Table 2. Univariate and multivariate analyses of overall survival.

Variables		Univariate	Multivariate	
		p-Value	Hazard Ratio (95% CI [1])	p-Value
Patient characteristics				
	Age	<0.01 *	1.02 (1.01–1.04)	0.02 *
	Male	<0.01 *	0.73 (0.50–1.06)	0.10
	Pack-year	0.11		
Prognostic nutritional index				
	Score < 50	0.02 *	0.74 (0.54–1.03)	0.08
Era				
	2006–2013	<0.01 *	0.50 (0.33–0.76)	<0.01 *
Clinical N stage				
	N1–2	0.27		
Histology				
	Adenocarcinoma	0.57		
Procedures				
	More than lobectomy	0.81		
Guideline				
	Inconsistent	<0.01 *	0.49 (0.34–0.71)	<0.01 *
Any mutation				
	Yes	<0.01 *	1.36 (0.94–1.97)	0.10
Pathological N status				
	Single involvement	0.39		

* Statistically significant p-value. [1] CI, confidential index.

3.5. Subgroup Analyses for OS

The study cohort was divided in four groups, as follows: no recurrence (NR), guideline-consistent, either ATSR or GMT-R (EAG), and guideline-inconsistent. The 5-year OS in the guideline-consistent group was significantly better than that in the EAG ($p = 0.03$) and guideline-inconsistent groups ($p < 0.01$). Nonetheless, the 5-year OS in the EAG groups was significantly better than that in the guideline-inconsistent group ($p < 0.01$; Figure 3a).

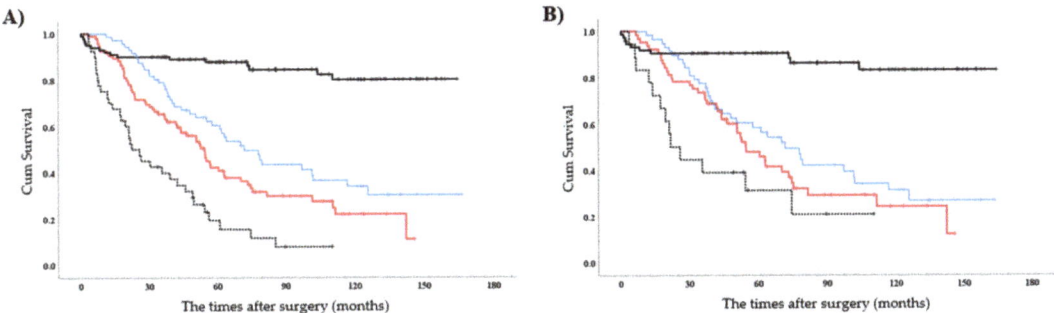

Figure 3. Kaplan–Meier curves in subgroup analyses. Overall survival curve after surgical tumour resection (A) before and (B) after propensity adjustment. Black, blue, red, and dotted lines represent no recurrence (NR group), both adjuvant treatments after surgical resection and guideline-matched first-line treatment for recurrence (guideline-consistent group), either treatment (EAG group), and neither treatment (guideline-inconsistent group).

Propensity adjustment was estimated using a logistic model including age, sex, era, pack-year, prognostic nutritional index, and any mutations, which were selected based on the results of univariate analyses (Table 3). The 5-year OS after propensity adjustment in the guideline-consistent group was significantly better than that in the guideline-inconsistent cases ($p < 0.01$), but not in the EAG group ($p = 0.24$; Figure 3b). However, a significant difference was not observed in the 5-year OS after propensity adjustment between the EAG and guideline-inconsistent groups ($p = 0.09$; Figure 3b).

Table 3. Clinicopathological characteristics after propensity adjustment.

Characteristics	Inconsistent $n = 106$	Consistent $n = 108$	p-Value
Age (years old), median	64	64	0.98
IQR	(60–68)	(58–69)	
Gender, male (%)	61 (57.5%)	59 (54.6%)	0.67
Era			0.97
2006–2013	69 (65.1%)	70 (64.8%)	
2014–2017	37 (34.9%)	38 (35.2%)	
Smoking history (pack-year), median	20.0	32	0.49
IQR	(0–49.1)	(0–50.8)	
Prognostic nutritional index, median			0.81
IQR	36 (34.0%)	35 (32.4%)	
Any mutation (EGFR/ALK/BRAF/ROS1) (yes, %)	50 (47.2)	50 (46.3%)	0.90

ALK, anaplastic lymphoma kinase; ATSR, adjuvant treatments after surgical resection; BRAF, v-raf murine sarcoma viral oncogene homolog B1; EGFR, epidermal growth factor receptor; IQR, interquartile range; NA, not available; ROS1, c-ros oncogene 1.

4. Discussion

According to the clinical guidelines, complete dissection of at least three mediastinal nodal stations is recommended for the treatment of NSCLC. After complete pulmonary resection with pN2 proven and negative margins, adjuvant chemotherapy is recommended, whereas for incomplete or complete unknown cases either re-resection or additional chemotherapy or radiotherapy is recommended. In clinical practice, therapeutic guidelines for advanced NSCLC can be substituted by those for metastatic NSCLC. This study was designed to explore whether adherence to therapeutic management guidelines could provide survival benefit for patients with stage III NSCLC. Multimodality staging may have led to superior patient outcomes by supporting more accurate staging and, subsequently, more appropriate treatment allocation. Nevertheless, one clinical question remains, "which of these two possibilities (adjuvant chemotherapy or therapeutic adherence) has a greater impact for metastatic NSCLC?" Herein, adherence to clinical guidelines for both ATSR and GMT-R showed promising potential to improve patient survival.

During the last decade, the development of molecular targets has dramatically evolved, enabling precision medicine and personalised treatment alternatives. The six currently approved U.S. Food and Drug Administration (FDA) EGFR inhibitors have demonstrated excellent efficacy regarding objective response rate and prognosis in EGFR-positive NSCLC, with fewer adverse effects [9,10]. Erlotinib was first approved in 2013 by the FDA as a first-line treatment, and afatinib was approved later on in the same year. In the present study, analysis of EGFR in all stage III NSCLC patients showed that 39.9% (123/308) harboured EGFR mutations. These patients were authorised to receive EGFR inhibitors as first-line treatment for tumour recurrence, in agreement with the guidelines. From 2006 to 2013, 92 (44.4%) patients were diagnosed with metastatic NSCLC, among whom 32 (34.8%) harboured EGFR mutations. First-line EGFR inhibitors were clinically used in 11 (34.4%) of these patients after approval by the institutional review board.

ALK rearrangement is widely recognized as being associated with NSCLC at younger age, never-to-light smoking, and a preference to affect the central nervous system, which contributes to a dismal prognosis [11]. Crizotinib was first approved by the FDA for metastatic NSCLC in 2011 [12]. Moreover, the ALFEX trial comprising 303 Asian advanced NSCLC patients harbouring the *ALK* rearrangement revealed a clinical benefit of alectinib as a first-line treatment [13]. In the present cohort of patients with surgically resected NSCLC from 2007 to 2012, *ALK* was assessed in 68.7% (136/198) of patients, among whom 0.6% (9/136) harboured an *ALK* rearrangement. In addition, our previous report revealed a significantly higher incidence of occult lymph node metastases in *ALK*-positive NSCLC, which makes these patients good candidates for adjuvant chemotherapy according to the clinical guidelines [14].

The *BRAF* and *ROS1* status in this cohort have been investigated since 2014 and 2016, respectively, but the BRAF inhibitors dabrafenib and trametinib were only approved by the FDA in 2017. No *BRAF*-positive patients were identified in this study, whereas 2.6% (1/43) of patients with stage III NSCLC were *ROS1*-positive; thus, crizotinib was used as per the guidelines as a first-line treatment for tumour recurrence.

Recently, immune checkpoint inhibitors (ICIs) have dramatically revolutionised the treatment of metastatic or advanced NSCLC, but their efficacy is limited to a well-equipped immune microenvironment [6]. Pembrolizumab was clinically approved in 2016 as a first-line treatment for metastatic NSCLC in patients with a total proportion score $\geq$ 50% and without *EGFR* or *ALK* mutations after the KEYNOTE 024 and 042 clinical trials [15,16]. In agreement, our previous study also suggested that ICI treatment was significantly less efficacious in patients with *ALK* rearrangement than in patients with *EGFR* mutations, and that PD-L1 expression was not a critical biomarker for ICI treatment in patients with one of these mutations [8]. Herein, six patients with recurrence (20.0%, 6/30) were treated with first-line ICI, according to the clinical guidelines stipulated since 2016.

Wilshire et al. reported that guideline-inconsistent diagnosis and staging occurred in 58% of clinical stage III cases, which was associated with incomplete staging, a higher number of additional procedures, and delayed management [17]. Moreover, absence of invasive mediastinal lymph node sampling in 43% of patients suspected of having clinical stage III disease before the initiation of treatment was associated with a higher number of additional procedures and delayed management [17]. In the present study, pathologically proven N2 cases were specifically selected, which may have contributed to obtaining precise efficacy in treatments after surgical resection. In addition, several prospective randomised trials in patients with stage I-IIIA NSCLC have demonstrated the survival efficacy of cisplatin-based adjuvant chemotherapy [18,19].

Herein, the single centre clinical data from before the establishment of various clinical guidelines were evaluated. Mutational information from operative specimens were assessed using direct sequencing, which allowed determination of the therapeutic statistics according to the mutational status of the patients, which also reflects the social changes over time. ATSR was established as a survival benefit of ~11% in DFS, but an additional benefit of 20% was identified in OS. Hence, guideline inconsistency, even in pathological stage III, might improve the survival outcome and allow application of precision medicine by introducing the new strategies established from newly acquired knowledge.

This study has several limitations. First, the data were collected and analysed retrospectively, which could have caused selection bias. Second, this study was based on data collected at a single centre with a relatively middle scale. Third, direct sequencing is not currently performed as a standard clinical tool because it only investigates a limited gene sequence portion. In addition, it should be also noted that the systematic process for identifying genomic mutations only recently was made available; for example, *ALK* since 2007, *BRAF* since 2014, and *ROS1* since 2016. Therefore, only few patients included in the present analysis were treated with more specific treatments. Nevertheless, targeted selection or exclusion of these patients did not seem reasonable as they would not represent the typical phases of medical application development or ongoing clinical investigation. Fourth, we restricted the therapeutic alternative to first-line treatment only.

5. Conclusions

This retrospective study suggests that a guideline-consistent treatment alternative comprising ATCR and GMT-R, depending on the genomic profiles and immune environments, can provide a survival benefit for patients with pathological stage III NSCLC. Both ATCR and GMT-R are optional in clinical practice, but at least one of them may be recommended to improve the outcome of these patients.

Author Contributions: Conceptualization, H.K. and Y.S.; methodology, Y.T.; software, R.Y.; validation, Y.T., T.N., and E.S.; formal analysis, K.M.; investigation, H.K.; resources, Y.S. and T.N.; data curation, R.Y.; writing—original draft preparation, H.K.; writing—review and editing, T.H.; visualization, N.S.; supervision, H.M.; project administration, T.H. All authors have read and agreed to the published version of the manuscript.

Funding: This research received no external funding.

Institutional Review Board Statement: The Institutional Review Board of the Aichi Cancer Centre approved this study (2020-1-614).

Informed Consent Statement: The requirement for informed consent obtained from the patients with cancer was waived because of the retrospective nature of this study.

Data Availability Statement: The data presented in this study are available in this article.

Conflicts of Interest: The authors declare no conflict of interest.

Appendix A

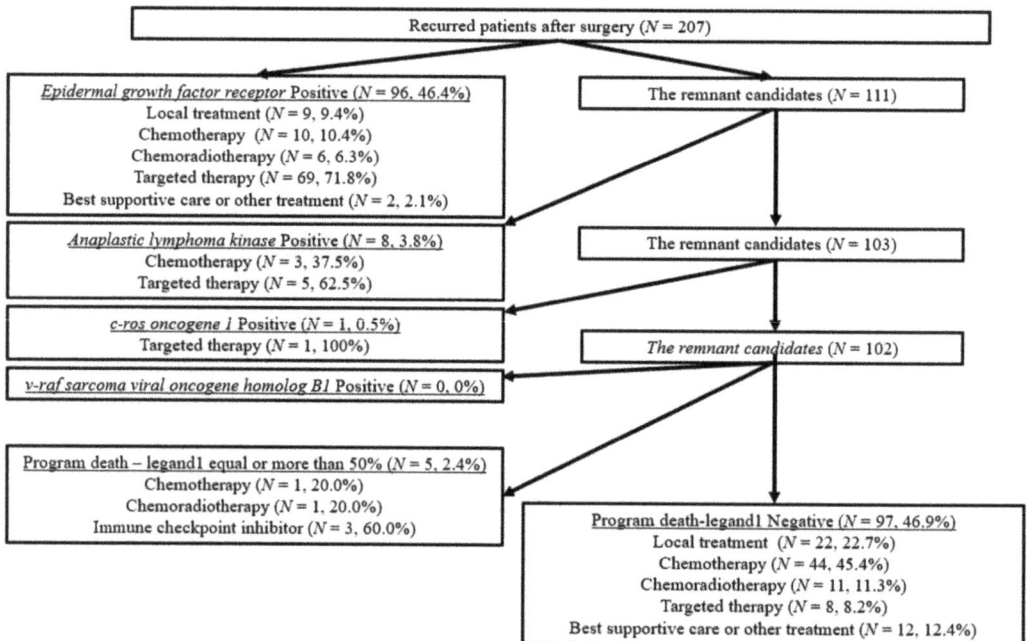

Figure A1. Patient flow diagram after recurrence according to the mutational information and program death—ligand 1 status.

References

1. Spiro, S.G.; Silvestri, G.A. One hundred years of lung cancer. *Am. J. Respir. Crit. Care Med.* **2005**, *172*, 523–529. [CrossRef] [PubMed]
2. Sakakura, N.; Mizuno, T.; Kuroda, H.; Arimura, T.; Yatabe, Y.; Yoshimura, K.; Sakao, Y. The eighth TNM classification system for lung cancer: A consideration based on the degree of pleural invasion and involved neighboring structures. *Lung Cancer* **2018**, *118*, 134–138. [CrossRef] [PubMed]
3. Le Chevalier, T.; Arriagada, R.; Pignon, J.; Scagliotti, G.V. Should adjuvant chemotherapy become standard treatment in all patients with resected non-small-cell lung cancer? *Lancet Oncol.* **2005**, *6*, 182–184. [CrossRef]
4. Mori, S.; Usami, N.; Fukumoto, K.; Mizuno, T.; Kuroda, H.; Sakakura, N.; Yokoi, K.; Sakao, Y. The Significance of the Prognostic Nutritional Index in Patients with Completely Resected Non-Small Cell Lung Cancer. *PLoS ONE* **2015**, *10*, e0136897. [CrossRef] [PubMed]
5. Goldstraw, P.; Chansky, K.; Crowley, J.; Rami-Porta, R.; Asamura, H.; Eberhardt, W.E.; Nicholson, A.G.; Groome, P.; Mitchell, A.; Bolejack, V.; et al. The IASLC Lung Cancer Staging Project: Proposals for Revision of the TNM Stage Groupings in the Forthcoming (Eighth) Edition of the TNM Classification for Lung Cancer. *J. Thorac. Oncol.* **2016**, *11*, 39–51. [CrossRef] [PubMed]
6. Ettinger, D.S.; Wood, D.E.; Aggarwal, C.; Aisner, D.L.; Akerley, W.; Bauman, J.R.; Bharat, A.; Bruno, D.S.; Chang, J.Y.; Chirieac, L.R.; et al. NCCN Guidelines Insights: Non-Small Cell Lung Cancer, Version 1 2020. *J. Natl. Compr. Canc. Netw.* **2019**, *17*, 1464–1472. [CrossRef] [PubMed]
7. Seto, K.; Haneda, M.; Masago, K.; Fujita, S.; Kato, S.; Sasaki, E.; Hosoda, W.; Murakami, Y.; Kuroda, H.; Horio, Y.; et al. Negative reactions of BRAF mutation-specific immunohistochemistry to non-V600E mutations of BRAF. *Pathol. Int.* **2020**, *70*, 253–261. [CrossRef] [PubMed]
8. Oya, Y.; Kuroda, H.; Nakada, T.; Takahashi, Y.; Sakakura, N.; Hida, T. Efficacy of Immune Checkpoint Inhibitor Monotherapy for Advanced Non-Small Cell Lung Cancer with ALK Rearrangement. *Int. J. Mol. Sci.* **2020**, *21*, 2623. [CrossRef] [PubMed]
9. Fukuoka, M.; Wu, Y.L.; Thongprasert, S.; Sunpaweravong, P.; Leong, S.S.; Sriuranpong, V.; Chao, T.Y.; Nakagawa, K.; Chu, D.T.; Saijo, N.; et al. Biomarker analyses and final overall survival results from a phase III, randomized, open-label, first-line study of gefitinib versus carboplatin/paclitaxel in clinically selected patients with advanced non-small-cell lung cancer in Asia (IPASS). *J. Clin. Oncol.* **2011**, *29*, 2866–2874. [CrossRef] [PubMed]
10. Soria, J.C.; Ohe, Y.; Vansteenkiste, J.; Reungwetwattana, T.; Chewaskulyong, B.; Lee, K.H.; Dechaphunkul, A.; Imamura, F.; Nogami, N.; Kurata, T.; et al. Osimertinib in Untreated EGFR-Mutated Advanced Non-Small-Cell Lung Cancer. *N. Engl. J. Med.* **2018**, *378*, 113–125. [CrossRef]
11. Yoshida, T.; Oya, Y.; Tanaka, K.; Shimizu, J.; Horio, Y.; Kuroda, H.; Sakao, Y.; Hida, T.; Yatabe, Y. Differential Crizotinib Response Duration Among ALK Fusion Variants in ALK-Positive Non-Small-Cell Lung Cancer. *J. Clin. Oncol.* **2016**, *34*, 3383–3389. [CrossRef] [PubMed]
12. Cho, B.C.; Chewaskulyong, B.; Lee, K.H.; Dechaphunkul, A.; Sriuranpong, V.; Imamura, F.; Nogami, N.; Kurata, T.; Okamoto, I.; Zhou, C.; et al. Osimertinib versus Standard of Care EGFR TKI as First-Line Treatment in Patients with EGFRm Advanced NSCLC: FLAURA Asian Subset. *J. Thorac. Oncol.* **2019**, *14*, 99–106. [CrossRef] [PubMed]
13. Wu, Y.L.; Lu, S.; Lu, Y.; Zhou, J.; Shi, Y.K.; Sriuranpong, V.; Ho, J.C.M.; Ong, C.K.; Tsai, C.M.; Chung, C.H.; et al. Results of PROFILE 1029, a Phase III Comparison of First-Line Crizotinib versus Chemotherapy in East Asian Patients with ALK-Positive Advanced Non-Small Cell Lung. *J. Thorac. Oncol.* **2018**, *13*, 1539–1548. [CrossRef] [PubMed]
14. Seto, K.; Kuroda, H.; Yoshida, T.; Sakata, S.; Mizuno, T.; Sakakura, N.; Hida, T.; Yatabe, Y.; Sakao, Y. Higher frequency of occult lymph node metastasis in clinical N0 pulmonary adenocarcinoma with *ALK* rearrangement. *Cancer Manag. Res.* **2018**, *10*, 2117–2124. [CrossRef] [PubMed]
15. Mok, T.S.K.; Wu, Y.L.; Kudaba, I.; Kowalski, D.M.; Cho, B.C.; Turna, H.Z.; Castro, G., Jr.; Srimuninnimit, V.; Laktionov, K.K.; Bondarenko, I.; et al. KEYNOTE-042Pembrolizumab versus chemotherapy for previously untreated, PD-L1-expressing, locally advanced or metastatic non-small-cell lung cancer (KEYNOTE-042): A randomised, open-label, controlled, phase 3 trial. *Lancet* **2019**, *393*, 1819–1830. [CrossRef]
16. Nosaki, K.; Saka, H.; Hosomi, Y.; Baas, P.; de Castro, G., Jr.; Reck, M.; Wu, Y.L.; Brahmer, J.R.; Felip, E.; Sawada, T.; et al. Safety and efficacy of pembrolizumab monotherapy in elderly patients with PD-L1-positive advanced non-small-cell lung cancer: Pooled analysis from the KEYNOTE-010, KEYNOTE-024, and KEYNOTE-042 studies. *Lung Cancer* **2019**, *135*, 188–195. [CrossRef] [PubMed]
17. Wilshire, C.L.; Rayburn, J.R.; Chang, S.C.; Gilbert, C.R.; Louie, B.E.; Aye, R.W.; Farivar, A.S.; Bograd, A.J.; Vallières, E.; Gorden, J.A. Not Following the Rules in Guideline Care for Lung Cancer Diagnosis and Staging Has Negative Impact. *Ann. Thorac. Surg.* **2020**, *110*, 1730–1738. [CrossRef] [PubMed]
18. Watanabe, S.I.; Nakagawa, K.; Suzuki, K.; Takamochi, K.; Ito, H.; Okami, J.; Aokage, K.; Saji, H.; Yoshioka, H.; Zenke, Y.; et al. Neoadjuvant and adjuvant therapy for Stage III non-small cell lung cancer. Lung Cancer Surgical Study Group (LCSSG) of the Japan Clinical Oncology Group (JCOG). *JPN J. Clin. Oncol.* **2017**, *47*, 1112–1118. [CrossRef] [PubMed]
19. NSCLC Meta-Analyses Collaborative Group; Arriagada, R.; Auperin, A.; Burdett, S.; Higgins, J.P.; Johnson, D.H.; Le Chevalier, T.; Le Pechoux, C.; Parmar, M.K.; Pignon, J.P.; et al. Adjuvant chemotherapy, with or without postoperative radiotherapy, in operable non-small-cell lung cancer: Two meta-analyses of individual patient data. *Lancet* **2010**, *375*, 1267–1277. [CrossRef] [PubMed]

MDPI
St. Alban-Anlage 66
4052 Basel
Switzerland
Tel. +41 61 683 77 34
Fax +41 61 302 89 18
www.mdpi.com

Cancers Editorial Office
E-mail: cancers@mdpi.com
www.mdpi.com/journal/cancers

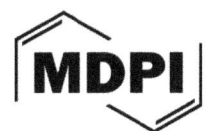

www.ingramcontent.com/pod-product-compliance
Lightning Source LLC
LaVergne TN
LVHW070157100526
838202LV00015B/1959